AYURVEDIC DRUGS AND THEIR PLANT SOURCES

AYURVEDIC DRUGS AND THEIR PLANT SOURCES

V.V. SIVARAJAN
Professor of Botany
University of Calicut, Kerala 673 635

and

INDIRA BALACHANDRAN
Research Officer
Herbal Garden, Arya Vaidya Sala
Kottakkal - 676 503, Kerala

Oxford & IBH Publishing Co. Pvt. Ltd.
New Delhi

CBS

(A Unit of CBS Publishers & Distributors Pvt Ltd)

New Delhi • Bengaluru • Chennai • Kochi • Kolkata • Mumbai
Hyderabad • Jharkhand • Nagpur • Patna • Pune • Uttarakhand

CBS Publishers & Distributors Pvt Ltd
204 FIE, Patparganj Industrial Area, Delhi-110 092
E-mail: delhi@cbspd.com, cbspubs@airtelmail.in

Last Reprint 2017

ISBN 81-204-0828-4

Printed at Chaman Enterprises, New Delhi.

8-Y17-05

DEDICATED TO THE MEMORY OF

Vaidyaratnam
P.S. Varier (1869–1944)

a great visionary and a great humanist
who thought and acted much ahead of his time

and founded

The Arya Vaidya Sala, Kottakkal

PREFACE

In his long struggle to achieve mastery over powerful forces of nature, man has always turned to plants for help. This is especially so, when he was struck with ailments, both physical and mental. Nearly all cultures, both ancient and recent, have used plants as source of medicine. We would never be able to say how exactly the ancients discovered the medicinal properties of herbs. Probably, it started with ancient beliefs, myths and lores, got involved with astrology and other occult practices, developed into folk-medicine and herbalism, and finally gave rise to traditional systems of herbal medicine.

After a period of disregard and decline, these traditional systems of 'green medicine' are, once again, back to the centre-stage of our health-care programmes. There has been a steady increase in demand for such medicine and these systems have now regained respectability among the scientific community, the world over. This new-found importance and enthusiasm have given great impetus to most such systems. That Ayurveda, the ancient Indian system of herbal medicine, is growing in popularity not only in India but also abroad, is a matter for great rejoicement for all of us.

But, this 'resurrection' also calls for a deep introspection on the part of all Ayurveda enthusiasts. We cannot afford to bask in the past glory of this prestine system and be complacent. It is time to look at our past failures and shortcomings and to strive to put Ayurveda back on rails, in a more objective and scientific manner avoiding past mistakes. Indeed, it is gratifying to note that there is a lot of research work being done on various aspects of Ayurvedic medicine. But, it is doubtful whether we have got our priorities right. Most such work revolve round pharmacological and clinical aspects. The need for standardisation of Ayurvedic medicines has attracted some attention in the recent times, but most people seem to forget that without standards in plant sources of drugs, we cannot evolve standards in Ayurvedic formulations.

This long-standing problem of accurate determination of drug sources is yet to receive adequate attention of Ayurvedic practitioners and researchers. In fact, the situation is rapidly deteriorating and is telling upon the credibility of the system with the public, in a big way. But, this is an area which requires collaborative efforts of men of Ayurveda and botanists, which unfortunately has not been very much forthcoming. To make matters worse, uncritical following of published literature on this matter has created more problems than it has solved. It is in this context that we thought of undertaking a resurvey of the whole scenario.

Since 1982, we have been working on this aspect—accurate and scientific identification of Ayurvédic medicinal plants with special reference to Kerala—with the intention of bringing out a state-of-art report on the diversity in this matter. We have, consistently refused to be (mis-)led by literature and have tried to see the actual materials in the market and the pharmacies, before identifying them. And our findings are revealing and even appalling at times. As we proceeded with the work, it was becoming increasingly clear that even within this tiny state, renowned for its unique Ayurvedic tradition, the situation is extremely chaotic.

So, we thought that it would be worthwhile to bring this problem to the attention of Ayurvedic practitioners and researchers. Eventhough, this would not, by itself, solve the problem of standardisation of drug sources, it is our hope that similar work in other parts of the country would finally provide us a realisitic idea about the extent of the rot at the national level, which could, in turn, be the basis for further studies to realise the final goal of a unified 'Materia Medica'.

This book is the end-product of about a decade's work. We don't make any tall claim about it. In fact, we are more conscious about its limitations. It is centred round Ayurvedic medicinal plants used in Kerala. Also, we could not study all drugs used by Kerala practitioners due to several constraints. Yet, if our good intentions would touch the right chords at the right places we would think that our mission is fulfilled.

Our readers are most welcome to appraise us of their critical appreciation of this work, so that we would be able to improve upon it in our future course of activities.

V.V. SIVARAJAN
INDIRA BALACHANDRAN

ACKNOWLEDGEMENTS

The number of persons and institutions to whom we owe a deep sense of gratitude for the various favours received during the course of this work, would virtually look like a WHO is WHO in Ayurveda. Unfortunately, for want of space, we would not be able to take the names of all of them here, which, we hope, will not be misconstrued. We offer them apologies for this inability. Yet, we would be failing in our duty, if we do not mention the few who stood by us all through, both in our triumphs and in our travails.

This work would not have been possible but for the unstinted support and encouragement we received from Dr. P.K. Warrier, Managing Trustee, and other members of the Trust Board of the Arya Vaidyasala (AVS), Kottakkal, for which we are very highly indebted. It gives us great pleasure to acknowledge that the Department of Botany, University of Calicut extended a long hand, by collaborating with this work. We feel highly previleged to have been able to have wide-ranging discussions on various aspects of Ayurvedic Medicine with Late Sri. S. Varier, Late Sri. Raghunatha Iyer, Late Sri N.S. Mooss and Sri. N.V. Krishnan Kutty Varier, all stalwarts in both philosophy and practice of Ayurveda. Dr. C. Raman Kutty, AVS, has always been generous with all kinds of assistance, particularly with proof-reading and transliteration, for which we owe him a special word of thanks. We are also grateful to Prof. Vasudevan Nair, Palghat for the drawings and to Dr. Murali and Dr. Ramesh, AVS, for their help during the course of the work.

The Scientists of CCRAS, Madras and Bangalore have rendered us valuable help with literature and other requirements. We are thankful to all of them, especially, Dr. Yoganarasimhan, Bangalore. We also take this opportunity to express our gratefulness to Dr. N.C. Shah, Director, Herbal Research and Development Institute, Gopeswar, Chamouli. Dr. O.P. Gupta, Asst. Director, CCRAS, Delhi and Dr. P.C. Sharma, Jawaharlal Nehru Medicinal Plants Garden, Pune, for their critical comments and suggestions for improvement of an earlier version of the text.

Finally, the staff of the Herbal Garden, AVS, Kottakkal, had to put up with lots of difficulties and hard work during this period, collecting and cultivating plants and helping us in various other ways. We have pleasure to acknowledge that they have done it with great grace and love. We thank each one of them for whatever they have done to help us in this task.

V.V. SIVARAJAN
INDIRA BALACHANDRAN

CONTENTS

INTRODUCTION

Āyurvēda, the Indian indigenous system of medicine, dating back to the Vēdic ages (1500–800 B.C.), has been an integral part of Indian culture (Weiss, 1987). The term comes from the Sanskrit root, *Āyu* (= life) and *vēda* (= knowledge). As the name implies, it is not only a science of treatment of the ill but covers the whole gamut of happy human life, involving the physical, metaphysical and the spiritual aspects. According to Suśruta, the foremost aim of Āyurvēda is to help people maintain health and treating the disease is only secondary.

Legend has it that Āyurvēda descended to earth from *Brahmā*, the creator of the universe, through ancient seers.

Brahmā smṛtvāyuṣō vēdaṃ
prajāpatimajigrahat
Sōśvinau tau sahasrākṣaṃ
sōtṛiputṛādikān munīn
Tēgnivēśādikāṁstē tu
pṛthak tantrāṇi tēnirē

(Aṣṭāṅgahṛdayam)

Caraka, one of the foremost exponents of Āyurvēda, has defined it as "*āyuṛvēdayanti iti āyuṛvēdaḥ*" (i.e., the science which instructs about life) and Suśruta, as "*āyurasmin vidyatē anēna vā āyuṛvindatīti āyuṛvēdaḥ*" (i.e., the science by which life is known or attained).

Over the centuries, Āyurvēda has developed (see Narayanaswamy, 1981) into a well-founded, time-tested, empirical science of life, based on three parameters: ***pratyakṣa*** (direct perception), ***anumāna*** (inference), and ***āptōpadēśa*** (seer's words). However, most of the texts being in Sanskrit, the education of which was firmly restricted to certain higher castes and communities of the Hindu society in the past, and which is a moribund language since long, Āyurvēda has been declining steadily, remaining an esoteric art, out of bounds for the common man. The disappearance of the traditional social patterns and *Gurukula* system of education (when the students acquired knowledge staying with the *Guru*, the teacher), on the one hand, and the increasing demand for medical care for the increasing population on the other, have also contributed, to a great extent, to the degeneration of the Āyurvēdic practice in the recent times. The present system of Āyurvēdic education, with its emphasis on the therapeutic part rather than on the conceptual basis, also leaves many things to be desired. As a result, we have now, innumerable practitioners throughout India, but have only few Āyurvēdists who are proficient in Āyurvēdic concepts.

Not that the authors are competent enough to discuss the basic premises of this pristine science of life, nor is the treatise on that subject. But, it seems important for any layman, who endeavours to study or discuss medicinal herbs used in the system, to have at least a basic understanding of certain important Āyurvēdic concepts, say for example, the concept of health, disease and medication.

Āyurvēdic concept of man and nature (The Pañcabhūtasiddhānta)

The entire edifice of ancient Indian medicine is based on the concept of a fundamental identity between man and nature (Khanna, 1987). Man is considered to be a microcosm of the macrocosm (Pal, 1989), both being constituted by the *pañcabhūtās* (five fundamental elements) namely, *pṛthvi* (earth), *ap* (water), *agni* or *tējas* (fire), *vāyu* (air) and *ākāśa* (space). Each of these can be perceived by their distinctive quality, such as *pṛthvi* by *gandha* (odour), *ap* by *rasa* (taste), *agni* by *rūpa* (form), *vāyu* by *sparśa* (touch) and *ākāśa* by *śabda* (sound). The vital man has three aspects: *ātman* (soul), *manas* (mind) and *śarīra* (body). Of these, *ātman* is not perceptible, but can only be realised through constant meditation. It emerges only through a unique union of *śarīra* and *manas*, and being a segment of the cosmic soul, is not subject to disease and destruction. Life is sustainable only to the period through which this union endures and afterwards the human being decays and disintegrates into the five basic elements it is formed of.

Concept of swāsthya (health) and rōga (disease)

During his life time, man derives everything essential for life through food. This, on being acted upon by *jaṭharāgni* (gastric juices and digestive enzymes) and consequent digestion, contributes to the development of the *saptadhātūs* (seven harbingers of life) namely, *rasa** (lymph), *rakta* (blood), *māmsa* (flesh), *mēda* (adipose tissue) *asthi* (bone), *majja* (bone marrow) and *śukḷa* (reproductive elements) that go into the biological structure and organisation of the body. During this process, however, some waste products like urine, faeces and sweat are also produced which are known as *maladhātūs*.

While Āyurvēda recognises these *dhātūs* as the structural basis of the living body, in functional terms, it recognises three different biological systems—*vāta*, *pitta* and *kapha*. *Vāta* is the controller of all movements in the body while *pitta* takes care of chemical reactions and biosynthesis of various compounds within the body system. *Kapha* is the one which deals with balanced growth, development and functioning of the body. When these three are well-harmonised and function in a balanced manner, it results in good nourishment and well-being of the individual. But when there is an imbalance or disharmony within or between them, it will result in *dhātuvaiṣamya* (elemental imbalance) leading to various kinds of ailments. Āyurvēdic concept of physical health revolves round these three *dōṣās* and hence is called *tridōṣasiddhānta* (philosophy of three morbidities). This humoral theory is not unique to ancient Indian medicine. The Yin and Yang theory in Chinese medicine and the Hippocratic theory of four humours in Greek medicine are also very similar.

So the primary purpose of Āyurvēda is to help people maintain *vāta*, *pitta* and *kapha* in the balanced state and thus to prevent disease. In cases where *dhātuvaiṣamya* has already occurred, it endeavours to restore the balance.

---

* *Rasa* is a complex term which denotes the readily absorbable essence of digested food, chyle, lymph, plasma etc.

There seem to be no exact English equivalents for many of the Āyurvēdic terminologies used here. In fact, we feel that this equation of *pañcabhūtās* with earth, water, fire, etc. is a gross over-simplification, incapable of conveying the subtle and exact meaning, a classical example where language fails. Yet, we use them here because there are no alternatives and because this is the way modern writers on Āyurvēda have treated them.

But, one should realise that Āyurvēda does not pertain only to bodily health. It takes care of the metaphysical and even spiritual needs of man, to acquire health and also healthy attitude towards life. Āyurvēda has defined health as:

Samadōṣaḥ samāgniśca samadhātu malakṛiyaḥ
Pṛasannātmēndriyamanāḥ svastha ityabhidhīyatē.

This means that besides a balance of body elements, one has to have an enlightened state of consciousness, sense organs and mind, if he has to be perfectly healthy. Āyurvēda has prescribed several ways to keep oneself healthy. They include a sound knowledge of *jīvitōddēśa* (the goal in life), *jīvitacarya* (a highly regulated mode of life), *hitāhitīyaṃ* (do's and don'ts in life), *āhāravivēcana* (good and bad aspects of different types of food articles), and *rōgapṛatirōdhōpāya* (methods of prevention of diseases). A man living according to the prescriptions would be able to attain all the four *puruṣārṭhās* (accomplishments)—*dharma* (duties), *artha* (wealth), *kāma* (desire), and ultimately *mōkṣa* (liberation).

Āyurvēda defines *rōga* (disease) as *duḥkhasaṁyōga*, the state of misery either of body or mind or both. Suśruta has recognised four different kinds of diseases:

1) *Āgantuja* : due to external reasons
2) *Śārīrika* : physical
3) *Mānasika* : mental
4) *Svābhāvika* : natural

Of these, *agāntuja rōga* are those caused by external reasons like accidents (cuts, burns, poisonous bites and other similar conditions). *Śārīrika rōga* by and large, manifest as diseases due to vitiation of *dōṣās* in the body system. There is an important difference in the approach of ancient Indian and western medicare systems. The latter places emphasis on pathogens and antibiotic philosophy of therapeutics, leaving the body system as such or even more vulnerable to similar pathogenic attacks. Āyurvēda, on the other, endeavours to modify the body system, so that it is rendered inhospitable for such pathogens. It is gratifying to note that the western medical scientists also now recognise that it is the body ecosystem that is to be treated rather than the pathogens. This has now given rise to the 'probiotic' concept of treatment as opposed to the antibiotic concept.

Svābhāvika rōga are those painful experiences that go with human life as a matter of natural course, such as birth, old age, death, urges of hunger, thirst and sleep.

Concept of drug

Āyurvēda holds that diseases can come in two different ways, by unwholesome diet and by sins and moral transgressions. "*Dvipṛakāra vyādhayah āhāranimittaḥ aśubhanimittaścēti, tatṛa āhārasamuthānaṃ vaiṣamya āyurvēdaṃ*" (*Kauśika sūtṛa*). Of these, the ones caused by sins and transgressions are dealt with in the *Atharvavēda*. This represents the "charms school", while Āyurvēda, the "drug school" is mainly concerned with diseases of the former kind. Many people consider the *Atharvavēda* and Āyurvēda to be two distinct disciplines of knowledge, but others consider the latter to be a supplement (*upavēda* or *upāṅga*) of *Atharvavēda*.

In any case, in practice, we find an admixture of the drug school and the charm school.

The concept of drug in Āyurvēda is slightly different from that in modern medicine. The term drug, derived from the French word "drogue" (a dry herb) is defined as "any substance or product used to modify or explore physiological systems or pathological states for the benefit of the recipient." The Āyurvēdic equivalent of the drug is *bhēṣaja* or *auṣadha*, that which overcomes *bhēṣaṃ* or *ōṣa*, diseases or even fear of diseases, and includes anything, material or means, used for this purpose. Thus, even food, fasting, penance, incantations, sleep, sunlight, shade and faith in physicians are prescribed in Āyurvēdic therapeutics for recuperation from ill-health. In fact, Āyurvēdic physicians prescribe not only medicines, but also a whole course of behaviour that would help the recuperation, because, the *dōṣās* which manifest as diseases will be aggravated by things, climate and activities not suitable to the constitution of the body and mind of the individual. Āyurvēdic texts mention four different types of treatment:

1) *Mantṛa:* Incantations. (Karnick (1983) found that certain plants when charged with certain *mantṛās* had better effect on patients.)
2) *Maṇi:* These are certain drugs, stones, beads or specially prepared forms of hardened mercury which are dynamised by great men.
3) *Auṣadha:* drugs.
4) *Pṛabhāva:* personal influence.

Mantṛa and *maṇi* operate at higher centres of consciousness and are used for psychological disorders, which were believed to be the handiwork of the evil spirits (Pandya, 1983). These are still popular among the tribal and rural folk, but do not come under the purview of the drug school with which we are concerned at present.

Āyurvēdic principle of medication:

As mentioned before, Āyurvēda, steeped in the *tridōsasiddhānta*, holds that diseases manifest themselves when there is *dhātuvaiṣamya*, i.e., elemental imbalance of *vāyu*, *pitta* and *kapha* and endeavours to alleviate these afflictions by restoring the balance, by promoting or depleting the ones that are causative, so that the root causes of the afflictions can be eliminated. In such a system, it is imperative for the practitioners to know the drugs which will strike the deal, the elemental composition of the drugs have to be known before they are administered.

According to Āyurvēda, this cannot be known directly, but can be inferred from the various attributes of the drugs, called *rasa*, *guṇa*, *vīrya* and *vipāka*. *Rasa* is generally defined as taste. In our food usually the actual tastes of materials are masked by mixing different items or by adding spices. Āyurvēda has classified all things into six classes, depending on their tastes; *madhura* (sweet), *lavaṇa* (saline), *amḷa* (sour), *kaṭu* (hot and acrid), *tikta* (bitter) and *kaṣāya* (astringent). While some substances have simple tastes (for example, sugar = sweet, salt = saline), others have composite tastes (garlic has all tastes except sour). The tastes of all food articles, drugs and other substances are given in the *nighaṇṭus* (lexicons), and their equations with the five elements (Pandya, 1983; 178-179) are as follows:

madhura = earth and water
aṁḷa = earth and fire
lavaṇa = water and fire
tikta = sky and air
kaṭu = fire and air
kaṣāya = earth and air

The basic principle is to choose the *rasa* which will rectify the imbalance of elements. *Guṇa* is the property of the drugs which is responsible for their pharmacological action. Seers have recognised 20 *guṇās* (for example, *guru*-heavy, *laghu*-light, *mṛdu*-soft, *kaṭhina*-hard). The term, *vīrya* in Āyurvēda has a different connotation from that in other systems of medicine. All things are classified broadly into two classes: *uṣṇa-vīrya* (heating) and *śīta-vīrya* (cooling), depending on the subtle influence of the sun and the moon respectively, on them. Great caution is necessary while prescribing these drugs, because of the different constitutional nature (*pṛakṛti*) of different people (e.g., *vāta-pṛakṛti*, *pitta-pṛakṛti*, *kapha-pṛakṛti*, etc.).

The ultimate effect of drugs on the body depends on *rasa* as they are digested and is what is called *vipāka*. There are three different kinds of *vipāka*. In some cases, the taste of the substance gets transformed in the stomach. Say, some acrid (*kaṭu*) substances change over to sweet (*madhura*) when acted upon by the digestive juices and the effect would be that of sweet and not acrid. This is called *rasa-vipāka*. In certain other cases, the *vīrya* of the substance gets transformed in the stomach. *Uṣṇa-vīrya* gets transformed into *śīta-vīrya* and vice-versa. This is called *vīrya-vipāka*. In *saṃskāra-vipāka*, the substances when subjected to certain processes get transformed with different properties or can be targetted to a specific site or organ. E.g. Papaya fruit is by nature, *uṣṇa-vīrya* but, when taken with lime juice, it becomes *sama-vīrya*. Guggulu (gummy secretion of *Commiphora mukul*) when purified with *gōkṣura* (*Tribulus terrestris*) acts on kidney and urinary tract while the same purified with *kāñcanāra* (*Bauhinia tomentosa*) acts on glands and glandular diseases (Pandya, 1983).

Besides all these, there are certain properties of substances which cannot be studied in terms of their *rasa*, *guṇa*, *vīrya* and *vipāka*. All such extraordinary properties are called *pṛabhāva* (characteristics). For example, certain drugs collected during full moon, new moon or particular constellations are reported to possess certain curative properties not found when collected at other times. Many like Suśruta hold that properties or efficacy of the drugs depend on all these factors.

The earliest works of Āyurvēda that we have today are the *samhitās* of Caraka and Suśruta (before 600 B.C.) modified and supplemented by later authors. In its pristine form, Āyurvēda was divided into eight subjects—*śalya* (surgery), *śālākya* (ENT and ophthalmology), *kāyacikitsa* (general medicine), *bhūtavidya* (curing influence of evil spirits, psychiatry), *kaumārabhṛtya* (paediatrics), *agadatantṛa* (toxicology), *rasāyana* (treatment for rejuvenation of the body) and *vājīkaraṇa* (treatment for acquiring virility).

Āyurvēda, by and large, is an experience with nature, and unlike in western medicine many of the concepts elude scientific explanation, in the modern sense of the term. Western medicine relies heavily on principles of physical sciences to explain various aspects of health science (see also Majumdar, 1989). This reductionist concept of science is an anathema to men of Āyurvēda. The concept of science cannot be limited to physical science alone, instead, it should explore physical, living and the conscious phenomena. The domain of science is more extensive than that of physical science (Sinha, 1984: 124). Jayantha, one of the ancient commentators, says that the very large number of medicines, their combinations and applications are of such an infinite variety that it would be absolutely impossible for anyone to know them by employing experimental methods (Dasgupta, 1922: 280). This has been concurred by recent authors as well, who hold that some of the concepts in Āyurvēda such as soul, and consciousness, cannot be operationally defined after making scientific measurement (Sinha, 1984). Despite, there have been isolated attempts in the recent times to explain and experimentally study some of the concepts e.g. the concept of three morbidities, (see Mahadihassan, 1980, 1986, 1989). Udupa (1983) has indicated that the morbidities can be easily estimated by biochemical studies and that they are neurohumours liberated by brain and its nerve endings. Thus, he has equated *vāta* with acetylcholine liberated by cerebral cortex and peripheral and para-sympathetic nerve endings, *pitta* with catecholamines liberated by the hypothalamus, sympathetic nerve endings and adrenal medulla and *kapha* with histamine secreted by brainstem. The drugs when administered, act by promoting or destroying the respective neurohumours or their precursors. He has also observed that a person of *vāta-prakṛti* is lean and thin with an excess of acetylcholine, that of *pitta-prakṛti* is muscular with a predominance of catecholamines and *kapha-prakṛti* has a heavy body with an excess of histamines. Udupa, unlike many others who equate *agni* with *pitta*, also holds that they are different and *agni* refers to hormones and equates *jaṭharāgni* with intestinal secretions, *bhūtāgni* with hormones regulating liver activities and *dhātvagni* with hormones produced by endocrine glands that regulate cellular metabolism. Such experimental studies in Āyurvēda, however, lead us to the trodden path of western medicine, leaving the much acclaimed "holistic approach" to total neglect (Laping, 1984; see also Singh and Singh, 1990).

With the unprecedented exposure that Āyurvēda and such other systems of traditional medicine are getting the world over and the consequent outbreeding of ideas and concepts of different systems, some of the men of Āyurvēda have called for an integrated system of medicine evolved through a "unification of theoretical concepts about the nature of human being, about illness and its etiology and about therapeutic management" (Parikh et al., 1984), losing sight of the fact that Āyurvēda and modern medicine are based on philosophical presuppositions and assumptions which are opposed to each other (see Sinha, 1984). Majumdar (1989), after a critical study of Āyurvēda and modern medicine, has highlighted some of the differences in their approach to the healing process. In fact, if Āyurvēda has to sustain itself, it is essential to retain its concepts and plurality of outlook on health and disease in the original form. Scientific studies in Āyurvēda have to be on its terms and not on those of western medicine. It is more important and necessary to collaborate rather than undermine each other's foundations and credibility (Laping, 1984; also see Sivarajan, 1985; Ravindran, 1986).

Disillusioned with the synthetic western medicines, more and more people are now realising that "natural is better" and are returning to the fold of traditional herbal system. This "green wave" (Tyler, 1986) is likely to gain momentum in the years to come. The immense possibilities of these systems in achieving the proclaimed goal of "Health for all by 2000 A.D." as enshrined in the Alma-Ata declaration, are now being realised by the international community. These systems are now groomed as sources of alternative medicine, even though it is difficult to find agreement as to how these systems, being synonymous with local medicine based on local resources, can best be utilised on a global basis (Farnsworth, 1984 a). Āyurvēda has already found patronage in some of the European and Latin American countries by now and it seems that it is on its way to be an international system. It is also the time for reflection, just as a builder re-examines the foundation before building an additional storey. The thrust of this treatise will be on raw drugs and pharmacognosy in Āyurvēda, as it would be of greater interest to us.

In Āyurvēda, drugs are, in general, called *auṣadha* or *bhēṣaja*, which means that which cures pain and sorrowful experience. The source plants of drugs are called *auṣadhi*, even though this term is sometimes used loosely for plants in general. There are three different types of drugs in Āyurvēda:

1) ***Audbhida*** : obtained from plants
2) *Jāṅgama* : obtained from animals (for example: honey, wax and lac)
3) *Pārthiva* : obtained from minerals, salts etc.

Of all these, plant drugs form the lion's share of Āyurvēdic drugs. With the rapid depletion of our forests, impairing the availability of raw drugs, Āyurvēda, like other systems of herbal medicine, has reached a very crucial phase. About 50 per cent of the tropical forests, the treasure-house of plant and animal diversity, has already been destroyed and the remaining half may not stand the onslaught of man for another decade. In India alone, about the 55,2000 sq. km. of forests we had in 1975 have been reduced to 45,7000 sq. km. by 1982 (Khoshoo, 1986). Forests in India have been disappearing at an average rate of 1.5 m ha every year, and what is left at present is only 8 per cent as against a mandatory 33 per cent of the geographical area. This wanton destruction has rendered almost 3–4 thousand species of Indian plants on the verge of extinction. Sivarajan (1991) has dealt with the causes and consequences of deforestation in India in some detail. This is the case in most of the developing countries which find themselves between the devil and the deep sea in matters of conservation of their forests. In spite of the public awareness, this is likely to continue in the coming years. There are no serious attempts being made for adequate regeneration of forests. Instead, the degraded land is very much sought after for various developmental needs.

This extensive forest destruction has resulted in the extinction of many valuable medicinal herbs along with many others which would have been potentially useful later. Even the extant ones are not available in sufficient quantities, nor do they yield to cost-effective procurement, as they have receded to inaccessible areas. Thus, we don't have the much renowned *rasāyana* (rejuvenative) drugs of the *aṣṭavarga* group which are now being substituted with various other herbs. In fact, we don't have even a rough estimate as to what the loss of such species mean in terms of national economy. However, Farnsworth and Soejarto (1985) have estimated that every single species that goes extinct will cost the exchequer to the tune of 203 million U.S. dollars.

Indiscriminate exploitation of medicinal herbs has also been responsible for the present state of affairs, in a large way. Some of them have been in great demand in the world market (Sivarajan, 1988 and given below), and many of them are becoming increasingly rare.

Name	Suppliers	Consumption per year
Rauvolfia serpentina	Thailand, India, Sri Lanka, Burma	11 tons
Digitalis lanata	Europe, India	1000 tons
Cinchona officianalis	India, Africa, S. America	500–1000 tons of bark
Glycyrrhiza glabra	Europe, W. Asia, USSR, China.	500 tons in Europe alone
Panax ginseng	China, USSR, Canada, Korea	2000 tons
Cassia angustifolia	S. India, Sudan, Egypt	5000–6000 tons
Plantago ovata	India, Gautemala,	15000 tons
Dioscorea floribunda	China, India	800 tons

So, unless we evolve a sound system for conservation of forests and for rational exploitation of medicinal herbs, it is going to be fatal for herbal medicine in future (see also Akerele et al, 1991).

Croom (1983), Farnsworth (1979, 1984 a & b) and Tyler (1986) have discussed in detail some of the problems facing medicinal plant research. But, by and large, they are led by their perceptions on western medicine which revolve round isolation and application of active principles. While this is certainly a useful approach, it does not reflect the problems of traditional herbal medicine, where plant and plant parts are used as such. So, here we shall try to discuss some of the problems which are unique to the latter, as perceived in an Āyurvēdic context.

Reflecting on the decline of Āyurvēda after the Brāhmaṇic period (800 B.C.–1000 A.D.) one would find that there are three broad, all-pervading reasons, for it:

1) a complacent attitude among men of Āyurvēda that everything is written in the ancient texts and there is little scope for further studies. This faith has, over the centuries, brought in a certain amount of lethargy among them and has taken away the spirit of questioning and experimentation;
2) a self-righteous feeling that their practice reflects the ancient wisdom; and
3) reluctance on their part to seek and get collaboration from people working in other allied fields.

The fallouts of these can be seen in pharmacognosy as well. One has to realise that, being a herbal system, the choice of herbs as sources of the various drugs have great bearing on the efficacy of the system and as such pharmacognosy is the foundation on which the survival of the system rests. Ironically though, as in western medicine (see Farnsworth, 1979, 1984 a; Farnsworth and Morris, 1976 and Farnsworth and Bingel, 1977), this is the most neglected area of medicinal plant research in Āyurvēda also. Over the years, it has become such a vicious circle that once somebody gets into it, it is very difficult to come out without losing one's common sense. This is especially ominous at a time when Āyurvēda is on its road to the international scene.

Even as plant resources are getting depleted, there is a steady decline in human expertise capable of recognising the various medicinal herbs. The ancient sages themselves suggested that they have to be known with the help of hermits, shepherds and tribals.

Ōṣadhīṛnāmarūpābhyāṃ jānatē hyajapā vanē
Avipāśċaiva gōpāśca yē canyē vanavāsinaḥ

(Caraka-Sutṛa).

But, these are also a vanishing lot. Our experience with nature and its flora and fauna have, with the increasing urbanisation, industrialisation and consequent changes in life-style, reached the rock bottom. Unlike in the olden days, when physicians themselves used to collect the herbs, prepare and administer the medicine, the newer generation of Āyurvēdic physicians, with prepared drugs in the market, have degenerated into prescription writers like their counterparts in western medicine, without much knowledge of the constituent herbs of the drugs that they are prescribing. As a result, professional plant collectors have taken over the floor and the industry is forced to accept the herbs they bring on their terms without question. Herb collectors on their part, unable to meet the increasing demand, adulterate the drugs with other plants, thereby undermining the quality of the drug and credibility of the system (Sivarajan and Balachandran, 1983a and b, 1986b). Pharmacists, trained as they are in the traditional way, to recognise the plants and plant parts by size, shape, texture, colour, smell and taste characters, are totally ill-equipped to meet the challenge posed by widespread adulteration. All check-points in between have vanished over the years.

The state of affairs with regard to pharmacognosy of Āyurvēdic drugs is extremely chaotic. There is an increasing realisation of the pitfalls of this among men of Āyurvēda and urgent steps for standardisation of raw drugs are being contemplated. However, even the scattered studies that have been trickling in are on standardisation of prepared drugs, forgetting the fact that without standards in the herbal sources of raw drugs there cannot be any standard in the prepared drugs. So, the first and foremost need of the hour is to have a uniform pattern in the selection of various herbal sources of drugs. This is an area in which plant taxonomy can be of considerable help, especially in a national or possibly a global perspective. But the problems are very formidable too.

In the first place, it is the non-availability of medicinal herbs and the lack of human expertise in recognising them, which have already been mentioned earlier, that leaves the arena free-for-all. The texts on which men of Āyurvēda swear, on the other hand, too are unhelpful in deciphering the identity of the genuine herbs because they give only names and no character details based on which we could have correctly spotted them out. Moreover, each plant will have a score of names some of which might figure among the names of other herbs as well. Āyurvēdic literature is replete with such *paryāyās* (synonyms) and *nānārṭhās* (homonyms).

Thus, *Tinospora cordifolia* which is widely used in various preparations and against a variety of ailments is known by the following names:

> Guḍūcī kuṇḍalī sōmā chinnā, chinnōtbhavāmṛtā
> Madhuparṇī chinnaruhā vayasthā cakṛalakṣaṇā

and the fruits of *Phyllanthus emblica* by:

> Āmalakī pañcarasā śṛiphalī dhātṛikā śivā
> Ākārāmṛta vayasthā ca vṛṣyātiṣyaphalā tathā

Some people are hopeful of discerning the identity of the actual herb intended in the texts by deciphering certain indications of characters provided in these names. But, this again, is often impossible. For example, *Dusparśa* is a medicinal herb. The name literally means, "difficult to touch", and as such, has been attributed to a variety of plants like *Fagonia cretica*, *Tragia involucrata* and *Mucuna pruriens*.

Sahacara is another widely used medicinal herb against rheumatic and many other complaints. Its various names and their implications are as follows:

Sairēyaḥ/sairēyakaḥ	= occuring in fully exposed habitats
Sahacarāḥ	= gregarious
Kuranṭakaḥ	= spiny
Rujākaraḥ	= pain-causing (refers to spine like structure)
Āṛtagalaḥ	= living in oppressive conditions
Bāṇaḥ	= refers to certain seedling establishment characters in some mangroves
Kakubhaḥ	= refers to certain air-sucking characters (probably the breathing roots in certain mangroves).

(Singh and Chunekar 1972: 445-447).

A variety of herbs including species of *Acanthus*, *Barleria*, *Strobilanthus*, *Ecbolium* and *Calacanthus* are used in different places as its plant source. And none of them exactly tallys with all the indications given in the synonyms. However, rejection of all of them would be highly preposterous, as they have been in use for so many years and every physician would vouchsafe that his choice has the desired effect. This problem is quite widespread in Āyurvēda. Thus, *Śaṅkhapuṣpī* has been equated with at least four plants namely, *Clitoria ternatea*, *Convolvulus pluricaulis*, *Evolvulus alsinoides* and *Canscora decussata* and *Vidārī* with *Pueraria tuberosa*, *Ipomoea mauritiana* and *Adenia hondala*. The list of *sandigdhadravya* (controversial drugs) is extremely formidable and is steadily increasing (see Singh and Chunekar, 1972; Vaidya Bapalal, 1982).

From this chaotic state, how can we proceed to evolve standards in the matter of plant sources of drugs? Can plant taxonomy be useful in this regard? No doubt, that plant taxonomy can provide unambiguous, universally accepted identification of plants that are in use and this is vital at present when Āyurvēda is finding increasing international acceptance. But unfortunately there is a subtle but firm resistance from men of Āyurvēda against this unsolicited offer of assistance. They are paranoid about the ancient Āyurvēdic texts and myopic in their approach to collaboration with other allied scientific disciplines (Sivarajan, 1988).

Botanists, on the other hand, will find their task to be extremely vulnerable and that with the present system of practice and overemphasis on Sanskrit nomenclature, there cannot be any order in this matter. Even as botany can provide them with correct identification of plants that they use, the verdict as to which of the various herbs is the genuine and which are spurious, have to come from pharmacologists and physicians after adequate investigations. So, the goal of standardisation in Āyurvēdic medicine is still a far cry. To our mind, it can be achieved only in stages:

1) preliminary surveys on a state or regional basis, compiling state-of-art reports on the various plant sources of different drugs, as are adopted now;
2) comparative pharmacological and clinical studies of these herbs to find out which one of them has the properties of the drug mentioned in the text and is more efficaceous; and
3) compilation of a final *Flora Medica* for Āyurvēda, on a national scale.

Some good work of the preliminary sort have been done by Nadkarni (1908), Kirtikar and Basu (1918), Chopra *et al.* (1956) and many others. But their subsequent utilisation by men of Āyurvēda in the determination of raw drugs leaves many things to be desired. They have, by and large, been followed uncritically, deriving botanical identifications from the Sanskrit or vernacular names given against each, without caring a bit for the fact that the herbs that they use are quite different from the ones described there. This has resulted in misidentifications with ridiculous effect. So the first and most important thing to remember before one proceeds with the work is that one has to go by materials and not by literature. The task, no doubt, is going to be extremely difficult. But sincere collaborative efforts are bound to yield results in course of time.

Higher plants are still "the sleeping giant of drug development" (Farnsworth and Morris, 1976), a virtually untapped reservoir of potentially useful sources of drugs (Farnsworth, 1984 b), that will continue to serve mankind in the 21st century as they have done since the dawn of history (Tyler, 1986). In India alone, out of 15,000 species of Higher plants that we have, the number of species used in medicine is well below one-fifth of it. In the light of current scarcity of several medicinal herbs, there is a great need to discover suitable substitutes for them (Sivarajan and Balachandran, 1987a). We may also have to spread our dragnet to the unutilised and underutilised species for drugs against various diseases, the cure of which have been so far elusive. While random screening methods have got several shortcomings (Spjut, 1985), folklore medicine and traditional medicine can well be the path-breakers (Spjut and Perdue Jr., 1976).

It is with this background that this work was undertaken. The treatise is a compilation of the state-of-the-art report on the various plant sources of different drugs, with special reference to the current Kerala practice. It is earnestly hoped that this will help not only in focussing the attention of men of Āyurvēda on the diversity of opinion that exists at present in the adoption of plant sources, but also in following it up with comparative studies on various plants, so that some unanimity as to what is right and what is wrong would emerge in the course of time.

Review of earlier work

The Indian system of herbal medicine and its plant drugs caught the attention of the west since the beginning of the colonial days. Garcia da orta, the personal physician of the then Portuguese Governor in India published his *Colloquies on the Simples and drugs of India* in 1563; and this was followed by Henrich Van Rheede, the Dutch Governor of Cochin, who published a 12-volume work on Kerala Medicinal Plants (1678–1703) from Amsterdam.

Since then, most of the systematic work on Indian medicinal plants has been done by north Indian authors such as Kirtikar and Basu (1918), Nadkarni (1908), Chopra *et al.* (1956), and many others. A comprehensive review of the voluminous literature is beyond the scope of this work. However, there are a few important recent studies on Kerala medicinal plants (see Anonymous, 1951, 1978; Kolammal, 1979; Aiyer and Kolammal, 1960–1966; Aiyer, *et al.*, 1957; Mooss, 1976, 1978, 1980; Nesamony, 1985; Nambiar *et al.*, 1986). Besides being incomplete, these works have been undertaken in a different perspective and hence this work.

Material and methods

The treatise is based on extensive field and laboratory studies covering a period of about five years. For this purpose market samples have been studied from selected centres throughout Kerala. When the market samples failed to give us concrete ideas about the identity of the source plant, we either got the plants collected by professional plant collectors, who supply to various pharmacies or accompanied them on collection trips to obtain the plant. Unfortunately, it was found that most of the samples we brought from the markets were not suitable for the preparation of herbarium specimens. However, we have prepared such voucher specimens for a few of them and some of them are being cultivated in the Herb Garden, Arya Vaidya Sala, Kottakkal.

Also, it has not been possible to consider all the drugs used in Āyurvēda, for the purpose of this work, due to several constraints. So we have selected a little more than 150, widely used drugs for the study. They are treated in the alphabetical order of their most popular Āyurvēdic (Sanskrit) names with their vernaculer names in brackets. The plants involved are provided with their correct names (updated using taxonomic literature) and important synonyms and a brief description together with notes on their distribution. Notes on or references to recent, important pharmacognostical, pharmacological and clinical studies are also provided. As far as possible, the plants described are illustrated, so that even non-botanists can know what is what.

Finally, we have no pretension that this is the last word on this topic. Probably, a more extensive exploratory study might reveal more of such variations, even within Kerala. We only hope that, as a pioneering effort, it is well begun.

DRUGS

AGASTI (Mal. AGATTI)

This plant, named after the great sage Agastya, is also called *munidruma* (*muni* = sage, *druma* = tree/plant - plant of the sage). *Agasti* is reported to be bitter, astringent, antihistaminic, febrifuge and tonic. It imparts strength to the body, cures intermittent fevers, catarrh, cough, discolouration of skin and diseases due to the discordance of *pitta* and *kapha*. The flowers of *agasti* are bitter, astringent, acrid on digestion and cure quartan fevers, nightblindness, catarrh, consumption and cough. The leaves are bitter, acrid and anthelmintic and cure haematemesis, itching, toxicosis and diseases caused by the excess of *kapha*. The pods are bitter, light, laxative and promote memory power. They cure tumours or glandular enlargement, anaemia, consumption and dispel toxins (Aiyer and Kolammal, 1964; 8: 5). A paste of the seeds is applied to hasten suppuration and healing of ulcers (Nesamony, 1985: 3). The bark, leaves, flowers and tender fruits are used in medicine.

The accepted plant source of this drug throughout India is *Sesbania grandiflora* of Papilionaceae. Rheede describes and illustrates the plant under the name *Agaty* (*Hortus Malabcricus* 1: 95-96. t. 51. 1678). The synonyms like *paṅktipatraḥ* (having compound leaves), *dīrghaphalā* (having long fruits) and *mṛduśiṁbī* (with smooth pods) go very well with this plant.

Sesbania grandiflora (*Linn.*) *Poiret* **(Papilionaceae)** (Fig. 1)
Robinia grandiflora Linn.
Agati grandiflora (Linn.) Desv.

Small tree; leaves pinnate, crowded towards the tip of branches; leaflets 25–30 pairs, linear-oblong, mucronate, 1-3.5 × 0.5–1 cm, glaucous beneath; flowers large, creamy white in lax axillary racemes; buds falcately recurved, calyx campanulate; corolla much exserted, petals clawed; stamens diadelphous; pod linear, the sutures thickened; seeds many.

Distribution: The plant is found in cultivation in various parts of South India. Probably a native of Indonesia, it is cultivated and naturalised in tropical Africa and Asia.

Note: The aqueous extract of the flowers of *Sesbania grandiflora* has been found to produce haemolysis of human and sheet erythrocytes even at low concentration. The active principle responsible for the haemolytic effect is characterised as the methyl ester of oleanolic acid (Kalyanagurunathan *et al.*, 1985).

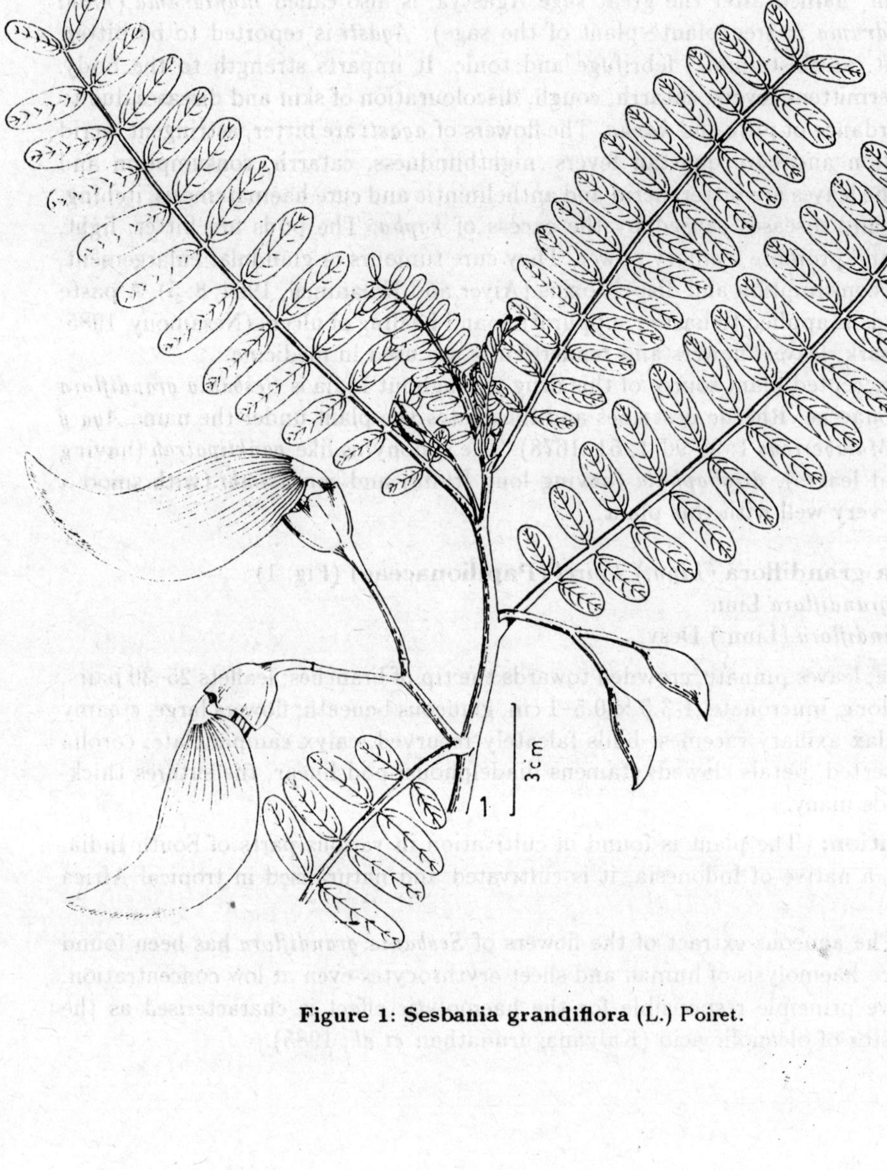

Figure 1: Sesbania grandiflora (L.) Poiret.

AGHŌRĪ (Mal. AGHŌRI)

There is no mention about this drug in any of the classic Āyurvēdic literature. But Kerala physicians use it in preparations like *Nirguṇḍyādi guḷika* and *Nirguṇḍyādi ghṛtaṃ*. The root is the officinal part. It is reported to be sweet, cooling, depurative, diuretic and is useful in bilious affections, rheumatism, poisonous bites, skin diseases urinary disorders and mental diseases. Fruit is used in cases of jaundice and enlarged spleen (Anonymous, 1956.4:44; Chopra *et al.*, 1956: 120).

Flacourtia indica (Burm.f.) Merr. of Flacourtiaceae is used as the drug source. Rheede describes this plant under the name *Couroumoelli* (Rheede V:77, t.39. 1685).

Flacourtia indica *(Burm.f.) Merr.* **(Flacourtiaceae)** (Fig. 2)
Gmelina indica Burm.f.
Flacourtia sepiaria Roxb.

Shrub or small tree with short, spiniferous branches; leaves (sub) opposite or alternate, obovate, obtuse 2.5–4 × 1.5–2.5 cms, coriaceous, glabrous, base attenuate, margin entire; flowers unisexual, clustered on spiniform branchlets, sepals 4 or 5, basally connate, ovate, ciliate; petals O; stamens in male many, unequal; ovary in female 3-celled with 2 ovules in each, styles 3, stout, stigma 3-fid; drupes globose, to 4 mm; seeds obovoid, 3–5.

Distribution: The plant is found in the scrub jungles in all districts in southern India especially on rocky hillocks. Also reported from Africa, Southeast Asia, Polynesia and Malesia.

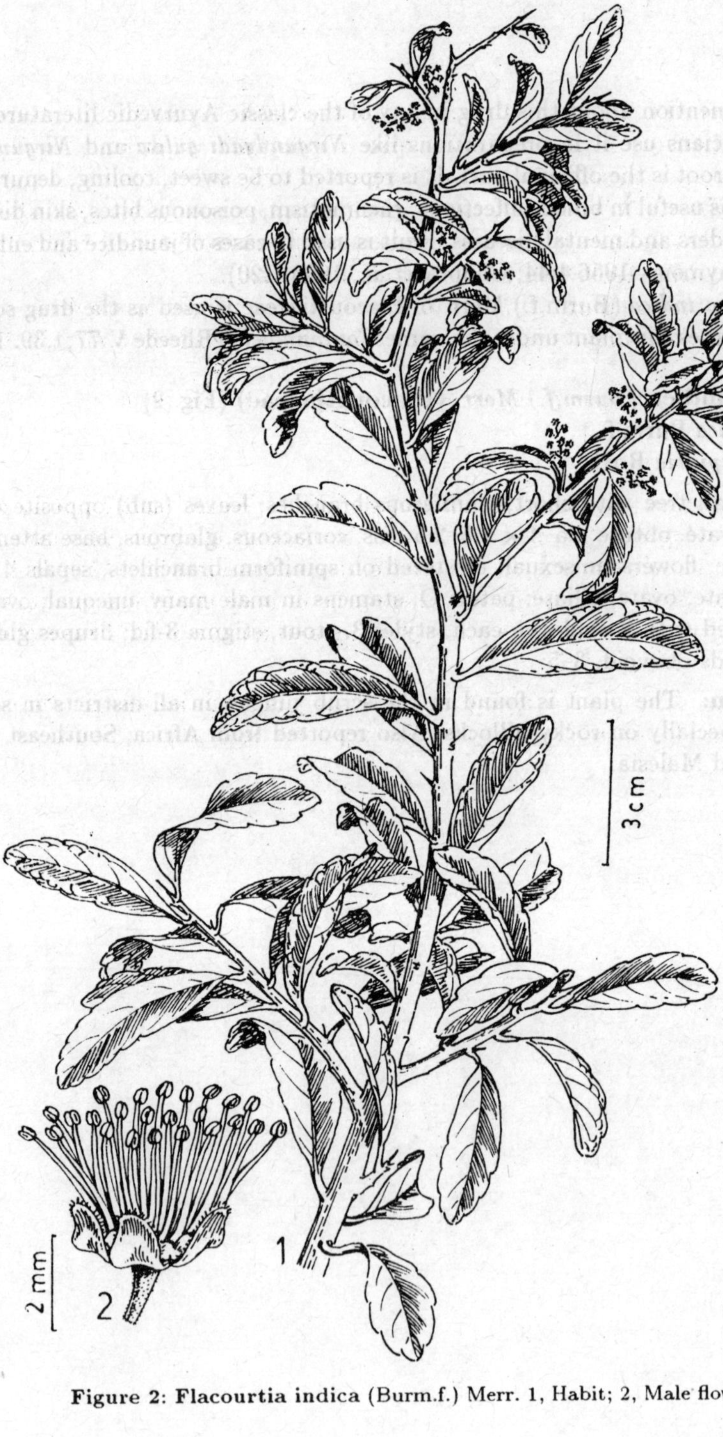

Figure 2: Flacourtia indica (Burm.f.) Merr. 1, Habit; 2, Male flower.

AGNIMANTHAḤ (Mal. MUÑÑA)

This is one of the ten drugs that constitute the group *daśamūla* (ten roots) which forms an ingredient of many important Āyurvēdic preparations like *Daśamūlāriṣṭaṃ*, *Dhānvantaraṃ kaṣāyaṃ*, *Agastyarasāyanaṃ*, *Sukumāraghṛtaṃ* etc. *Agnimanthaḥ* is reported to be acrid, bitter, astringent, cardiotonic, carminative, laxative, stomachic and tonic. It improves digestive power and is useful in constipation, fever, heart diseases, neurological diseases and rheumatism. It overcomes *kapha* and *vāta* disorders, anemia, piles, oedema, poison, anasarca and abdominal diseases. Traditionally, this drug is highly valued for its anti-inflammatory property. Infusion of the leaves is used in eruptive fevers, colic and flatulence (Nadkarni, 1954: 1010; Kolammal, 1978. 2:23; Kurup *et al.*, 1979:2) Root, rootbark and leaves are used in medicine.

As the synonyms *agnimanthaḥ*, *vahnimanthaḥ*, *haviṛmanthaḥ* etc. indicate, the tree is believed to have been used to produce fire in the sacrificial ceremonies by rubbing the sticks together. Two types of *agnimanthaḥ* - *laghu* (small) and *bṛhat* (big) are mentioned in the *nighaṇṭus*, having somewhat similar properties. Caraka and Suśrutha have mentioned them separately as *agnimanthaḥ* and *taṛkārī* respectively. Later authors have identified *Clerodendrum phlomides* and *Premna corymbosa* (= *P. serratifolia*, *P. integrifolia*), both belonging to Verbenaceae, as the respective sources of these two varieties, *laghu* and *bṛhat* (Chunekar, 1982:281; Vaidya Bapalal, 1982:267). Āyurvēdic formulary of India suggests *Clerodendrum phlomides* as the real source of the drug and *Premna serratifolia* as the substitute (Anonymous, 1978a: 241). In his commentary on *Bhāvapṛakāśa nighaṇṭu*, Chunekar (1982:281) also opines that these two can be used as substitutes for each other, as they have similar properties. Most of the authors also equate the drug with *Premna serratifolia* (Kirtikar and Basu, 1918:992; Vaidya, K.M. 1936:5; Kurup, *et al.*, 1979: 29; Dey 1980:1. Mooss, 1980:56). In Kerala also this is the accepted source of the drug. Rheede has illustrated this plant but under a different vernacular name (*Hort. Malab.*I:99–100, t.53. 1678. *Appel*).

Premna corymbosa Rottl. (Verbenaceae) (Fig. 3)
Premna serratifolia Linn.
Premna integrifolia Linn.

Small-sized tree; leaves highly aromatic, simple, opposite, elliptic-ovate, acute, 5–9 × 3–6 cm, irregularly toothed, thin coriaceous, dark green and shining above, dull below; flowers small, greenish white in many flowered, terminal, short-peduncled, corymbiform, cymose panicles; calyx cupular, persistent, becoming slightly larger and saucer-shaped in fruit; corolla obliquely funnel-shaped, 4- or 5-lobed; stamens 4, filaments hairy at base; ovary 2- or 4-celled, 4-ovuled, style linear, ending in a shortly bifid stigma; fruit a globose drupe, 4 mm across, black when ripe.

Distribution: The plant is common in many parts of India, Sri Lanka and Malaya.

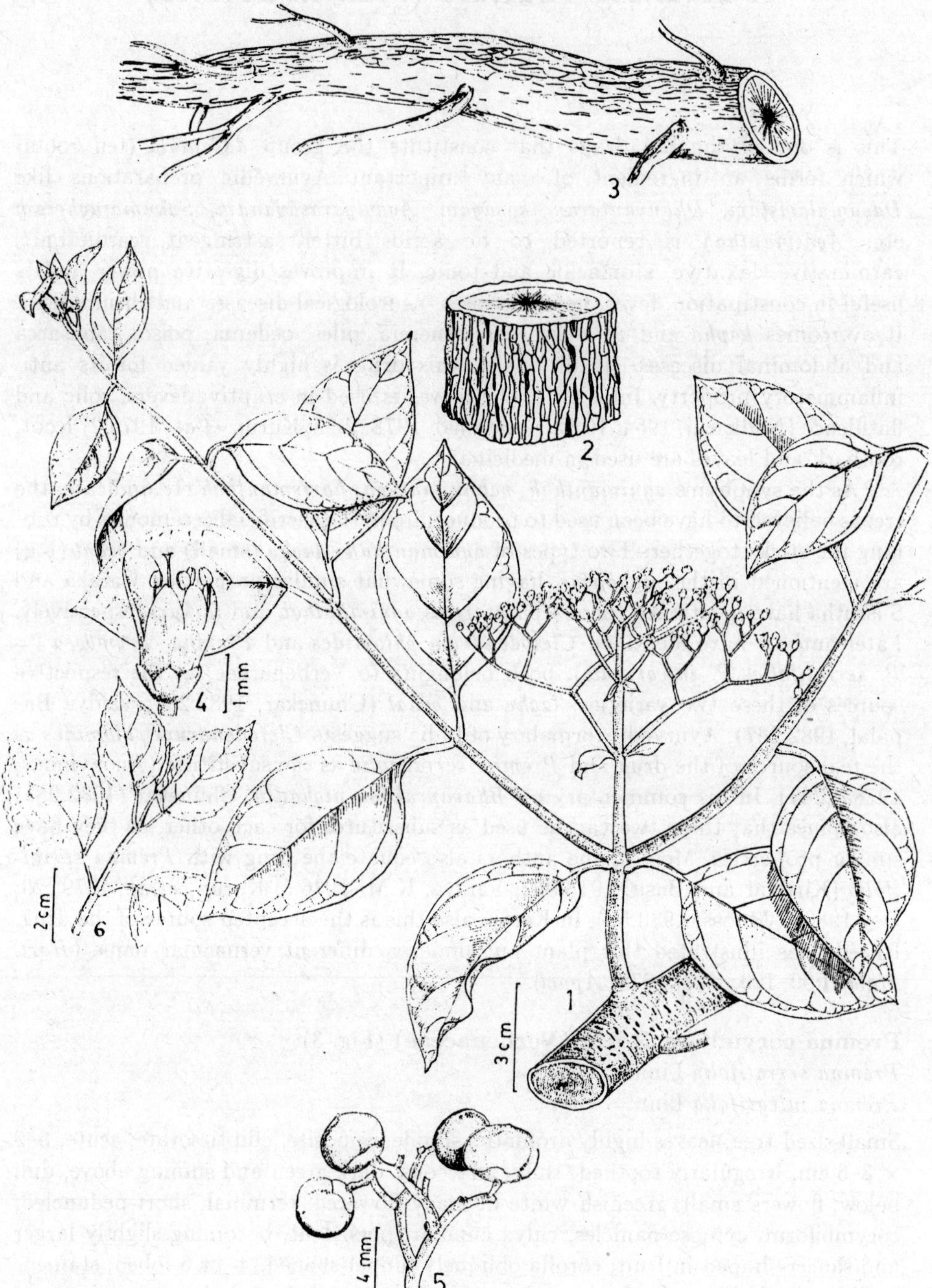

Figure 3: Premna corymbosa Rottl. 1, Habit; 2–3, Root; 4, Single-flower: 5, Fruits; 6, Young shoot.

ĀKHUKARṆĪ (Mal. ELICCEVI)

As the name indicates, the plant has leaves which resemble the ears of a rat or mouse (*ākhukarṇī, ākhuparṇī, mūṣakarṇī*, etc.). Caraka includes this among anthelmintics. According to *Bhāvaprakāśa nighaṇṭu*, it is acrid, bitter, astringent, cooling and light and overcomes urinary afflictions, diseases due to the morbidity of *kapha*, worms, fever and gastric problems. A decoction of the plant is said to act as deobstruent, diuretic and alterative, useful in rheumatism, neuralgia and headache. Leaf juice is given for migraine, headache and bites of rats and snakes. It is used as an eardrop in cases of ulcers, abscesses, etc. (Nadkarni, 1954:690; Aiyer and Kolammal, 1962.5:29). The whole plant is used medicinally. The drug is an ingredient of *Surasādi tailaṃ*.

According to the description in the texts, the plant is a creeper (*dravantya*) with its leaves and flowers occurring at regular intervals on the stem and with numerous roots arising from the nodes (*parṇikā, pratyakpuṣpī, pratyakśrēṇī, sutaśrēṇī, bahukarṇikā, bahupādikā*) (Aiyer and Kolammal, 1962.5:28). This description suits well with the plant *Merremia emarginata* (= Ipomoea reniformis) (Convolvulaceae) which is equated with the drug by most of the authors (Kirtikar and Basu, 1918: 879; Nadkarni, 1954:690; Chopra *et al.*, 1956:142; Aiyer and Kolammal, 1962.5:30; Kapoor and Mitra, 1979:78; Chunekar, 1982:477; Sharma, 1983:525). However, some practitioners in Kerala take a fern, *Hemionitis arifolia* (Burm.) Moore (Cheilanthaceae) as the drug source. But this is not mentioned in any of the authentic publications as the source of the drug. As far back as in 1693, Rheede has recorded that this plant has been in use with the local name *Pattitsjivi-Maravara* (Hort. Malab. XII:21, t.10.1693).

The important features of the two plants are described below:

Merremia emarginata (*Burm.f.*) *Hall.f.* **(Convolvulaceae)** (Fig. 4)
Ipomoea reniformis (Roxb.) Choisy
Merremia gangetica (Linn.) Cuf.

Slender, prostrate herb, rooting at nodes; stem creeping, softly hairy; leaves simple, alternate, long-stalked, reniform, subentire, 3 × 2.5 cms, glabrous; flowers small, yellow, solitary, on short axillary peduncles; sepals 5, unequal, ciliate on the margins, persistent; corolla gamopetalous, campanulate; stamens 5, epipetalous, filaments filiform, unequal, often villous at base; ovary 2–4 loculed, conical, style filiform, stigma capitate; fruit a subglobose capsule; seeds glabrous.

Distribution: The plant is found in most parts of tropical India in slightly moist areas in the plains as well as in the hills upto an elevation of about 3,000 ft. It is also reported from tropical Asia, Malesia and tropical Africa.

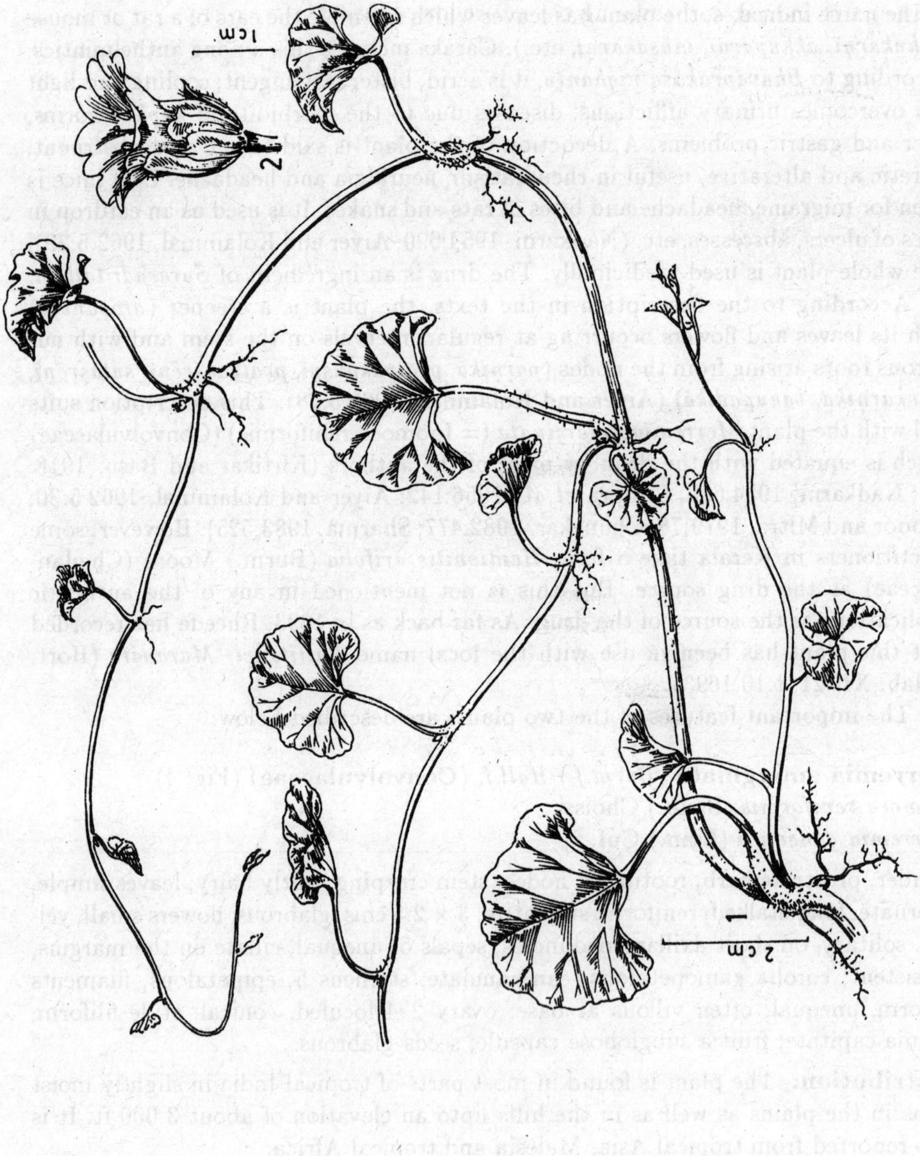

Figure 4: Merremia emarginata (Burm.f.) Hallf. 1, Habit; 2 Flower.

Hemionitis arifolia (*Burm.*) *Moore* **(Cheilanthaceae)** (Fig. 5)
Asplenium arifolium Burm.

A small, terrestrial, rhizomatous fern; rhizomes short, 5–10 cms long, suberect, covered with persistent leaf bases; scales lanceolate-acuminate; leaves dimorphic, sterile ones deeply cordate, fertile ones sagitate, stiped, shining green, coriaceous, reticulately veined; sori covering the entire lower surface.

Distribution: N.E. and southern India, Burma, Malesia and Philippines.

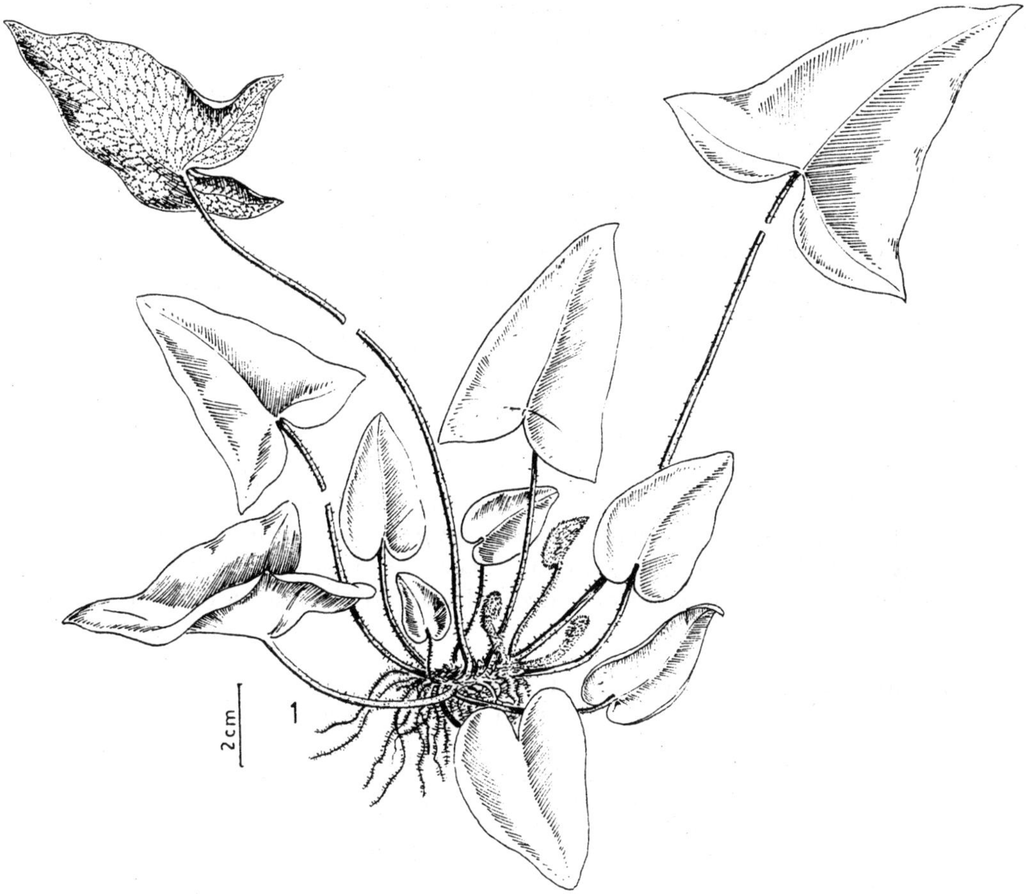

Figure 5: Hemionitis arifolia (Burm.) Moore.

ALAṀBUṢĀ (Mal. MUKKUṬṬI)

This is one of the ten auspicious herbs that constitute the group *Daśapuṣpās.* The whole plant is reportedly cooling, bitter, astringent, antipyretic, antiseptic and alleviative of *pitta* and *kapha.* It is useful in fever, burning sensation, haemorrhages, chronic cough, dysentery, urinary calculi and vaginal disorders. It cures piles and hydrocele. The leaves are antiseptic and styptic and hence very useful in healing wounds and ulcers. The leaves act as diuretic when given internally (Mooss, 1978:48; Chunekar, 1982:458). *Ceṁparutyādi tailaṃ* is an important preparation using the drug.

Many authors consider *alaṁbuṣā* and *lajjālu* to be the same and attribute the same synonyms to both. Thus, it is described as having reddish roots (*raktapādī*) and behaving like a bashful person (*lajjālu*) folding its sensitive leaves on touch (*sparśasaṅkōcaparṇikā*) resembling the folded hands of a person greeting somebody (*añjalikārikā, namaskarī*) (Aiyer and Kolammal, 1963.6:27). These synonyms suit both these plants to a great extent. Yet, in Kerala, *alaṁbuṣā* and *lajjālu* are considered different. Bhāvamiśra has already described *alaṁbuṣā* as a distinct variety of *lajjālu* (*lajjālubhēda*) (Chunekar, 1982:457). In common practice, in Kerala, *lajjālu* (Mal. *toṭṭāvāḍi*) has been equated with *Mimosa pudica* (Mimosaceae) and *alaṁbuṣā* with *Biophytum candolleanum* (Oxalidaceae). Rheede's description of the latter as *toṭṭāvāḍi* (Hort. Malab. IX:33-34.t.19.1689) does not go well with the current Kerala practice. This is most widely known by the name *mukkuṭṭi* in Kerala.

This drug has been equated with *Biophytum sensitivum* by many authors (Vaidya, K.M., 1936:29; Chopra, *et al.*, 1956:37, Chunekar, 1982:457; Nesamony, 1985:409). But the most commonly accepted source of the drug in Kerala is *B. candolleanum.*

Biophytum candolleanum *Wt.* **(Oxalidaceae)** (Fig. 6)
B. sensitivum var. candolleanum (Wt.) Hook.f. & Edgew.

Erect herb; stem simple, hispid; leaves crowded into a rosette at the tip of the stem, 8 to 12 cm long, paripinnate; leaflets 8–15 pairs, sensitive to touch, subsessile, glabrous above, pale beneath, smaller ones towards the base; flowers small, yellow on long-peduncled umbels; sepals 5, lanceolate, glandular-pubescent, 5-nerved; petals 5, laterally cohering to form a salver-shaped corolla; stamens 10, free, dimorphic; ovary 5-chambered with many ovules on axile placenta, styles 5, ending in notched or bifid stigmas; fruit a small ellipsoid, loculicidal capsule.

Distribution: Widespread in tropical Indo-Malesia. The plant is found throughout the hotter parts of India, ascending to 1800 m. It is very common in shady moist places, roadsides, river banks and also on cultivated ground.

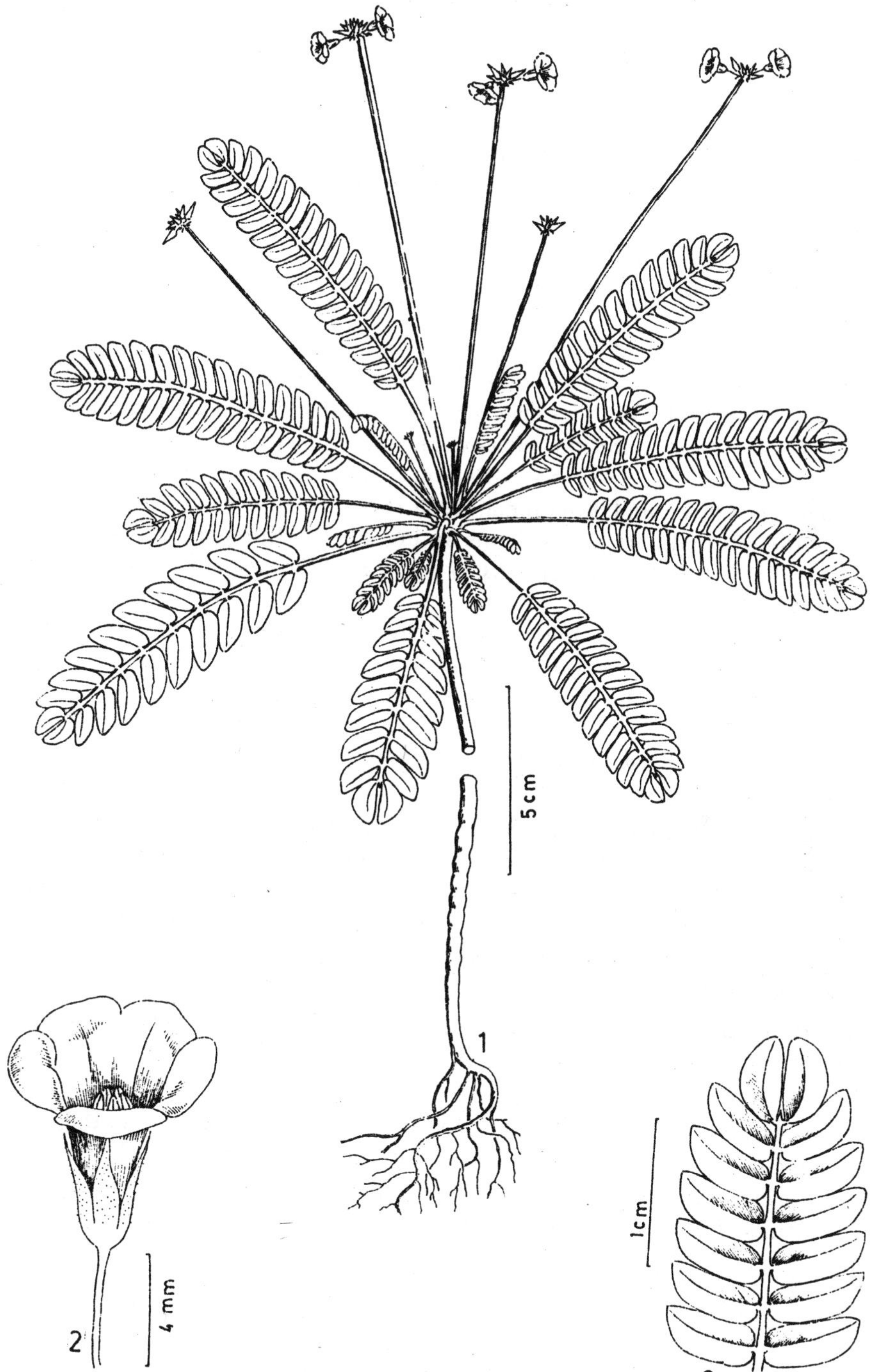

Figure 6: Biophytum candolleanum Wt. 1, Habit; 2, Single flower; 3, Portion of leaf enlarged.

ĀMALAKĪ (Mal. NELLIKKA)

Āmalakī, one of the three constituents of the group *tṛiphala* (three fruits, others being *harītakī* and *vibhītakī*), is an important *rasāyana* drug, capable of imparting youthful vigour and strength to the consumer and hence the synonyms *vayasthā* and *amṛtā*. A very important source of vitamin C, this is one of the major ingredients of the famous tonic *Cyavanapṛāśaṃ* and can also help improve intelligence and memory power.

Āmalakī is astringent, bitter, digestive, aphrodisiac, laxative, diuretic and tonic. It cures diseases due to morbid *vāta*, *pitta* and *kapha* and is especially good for the abundant growth of hair. The drug also cures thirst, burning sensation, vomiting, diabetes, emaciation, anorexia, toxicoxis, fever, impurity of blood and haemorrhage. It is useful in cough, dyspnoea, inflammation of eyes, jaundice, leucorrhoea and menorrhagia (Aiyer and Kolammal, 1963.7:122; Kurup, *et al* 1979:5). The ripe fruit is the officinal part and it forms an ingredient of preparations like *Dhātryādi ghṛtaṃ*, *Tṛiphalādi tailaṃ*, *Mahātiktaka ghṛtaṃ*, *Kayyanyādi tailam*, etc. besides *Cyavanapṛāśaṃ*.

Phyllanthus emblica (Euphorbiaceae), locally called *Nelli*, has been the accepted source of the drug. Rheede (*Hort. Malab.* I:69-70, t.38.1678) has dealt with its wide application in Āyurvēdic medicine in Kerala of his times.

Phyllanthus emblica *Linn.* **(Euphorbiaceae)** (Fig. 7)
Emblica officinalis Gaertn.

Deciduous tree with the ultimate branches pyllanthoid; leaves simple, many in each branchlet, small, linear-oblong, 15 × 3 mm, entire; flowers unisexual, greenish yellow in dense axillary fascicles along the branchlets; tepals 6, oblanceolate; in male flowers stamens 3, filaments connate to form a short column; in females ovary globose, 3-chambered with 2 ovules in each; fruit depressed globose, fleshy, 3 cm across, shining yellowish green when ripe; seeds trigonous.

Distribution: The plant is found both in the wild and cultivated state throughout tropical India. Also distributed in North Burma, South China, Indo China and Malesia.

Note: *Āmalakī* (*Emblica officinalis*) has been found to be effective in the treatment of *amḷapitta* (peptic ulcer) (Singh and Sharma, 1971; Banu *et al.*, 1982) and in dyspepsia (Chawla *et al.*, 1987). The anticholesterolaemic and antiatherogenic effect of the fruits of *Emblica officinalis* have been studied by Thakur and Mandal (1984).

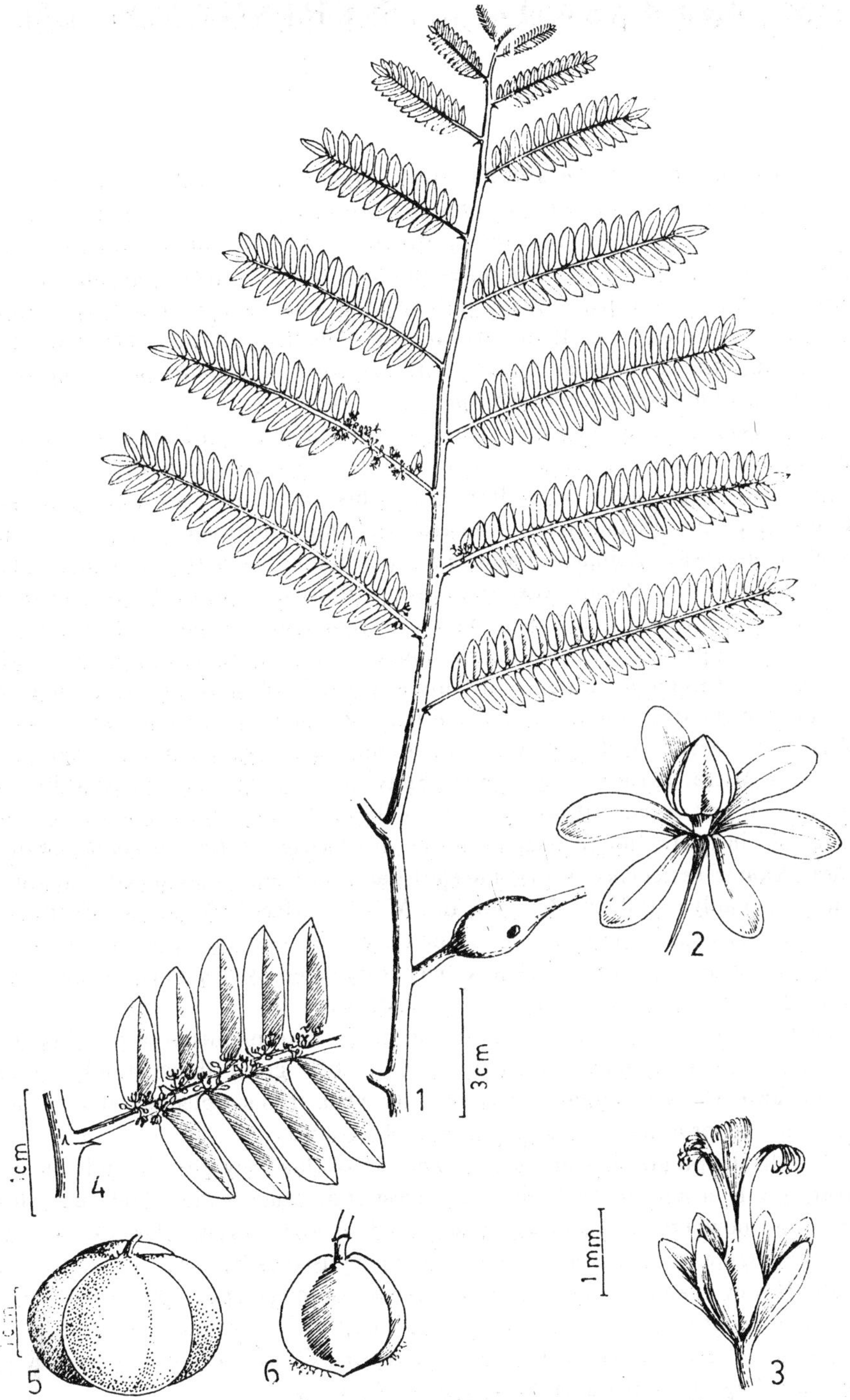

Figure 7: Phyllanthus emblica L. 1, Flowering shoot; 2, Male flower; 3, Female flower; 4, Short shoot enlarged; 5–6, Fruits.

AṀḶAVĒTASAḤ (Mal. ÑERIÑÑĀṀPUḶI)

Aṁḷavētasa is included in the group of fruit drugs (*phalavaṛga*) by Caraka. The fruit is antiscorbutic, astringent, carminative, cardiotonic, cooling, emollient and is used in anorexia, colic, dyspepsia, heart diseases, piles, difficult micturition, skin diseases, thirst and ulcers. It overcomes diseases due to *kapha* and *vāta*, loss of appetite, indigestion, flatulence, liver and spleen diseases, cough and other respiratory disorders (Kurup *et al.*, 1979:7; Chunekar, 1982:599; Sharma, 1983:339). The drug enters into the composition of preparations like *Pañcāṁḷatailaṃ*, *Hiṅguvacādi cūṛṇaṃ*, *Pūtīkarañjāsavaṃ*, *Abhṛabhasmaṃ* (101) etc.

Aṁḷavētasa has been classified variously by different authors and has been included under *vṛkṣavaṛga* (*vṛkṣa* = *tree, vaṛga* = group), *phalavaṛga* (*phala* = fruit) and *aṁḷavaṛga* (*aṁḷa* = acidic). From this, one can easily infer that it is a tree and that the officinal part is its fruits having sour taste. The drug is also described as *dīpanīya* (stomachic) and *hṛdya* (cardiac). The active part of the drug has been described as *phalaniryāsa* (exudation from the fruits) (Togunashi *et al.*, 1976). Caraka has mentioned a drug called *vṛkṣāṁḷa* (now equated with *Garcinia indica* by some authors), but this, unlike *aṁḷavētasa*, is purgative in action and is hence considered different. Singh and Chunekar (1972:21) have observed that the plant source of the drug *aṁḷavētasa* is the fruit of either a *Citrus* or a *Garcinia*.

Many of the earlier authors have equated *aṁḷavētasa* with *Garcinia pedunculata* (Kapoor and Mitra, 1979:76; Dey, 1980:6; Sharma, 1983:339) and this is still being used in Bengal and Assam. However, Vaidya Bapalal (1982:195) has reported that the drug sold in north Indian bazaars is the dried twigs of *Rheum emodii* (Polygonaceae). *Rumex vesicarius* (Polygonaceae) has also been equated with this drug by some (see Vaidya, 1936:22, Kapoor and Mitra, 1979:81). Āyurvēdic Formulary of India (Anonymous, 1978a:241) has concluded that *Garcinia pedunculata* is the actual source of the drug (This has also been supported by Togunashi *et al.*, 1976) and that *Rheum emodii* can be used as a substitute.

In fact, this is a classic case of confusion in the determination of plant sources of the drugs used in Āyurvēdic medicine. The picture given above is only partial. One could have a more complete scenario only when it is supplemented with facts from the current practice in various parts of the country.

In Kerala the plants that are used as sources of this drug and the indication of its nature given in ancient texts do not correspond. None of the plants used here is a tree, and nowhere the fruits are being used. A wide variety of weak-stemmed climbers belonging to the family Vitaceae are being used as the source of *aṁḷavētasa* in Kerala. However, since we are not the people to comment upon the authenticity of the choice, we confine ourselves to provide means of identification of plants that are being used here. The plants used are *Cissus repens*, *Cissus vitiginea*, *Ampelocissus latifolia* and *Cayratia trifolia*, all belonging to Vitaceae.

Cissus repens *Lamk.* **(Vitaceae)** (Fig. 8)
Vitis repens (Lam.) Wt. & Arn.

Tendril climbers; stem glaucous-white; leaves simple, alternate, ovate-acuminate, cordate at base, serrate, basally 5-nerved, glabrous, 15 × 10.3 cm; flowers small, greenish-pink in leaf-opposed umbellate cymes; calyx campanulate, truncate; petal 4, ovate; stamens 4, filaments short; ovary 2-celled; berry globose; seeds smooth.

Distribution: The plant is found in the West Coast and Western Ghats from South Canara to the Anamalais and Travancore upto 4,000 ft. Also distributed in the Himalayas, Northeast India and Malesia.

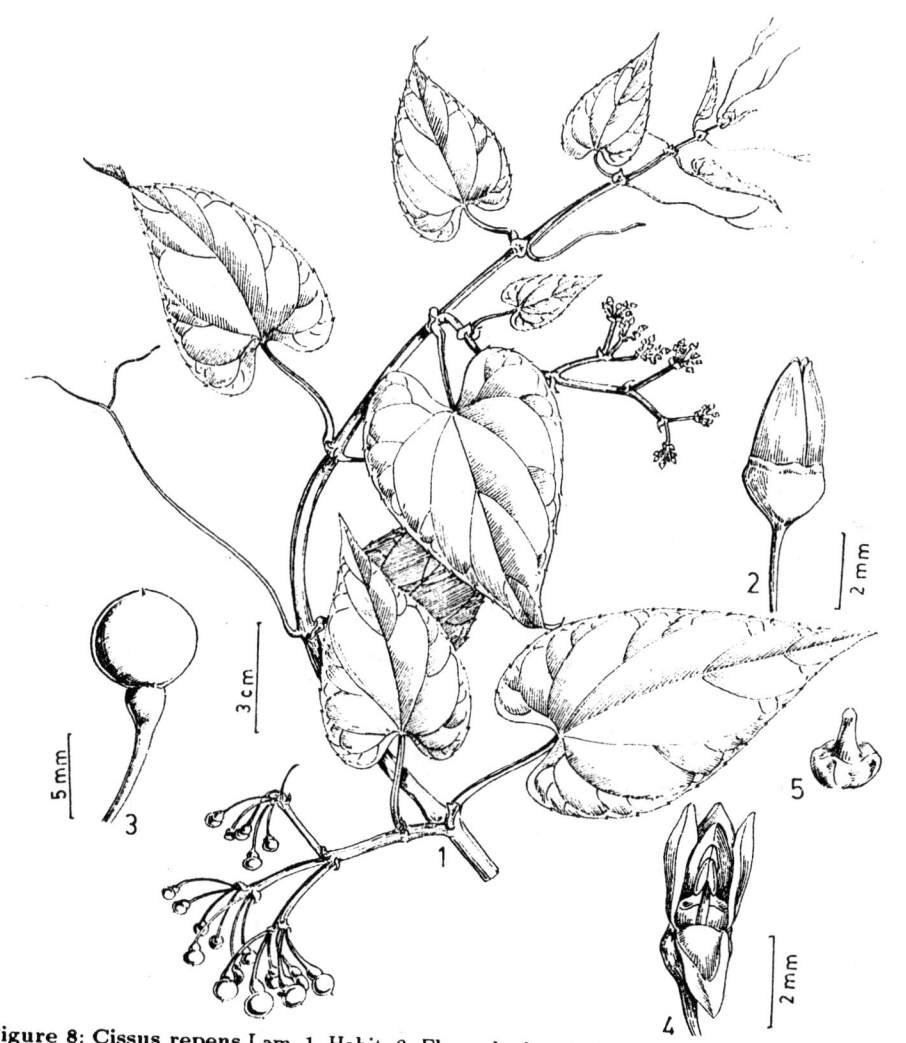

Figure 8: Cissus repens Lam. 1, Habit; 2, Flower bud; 3, Fruit; 4, Flower showing stamens; 5, Pistil.

Cissus vitiginea *Linn.* **(Vitaceae)** (Fig. 9)

Vitis linnaei Wallich ex Wt. & Arn.

Tendril climber; stem and petioles soft-tomentose; leaves simple, alternate, broadly ovate-cordate, 5-angled, to 12 × 13.3 cm, basally 3-nerved, margin dentate, pubescent; tendrils simple, opposite to leaves; flowers pale yellow in umbellate cymes; calyx tube obscurely lobed; petals 4, ovate; stamens 4, ovary 2-celled; berries blue, pyriform, rugose; seeds tessellate.

Distribution: Peninsular India and Sri Lanka

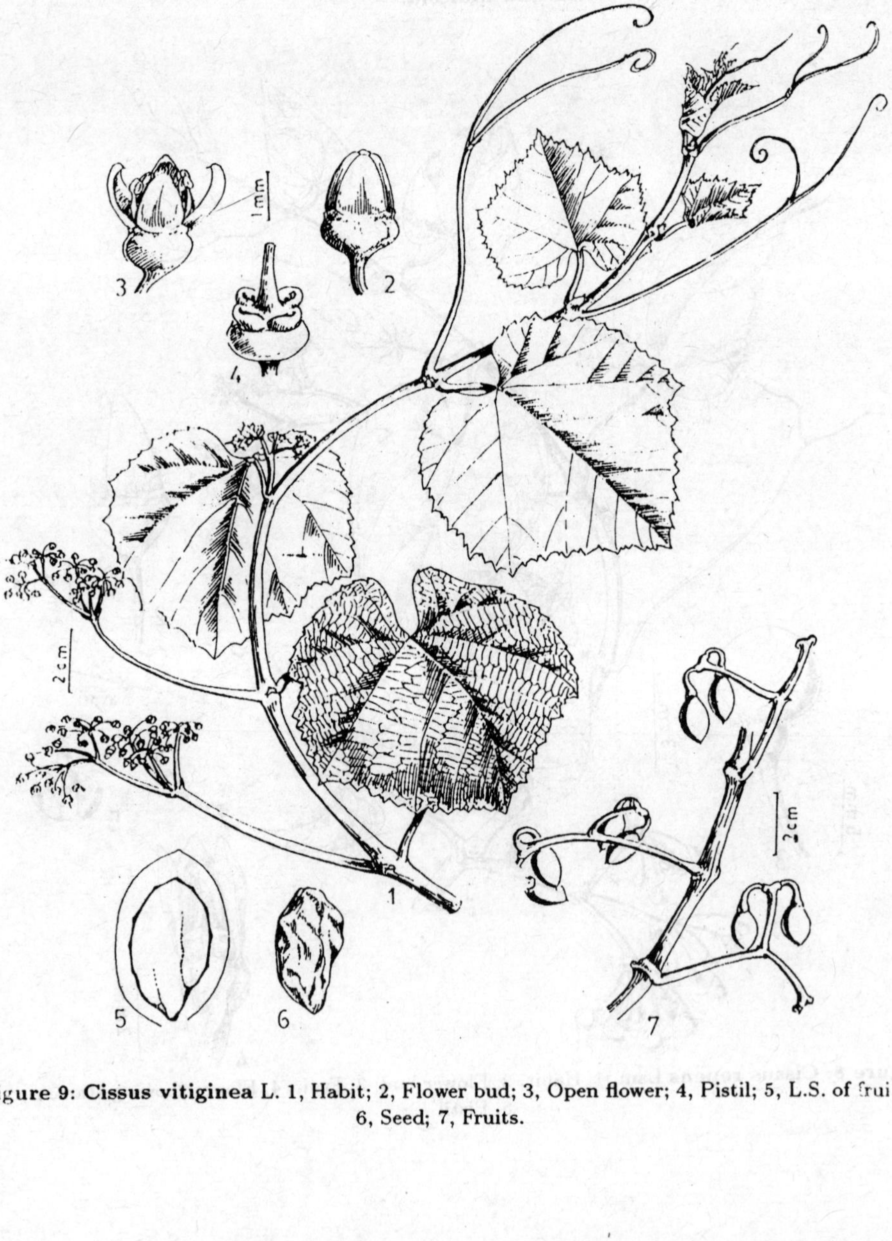

Figure 9: Cissus vitiginea L. 1, Habit; 2, Flower bud; 3, Open flower; 4, Pistil; 5, L.S. of fruit; 6, Seed; 7, Fruits.

Ampelocissus latifolia (*Roxb.*) *Planch.* **(Vitaceae)** (Fig. 10)
Vitis latifolia Roxb.

Tendril climber; stem glaucous; leaves orbicular-cordate, 3–5 lobed or angled, serrate, glabrous; tendrils forked; flowers small in axillary peduncled umbellate inflorescence; calyx cupular, teeth obscure; petals 4–5, recurved in flower; stamens 4–5, inserted without the disk, disk short, thick, 5-furrowed; ovary 2-celled, immersed more or less in the disk; fruit a succulent berry; seed oblong, crenate on the margin.

Distribution: Peninsular India

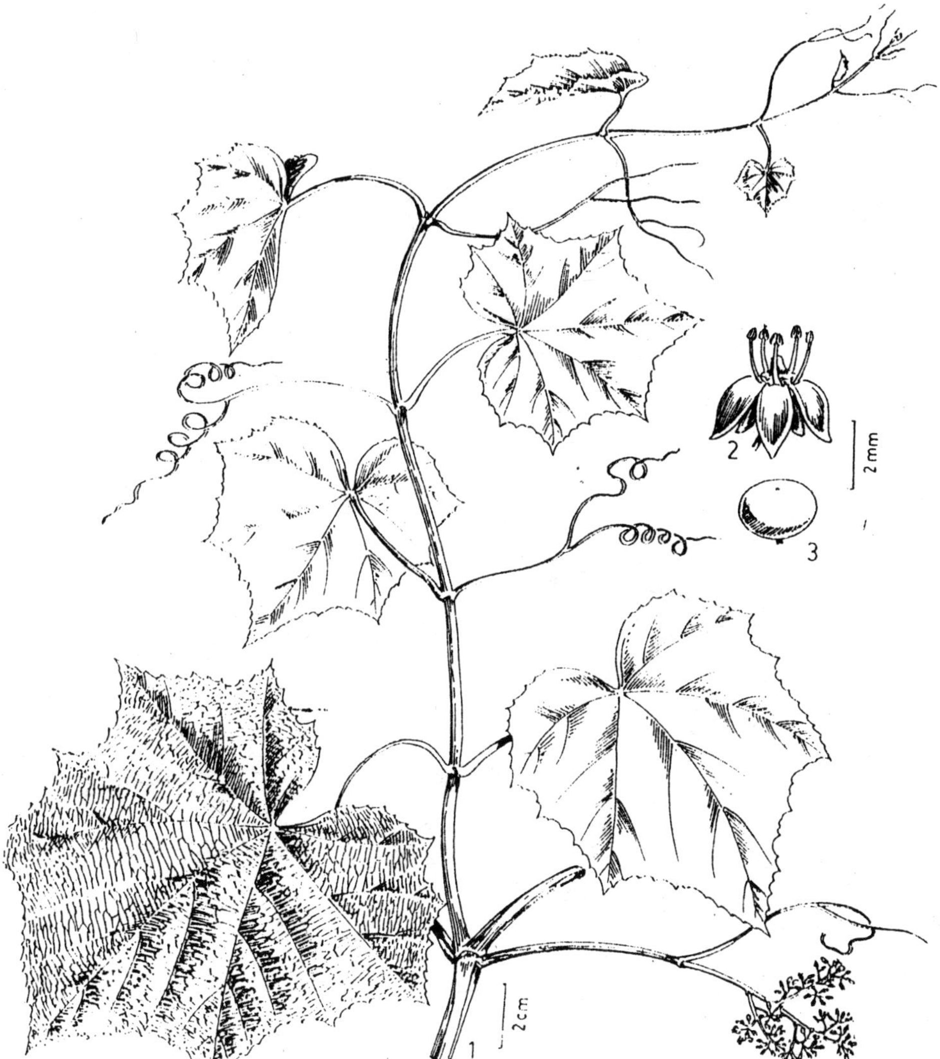

Figure 10: Ampelocissus latifolia (Roxb.) Planch. 1, Habit; 2, Flower; 3, Fruit.

Cayratia trifolia (*Linn.*)*Domin* **(Vitaceae)** (Fig. 11)
Vitis trifolia Linn.

Tendril climber; leaves alternate, pedately trifoliate; leaflets ovate or elliptic-obtuse, serrate, glabrous, 10 × 6 cm, laterals unequal-sided and smaller, 7 × 5 cm; flowers green in corymbose panicles; calyx tube 0.5 mm; petals 4, greenish white; disc obscurely lobed, apically crenulate; stamens 4, filaments short; ovary 2-celled; berry obovoid; seeds 2, pyriform.

Distribution: Peninsular India, Sri Lanka, China, Indo-China & Malesia.

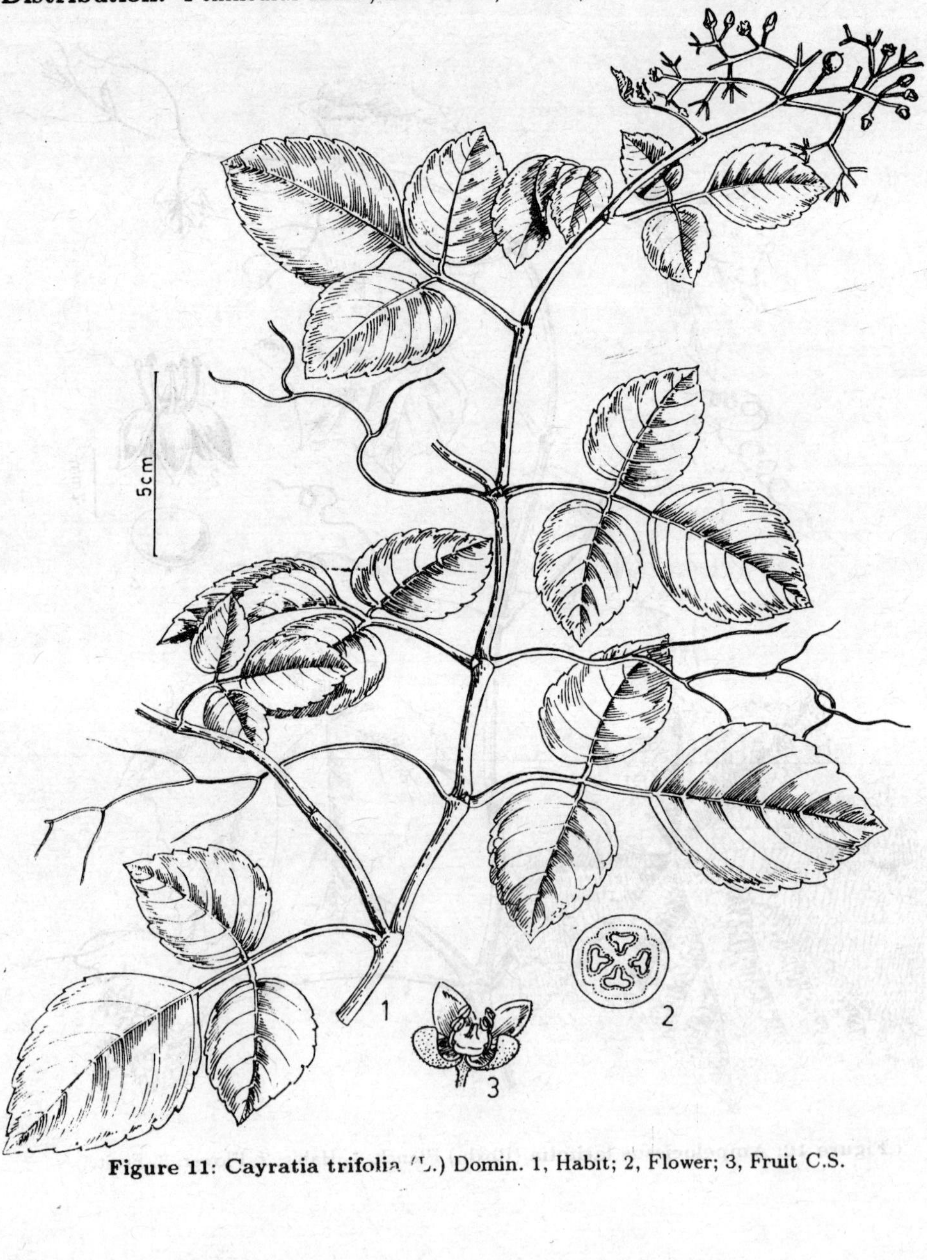

Figure 11: Cayratia trifolia (L.) Domin. 1, Habit; 2, Flower; 3, Fruit C.S.

Garcinia pedunculata *Roxb.* **(Clusiaceae)**

Tree about 60 feet tall, leaves to 30 × 15 cm, subcoriaceous, base acute or acuminate; flowers unisexual, male flower large, pale green in 8–12 flowered cymes; sepals orbicular, fleshy, inner pair narrower, oblong; stamens many in a 4-angled, truncate, shortly stipitate mass; anthers 2-celled, female flower larger than the male, solitary on a thick 4-angled peduncle; ovary globose, stigma sessile, 8–10 rayed, spreading; fruit large, yellow with a copious yellow exudate; seeds reniform.

Distribution: The tree is cultivated for its acid fruit in Silhet. It is found in the forests of Northeast Bengal, near Rungpore and Goalpara.

ĀMṚĀTAKAḤ (Mal. AṀPAḺAṂ)

This drug, included in the *Ambaṣṭhādigaṇa*, is reported to be sour in taste, hot and heavy. It cures *vāta* and promotes appetite. Leaves and bark are astringent and are good for dysentery; the bark is used in bilious dyspepsia. Juice of the leaves is applied locally in ear-ache. Pulp of the fruit is acid, astringent, antiscorbutic, aphrodisiac and tonic and cures *vāta, pitta,* thirst, dyspepsia, tuberculosis and hemopathy (Nadkarni, 1954:1166; Chunekar, 1982:553). The important formulations using the drug are *Pāṭhādi guḷika, Pañcāmḷa tailaṃ, Annabhēdisindūraṃ, Puṣyānugacūrṇaṃ, Vārāhyādi ghṛtaṃ,* etc.

Some of the synonyms attributed to this indicate that the plant has got a colour resembling that of monkeys (*kapītanaḥ*), fruits resemble mangoes (*āmṛātakaḥ*) and that it is provided with a yellow exudate (*pītanaḥ*) (cf. Moosad, 1983:290).

Spondias mangifera (Anacardiaceae), locally called *aṁpaḻaṃ* is the accepted source of the drug. (Kirtikar and Basu, 1918:393; Vaidya K.M., 1936:48; Nadkarni, 1954:1166; Chopra *et al.*, 1956:233; Chunekar, 1982:553).

Some people erroneously treat *ambaṣṭhā* and *aṁpaḻaṃ* as same, probably due to superficial similarity in the names and equate both with *Spondias pinnata* (See Mooss, 1980:96) but actually *ambaṣṭhā* is a synonym of *pāṭhā* which is discussed elsewhere.

Spondias pinnata (*L.f.*) *Kurz.* **(Anacardiaceae)** (Fig. 12)
S. mangifera Willd.

Deciduous tree; bark grey; leaves clustered towards branch apices, imparipinnate; leaflets ovate-oblong, acuminate, 20 × 8 cms, glabrous, nerves close, parallel, connected by a prominent intramarginal nerve; flowers yellowish, polygamous in terminal panicles on bare branches; calyx lobes 5, caducous; petals 5, disc cupular, 10-toothed; stamens 10, free, inserted below the disc; ovary 5-celled, style 5, connivent, drupe oblong-ovoid, furrowed.

Distribution: The tree is distributed in Indo-Malesia, especially in Java and the Philippines. It is found in the deciduous forests in almost all districts in India, upto about 2000 ft.

Taxonomic notes

Rheede (1.92–93. 1678) has described two types of '*Ambalam*' (= Ambazham) viz. *ambalam* and *cat-ambalam/pee-ambalam.* The former is seen wild as well as cultivated for its edible fruits, while the latter is wild and fruits bitter. He has rightly portrayed *Spondias pinnata* as *ambalam*, but has given only a description for the latter.

Nicolson *et al.* , (1988:49) have presumed that Rheede's *cat-ambalam* may be a wild form of *Spondias pinnata.* However, this vernacular name is still prevalent and is applied to a different, but closely related taxon, *Spondias indica* (Wt. &

Arn.) Airy Shaw & Forman (Syn. *Solenocarpus indica* Wt. & Arn.). The two can be distinguished as follows:

Leaflets entire, flowers yellow, styles 4–5 . . . . *S. pinnata.*

Leaflets serrulate, flowers white, style single . . . . . . *S. indica.*

Only *S. pinnata* is used in medicine.

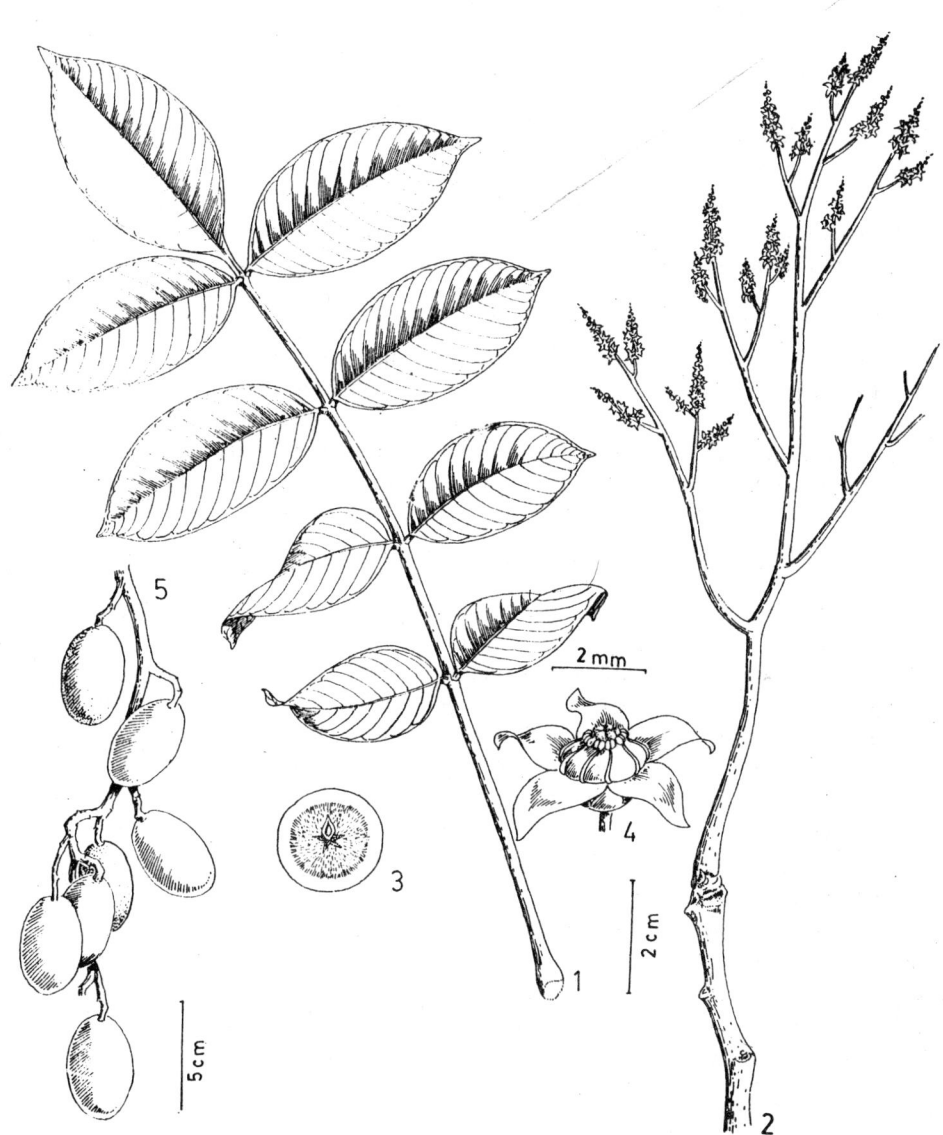

Figure 12: Spondias pinnata (L.f.) Kurz. 1, A leaf; 2, Inflorescence; 3, Fruit T.S.; 4, Flower; 5, Fruits.

AMṚTĀ (Mal. AMṚTU, CIṬṬAMṚTU)

Amṛtā is a Hindu mythological term which refers to the heavenly 'elixir' which saved the celestial people from senescence and kept them eternally young. This term is attributed to this drug in Āyurvēda in recognition of its capacity to impart youthfulness, vitality and longevity to the consumer. The officinal part i.e. the mature stem of this widely used herb is reported to be acrid, bitter, hot, restorative, aphrodisiac, alleviative of all the three *dōṣās* or morbidities and a digestive tonic. It cures fever, jaundice, thirst, burning sensation, diabetes, piles, skin ailments, respiratory disorders, neurological diseases and improves intellect. Externally the drug is used against rheumatic complaints (Iyer & Kolammal 1963.7:21). *Amṛtā* is a constituent of several preparations like *Amṛtāriṣṭaṃ, Dhānvantaraṃ tailaṃ, Ceṟiya Rāsnādi kaṣāyaṃ, Valiya Maṟmaguḷika*, etc.

Āyurvēdic texts have provided some useful indications for the identification of the plant source. This herb, which can impart youthful vitality to the consumer (*amṛtā, amṛtavallarī*), is a twiner (*kuṇḍalī*) with sweet leaves (*madhuparṇī*) and without any hurting structures like spines or prickles (*viśalyā*). It is capable of regenerating from stem cuttings (*chinnā, chinnaruhā, chinnōtbhavā*) and the stem when cut, displays the configuration of a wheel (*cakṛalakṣaṇā*) (Iyer & Kolammal, 1963:7:21).

According to Āyurvēdic lexicons, there are two varieties of *amṛtā*: viz. *amṛtā*, also called *ciṭṭamṛta* and *kanda-amṛta*, also called *kanda-guḍūcī, padmaguḍūcī* or *pee-amṛta*. The accepted source of the former throughout India is *Tinospora cordifolia* (Willd.) Hook f. & Thoms. (Menispermaceae). The latter has been equated with *T. sinensis* (Lour.) Merr., a much larger species with thicker stem and larger, densely pubescent leaves (Mooss, 1976:144, Chunekar; 1982:270; Sharma, 1983:761). *T. cordifolia* is considered more potent and hence preferred by practitioners. However, the latter variety is often used as a substitute. Sharma (1983:761) mentions yet another species *T. crispa* Hook.f. & Thoms. which is used as a specific for fevers in North Western India. However, this species is not available down south and has never been in use here.

Kerala physicians use *T. cordifolia* eventhough sometimes *T. sinensis* is also occasionally used as a substitute. Rheede has portrayed both *Chittamrdu* (Hort. Malab. 7: 39.t. 21. 1688) and *Pee-Amrdu* (Hort. Malab. 7. 37–38, t. 19–20. 1688) and they correspond to these species respectively, pointing to the fact that these were widely used by practitioners in Kerala since long.

Tinospora cordifolia (*Willd.*) *Hook.f.* & *Thoms.* **(Menispermaceae)** (Fig. 13)
Menispermum cordifolium Willd.
Tinospora glabra (N. Burm.) Merr.

Glabrous twiners, stem terete, sparcely lenticellate and often producing filiform aerial roots, green when young with a loose greyish bark when mature; leaves simple, alternate, long-petioled, lamina broadly ovate-cordate, shortly acuminate at apex, to 9 × 8 cms; flowers green, unisexual in dioecious spikes, mostly in the axils of fallen leaves; sepals 3 + 3, free; petals 6; stamens in male 6; in female flowers carpels 3, with 6 subulate staminodes; fruit drupaceous, ovoid or ellipsoid.

Distribution: This species occurs in India, Bangladesh and Ceylon. In India it is distributed almost throughout, extending from the Himalayas down to southern part of Peninsular India. It usually grows in waste lands and in deciduous forests and scrub jungles, growing over hedges and bushes.

Note: Recent clinical and pharmacological studies have revealed that an aqueous extract of the stem helps in reducing the blood sugar in alloxan induced hyperglycaemic rats and rabbits (Raghunathan & Sharma, 1969). Mhaiskar *et al.*, (1980) found the stems as an effective remedy for *āmavāta* and *sandhigata vāta*, two types of rheumatic afflictions. The anti-pyretic and anti-inflammatory actions of the drug have been studied by Pillai *et al.*, (1980) and Gulati and Pandey (1982) respectively.

Detailed pharmacognostic studies on this plant have been made by Khosla and Prasad (1971).

Tinospora sinensis (*Lour.*) *Merr.* **(Menispermaceae)** (Fig. 14)
Campylus sinensis Lour.
Tinospora malabarica (Lam.) Hook.f. & Thoms.
T. tomentosa (Colebr.) Hook.f. & Thoms.

Pubescent twiners or climbers, much larger than the earlier species; stem terete with scattered lenticels and prominent leaf scars, bark loose, grey, papery when mature; leaves long-petioled, alternate, broadly ovate-cordate, entire or sinuately 3–5 lobed, to 15 × 12 cm, densely pubescent on both sides; flowers unisexual in long, pendant, dioecious spikes mostly from the axils of fallen leaves, sepals 3 + 3 free; petals 6; stamens 6 in male flowers; carpels 3 in female flowers; fruit an aggregate of 1–3 ovoid drupelets which turn reddish when ripe.

Distribution: Distributed in South and South East Asia, this species runs wild in most parts of India, both in forests and plains. The Indo-Chinese use its stem as a muscle relaxant. In Chinese, it has got a name which means "muscle-relaxing vine" (cf. Forman 1981).

Note: The details about the macro and micro-scopical characters, physical constant values, fluorescence analysis and phytochemical studies of *Tinospora cordifolia* and *T. sinensis* are discussed by Raghunathan & Mitra (1982:322–347).

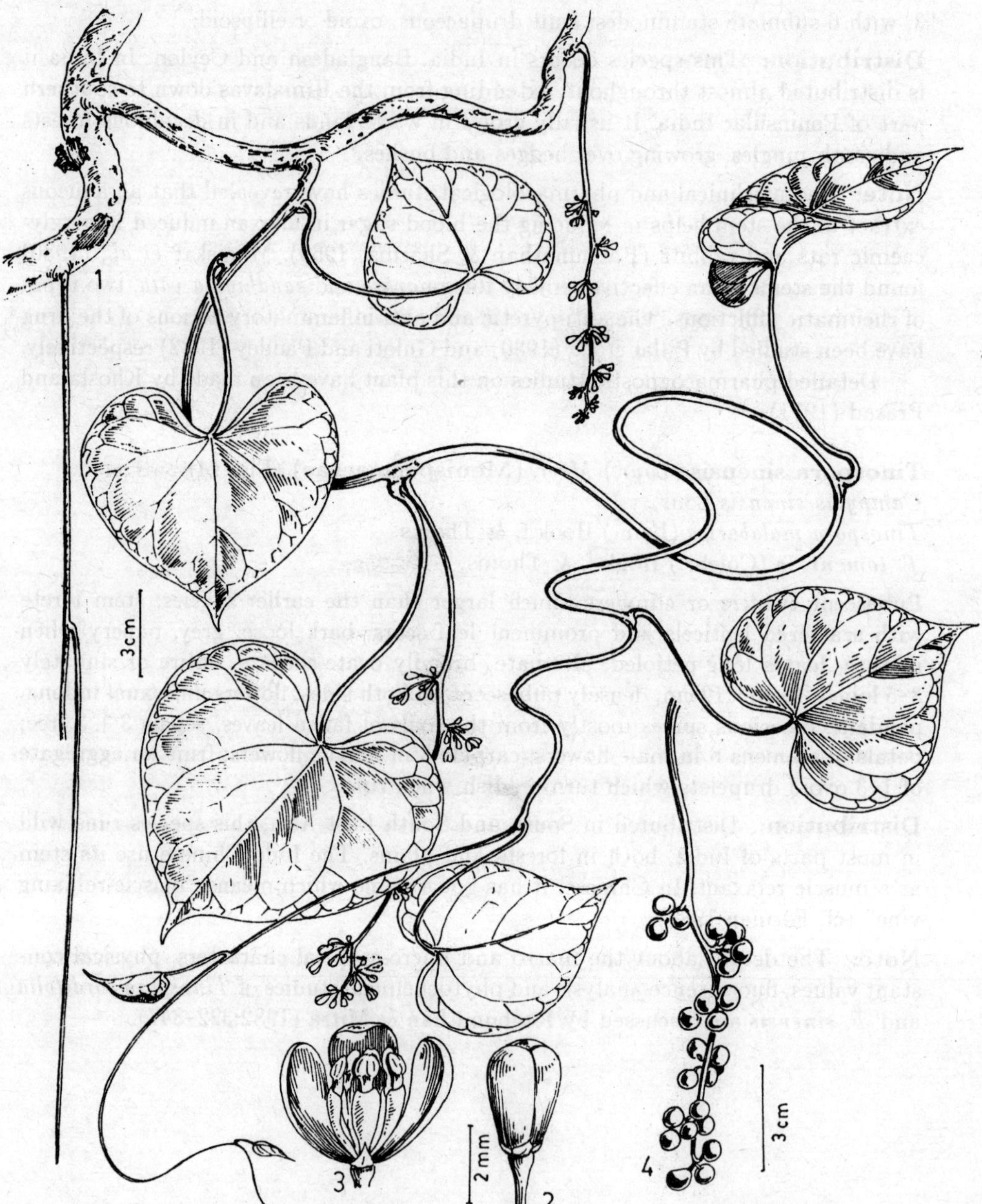

Figure 13: Tinospora cordifolia (Willd.) Hook.f. & Thoms. 1, Habit; 2, Flower bud; 3, Male flower showing stamens; 4, Fruits.

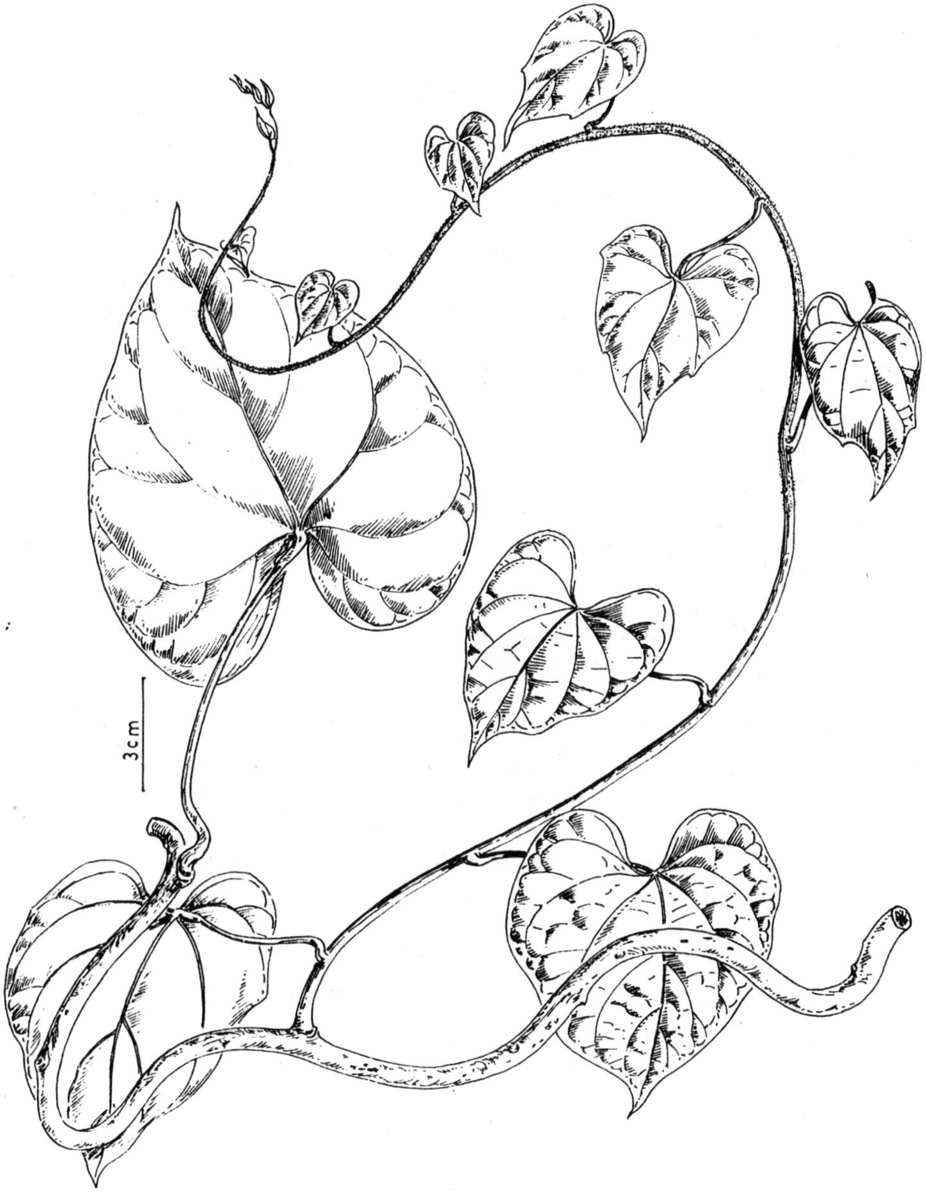

Figure 14: Tinospora sinensis (Lour.) Miers.

AṄKŌLAḤ (Mal. AṄKŌLAṂ)

This is a reputed single drug in Āyurvēda for the treatment of rabies. The root bark is administered both internally and externally in cases of rabid dog-bites and also as an antidote for other poisonous bites including snake bites. The drug is reported to be bitter, alterative, anthelmintic, astringent, laxative, easily digestible and unctuous and is emetic in large doses. It is useful in diarrhoea, simple continued fevers, worms, colic, hemopathy and inflammation. It is a reputed remedy for leprosy and other skin diseases and syphilis. The fruit is laxative, antiphlegmatic and tonic and is useful in burning sensation, emaciation, haemorrhages and morbidity of *tridōṣās—vāta, pitta* and *kapha* (Nadkarni, 1954:59, Mooss, 1978:21). The drug is an ingredient of *Mahābhūtarāvaghṛtaṃ*.

Alangium salvifolium (Linn.f.) Wangerin of Alangiaceae, locally called *Aṅkōlaṃ*, is the accepted source of the drug. (See Kirtikar and Basu, 1918:637; Nadkarni, 1954:58; Chopra *et al.*, 1956:10; Mooss, 1978:19; Kapoor & Mitra, 1979:71; Chunekar, 1982:365; Sharma, 1983:779). Rheede has described two different varieties of this drug namely *angolam* (Hort. Malab. 4:39–40.t.17.1682) and *karaangolam* (Hort. Malab. 4:55–56.t.26.1683). They correspond to *Alangium salvifolium* subsp. *salvifolium* and subsp. *hexapetalum* respectively (See Nicolson *et al.*, 1988:42–43). Known as *kurukkuṭṭi* in Travancore, the latter is seldom used in medicine, but its fruits are usually eaten by children (cf. Mooss, 1978:19).

Alangium salvifolium (*Linn.f.*) *Wang.* ssp. **salvifolium (Alangiaceae)** (Fig. 15)

Tree; leaves alternate, petiolate, oblong or elliptic-lanceolate, 5–14 × 2–2.25 cm, chartaceous, 3–5 nerved at base, glabrous above, glabrescent or puberulous below, base oblique, margin entire, apex acuminate, petiole to 1 cm, tomentose; flowers white, scented, in axillary clusters, pubescent outside; calyx tube cupular, adnate to the ovary, tomentose; petals 10, linearly oblong, reflexed; stamens 20, filaments villous at base, subconnate, anthers linear; ovary turbinate, 1-celled, stigma capitate; fruits ovoid, 2–2.5 cm long, rusty tomentose.

Distribution: The plant is distributed in dry regions, in the plains and lower hills in India and also in Africa, Sri Lanka, Indochina and China.

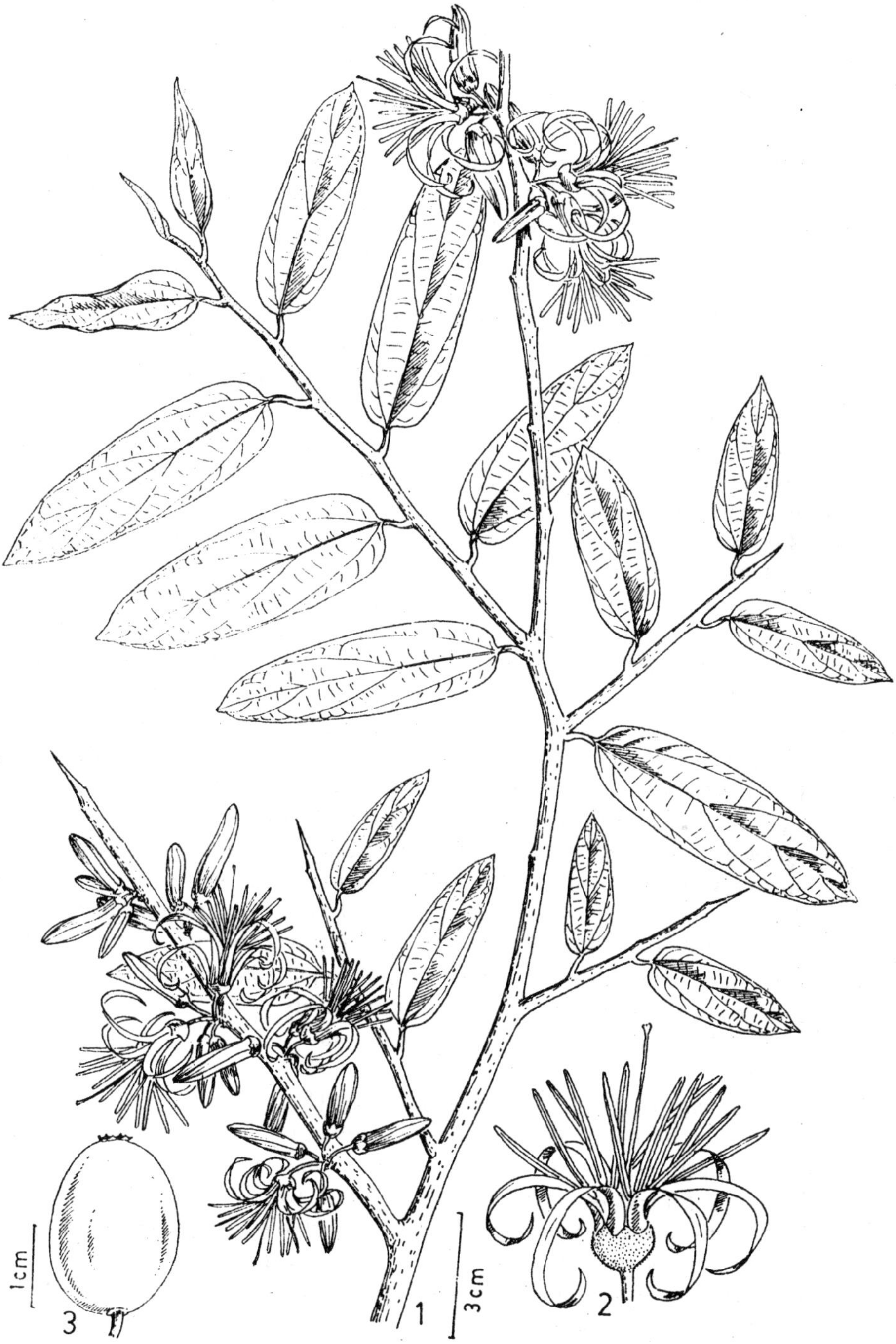

Figure 15: Alangium salvifolium (L.f.) Wang. ssp. salvifolium. 1, A flowering shoot; 2, Flower; 3, Fruit.

APĀMĀṚGAḤ (Mal. KAṬALĀṬI)

As the name *Apāmāṛgaḥ* indicates, it hinders the path of the pedestrians. The drug is bitter, acrid, cardiotonic, astringent, carminative, diuretic, alleviative of *kapha* and *vāta* and is useful as an errhine. It cures hiccough, ascites, enlargement of cervical glands, skin diseases, piles, pruritus, anorexia and urinary diseases. It overcomes the troubles due to worms and pathogenic organisms, arrests bleeding and dysentery (Aiyer & Kolammal, 1963.6:60; Mooss, 1976:6; Kurup *et al.*, 1979:10). The whole plant is used in medicine. The important formulations using the drug are *Surasādi tailaṃ, Āviltōlādi bhasmaṃ, Suvarṇamuktādi guḷika, Jātyādi tailaṃ, Aṛdhavilvaṃ kaṣāyaṃ*, etc.

The texts describe the plant as one having leaves which are borne at right angle to the stem (*pṛatyakparṇī*) and which possesses hairs like that of a monkey (*kīśaparṇī*), with an inflorescence resembling the crest on the head of a peacock (*mayūrakaḥ*) and which is sharp-pointed (*kharamañjarī, paṅgtikaṇṭakaḥ*) (Kolammal, 1963.6:60).

Most of the authors equate the drug with *Achyranthes aspera* Linn. (Amaranthaceae) (Vaidya, 1936:18; Nadkarni, 1954:21; Kurup *et al.*, 1979:10; Sharma, 1983:542) and this goes well with the name *apāmāṛga*, because its fruiting spikes with barbed prickles stick to the clothes of human beings and body of the animals passing its way. The *nighaṇṭus* mention a red variety also, called *raktāpamāṛgaḥ* and this is equated with *Achyranthes bidentata* Bl. by some (Chunekar, 1982:416).

Kerala Physicians do not make a distinction between *apāmāṛgaḥ* and *raktāpamāṛgaḥ*. Nevertheless, they have two varieties of their own, a larger variety and a smaller variety, called *kaṭalāṭi* and *ceṛukaṭalāṭi* in vernacular, respectively. As far back as in 1960, Rheede has portrayed them separately (Hort. Malab. 10:155.t.78. *Cadelari* and 10:157.t.79. *Scherucadelari*) testifying to the fact that it has been so since long. These two are invariably equated with *Achyranthes aspera* and *Cyathula prostrata* of Amaranthaceae respectively.

The two plants can be distinguished as follows:

Achyranthes aspera *Linn.* **(Amaranthaceae)** (Fig. 16)

Erect pubescent herb; leaves opposite, short-petioled, exstipulate, obovate-orbicular or elliptic, obtuse or shortly acuminate, entire or slightly flexuous, upto 12 × 8 cms, soft-tomentose; flowers small, greenish-white, sessile, deflexed on terminal spikes; bracts membraneous, persistent; bracteoles 2, persistent, spinescent; perianth persistent, segments 5, spinous-tipped; stamens 5 with filiform filaments and 2-celled anthers; ovary one-celled with a solitary pendulous ovule, style filiform, stigma capitate; fruit an ovoid utricle.

Distribution: The plant is found throughout India in all plains districts and also in other tropical and warmer regions of the world. It is a gregariously growing troublesome weed of waste places, roadsides, grasslands, etc.

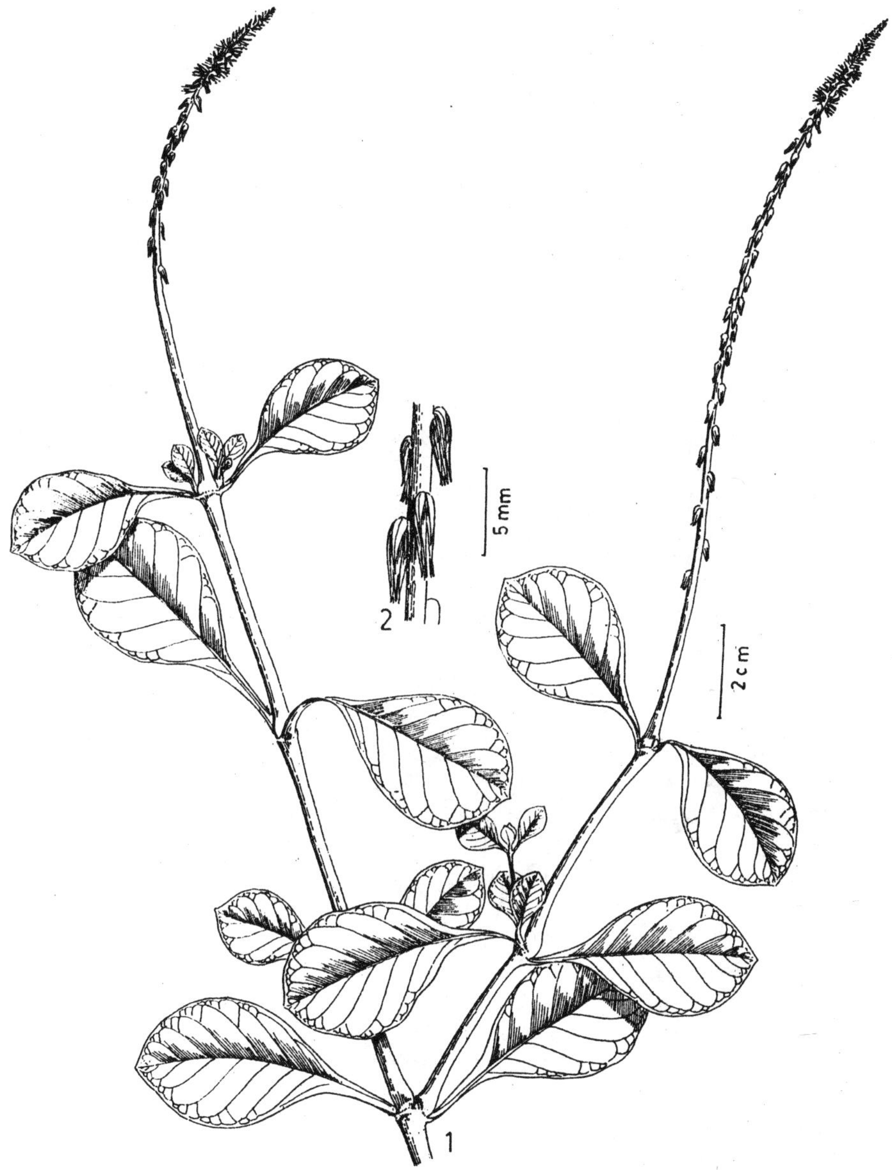

Figure 16: Achyranthes aspera L. 1, Habit; 2, Portion of inflorescence.

Cyathula prostrata (*Linn.*) *Blume* (**Amaranthaceae**) (Fig. 17)
Achyranthes prostrata Linn.

Diffuse herb; stem and branches reddish, clothed with fine hairs; leaves opposite, exstipulate, short-petioled, broadly elliptic-acute, entire, 7 x 4 cms, slightly hairy on both surfaces; flowers pale violet in clusters of 2–4 in interrupted terminal spikes;

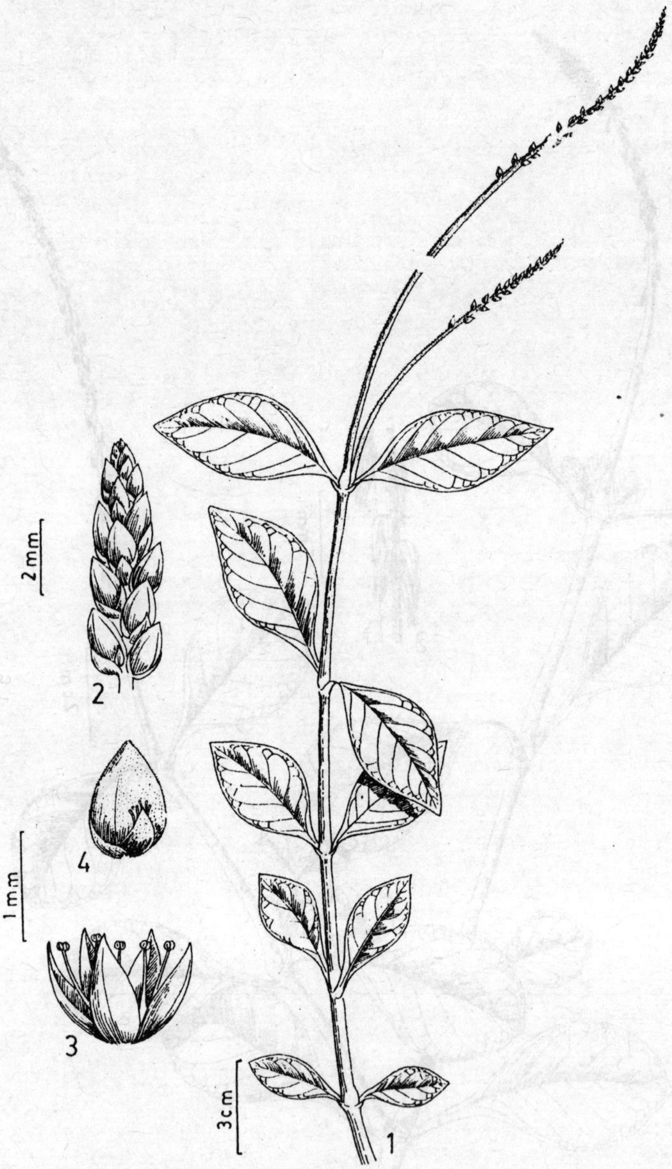

Figure 17: Cyathula prostrata (L.) Blume. 1, Habit; 2, Inflorescence; 3, Flower; 4, Fruit.

bracts and bracteoles ovate, acuminate, pubescent; perianth segments of the sterile flowers get reduced to hooked awns helping in dispersal; perianth segments of perfect flowers 5, calycine, scarious, one-nerved; stamens 5, staminal flowers connate at base with the staminodes forming a cup; ovary obovoid, unilocular with a solitary pendulous ovule, style short, filiform, ending in a capitate stigma; fruit an ovoid, thinly membraneous indehiscent utricle enclosed in the perianth; seeds oblong, yellowish brown.

Distribution: The plant grows in moist shady localities of all the plain districts in India.

Note: Sidha physicians use *Achyranthes aspera* effectively against bronchial asthma (Suresh *et al.*, 1985). The drug is also found to have contraceptive property in rats and hamsters (Wadhwa *et al.*, 1986).

ĀRAGVADHAḤ (Mal. KAṆIKKONNA)

Āragvadhaḥ is a reputed drug employed in the treatment of skin diseases. The stembark is the main officinal part though other parts are also occasionally used. *Āragvadhaḥ* is sweet, cold, germicidal and a good purgative. It promotes digestion and appetite, cures fever, haemetemesis, leucoderma, eczema, ascites, diabetes, dysuria, arthritis and cardiac disorders. Leaves of the tree bring down *kapha* and *mēdas* and are specially indicated in various kinds of fevers. Root cures arthritis and ringworm troubles. (Aiyer & Kolammal, 1964.8:51). The important formulations using the drug are *Āragvadhāriṣṭaṃ, Māṇibhadraṃ lēhaṃ, Valiya Rāsnādi kaṣāyaṃ, Vasiṣṭarasāyanaṃ* etc.

According to the texts, the tree is characterised by beautiful golden-coloured flowers (*hēmapuṣpī, suvarṇakaḥ, svarṅabhūṣaṇaḥ, svarṇavṛkṣaḥ*) which attract bees (*śēphāḷikaḥ*) and which are generally used in garlands (*kṛtamālaḥ*). Having long fruits (*dīrghaphalaḥ*), this considered as the king of trees (*rājavṛkṣaḥ, nṛpadrumaḥ*). *Āragvadhaḥ* and *śaṁpākaḥ* denote its therapeutic prowess (Aiyer & Kolammal, 1964.8:51). These synonyms agree well with the plant that is being used as the source of the drug namely *Cassia fistula* Linn. of Caesalpiniaceae, locally called *konna* or *kaṇikkonna*. Rheede has also described this plant under the name *conna* (Hort. Malab. 1:37–38, t.22.1678).

Cassia fistula *Linn.* **(Caesalpiniaceae)** (Fig. 18)

A medium-sized deciduous tree; leaves alternate, paripinnate, stipulate; leaflets 3–8 pairs, large, ovate-lanceolate, acute or acuminate, to 16 × 6 cms, glabrous green above, pale beneath; flowers bright yellow, fragrant, in long axillary pendulous racemes, long-pedicelled; sepals 5, green, pubescent, ovate or oblong obtuse, caducous; corolla of 5, free, subequal, shortly clawed, reddish-veined petals; stamens 10, unequal; ovary stalked, ovules many, style long and curved, ending in a smooth, conic stigma; pods upto 80 cms long, cylindric, pendulous; seeds immersed in a pulp.

Distribution: The tree is found throughout India in all deciduous forests and hilly tracts. Also in Sri Lanka and Burma.

Note: *Cassia fistula* has been found to be effective in the treatment of pyoderma (Nair, *et al.*, 1977) and other skin diseases (Nair, 1984).

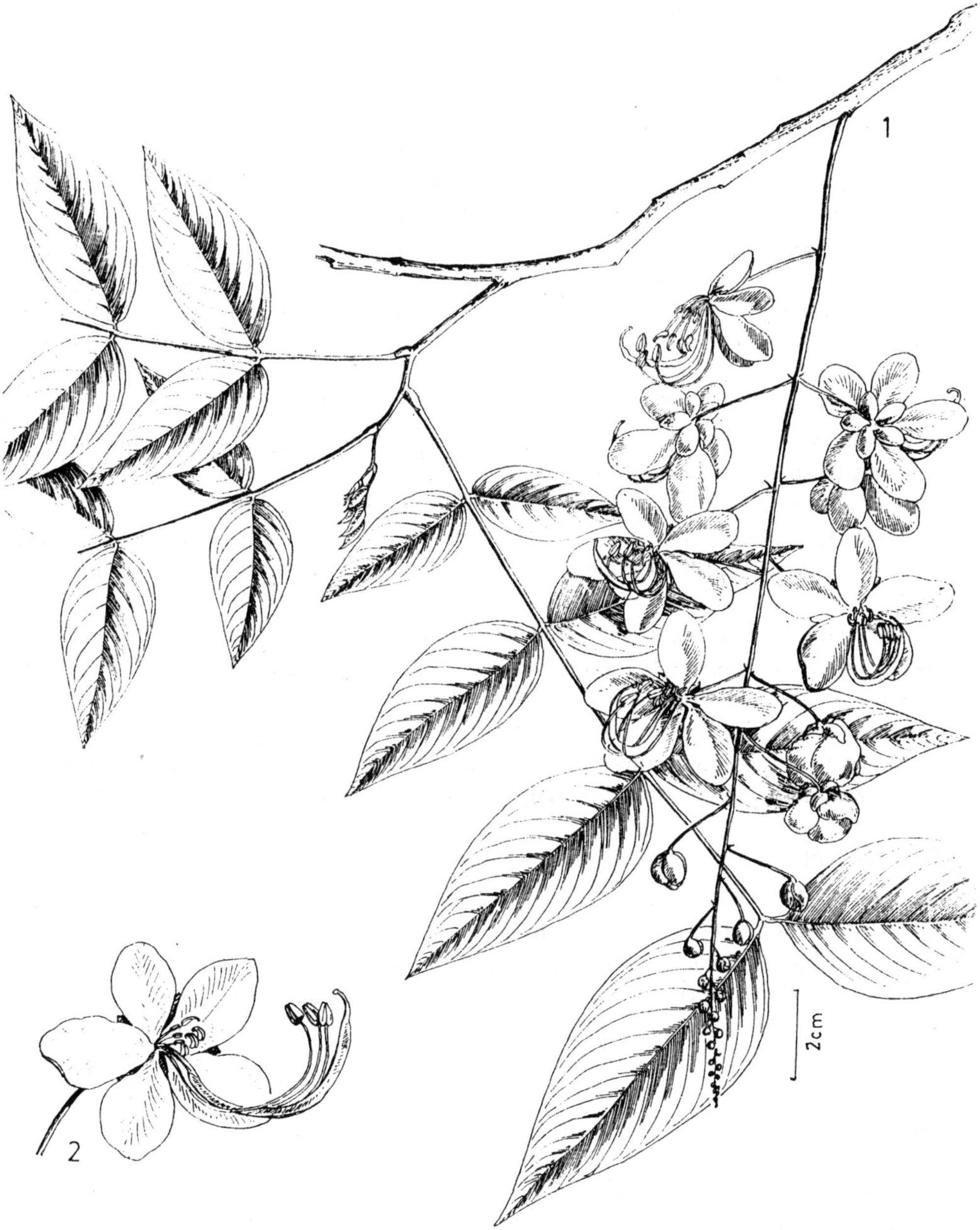

Figure 18: Cassia fistula L. 1, Flowering twig; 2, Flower.

ĀṚDRAKAḤ (Mal. IÑCI, CUKKU)

This is an important spice used in the preparations of condiments, curries, pickles and syrup. It is one of the reputed drugs of Āyurvēdists and is employed in Indigenous systems of medicine for very long period. Almost similar properties and uses have been attributed to the fresh rhizome called *ārdraka* and also to the dried one, known as *śuṇṭhī*. It is acrid, hot, anodyne, antirheumatic, carminative, cooling, cordial, diuretic and aphrodisiac. It promotes digestive power, cleanses the throat and tongue, dispels cardiac disorders and cures vomiting, ascites, cough, dyspnoea, anorexia, fever, anaemia, flatulence, colic, constipation, swelling, elephantiasis and dysuria. It is also used in diarrhoea, cholera, dyspepsia, neurological diseases, diabetes, eye diseases and tympanitis. In traditional medicine, *ārdraka* is extensively used for its specific action in rheumatism and inflammation of liver (Aiyer & Kolammal, 1966, 9:122; Kurup, *et al.*, 1979:200). The fresh rhizome is used to prepare *Ārdrakaghṛtaṃ, Sūraṇādi ghṛtaṃ, Valiya Ciñcādi lēhaṃ, Mahākukkuṭamāṁsatailaṃ* etc. The dried ginger forms an ingredient of preparations like *Indukāntaṃ kaṣāyaṃ, Sūraṇādi lēhaṃ, Tālīsapatravaṭakaṃ, Viśvāmṛtaṃ*, etc.

According to the texts, the plant grows in sandy places (*saikatēṣṭaṃ*) and it has spongy roots (*rhizomes—gulmamūlaṃ*) which resemble in shape the horns of animals (*śṛṅgivēraṃ, śārṅgaṃ, śṛṅgikaṃ*) (Aiyer & Kolammal, 1966.9:111). All other synonyms indicate only the properties of the drug. *Zingiber officinale* (Zingiberaceae), the common ginger, locally known as *iñci* is the plant source of the drug throughout the country (See also Rheede, Hort. Malab. 11:23–25, t.12.1692).

Zingiber officinale *Rosc.* **(Zingiberaceae)** (Fig. 19)

Perennial herb with a stout, horizontal, tuberous, jointed, aromatic root-stock having several sessile lateral tubers; stem erect; leaves subsessile, 12–30 × 1.8–2.5 cms, bifarious, ovate-lanceolate or linear-lanceolate acute, glabrous with a prominent midrib; flowers yellowish green in solitary, lateral, pedunculate, oblong cylindric spikes; bracts obtuse, scarious; calyx gamosepalous, 3-toothed at apex, splitting open on one side; corolla tube cylindric, lobes 3, greenish, subequal, lanceolate, the upper concave; lip small, 3-lobed and of a purplish black colour spotted with yellow, mid-lobe orbicular or oblong-obovate, laterals short, ovate obtuse; fertile stamen 1, anther oblong, 2-celled, the cells contiguous, crowned with a grooved crest; ovary inferior, 3-chambered with many ovules on axile placenta, style filiform, stigma subglobose; fruit an oblong capsule; seeds globose.

Distribution: The plant is widely cultivated all over the warm parts of India.

Note: Clinical studies made by Singhal and Joshi (1982) and Girij *et al.*, (1984) prove that *Zingiber officinale* reduces the serum cholesterol level considerably in hypercholesterolemic rats. *Śuṇṭhī* (dried ginger) has been found to be effective in the treatment of *grahaṇirōga* (Nanda *et al.*, 1985). The drug significantly improved body weight, appetite and haemoglobin percentage and controlled number of motions.

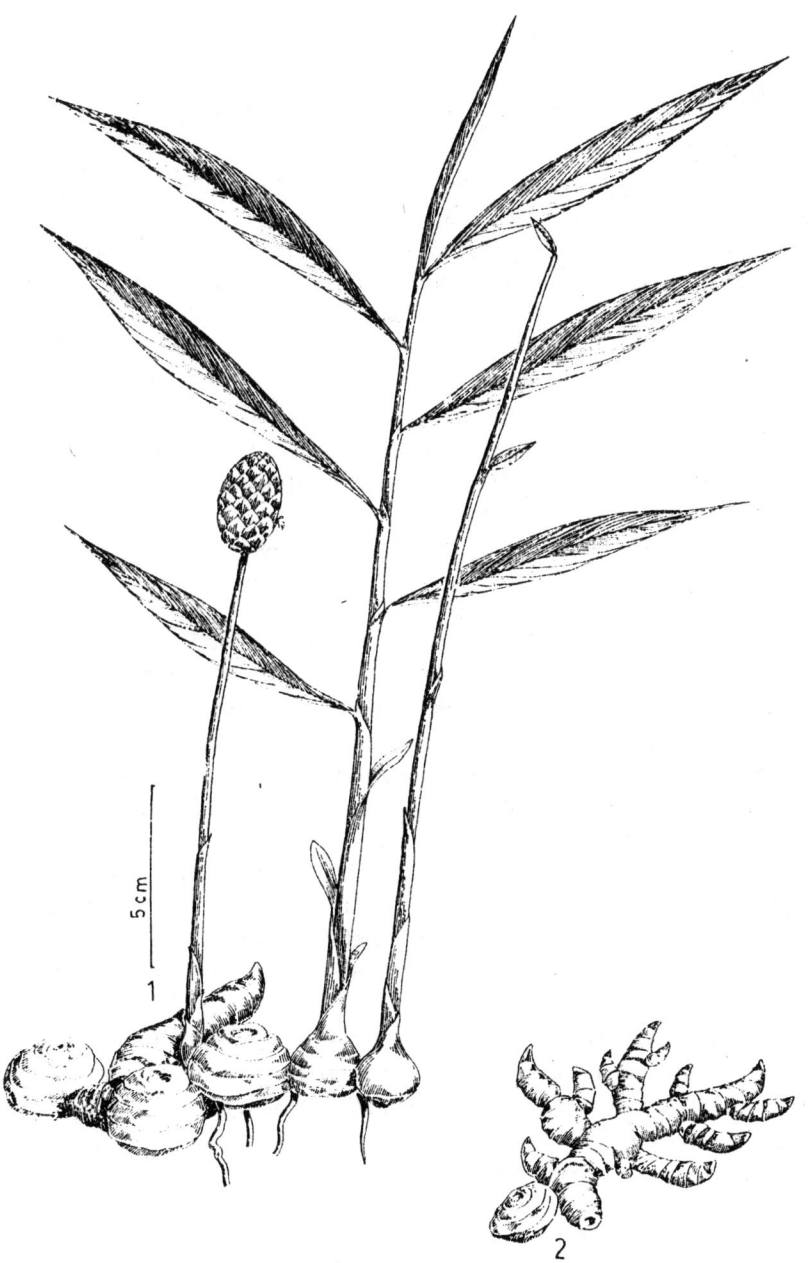

Figure 19: Zingiber officinale Rosc. 1, Habit; 2, Rhizome.

AṚKAḤ (Mal. ERIKKU)

The term *'Aṛkaḥ'* meaning 'sun' possibly refers to the caustic nature of the plant especially of its milky latex. Included among the *virēcana* (purgatives) group, it cures morbid *vāta*, skin diseases, pruritus, poison, ulcers, enlargement of spleen, liver and abdominal glands, colics, piles and worms. *Aṛkaḥ* is hot, acrid and laxative. It promotes digestion and is useful in anasarca. The latex is useful in skin ailments, *gulma* and ascites. Slightly roasted leaves are externally applied to painful joints, swellings and in cases of enlarged abdominal viscera. The officinal parts are leaves, roots, flowers and the latex. It enters into the composition of many preparations like *Kaccōrādi oil, Dhānvantaraṃ ghṛtaṃ, Vajṛakatailaṃ, Nāgarādi tailaṃ, Āviltōlādi bhasmaṃ*, etc.

Most of the synonyms of this plant (*aṛkaḥ, vasukaḥ, pṛatāpaḥ, vikīraṇaḥ*) refer to its strong caustic action. With very virulent leaves (*aṛkapaṛṇaḥ*), and white seeds (*śukaphalaṃ, tūlāṛkaḥ*), this plant blossoms throughout the year (*sadāpuṣpaḥ, sadāsumaḥ*) (cf. Kolammal, 1978, 2:17).

The drug *aṛkaḥ* is invariably equated with the genus *Calotropis* Linn. (Asclepiadaceae). But mention of different types of *aṛkaḥ* in some of the texts have caused some confusion in determining their actual plant source. Caraka mentions only one *aṛka* whereas Suśruta refers to two types: *aṛkaḥ* and *aḷaṛkaḥ*. There is mention of three varieties viz. *rājāṛkaḥ* (*aḷaṛkaḥ*); *śukḷāṛkaḥ* and *śvētamandāraḥ* in *Dhanvantari nighaṇṭu* and of four varieties viz. *aṛkaḥ, rājāṛkaḥ, śukḷārkaḥ* and *śvētamandāraḥ* in *Rājanighaṇṭu*. (cf. Kolammal, 1978: 2:16; Bapalal Vaidya, 1982:284).

In practice, however, physicians distinguish only two varieties, namely white (*aṛkaḥ*) and red (*aḷaṛkaḥ*), presumably recognised on the basis of flower colour. They are also reported to have different properties. The white variety is hot, bitter and cures difficult micturition, ulcers and expels worms. Its flowers are aphrodisiac, promote digestion, remove excessive secretion in the mouth and cure piles, difficult breathing and cough. Flower of the red variety is sweet, useful in skin diseases, worms, *kapha* and haemorrhagic disease caused by the vitiation of blood and bile, rat poison, *gulma* and swellings.

The botanical identity of these two varieties of *aṛkaḥ* is in some doubt. While some pundits equate *aṛkaḥ* with *Calotropis gigantea* and *aḷaṛkaḥ*, also called *śvētāṛkaḥ*, with *C. procera* (Kirtikar & Basu, 1918.2:810, 812; Nadkarni, 1954; 237, 242; Chopra *et al.*, 1956:46), others consider them vice-versa (Chunekar, 1982:304; Sharma, 1983:433–34). Mooss (1976:29) is not in favour of treating *C. procera* as *śvētāṛkaḥ* because it has pink flowers with purple spots on them.

Kerala physicians have never accepted this treatment, particularly because *C. procera* is not available in this part. *C. gigantea* which is commonly seen in southern India, has two forms, one with lilac or purple flowers which is very common and the other having white flowers which is not so common. These two forms are the accepted sources of *aṛkaḥ* and *aḷaṛkaḥ* respectively here (Mooss, 1976:31).

As far back as in 1679, Rheede has portrayed *C. gigantea* under the vernacular name *Ericu* (Hort. Malab. 2:53–56, t.31:1679) and has stated that *Bel Ericu* (*śvētāṛkaḥ*) is the white-flowered form of the same species. In other parts of India, where *C. procera* is abundant, it is this species which is used as the source of both.

Calotropis gigantea (*Linn.*) *R. Br.* **(Asclepiadaceae)** (Fig. 20)
Aselepias gigantea Linn.

Erect, pale greyish, subsucculent, laticiferous shrub covered with white cottony pubescence; leaves simple, opposite-deccussate, subsessile, obovate-oblong, obtuse, slightly cordate and auricled at base, to 9–15 × 4–9 cms, pale green above, white tawny beneath; flowers lilac or dull white in lateral or terminal panicles of umbellate cymes; calyx lobes 5, ovate; corolla lobes 5, spreading, corona lobes 5, compressed, adnate with the staminal column; ovary of 2 distinct carpels; follicles large, inflated, 8 × 4 cms, the apex surmounted by a coma of long slender silky hairs.

Distribution: The plant is found distributed throughout India, especially in the south. It is very common on roadsides and in waste places in all plain districts. Also distributed in Sri Lanka, China and Malesia.

Calotropis procera *R. Br.* **(Asclepiadaceae)**

A shrub, smaller in size than *C. gigantea*; leaves as in the former species, but more oblong and acute; flowers pink, spotted with purple, in long-peduncled umbels; corona scales equal to or longer than the staminal column, glabrous on the back, the apex bifid without auricles; follicles recurved; seeds ovoid.

Distribution: Though common in the drier parts of India, it is conspicuously absent in Kerala.

Note: The terminal leaves of *C. procera* have been found to be effective in the treatment of migraine (Prasad, 1985). The root bark of *C. procera* has been found to produce marked improvement in cases of diarrhoea and dysentery (Jain, *et al.*, 1985). The ethanol extract of *C. procera* applied to cancer ulcers showed 60° growth regression (Bhatnagar & Verma, 1986). 'Calotropin', isolated from the roots of this species, has also been found to be effective in fertility control (Gupta *et al.*, 1990)

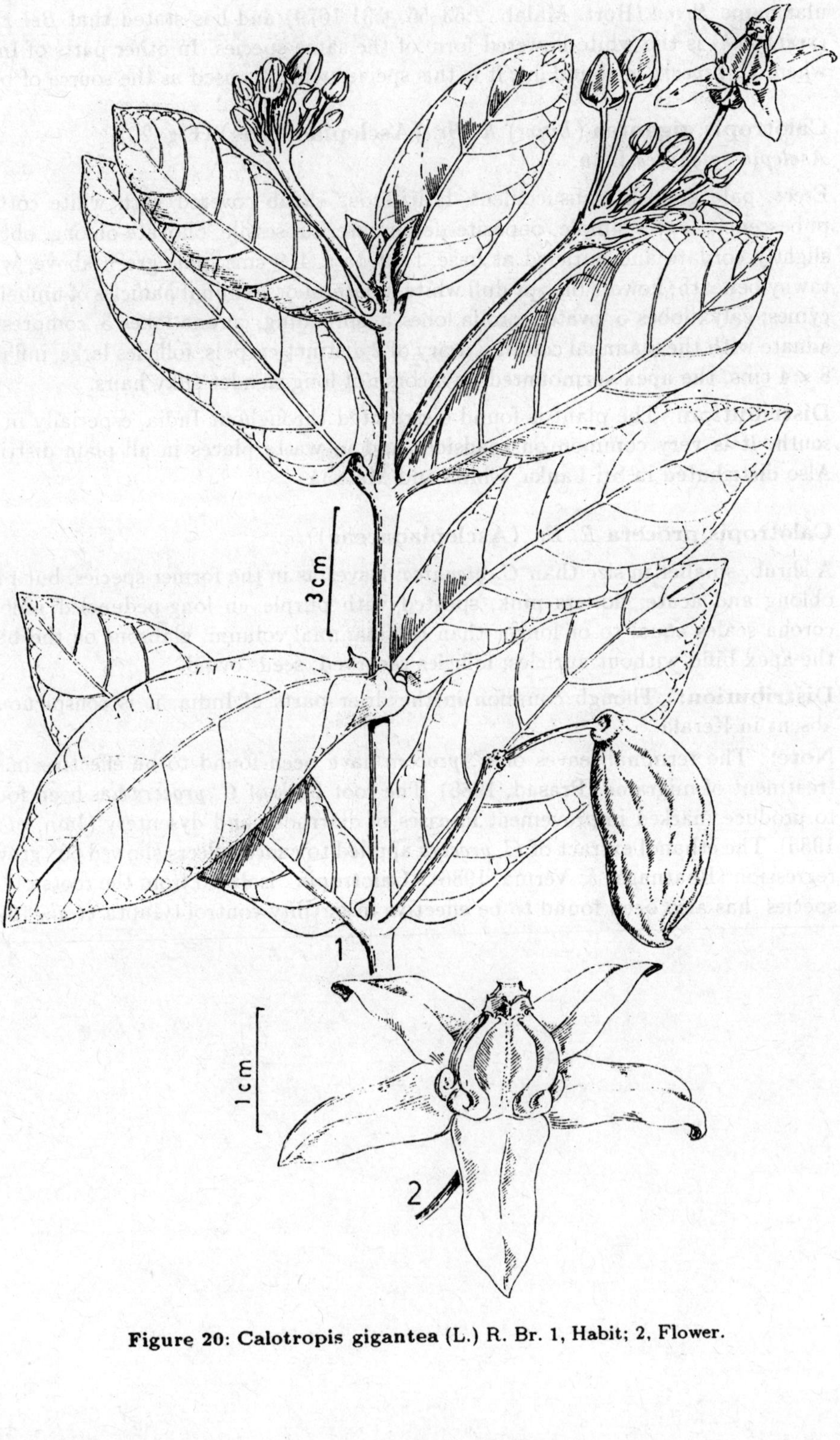

Figure 20: Calotropis gigantea (L.) R. Br. 1, Habit; 2, Flower.

ASANAḤ (Mal. VĒṄṄA)

Asanaḥ is a reputed drug for the treatment of leprosy and other skin diseases. It is also considered as an esteemed remedy for diabetes, and is an important ingredient of the *Asanādigaṇa* of Vāgbhaṭa which cures leucoderma, skin diseases, morbid *kapha*, diabetes, anaemia, parasites (*kṛmi*) and disorders due to deranged fat (Mooss, 1980:51). The heart wood is the officinal part. It is cool, bitter, astringent and acrid and cures morbid *kapha* and *pitta*, dysentery, diarrhoea, and haemophilic disorders (*raktapitta*). The bark and leaves form a good application to itches, scabies, leucoderma, leprosy and other skin diseases. The gum is useful in tooth ache and pyorrhoea. This tree is the source of the 'kino' of European pharmacopoeas, which is an astringent administered in diarrhoea (Nadkarni, 1954:1025; Sharma, 1983:682; Nesamony, 1985:468). The drug is a constituent of preparations like *Asanavilvādi tailam̥, Ayaskṛti, Varādi kaṣāyam̥, Khadirasārādi ghṛtam̥*, etc.

According to the texts, the tree possesses a yellow wood (*pītasāraḥ, pītasālakaḥ*) which exudes a gum (*sarjakaḥ*) and have flowers which resemble those of *bandhūka* (*bandhūkapuṣpa*) i.e. *Pentapetes phoenicea* (Sterculiaceae), known as *uccamalari* in vernacular (Moosad, 1983:302).

Pterocarpus marsupium Roxb. of Papilionaceae, locally called *vēṅṅa*, is the accepted source of the drug.

Pterocarpus marsupium *Roxb.* **(Papilionaceae)** (Fig. 21)

Large, deciduous tree; branchlets pubescent; leaves odd-pinnate; leaflets 5–7, elliptic or oblong, 7–14 × 4.5–9.5 cm, coriaceous, pubescent below, base obtuse or truncate, apex emarginate, margin entire; flowers golden-yellow in terminal panicles; calyx tube 8 mm; corolla papilionaceous; stamens 10, filaments subequal; ovary tomentose; pod stipitate; broadly winged.

Distribution: The plant is seen in all forest districts of India chiefly in deciduous forests, upto 4,500 ft. Also distributed in Sri Lanka.

Note: The pharmacognostical and clinical studies of *P. marsupium* have been discussed by Satyavati *et al.* (1987: 530–536).

The hypoglycaemic effect of *Pterocarpus marsupium* had been clinically tried by Ojha *et al.* (1978), Chakravarthy *et al.* (1981), Sheehan *et al.* (1983) etc. The bark of this tree is found to have significant hypocholesterolemic action (Anonymous, 1978c). The antifungal activity of the wood of *P. marsupium* has been clinically tried by Dhir *et al.*, (1982).

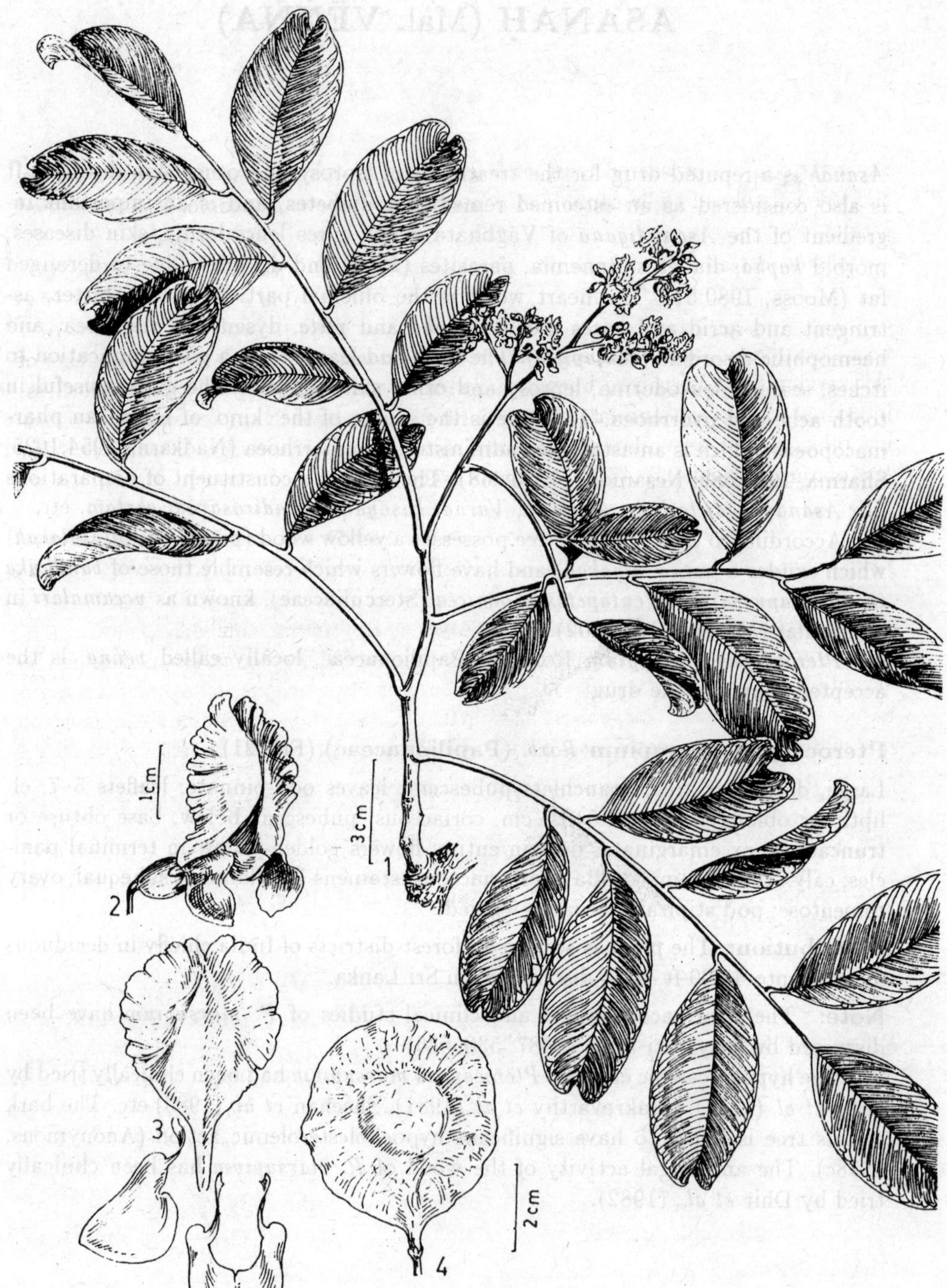

Figure 21: Pterocarpus marsupium Roxb. 1, Flowering twig; 2, Flower; 3, Petals; 4, Fruit.

AŚŌKAḤ (Mal. AŚŌKAṂ)

Aśōka is one of the sacred trees of Hindus and Buddhists. As the name signifies, the tree is believed to be capable of relieving the sorrows of people. It is considered as a symbol of love and is dedicated to 'Kāma', the Indian God of love.

Aśōka bark has been very widely used in Indian medicine from time immemorial for the treatment of uterine disorders, particularly in uterine haemorrhages, dysmenorrhoea and menorrhagia. According to *Bhāvaprakāśa*, the bark is bitter, cool, astringent and constipative and can cure inflammation and enlargement of the cervical glands, thirst, burning sensation, emaciation, dyspepsia, biliousness, intestinal worms and animal poisoning. Flowers are used in the treatment of bleeding piles, scabies in children and other skin diseases (Nadkarni, 1954:1105; Aiyer & Kolammal, 1960.4:3) *Aśōkaghṛtaṃ, Aśōkāriṣṭaṃ*, etc. are some of the important preparations using the drug.

According to the description in the text, the tree has copper-coloured tender leaves (*tāmṛapatṛaḥ*) and red, odorous, flowers (*hēmapuṣpaḥ, gandhapuṣpaḥ*) which are borne in dense inflorescences (*piṇḍīpuṣpaḥ, stabakapuṣpaḥ*), beautifully coloured like a butterfly (*citṛaṣaḍpadamañjarī*) (Aiyer & Kolammal, 1960.4:2).

Saraca asoca (Roxb.) de wilde of Caesalpiniaceae, locally called *aśōkaṃ* is the accepted source of the drug. Rheede describes and portrays the plant under the same name *Asjogam* (Hort. Malab. 5:117,t.59.1685). *Polyalthia longifolia* (Annonaceae) is equated with the name *aśōka* by some (Kapoor & Mitra, 1979:60; Chunekar, 1982:500) and is often used as an adulterant of the genuine *aśōka* bark or as a substitute. The detailed pharmacognosy and pharmacology of the two barks have been studied and discussed (Anonymous, 1982:122–136).

Saraca asoca (*Roxb.*) *De Wilde* **(Caesalpiniaceae)** (Fig. 22)
Jonesai asoca Roxb.
Saraca indica sensu Baker

Medium-sized evergreen tree; leaves alternate, pinnate, copper-red when young, green later; leaflets 4–6 pairs, short-petioled, oblong-lanceolate, upto 20 × 6 cm, glabrous; flowers orange-red in dense axillary corymbose cymes; bract small, deciduous; bracteoles reddish, oblong-spathulate, ascending amplexicaul; calyx tube cylindric, lobes 4, unequal, petaloid, orange red; petals absent; stamens usually 7, filaments filiform, anthers reniform-oblong; ovary superior, unilocular, many-ovuled, style long, filiform, ending in a minute, capitate stigma; fruit a scimitar-shaped, dehiscent, woody pod, tapering at both ends; seeds obovate or orbicular, slightly compressed, smooth.

Distribution: The tree is distributed throughout India, particularly N. Circars, in hill forests, S. Canara, Mysore and Travancore. It is scarce in the wild, but is widely cultivated.

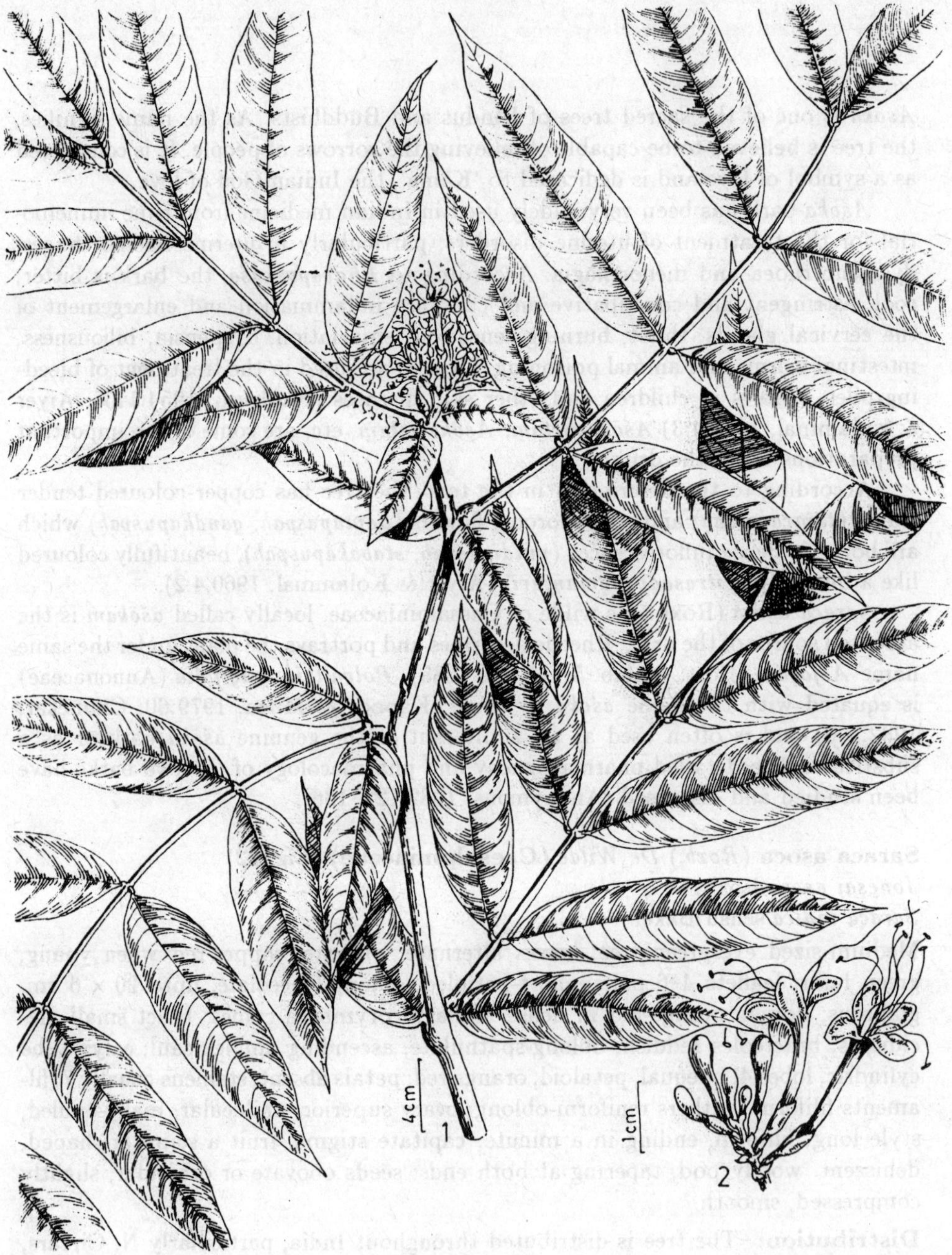

Figure 22: Saraca asoca (Roxb.) De Wilde. 1, Flowering twig; 2, Flowers.

Note: Satyavati *et al.* (1969) have demonstrated its curative efficacy on various uterine disorders. Ray and Datta (1981) have studied the pharmacognostic characters of the bark of *Saraca indica*.

This plant is referred to as *Saraca indica* in our earlier Floras. However, in a revision of this genus, De Wilde (1967) has treated the Indian material as a different species, *S. asoca*, which can be distinguished from *S. indica* as follows:

Bracteoles erect, clasping the pedicel, persistent .... *S. asoca*
Bracteoles spreading, persistent or fugacious .... *S. indica*

S. indica does not occur in India

Polyalthia longifolia (*Sonn.*) *Thwaites* (**Annonaceae**)
Uvaria longifolia Sonn.
Gautteria longifolia Wallich

Tree; leaves simple, alternate, narrowly lanceolate, acuminate, glabrous, margins flexuous, upto 24 × 4.5 cms; flowers greenish white, fascicled on the older parts of branches; sepals free; petals 6, 2-seriate, lanceolate; stamens many, cuneate; carpels many; berriers one-seeded.

Distribution: The plant is introduced from Sri Lanka. Now cultivated throughout India in gardens and avenues.

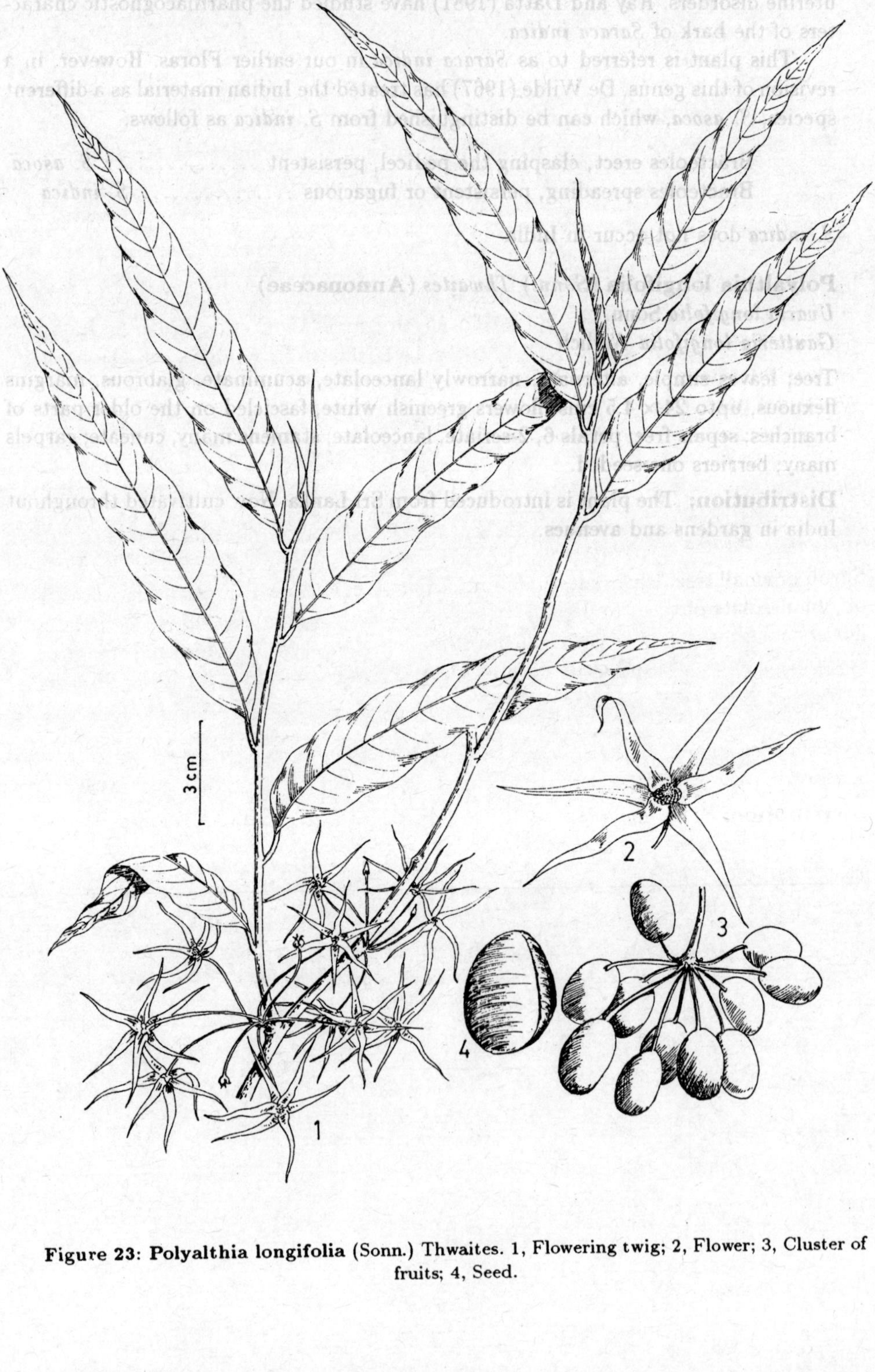

Figure 23: Polyalthia longifolia (Sonn.) Thwaites. 1, Flowering twig; 2, Flower; 3, Cluster of fruits; 4, Seed.

AŚVAŚĀKHŌṬAḤ (Mal. PĀṆAL)

The plant is used in indigenous medicine for cough, rheumatism, anaemia and jaundice. The whole plant is bitter, astringent, vermifuge, anti-inflammatory and expectorant. The juice of the leaves is used in fever and liver complaints. A paste of the leaves with ginger is applied in eczema and skin affections. A decoction of the root is given for facial inflammations. The drug is a component of preparations like *Nirguṇḍyādi guḷika* and *Nirguṇḍyādi ghṛtaṃ*.

The Āyurvēdic texts do not make any mention about this drug. In Kerala *Glycosmis pentaphylla* (Retz.) DC. (Rutaceae), known as *Pāṇal* in vernacular, is used as the source of the drug. Rheede's description of this plant under the same vernacular name (Hort. Malab. 2:9–10, t.9.1679, *Panel*) also indicates that this has been in use in Kerala since long.

Glycosmis pentaphylla (*Retz.*) *DC.* **(Rutaceae)** (Fig. 24)
Limonia pentaphylla Retz.
Glycosmis arborea (Roxb.) DC.

Shrub or small tree; leaves alternate, imparipinnate; leaflets 3–5, aromatic, obovate or oblanceolate-obtuse, to 18 × 7 cms, base cuneate, margin entire to crenulate; flowers small, white in axillary spiciform panicles; sepals 5, ovate-rotund, margins scarious, ciliate; petals obovate-elliptic, glandular; disc obscurely lobulate; stamens 8–10, free, inserted round a disc, filaments flat, anthers ovate to elliptic-cordate with 1 prominent dorsal gland on the connective; ovary 2–5 celled, coarsely pustulate, style short, stigma flat, obscurely angled; fruit 1–3 seeded, white or pink subglobose berry.

Distribution: The plant is seen in all districts in India as forest undergrowths. Also known from Sri Lanka, S.E. Asia & W. Malesia.

Note: For pharmacognostic information refer Santha et al. (1988).

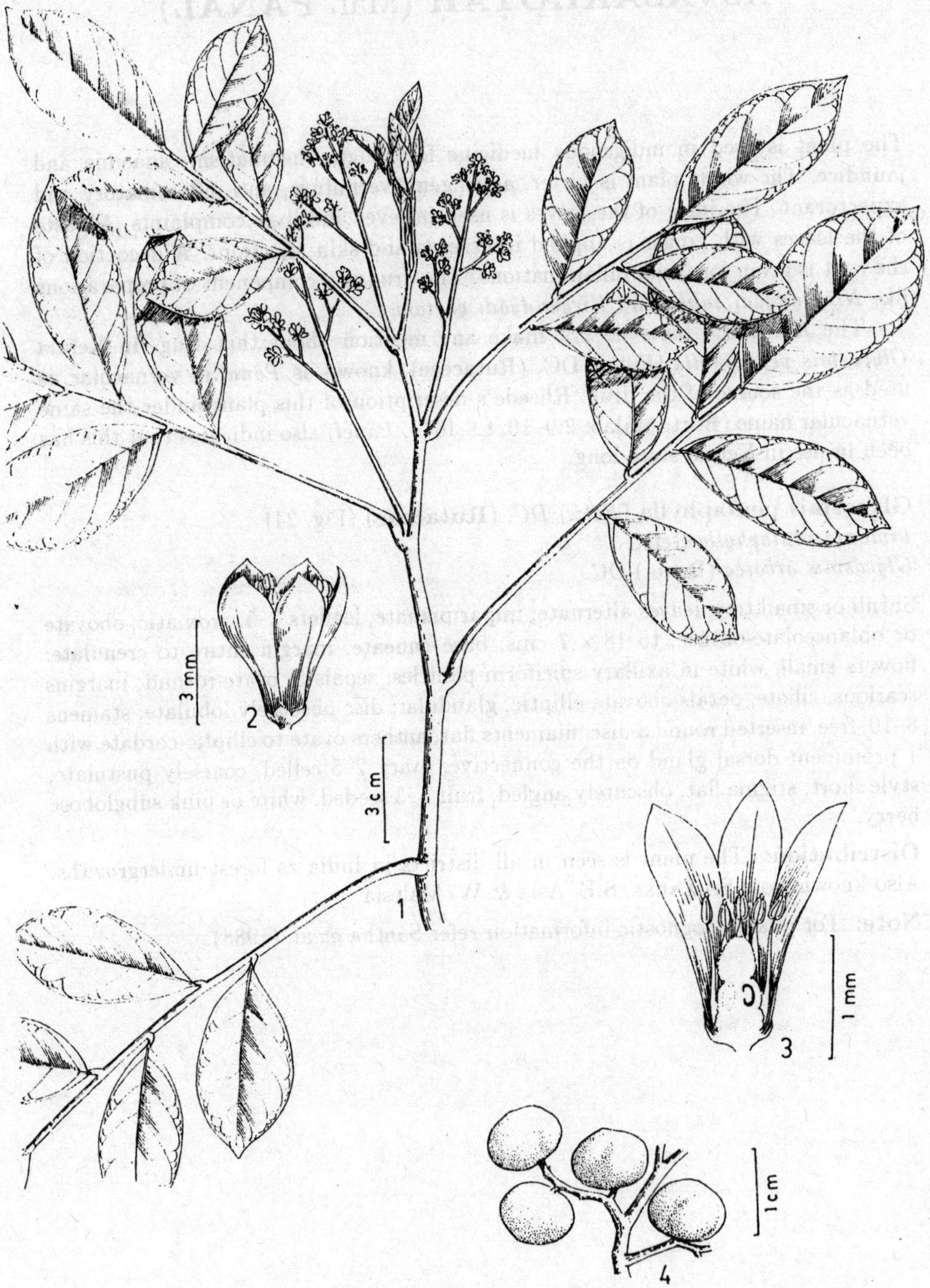

Figure 24: Glycosmis pentaphylla (Retz.) DC. 1, Flowering twig; 2, Flower; 3, L.S. of Flower; 4, Fruits.

AŚVATTHAḤ (Mal. ARAYĀL)

The tree, venerated by the Hindus, is one of the four trees which constitute the group *Nālpāmaraṃ* (the four trees with milky latex), and the barks form an important ingredient in many Āyurvēdic formulations. The bark is astringent, heavy, alterative, cooling in action, haemostatic, laxative, alleviative of *pitta* and *kapha*, improves complexion and cleans vagina. It is used in diabetes, diarrhoea, leucorrhoea, menorrhagia, nervous disorders and vaginal diseases. Also used in hemopathy, earache, fracture, glandular diseases especially suppurating glands in the neck, scabies and other skin diseases, ulcers, soreness in the mouth and urinogenital disorders. Decoction of the bark if taken in with honey subdues *vātarakta* (Nadkarni, 1954:552; Aiyer & Kolammal, 1957:3.78; Mooss, 1976:73, Kurup *et al.*, 1979:19). The bark, leaf buds and seeds are medicinal. The important preparations using the drug are *Nālpāmarādi tailam, Candanāsavaṃ, Śāribādyāsavaṃ, Karṇaśūlāntakaṃ, Valiya Marmaguḷika, Kaccōradi tailaṃ*, etc.

This tree, with characteristic milky latex (*kṣīravṛkṣaḥ*) and deltoid, papery leaves producing restling sound at the slightest breeze (*chalapatraḥ, chaladaḷaḥ*) has been equated with *Ficus religiosa* of Moraceae, by all. (See also Rheede, Hort. Malab. 1:47–48.t.27.1678).

Ficus religiosa *Linn.* **(Moraceae)** (Fig. 25)
Urostigma religiosum (Linn.) Gasp.

Large tree, leaves alternate, long-petioled, petiole to 12 cm, lamina broadly ovate, with a long lanceolate cuspidate tip, base truncate, margin sinuate, upto 16 × 13 cm, cusp to 8 cm, (sub) coriacious, 3-nerved from base; figs monoecious, axillary, paired, sessile, obovoid or globose, 4–6 mm across, purplish when ripe, male osteolar, sessile; tepals 2, free, ovate-lanceolate; stamen 1; female sessile, tepals 3–4, free, linear-lanceolate, brownish, glabrous; ovary ovoid-oblong; 1 mm, style dilated above, gall flowers similar; achenes smooth.

Distribution: The tree is common in most parts of India, often planted in the vicinity of the temples. Also known from S.E. Asia.

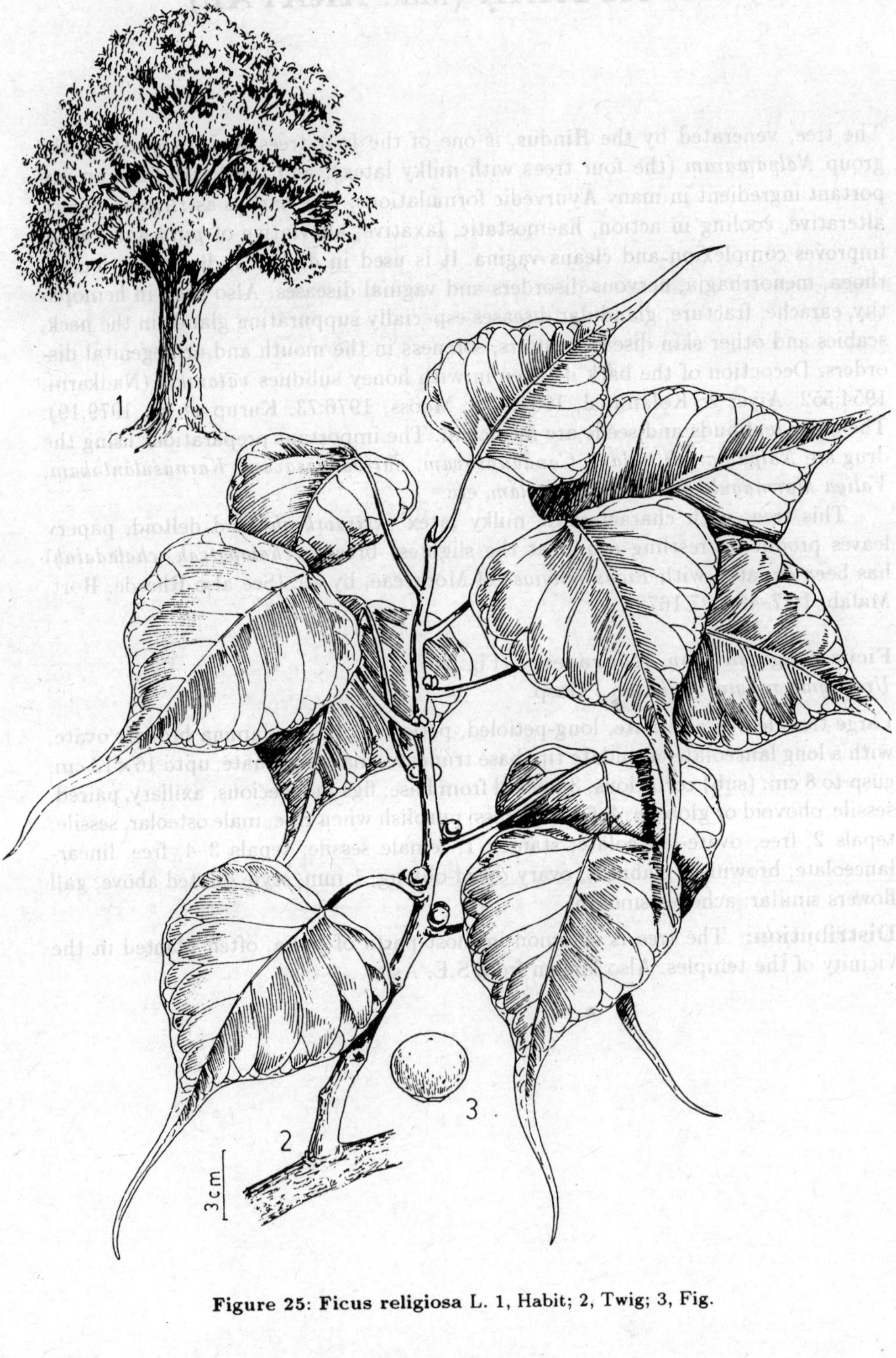

Figure 25: Ficus religiosa L. 1, Habit; 2, Twig; 3, Fig.

AŚVAGANDHĀ (Mal. AMUKKURAṂ)

Aśvagandhā is highly esteemed as a *rasāyana* drug by Āyurvēdists which is capable of imparting long life, youthful vigour and good intellectural powers. The root is the officinal part and it is bitter in taste, hot in action, germicidal, aphrodisiac, diuretic and alleviative of *vāta* and *kapha*. It cures ulcers, fever, cough, dyspnoea, consumption, dropsy, impotence, rheumatism, toxicosis and leucoderma. The drug is a good tonic. It improves physical strength and is prescribed in all cases of general debility. The paste made out of the leaves of *aśvagandhā* cures tumour and scrofula (Aiyer & Kolammal, 1964.8:34; Kurup *et al.* 1979:18). *Aśvagandhāriṣṭaṃ, Cyavanaprāśaṃ, Valiya Nārāyaṇa tailaṃ* etc. are some of the important preparations using the drug.

Most of the synonyms given in the text like *balya, varadā, vājīkarī, baladā,* etc. indicate only the prowess of the drug in giving strength, health and longevity. Though other terms are not of much help in identifying the plant, there is no confusion regarding the botanical source of the drug. *Withania somnifera* (Linn.) Dunal of Solanaceae, locally called *amukkuraṃ*, is the accepted source throughout India.

Withania somnifera (*Linn.*) *Dunal* **(Solanaceae)** (Fig. 26)
Physalis somnifera Linn.

Erect, greyish tomentose, undershrubs with fairly long tuberous roots; leaves alternate or sub-opposite, broadly ovate, subacute, entire, 5–10 × 2.5–7 cm; flowers small, greenish, axillary, solitary or in few-flowered fascicles; calyx gamosepalous, campanulate, 5-lobed, lobes acute from a broad base, accrescent and inflated in fruit; corolla campanulate, greenish yellow, lobes 5, triangular-oblong; stamens 5, included; ovary ovoid or globose, glabrous, many ovuled, style filiform, stigma two-lobed; fruit a globose berry, orange-red when ripe and enclosed within the enlarged calyx; seeds many, discoid.

Distribution: The plant is distributed throughout the drier subtropical regions of India. Not common in Kerala. The plant is also recorded as occuring in Mediterranean, Canary Isls and Cape of Good Hope.

Notes: Singh and Malaviya (1978) and Singh and Tripathy (1982) have demonstrated the psychotropic efficacy of the drug and found that the drug is very effective in the treatment of anxiety neurosis. The drug has also been found to possess significant antitumour activity (Singh *et al.*, 1986) while the leaves have been reported to be an anti-inflammatory agent (Sudhir *et al.*, 1986).

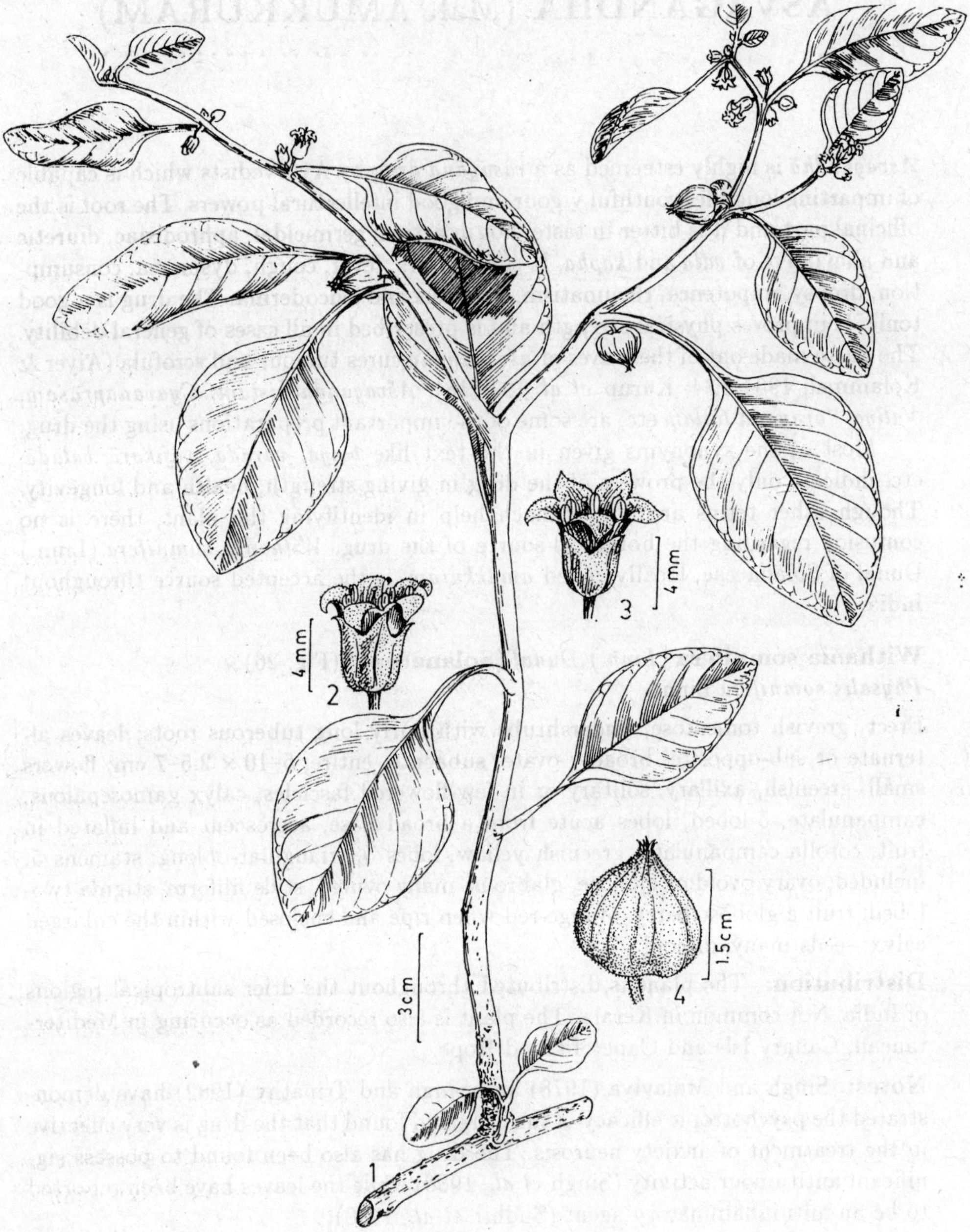

Figure 26: **Withania somnifera** (L.) Dunal. 1, Twig; 2–3, Flowers; 4, Fruit enclosed in the accrescent calyx.

ĀTMAGUPTĀ
(Mal. NĀIKORAṆA, NĀIKKURUṆA)

This is considered to be an important *vājīkaraṇa* drug, capable of promoting the semen and sexual vigour. It is mentioned in the texts that the ascetics are reluctant even to utter its name on account of its powerful aphrodisiac (*vṛṣya*) properties (*maharṣibhiḥ, ārṣabhī, ṛṣyaprōktā*). The drug is also reported to be anthelmintic, diuretic, purgative and a nervine tonic. It promotes strength and overcomes *vāta, pittarakta* and malignant ulcers. It is also used in cholera, delirium, impotence, leucorrhoea, spermatorrhoea, urinary troubles and in expelling round worms. Seeds and hairs covering the pods are the officinal parts. A paste of the seeds is applied on the body in dropsy (Nadkarni, 1954:819; Aiyer & Kolammal, 1962.5:3; Kurup *et al.*, 1979:22). The important formulations using the drug are *Aśvagandhādi lēhaṃ, Vidāryādi kaṣāyaṃ, Amṛtaprāśaghṛtaṃ, Stanyajananarasāyanaṃ, Ātmaguptācūrṇaṃ*, etc.

According to the texts, the plant is a perennial (*vyaṇgā*), densely hairy vine (*rōmālu, rōmavallī*) which cannot be handled or touched (*dusparśā, durālabhā, durabhigrahā*), due to the bristly hairs on the pods (*śukavati, śūkaśiṁbi*) resembling the hair of monkeys (*kapirōmaphalā, kīśarōmā*) which cause severe itching and irritation (*kaṇḍūkarī, kaṇḍurā, Kaṇḍulā*) even to monkeys (*kapikacchūḥ*), resulting in the blistering of the skin (*brahmaṇī, sadyaśōdhā*). The plant is capable of self protection (*ātmaguptā, svayamguptā*) on account of these hairs (Aiyer & Kolammal, 1962.5:2). All the features attributed point only one source plant viz. *Mucuna pruriens* (Linn.) DC. of Papilionaceae which is the accepted source of the drug throughout the country. This plant, locally called *nāicoraṇa* is illustrated and described by Rheede also (Hort. Malab. 8:61–62, t.35.1688).

Mucuna pruriens (*Linn.*) *DC.* **(Papilionaceae)** (Fig. 27)
Mucuna prurita Hook.

Perennial twining shrub clothed with dense hairs when young; leaves alternate, trifoliolate, long-petioled, leaflets ovate-rhomboid, acute, mucronate, terminal leaflet upto 10.5×5.5 cm, laterals unequal-sided at base, appressed white-pubescent above, densely covered with silvery grey hairs beneath; flowers purple, in axillary pendulous racemes; calyx 2-lipped, tube pubescent; corolla papilionaceous, exserted; stamens diadelphous; fruit a turgid, falcately curved pod, densely covered with irritant bristles.

Distribution: Found wild throughout India upto 3,000 ft. Also reported from Sri Lanka, S.E. Asia and Malesia.

Note: In addition to its aphrodisiac property, *ātmaguptā* has been found to produce antidepressent effect in patients suffering from depressive neurosis (Singh & Tripathy, 1982).

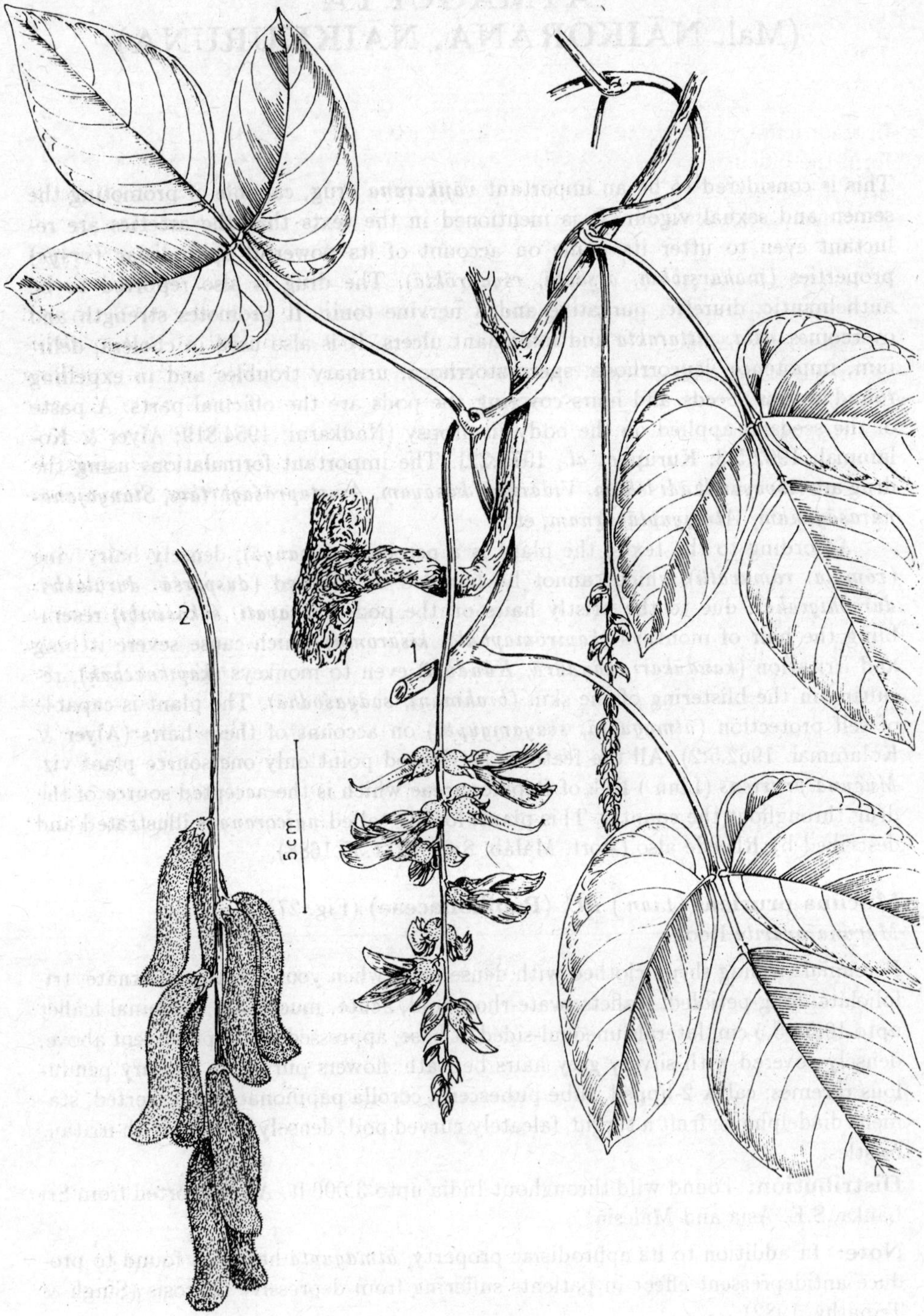

Figure 27: Mucuna pruriens (L.) DC. 1, Flowering Branch; 2, A bunch of fruits.

BĀKUCĪ (Mal. KĀṚKŌKIL)

In traditional medicine, *bākucī* is extensively used in all forms of leucoderma. Seeds form the officinal part. It is sweet, bitter, astringent, stomachic, anthelmintic, diuretic, germicidal and easy of digestion. It imparts vigour and vitality, improves digestive power and receptive power of mind, improves the texture and complextion of skin and helps growth of hair. It overcomes diseases due to the morbidity of *vāta* and *kapha* and cures haemetemesis, leprosy, diabetes, fever, cough, oedema, anaemia, piles, dysuria and poisonous affections and help in healing ulcers (Aiyer & Kolammal, 1966. 9: 97; Kurup *et al.*, 1979: 224). The drug is an ingredient of preparations like *Khadirāriṣṭaṃ, Gōpīcandanādi guḷika, Mañjiṣṭhādi kaṣāyaṃ, Āvalgujabījādi cūrṇaṃ*, etc.

The synonyms only indicate that the plant has black (*kṛṣṇaphalā*), bad-smelling fruits (*pūtiphalī*). The botanical source of the drug throughout India is *Psoralea corylifolia* Linn. of Papilionaceae, known as *kāṛkōkil* in Malayalam.

Psoralea corylifolia *Linn.* **(Papilionaceae)** (Fig. 28)

Erect, coarse, annual herb; stem and branches striated; leaves simple, alternate, long-petioled, ovate-acute, to roundish, serrate-dentate, upto 9.5 × 7.5 cms; flowers small, pale lilac in axillary, dense racemes; calyx glandular, 5-lobed, lobes lanceolate, upper ones connate; corolla papilionaceous, exserted, petals clawed; stamens 10, diadelphous; ovary sessile, unilocular with one ovule, style long, filiform, incurved with a minute terminal stigma; pod ovoid, one seeded, indehiscent; seed ovoid, blackish with a bitter taste.

Distribution: The plant is distributed in most of the plains districts of India, Pakistan, Sri Lanka, Burma, China, Yunnan, Arabia and Socotra. In India, it is a weed of roadsides, cultivated fields and waste-places, growing during the rainy season.

Note: The anthelmintic activity of *Psoralea corylifolia* seeds is clinically proved by Srivatsava *et al.*, (1967) on flat worms and round worms. *Bavachinin* isolated from *P. corylifolia* seeds was found to possess marked anti-inflammatory, antipyretic and mild analgesic properties (Anand, *et al.*, 1978) Ethnobotanical studies conducted by Khan and Chaghtai (1982) reveal that the powdered seeds of *Psoralea corylifolia* administered orally is beneficial in eczema.

The pharmacognostical, chemical, pharmacological and clinical studies of the seeds of *Psoralea corylifolia* have been discussed in detail by Satyavati *et al.*, (1987: 518–525).

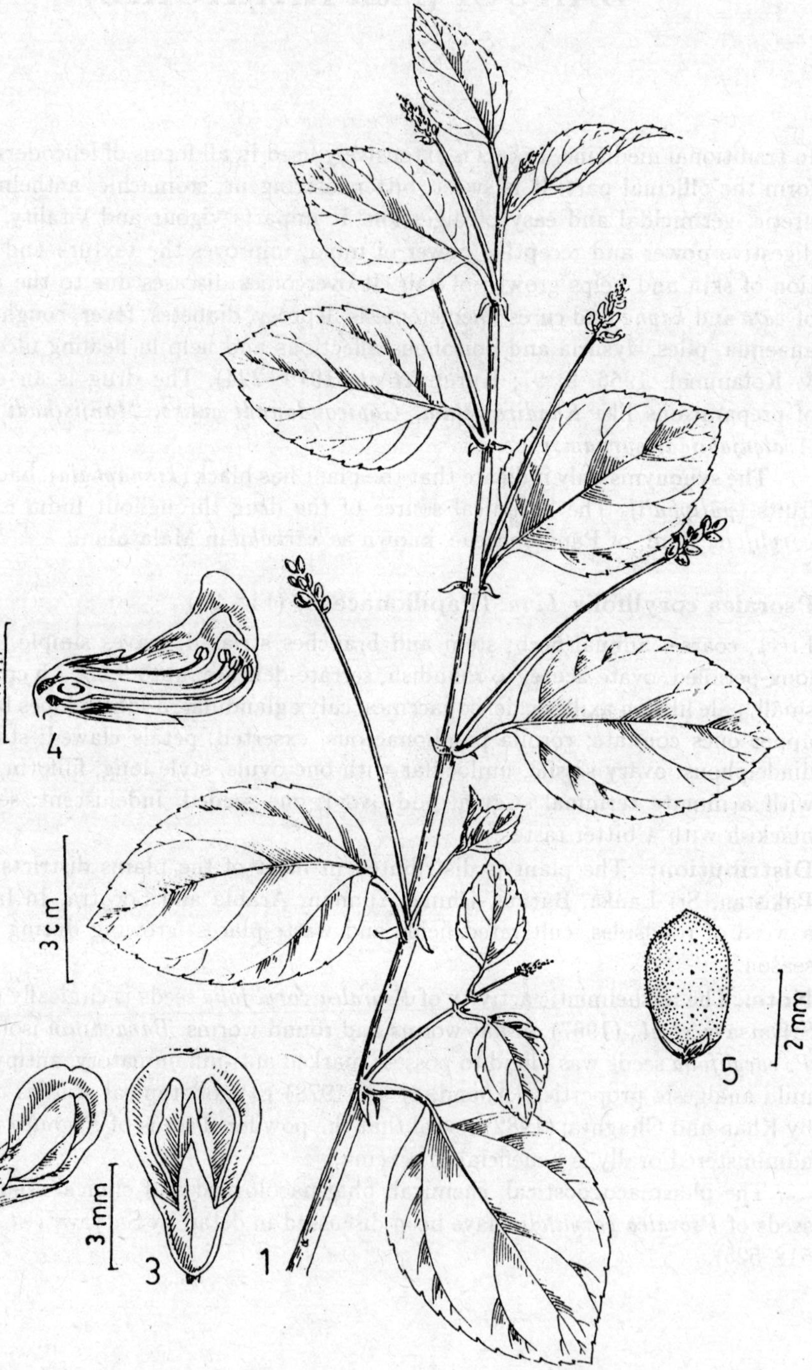

Figure 28: Psoralea corylifolia L. 1, Flowering twig; 2–3, Flower, different views; 4, L.S. of Flower; 5, Fruit.

BALĀ (Mal. KUṚUNTŌṬṬI)

The drug is held in great repute by Āyurvēdic physicians for the treatment of rheumatism and it forms a chief ingredient of several important preparations like *Kṣīrabala, Dhānvantaraṃ, Balāriṣṭaṃ, Rāsnādi kaṣāyaṃ, Aśvagandhādi lēhaṃ*, etc. Root is the officinal part. It is reported to be cool, sweet, demulcent, aphrodisiac and tonic. It produces strength, imparts beauty to the body and cures *vātarakta, raktapitta*, consumption, polyuria and ulcers. The drug is also useful in neurological disorders like hemiplegia, facial paralysis and sciatica, general debility, headache, opthalmia, dysuria, leucorrhoea, tuberculosis, diabetes, fever and uterine disorders. (Dey, 1980: 22; Chunekar, 1982: 368; Sharma, 1983: 736).

Four varieties namely *balā, atibalā, nāgabalā* and *mahābalā* are mentioned in *Bhāvaprakāśa nighaṇṭu*, which constitute the group *Balācatuṣṭayaṃ* (cf. Chunekar, 1982: 366). The other two varieties, i.e. *rājabalā* mentioned in *Rājanighaṇṭu* (cf. Sharma, 1983: 735) and *bhūmibalā* in *Ouṣadhinighaṇṭu* (cf. Aiyer & Kolammal, 1962. 5: 70) are not in vogue in practice.

Of the 4 types of *balā* mentioned above, *balā* is the most widely used. This has been equated with *Sida cordifolia* Linn. of Malvaceae (Kirtikar & Basu, 1918: 173 Vaidya, K.M. 1936: 385; Nadkarni, 1954: 1134; Kurup *et al.*, 1979: 28; Dey, 1980: 21; Chunekar, 1982: 367; Vaidya Bapalal, 1982: 214; Sharma, 1983: 735). Āyurvēdic formulary of India (Anonymous, 1978a: 252) has also accepted this. While this is the widely used source of *balā* in northern parts of India, Kerala physicians have adopted *Sida rhombifolia* ssp. *retusa*. for this drug (See also Rheede, Hort. Malab. 10: 35, t. 18. 1690; Aiyer & Kolammal, 1962. 5: 71; Mooss, 1976: 124), but *S. acuta* is also used widely to adulterate this. These species can be identified as follows:

Sida cordifolia *Linn.* **(Malvaceae)** (Fig. 29)

Erect, bushy plant, densely pubescent all over; leaves simple, alternate, orbicular, ovate, obtuse, cordate at base, 1.5–4 × 1–3 cms, tomentose, margin serrate-crenate; flowers pale yellow, solitary or in few-flowered clusters in axils; calyx gamosepalous, persistent, 5-lobed; petals united with the staminal column at base; stamens many, modnadelphous, filaments free towards the top; ovary 10-chambered with one ovule in each; fruit a depressed globose schizocarp; seeds smooth.

Distribution: A pantropical weed found throughout the tropical and subtropical regions of India, chiefly in Bengal, Bombay, Coromandel, Carnatic and Kerala.

Sida rhombifolia *Linn. ssp.* **retusa** (*Linn.*) *Borss.* **(Malvaceae)** (Fig. 30)
S. rhombifolia var. retusa (Linn.) Mast.

Erect, minutely stellate-hairy herb; leaves simple, alternate, short-petioled, rhomboid or obovate-retuse, cuneate at base, coarsely toothed, 2 to 3.5 cms long, stellate-

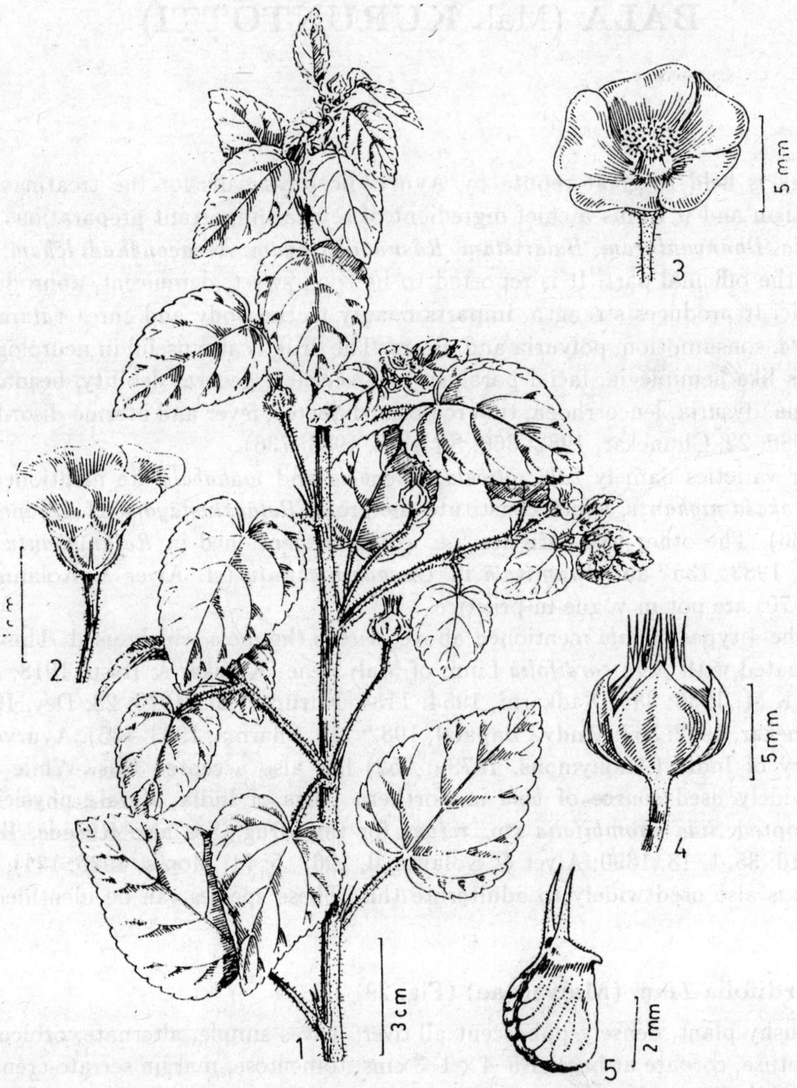

Figure 29: Sida cordifolia L. 1, Twig; 2–3, Flowers; 4, Entire fruit; 5, A single mericarp.

hairy beneath; flowers yellow, solitary, axillary; calyx gamosepalous, persistent, broadly campanulate, 5-lobed; corolla of 5 petals united at the base with the staminal column; stamens many, filaments united to form the tube, but free above, anthers kidney-shaped; fruit depressed-globose, enclosed in the persistent calyx; cocci usually 10, reticulate, awns 2.

Distribution: The plant is found throughout the warmer parts of India, chiefly in Bengal, Konkan, Bombay, Carnatic and Kerala.

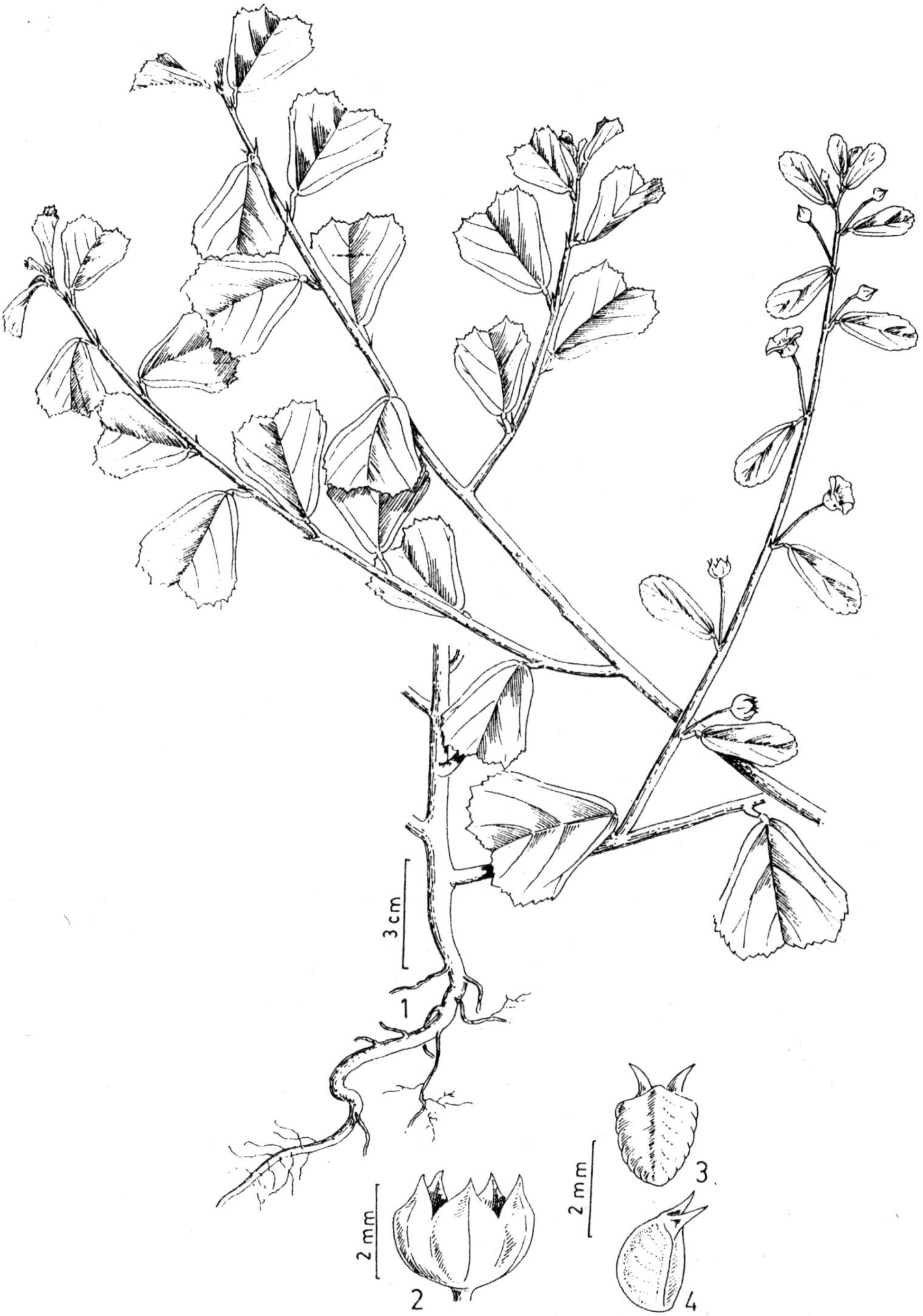

Figure 30: **Sida rhombifolia** L. ssp. retusa (L.) Borss. 1, Habit; 2, Calyx; 3–4, Mericarp. different views.

Sida acuta *Burm. f.* **(Malvaceae)** (Fig. 31)

Much branched subshrub; branchlets minutely stellate-pubescent; leaves simple, alternate, oblong-lanceolate or elliptic, 1.5–7 × 0.5–2 cm, inequilateral, basally 3–5 nerved, glabrescent, base obtuse, margin serrate, apex acuminate; flowers pale yellow, solitary; calyx gamosepalous, persistent, 5-lobed, lobes triangular, acuminate; petals 5, obliquely ovate, emarginate, ciliate at base; staminal column hispid; ovary ovoid, 6-celled; schizocarp enclosed within the calyx, mericarps 6, 4-hedral, awns 2, linear; seeds 3-gonous.

Distribution: The plant is found distributed throughout the hotter parts of India and Malesia.

Mahābalā

Mahābalā is also attributed the same qualities of *balā*. It cures dysuria, vitiated *vāta*, heart disease, piles, oedema, and irregular fevers. (Aiyer & Kolammal, 1962. 5: 76). Most of the authors equate this drug with *Sida rhombifolia* ssp. *rhombifolia* (Malvaceae) (Nadkarni, 1954: 1137; Anonymous, 1978a: 253; Vaidya Bapalal, 1982: 218; Chunekar, 1982: 367; Sharma, 1983: 737).

Sida rhombifolia *Linn. ssp.* **rhombifolia (Malvaceae)** (Fig. 32)

Erect, woody hoary-pubescent herb with strong, wiry, flexuose branches; leaves simple, alternate, rhomboid or elliptic-oblong, obtuse or truncate, 1.5–4 × 0.5–3.5 cm, basally 3-nerved, sparsely stellate-hairy above, woolly below; flowers yellow, axillary, solitary or in cymose clusters; calyx tube shortly stellate-pubescent, 5-lobed; staminal column hairy; ovary 10-celled; schizocarp rugulose, mericarps 7–10, tomentose at apex.

Distribution: Tropical and subtropical regions of the Old and the New World, Malesia and throughout tropical India.

Nāgabalā

Nāgabalā is reported to be sweet, sour, astringent, hot and heavy and cures *vāta* ulcers, disorders due to morbid *pitta* and skin diseases. (Aiyer & Kolammal, 1962. 5: 76). The drug has been equated with *Sida spinosa* (Kirtikar & Basu, 1918: 169; Nadkarni, 1954: 1138; Chunekar, 1982: 371) by some and with *S. veronicaefolia* (now *S. cordata*) by others (cf. Chunekar, 1982: 371; Vaidya Bapalal, 1982: 216).

Sida spinosa *Linn.* **(Malvaceae)**

Subshrub; branchlets shortly stellate-tomentose; leaves ovate-elliptic or oblong, 1.5–3 × 1–2 cm, chartaceous, basally 3 nerved, minutely stellate-tomentose above, cinereous beneath, base and apex obtuse-rotund or acute, margin serrate; flowers solitary or 2–5 in a cluster, yellow; calyx tube cinereous, lobes 5, triangular; petals yellow, obovate; ovary ovoid, 5-celled; schizocarp wrinkled, mericarps 5, 3-gonous, stellate, stiff-tomentose at apex, awns 2; seeds ovoid or 3-gonous.

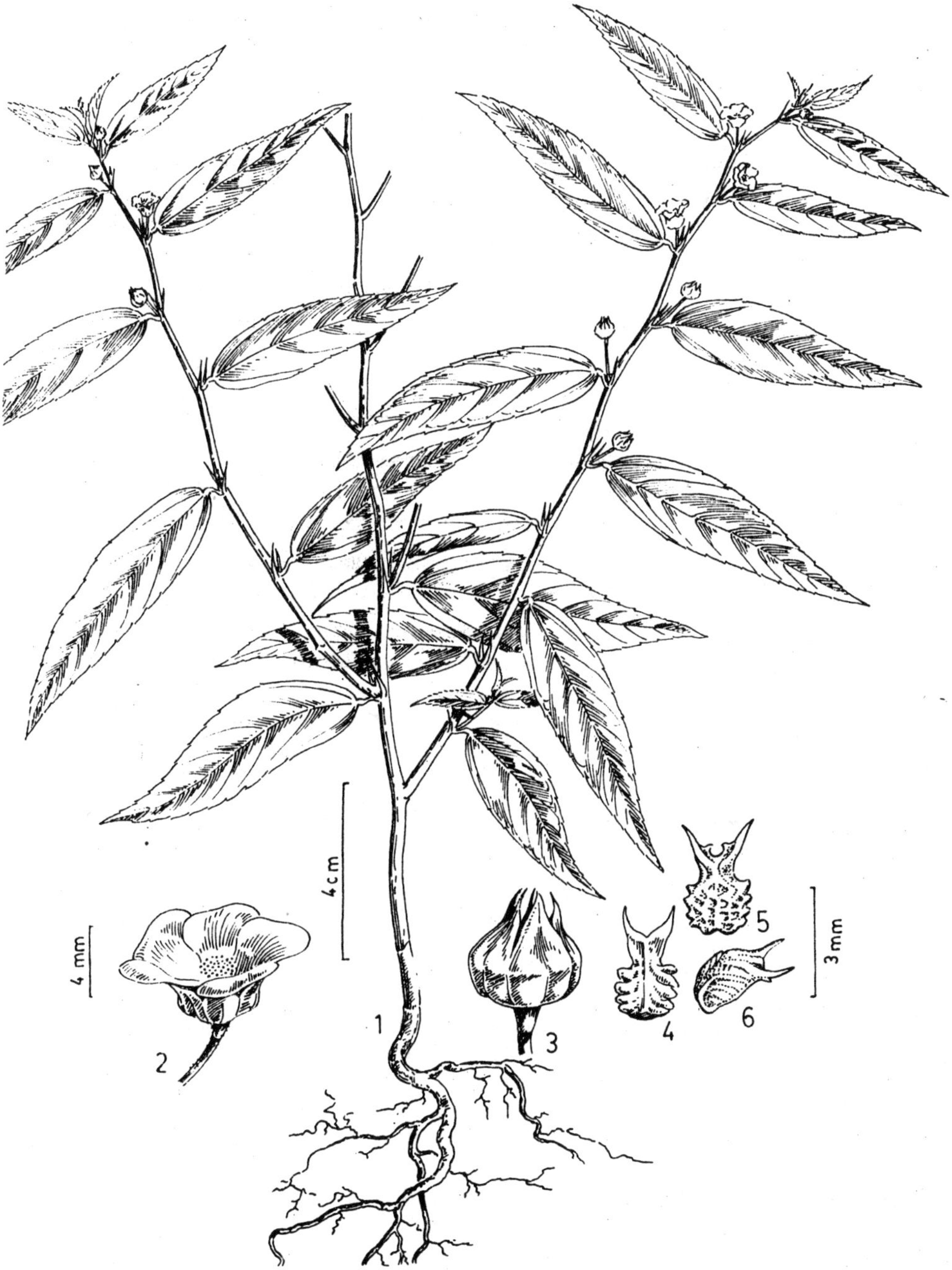

Figure 31: Sida acuta Burm. f. 1, Habit; 2, Flower; 3, Accrescent calyx enclosing fruits; 4–6, Different views of the mericarp.

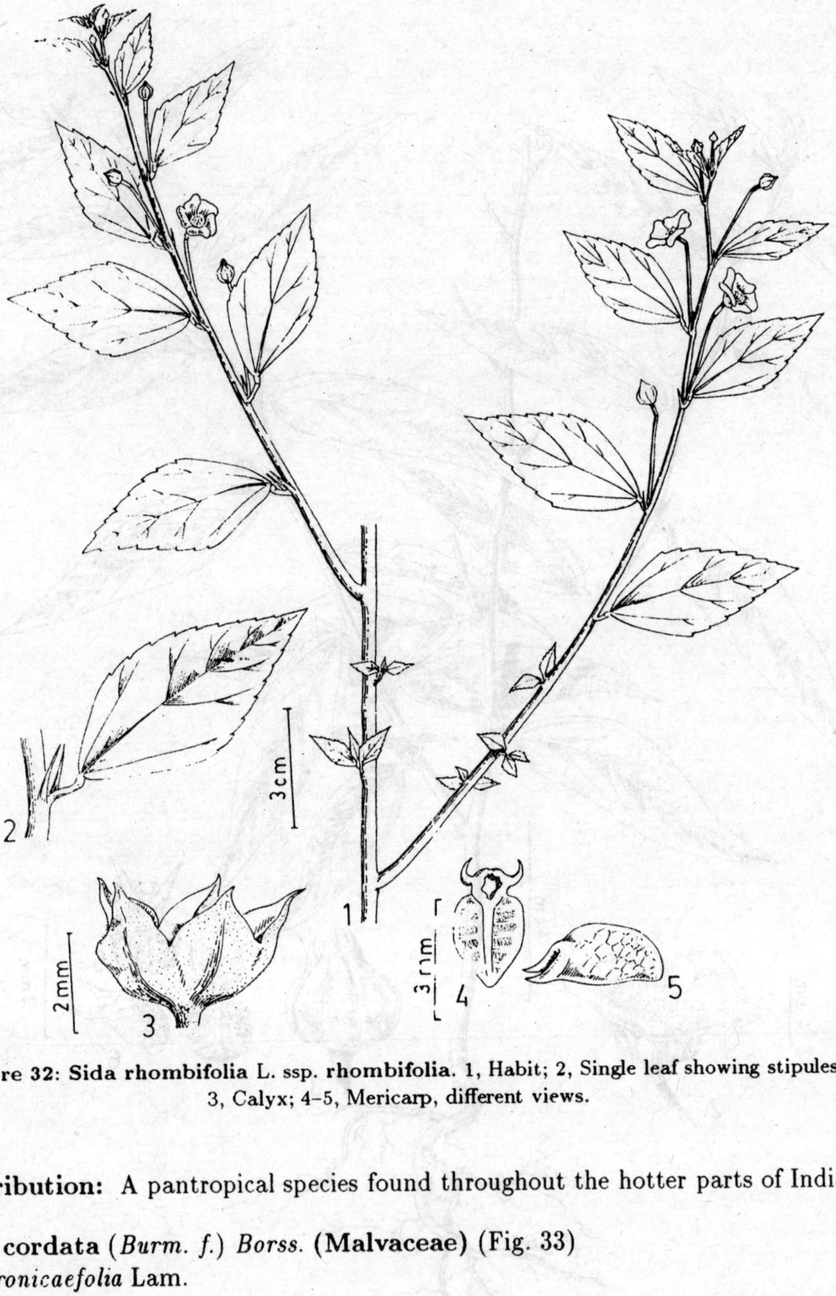

Figure 32: Sida rhombifolia L. ssp. **rhombifolia**. 1, Habit; 2, Single leaf showing stipules; 3, Calyx; 4–5, Mericarp, different views.

Distribution: A pantropical species found throughout the hotter parts of India.

Sida cordata (*Burm. f.*) *Borss.* **(Malvaceae)** (Fig. 33)

S. veronicaefolia Lam.

S. humilis Cav.

Trailing hispid herb; leaves simple, alternate, ovate-cordate, crenate-serrate, clothed with stellate hairs on both surfaces, 0.5–3.5 × 1–3 cm, flowers small, yellow, axillary, solitary on jointed peduncles; calyx gamosepalous, hairy, persistent, 5-lobed; ovary 5-chambered, with one ovule in each; fruit a schizocarp enclosed within the calyx; seeds glabrous, brownish.

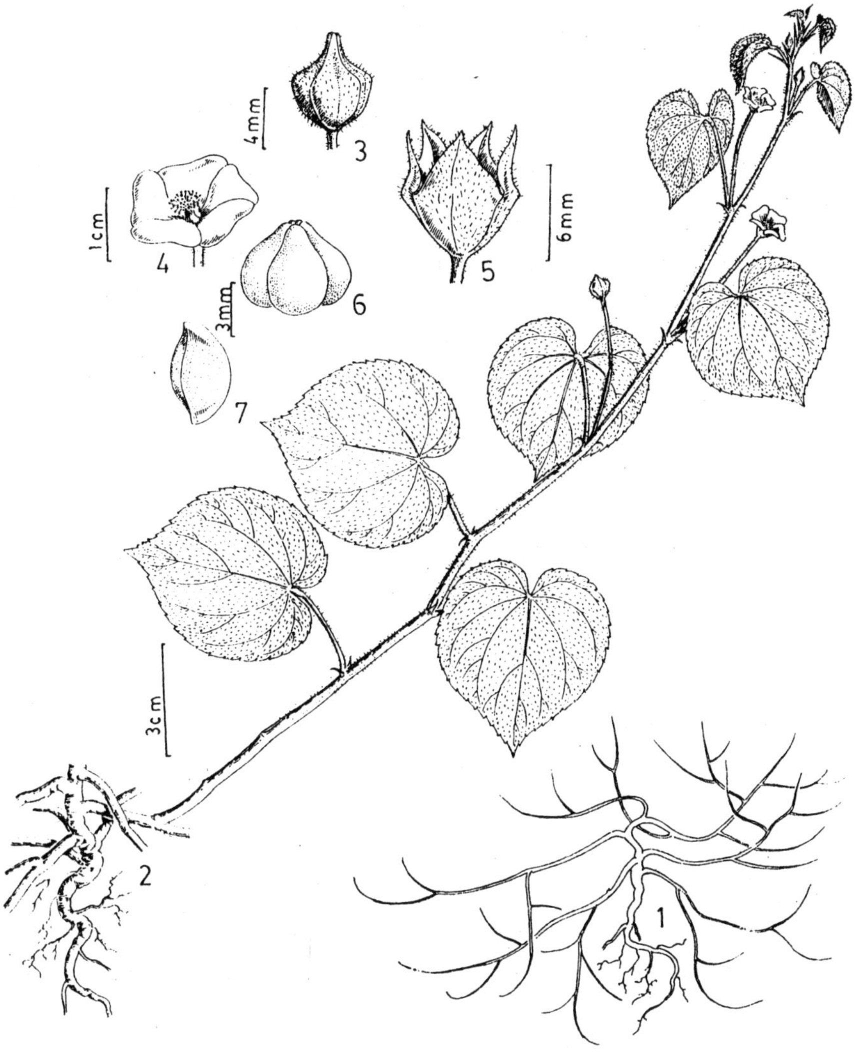

Figure 33: Sida cordata (Burm. f.) Borss. 1, Habit (diagrammatic); 2, Flowering Branch; 3, Flower bud; 4, Flower; 5, Calyx; 6, Fruit; 7, Mericarp.

Distribution: Pantropical weed distributed throughout the hotter parts of India, Malesia and Philippines.

Atibalā

This is supposed to be one of the two constituents of *balādvayaṃ* (i.e. pair of *balās*). *Atibalā* root is reportedly aphrodisiac, diuretic, tonic and cures cough, dysuria, diabetes, fever, thirst, dysmenorrhoea, piles, diarrhoea and worms. (Chunekar, 1982: 370). This is equated variously with *Abutilon indicum* (cf. Kirtikar & Basu, 1918; 174; Nadkarni, 1954: 8; Anonymous, 1978a: 241; Chunekar, 1982: 370; Vaidya Bapalal, 1982: 216; Sharma, 1983: 736), *Abutilon hirtum* (cf. Chunekar, 1982: 370:

Sharma 1983: 737) and *Urena lobata* (cf. Aiyer & Kolammal, 1962. 5: 108), all belonging to the family Malvaceae.

Abutilon indicum (*Linn.*) *Sweet* (Malvaceae) (Fig. 34)

Soft-pubescent shrub; leaves simple, alternate, long-petioled, broadly ovate-cordate, acuminate, 2.5–8 × 2.7 cm, minutely stellate-hairy above, glaucous beneath, margin crenate-dentate; flowers yellow, axillary, solitary; staminal column stellate-hairy at base; schizocarp globose, mericarps 14–20, densely stellate-hairy; seeds ovoid or suborbicular.

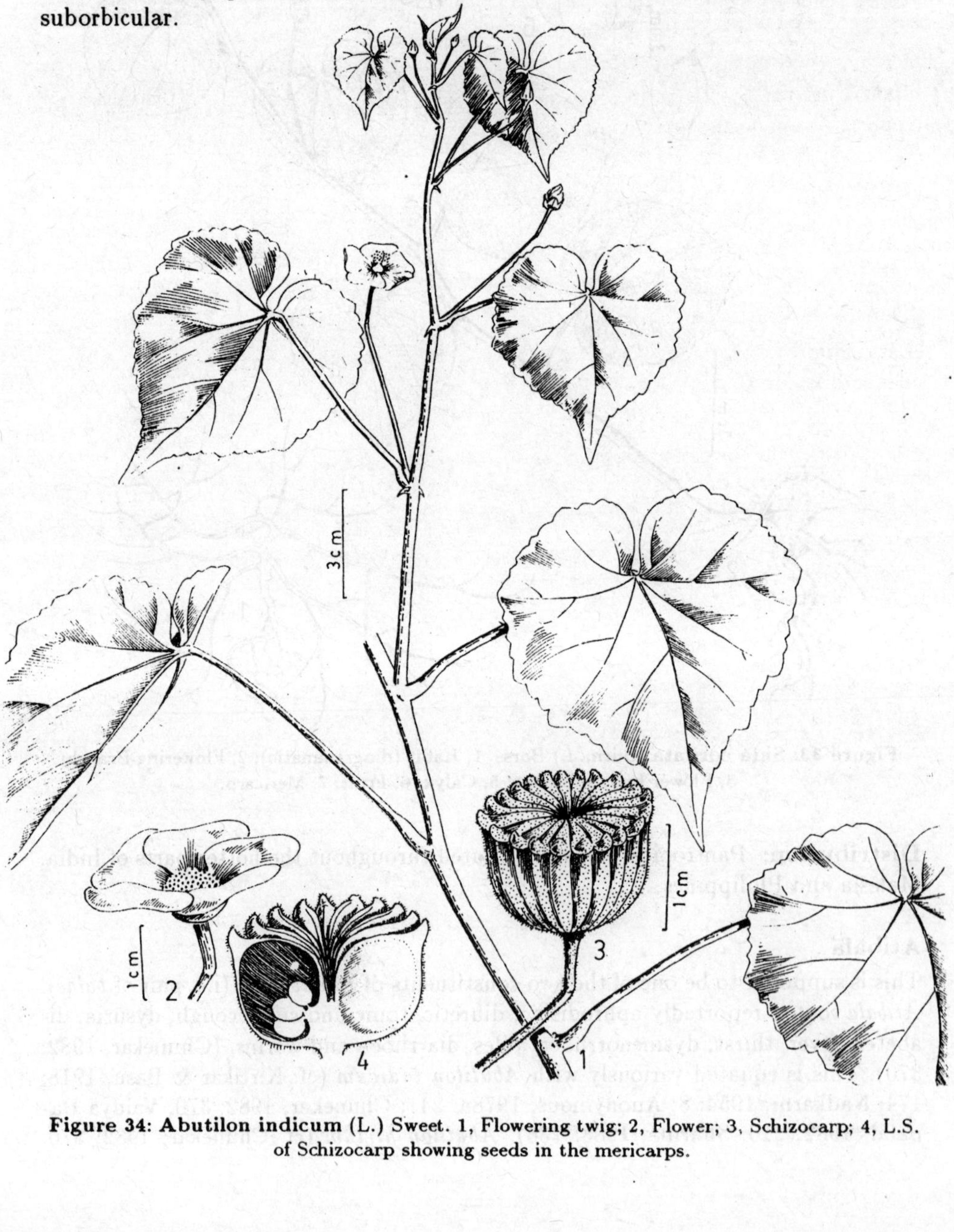

Figure 34: Abutilon indicum (L.) Sweet. 1, Flowering twig; 2, Flower; 3, Schizocarp; 4, L.S. of Schizocarp showing seeds in the mericarps.

Distribution: Widely distributed throughout the tropics and subtropics of both hemispheres. In India it is a common weed of roadsides and waste places.

Abutilon hirtum (*Lam.*) *Sweet* **(Malvaceae)**
Sida hirta Lam.

Subshrub; branchlets viscid, indumentum stellate and tomentose; leaves broadly ovate-suborbicular, 4–8 × 3–6 cm, tomentose above, woolly below, base cordate, margin dentate-crenate, apex acute-acuminate; stipules falcate; flowers solitary, yellow; calyx of 5 ovate sepals; petals 5, inside base purplish, obovate; staminal column stellate-tomentose below, glabrous above; ovary 20–25 celled; schizocarp globose, densely stellate; mericarps 20–25; seeds reniform, stellate-pubescent.

Distribution: Common in all districts in India, tropical regions of the Old World-tropical America and Malesia.

Urena lobata *Linn.* **(Malvaceae)** (Fig. 35)

Woody herb, stellate-tomentose all over; leaves simple, alternate, digitately lobed, lobes again pinnately toothed or incised, stellate-tomentose on both surfaces; flowers pink, axillary, solitary; ovary 5-celled, stiff-hirsute; schizocarp globose, mericarps 5, covered with glochidiate bristles.

Distribution: Circumtropical, throughout Malesia. The plant is a weed of roadsides and waste places in most districts of India.

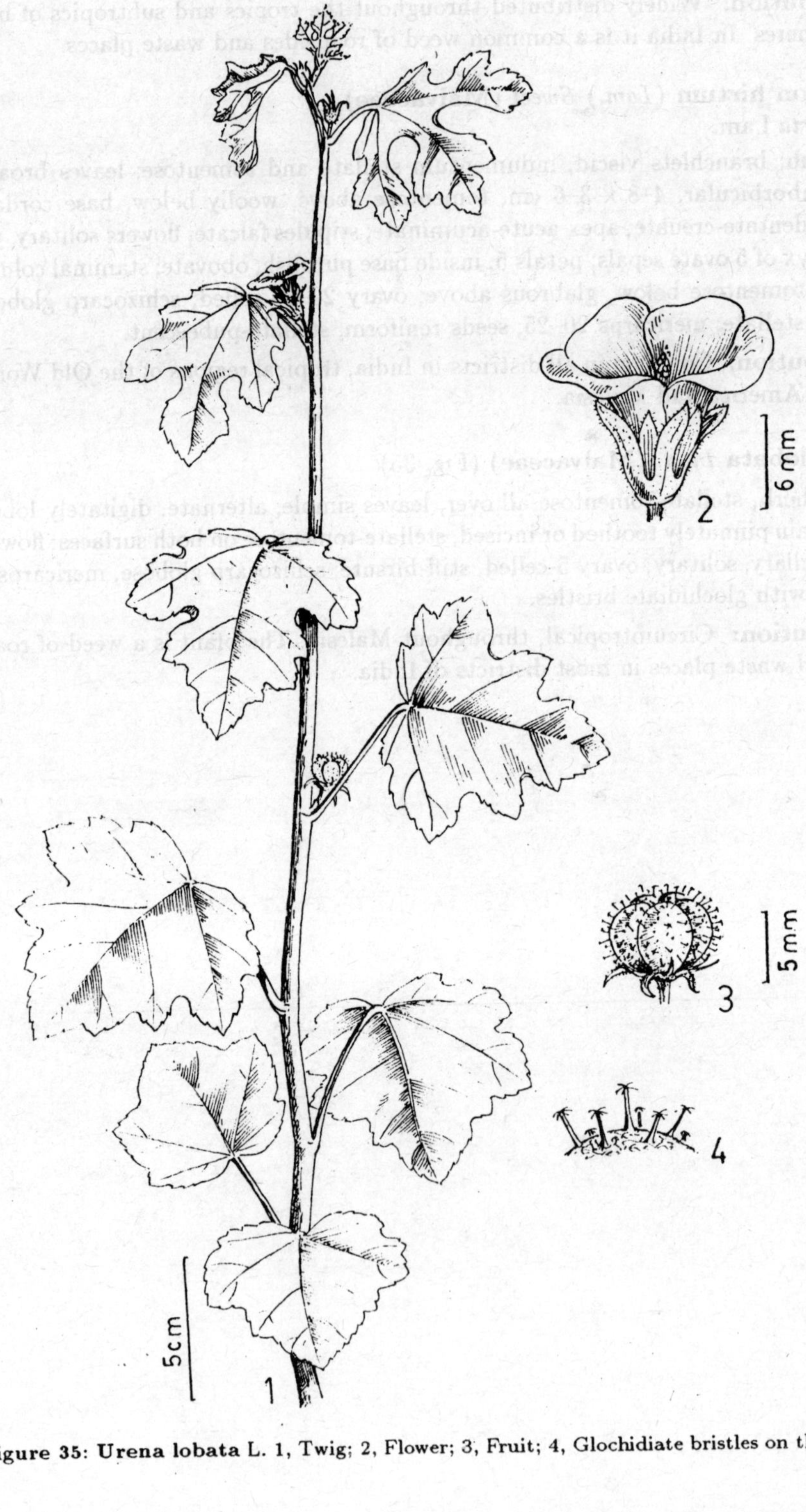

Figure 35: Urena lobata L. 1, Twig; 2, Flower; 3, Fruit; 4, Glochidiate bristles on the fruits.

BAṚBARĪ (Mal. RĀMATUḶASI)

This is an ingredient of the *Surasādi gaṇa* of Vāgbhaṭa which eradicates disorders born of *kapha* and fat, intestinal worms, rhinitis, anorexia, dyspnoea, cough and ulcers (Mooss, 1980: 77–79). *Baṛbarī* is reported to be light, bitter, hot, acrid, anthelmintic, diuretic and carminative. It cures disorders due to *kapha* and *vāta*, dyspepsia, constipation, hemopathy, cough, bronchitis, intermittent fevers, poisonous affections, itching and other skin diseases. Leaf paste is applied to inflammatory swellings. Leaf juice is administered through nostrils in cases of cold and unconsciousness. The seeds are useful in curing morbid *vāta* and *pitta*, chronic diarrhoea, dysentery, bleeding piles, dysuria, excessive thirst, ulcers and general debility. Root, leaves and seeds are medicinal (Sharma, 1983: 517).

Ocimum basilicum Linn. of Lamiaceae is the plant source of this drug (see also Chunekar, 1982: 512; Sharma, 1983: 516). Rheede describes this plant (Hort. Malab. 10: 173, t. 87. 1690) under the name *Solati-tirtava*, but now it is known as *rāmatuḷasi.*

Ocimum basilicum *Linn.* **(Lamiaceae)** (Fig. 36)

Glabrous, strongly aromatic shrub; leaves simple, opposite, elliptic-ovate or lanceolate-acute, cuneate at base, 5–7 × 2.5–3 cm, margin entire to serrulate, nearly glabrous; flowers white on terminal, closely whorled racemes; calyx 2-lipped, enlarged in fruit, hairy outside, upper lip broad and rounded, lower lip 4-lobed; stamens 4, exserted, white; nutlets black, very mucilaginous when wetted.

Distribution: The plant is found in Carnatic and throughout the warmer parts of Asia, Africa and America, widely cultivated.

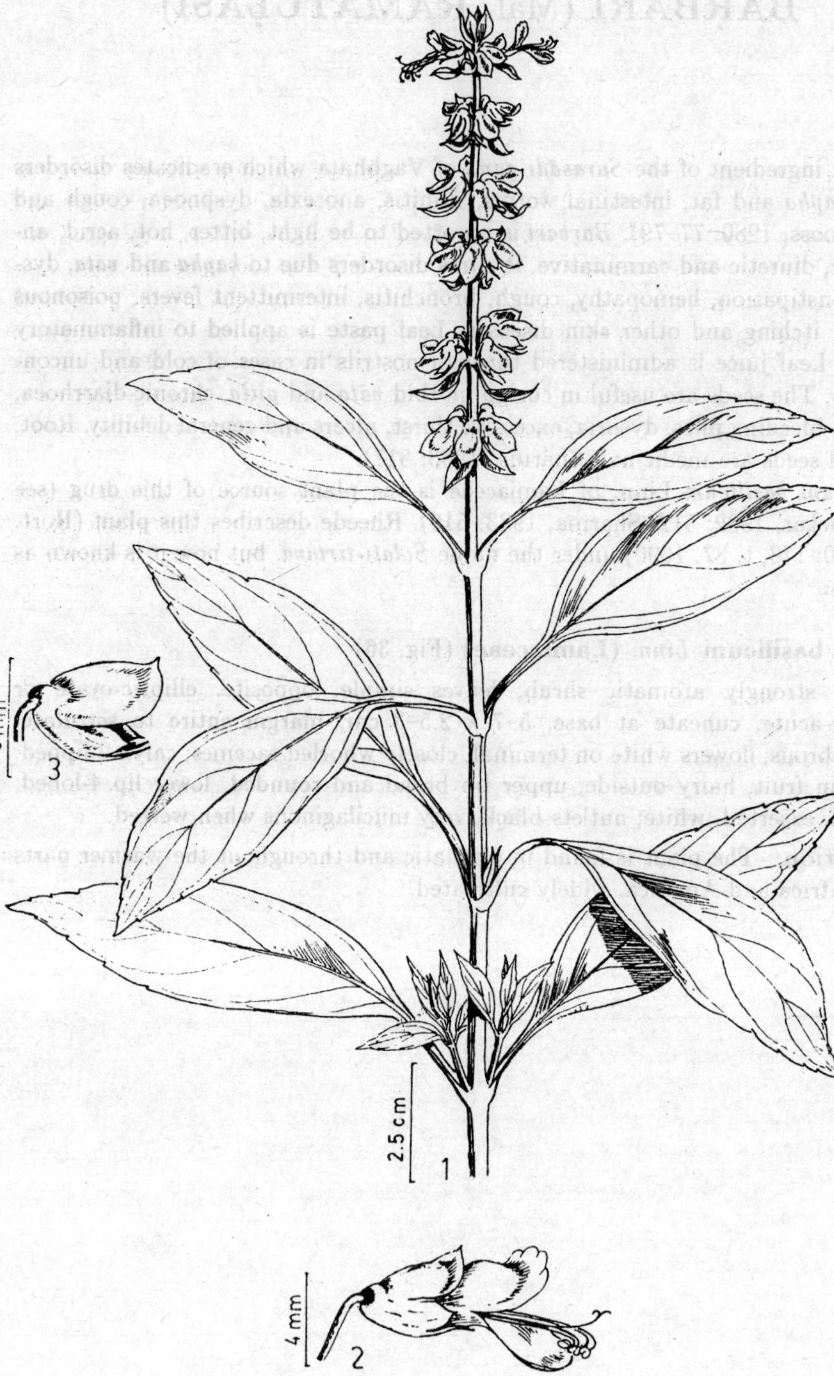

Figure 36: Ocimum basilicum L. 1, Flowering twig; 2, Flower; 3, Calyx.

BHADRĀ (Mal. CEṚŪḶA)

This is one of the ten auspicious herbs that constitute the group *Daśapuṣpaṃ* (i.e. ten flowers), the members of which are believed to curb the incentive for sinful acts, destroy the causative factors of all unhealthy features and bestow good health and prosperity. *Bhadrā* is cooling, diuretic, lithontriptic and is used in haemetemesis, diabetes and lithiasis. It helps to arrest haemorrhage associated with pregnancy. The roots are demulcent and are used in the treatment of headache and strangury. This whole herb is medicinal, though the roots are often preferred (Aiyer & Kolammal, 1963: 6: 24).

Aerva lanata (Linn.) Juss. (Amaranthaceae) is the plant used as the drug source (Aiyer & Kolammal, 1963. 6: 23; Mooss, 1978: 16; Nesamony, 1985: 247). In some parts of Kerala, it is used as an unauthorised substitute for *śvētabṛhatī* which forms an ingredient of the *bṛhatīdivayaṃ* of *daśamūla* group. But most of the authors equate this plant with the drug *pāṣāṇabhēda* or *aśmabhēda* (Kirtikar & Basu, 1918: 1060; Vaidya, K.M. 1936; 34; Nadkarni, 1954: 49; Chopra *et al.*, 1956: 8; Kurup *et al.*, 1979: 163; Chunekar, 1982: 105). This equation may be due to the diuretic and lithontriptic properties of the drug. However, in Kerala, it is not used for this purpose. Rheede's description of this plant (Hort. Malab. 10: 57, t. 29. 1690 *Scheru-bula*) substantiates the fact that it has been in use in Kerala since his time.

Aerva lanata (*Linn.*) *Juss.* (Amaranthaceae) (Fig. 37)
Achyranthes lanata Linn.

Much branched woody herb, pubescent when young; leaves simple, alternate, short petioled, ovate to orbicular, 2–3.5 x 1–2.5 cms, gradually smaller towards apices, base attenuate to cuneate, apex obtusely apicullate, glabrate or finely pubescent above, white woolly beneath; flowers minute, sessile, bisexual, greenish or hoary-white in axillary spicate clusters; bracts and bracteoles ovate, membraneous; perianth calycine, membraneous, of five free keeled segments, covered outside with white woolly hairs; stamens 5, filaments connate at base with alternating linear staminodes, anthers 2-celled; ovary ovoid or subglobose, unilocular with one ovule; fruit greenish, compressed, membraneous utricle or circumscissile capsule; seed reniform.

Distribution: A common weed found in all plains districts and upto 900 metres elevation. It is widespread in the drier parts of the tropics and subtropics of the Old World, Africa and Asia.

Note: The pharmacological studies conducted by Prasad *et al.*, (1986) reveal that the roots of *Aerva lanata* possess diuretic, anti-inflammatory, anthelmintic, antibacterial and mild analgesic effects.

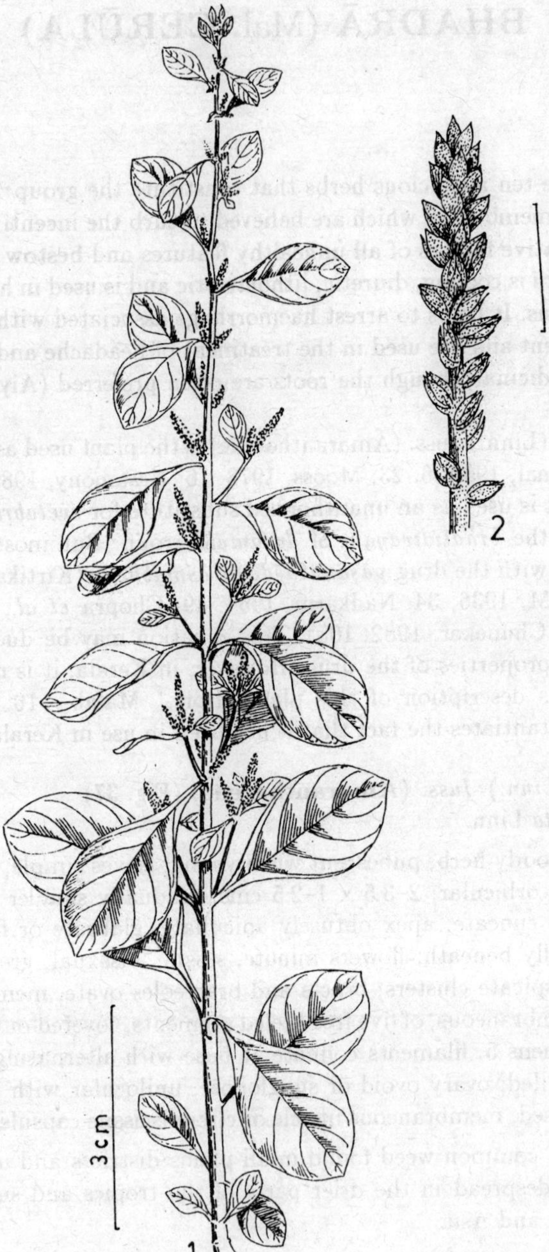

Figure 37: Aerva lanata (L.) Juss. 1, Habit; 2, Inflorescence.

BHALLĀTAKAḤ (Mal. CĒRU)

Bhallātakaḥ is a powerful drug used in Āyurvēda against several types of ailments, since long. It is considered to be one of the toxic drugs and so is used after curing. Fruit is the major officinal part and it enters into many important formulations like *Guggulutiktaka ghṛtaṃ, Niṁbāmṛtāsavaṃ, Nārasiṁharasāyanaṃ, Mahārājapṛasāraṇītailaṃ, Varaṇādi kaṣāyaṃ* etc. The juice of the bark and oil from the fruits are vesicant (*agnimukhī, aruṣkaraḥ*) and cause severe itching, redness, oedema, swelling of the eyelids and produce eczematous vesicles on the skin. It may be because of this property that people are scared to go near the tree and hence the name *vīravṛkṣaḥ* (Moosad, 1983: 301).

In traditional medicine, *bhallātakaḥ* is highly valued for the treatment of tumours and malignant growths. Recent studies carried on the drug have also shown promising results in the treatment of cancer (See Raghunathan & Mitra, 1982: 193). The fruit is reported to be caustic, astringent, alterative, antirheumatic, carminative, counterirritant, rubefacient and vesicant. It is used in cough, asthma, indigestion, enlargement of spleen, alopacia, ulcers, corns, leprosy, leucoderma, rheumatism and piles. The drug is also recommended in the treatment of insanity, fever, dysentery, loss of appetite, neurological diseases and cardiac troubles (Kurup *et al.*, 1979: 32; Raghunathan & Mitra, 1982: 185). *Semecarpus anacardium* Linn. f. (Anacardiaceae), locally called *cēru* is the accepted source of the drug.

Semecarpus anacardium *Linn. f.* **(Anacardiaceae)** (Fig. 38)

Medium-sized tree with a rough bark yielding acrid juice; leaves simple, oblong-elliptic or ovate, 20–35 x 8–15 cm, thick, rusty villous below, base obtuse, subacute or cordate, margin entire, apex rotund, retuse-emarginate; flowers unisexual or bisexual, greenish in terminal panicles. Male: calyx 5-lobed; petals 5; stamens 10, inserted below the annular disc; pistillode hairy with 3-fid styles. Bisexual: ovary 1-celled, styles 3, stigmas subclavate; drupe globose-ovoid, reniform.

Distribution: Distributed throughout the hotter parts of the country and in the deciduous forests in all districts, N. Australia and Malayan Archipelago.

Note: The pharmacognosy and pharmacology of *Semecarpus anacardium* have been discussed in detail by Raghunathan & Mitra (1982: 187–194).

The anti-inflammatory and antiarthritic activity of *Semecarpus anacardium* have been studied by Tripathi *et al.* (1979). Rao, (1981) and Upadhyay *et al.* (1986) found that the drug is effective in the treatment of *āmavāta* (rheumatoid arthritis). The seed kernel of *Semecarpus anacardium* has been found to exhibit antitumour activity (Indap *et al.*, 1983) and to regulate the male sterility in albino rats (Singh, 1985). The toxicity of the drug is studied by Patwardhan, (1988).

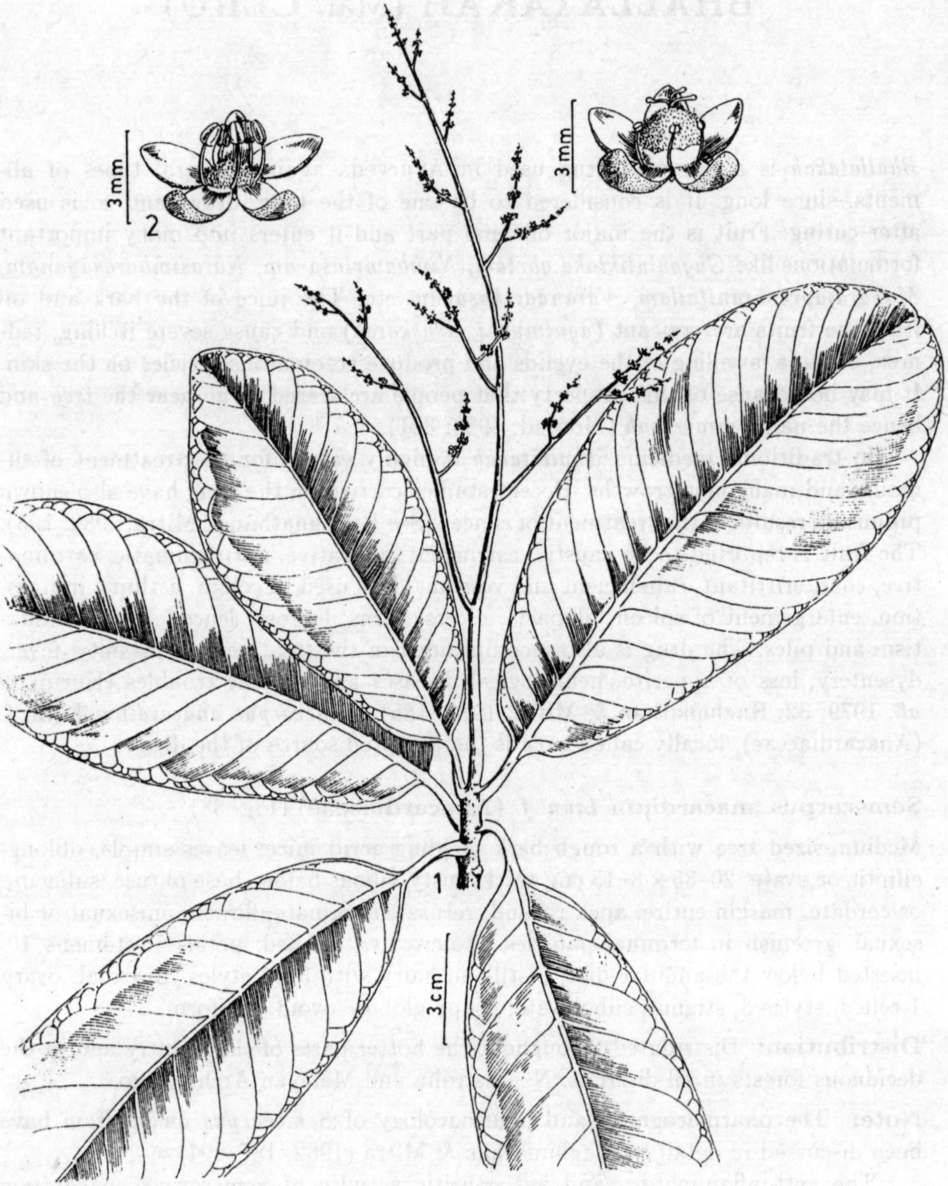

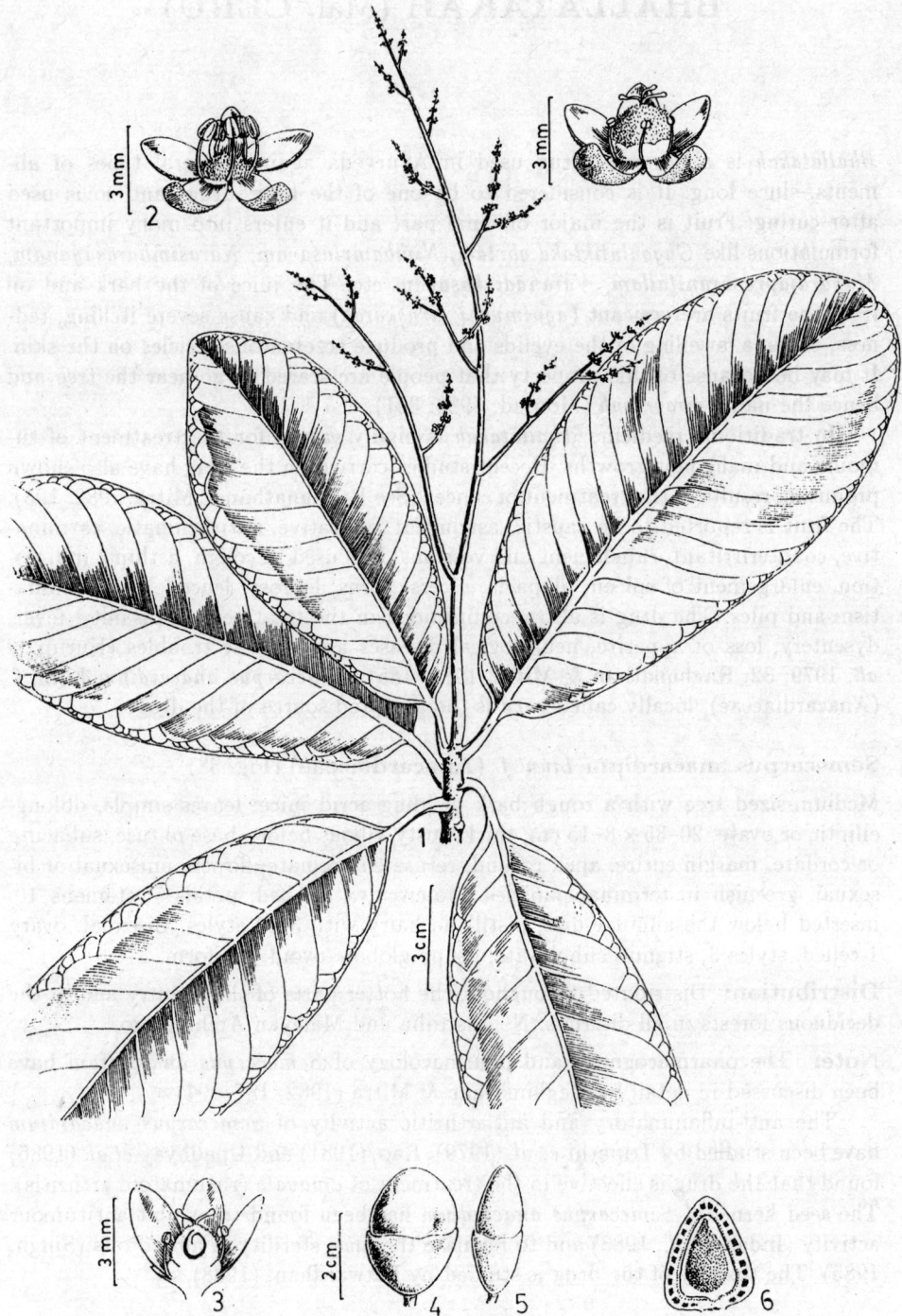

Figure 38: Semecarpus anacardium L. f. 1, Flowering twig; 2, Flower; 3, Flower L.S.; 4–5, Fruits; 6, Fruit T.S.

BHĀṚṄGĪ (Mal. CEṚUTĒKKU)

As the name *bhāṛṅgī* indicates, the drug dispels *kapha* and is hence considered as a specific remedy for all respiratory diseases that are caused by the morbidity of *kapha*. Root, which is the officinal part, is reported to be antispasmodic, carminative, expectorant, febrifuge and tonic and is useful in anasarca, coryza, cough, dyspnoea, catarrhal affections, epilepsy, febrile conditions simulating malaria, indigestion and dropsy. Leaves are suppurative (cf. Kurup *et al.*, 1979: 34; Dey, 1980: 29; Moosad, 1983: 333). The important formulations using the drug are *Ayaskṛti, Bhāṛṅgyādi kaṣāyam, Yōgarājaguggulu vaṭika*, etc.

Clerodendrum serratum (L.) Moon of Verbenaceae is equated with *bhāṛṅgī* by almost all authors on materia medica of Āyurvēda. In Kerala also this plant, locally called *ceṛutēkku* has been the accepted source of the drug. (Hort. Malab. 4: 61–62, t. 29. 1683 *Tsjerou-theka*). Some authors, however, consider *Clerodendrum indicum* (Linn.) Kuntze (= *C. siphonanthus* R. Br.) also as the source of *bhāṛṅgī* (Nadkarni, 1954: 354; Chopra *et al.*, 1956: 71; Singh & Chunekar, 1972: 284; Vaidya Bapalal, 1982: 252). Ayurvedic formulary of India (Anonymous, 1978a: 252) suggests *C. serratum* as the actual drug and *C. indicum* as a substitute, as the latter reportedly has the same properties of *C. serratum* (Singh & Chunekar, 1972: 284). It has been found that the stem bark of certain tree species such as *Gardenia turgida* Roxb., *Gardenia latifolia* Ait. (Rubiaceae), *Picrasma quassioides* Benn. (Simaroubaceae) and *Premna herbacea* Roxb. (Verbenaceae) are sold as *bhāṛṅgī* in north Indian markets. (cf. Singh & Chunekar, 1972: 285; Dey, 1980: 29; Chunekar, 1982: 103; Sharma, 1983: 300). However, on their own merits of possessing antispasmodic and febrifuge properties, they may serve as substitutes of real *bhāṛṅgī* (Singh & Chunekar, 1972: 285).

Studies on south Indian market samples made by Nair *et al.*, (1982) reveal that the root and root nodules of *Pygmaeopremna herbacea* (Roxb.) Mold. (Verbenaceae) are used as *bhāṛṅgī* in Āyurvēdic preparations in some south Indian pharmacies. This is found to promote digestion, cure *gulma, kapha*, dyspnoea and fever. The various plant sources used in southern India can be identified as follows.

Clerodendrum serratum (*Linn.*) *Moon* **(Verbenaceae)** (Fig. 39)
Volkameria serrata Linn.
Shrub; stem 4-angled; leaves simple, or in whorls of 3, subsessile, obovate-oblong, shortly acuminate, base cuneate, coarsely serrate, thick, coriaceous, 25–32 × 10–12 cms; flowers blue, showy, in terminal bracteate thyrsoid panicle; calyx subtruncate, lobes short; corolla tube 1 cm, lobes 5, unequal, oblong-obtuse or (sub) orbicular; stamens 4, didynamous, long exserted, filaments incurved in bud; ovary globose, 4-celled, 4-ovuled, style filiform, stigma bifid; drupe obovoid, purple, partly enclosed in the persistent calyx.

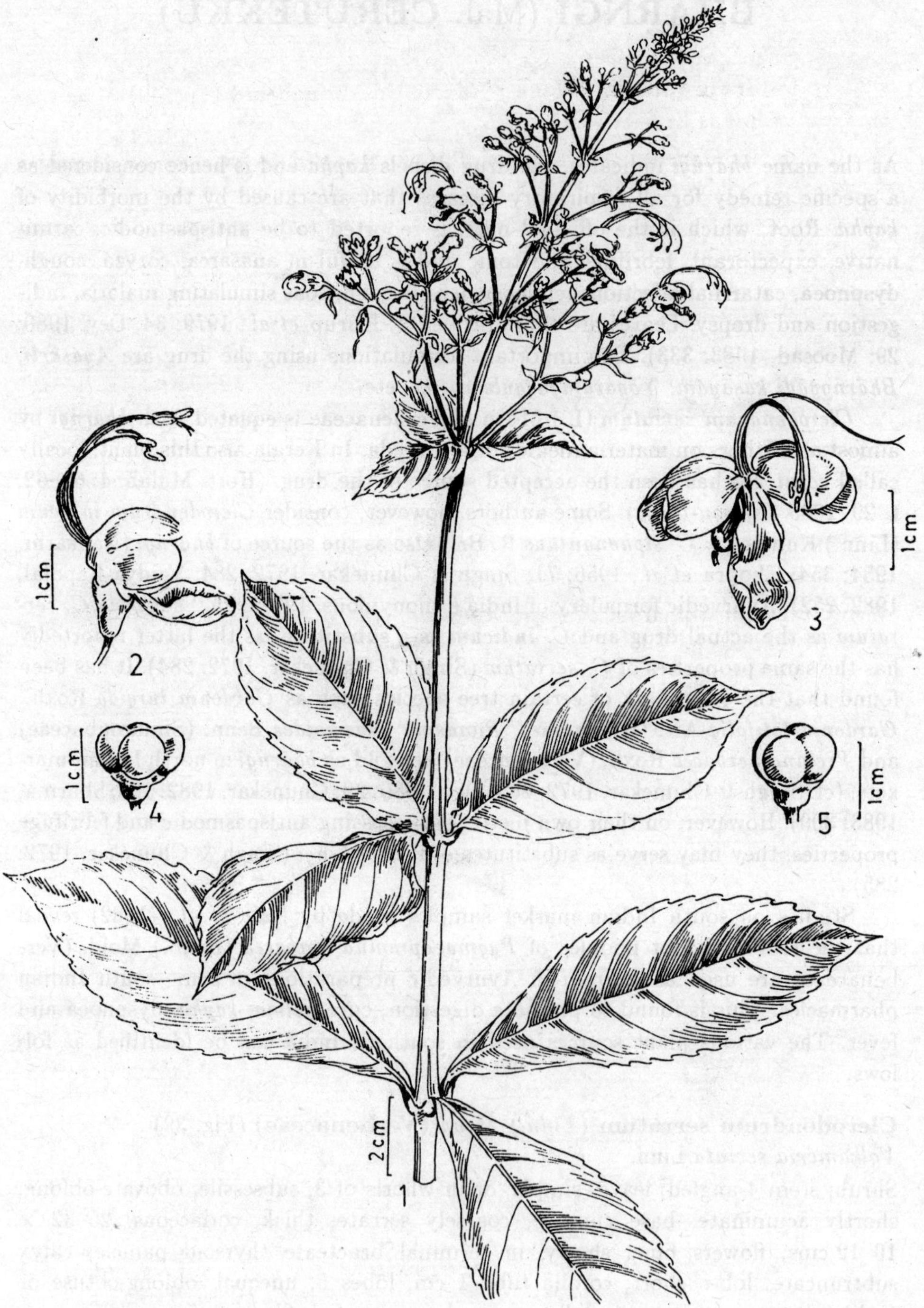

Figure 39: Clerodendrum serratum (L.) Moon. 1, Flowering twig; 2–3, Flowers; 4–5, Fruits.

Distribution: The plant is found in all forest districts in India, chiefly in damp places. It is distributed in Sri Lanka and Burma also.

Clerodendrum indicum (*Linn.*) *Kuntze* **(Verbenaceae)** (Fig. 40)
C. siphonanthus R. Br.

Tall, scarcely branched shrubs; stem obtusely 4-angled; leaves whorled, lanceolate-acuminate, glabrous, upto 38 × 4 cms; flowers white in cymes in the upper axils, forming an apparent terminal panicle; calyx lobes lanceolate-acute; corolla tube narrow, long and drooping, to 15 cms long; stamens 4, didynamous; drupes purple when ripe, enclosed partly in the calyx.

Distribution: The plant is distributed in Deccan, Carnatic and W. Coast district in India.

Pygmaeopremna herbacea (*Roxb.*) *Mold.* **(Verbenaceae)**

Herbs with perennial root stock and root nodules; leaves sessile, in whorls of 2–3, obovate, serrate on upper half; flowers small, pale yellow, in terminal corymbose cymes; drupes small, globose, seated on persistent calyx.

Distribution: The plant is found in the forests of Andhra Pradesh, Tamil Nadu and Orissa and some parts of Kerala.

Note: Detailed pharmacognostic studies on the root of *Clerodendrum serratum* and *C. indicum* have been carried out by Prasad *et al.* (1967).

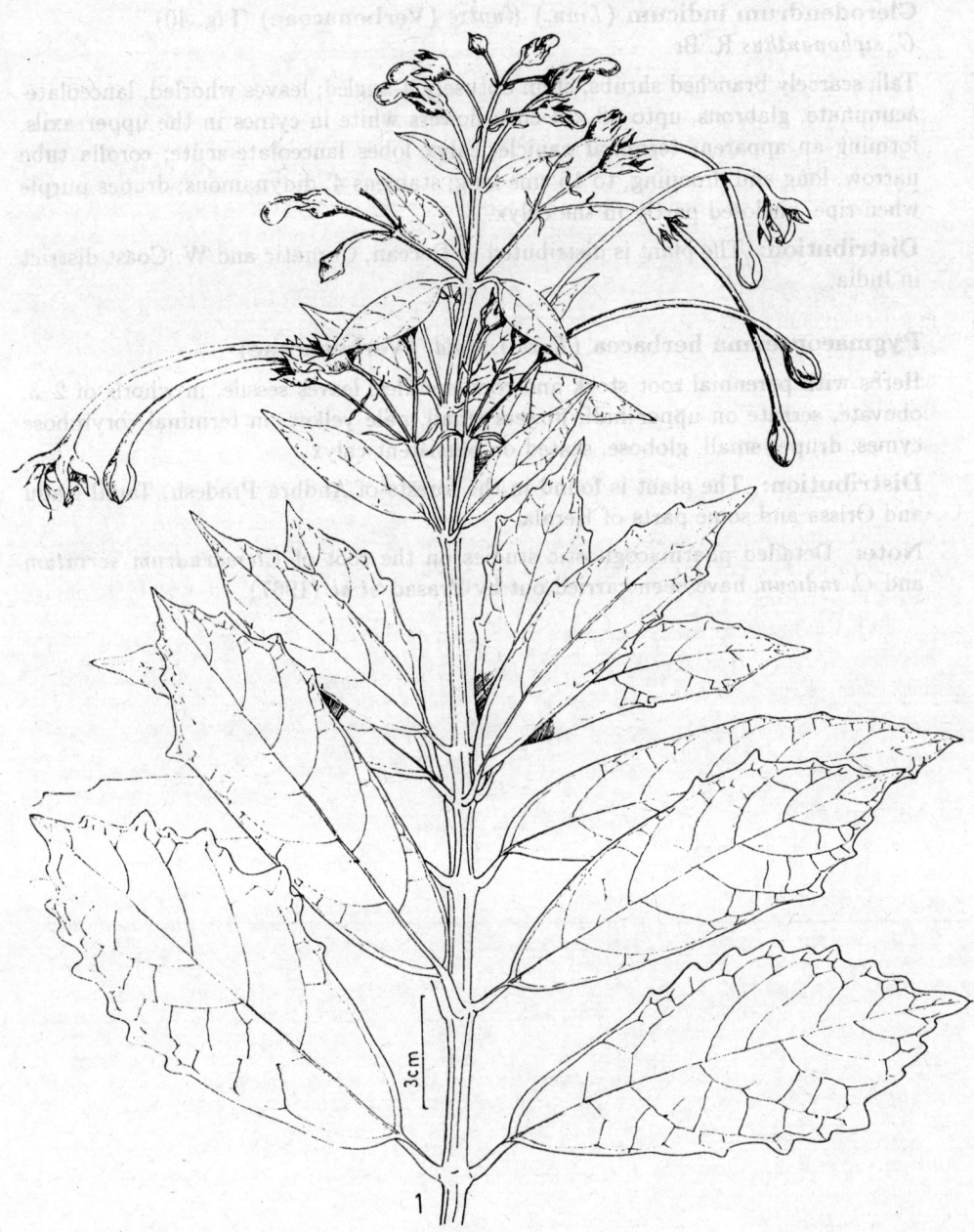

Figure 40: Clerodendrum indicum (L.) Kuntze.

BHṚṄGARĀJAḤ
(Mal. KAYYUṆṆI, KAÑÑUṆṆI)

This is one of the ten auspicious herbs that constitute the group *Daśapuṣpaṃ* (= ten flowers) which is considered to destroy the causative factors of all unhealthy and unpleasant features and bestow good health and prosperity. The members of this group cure wounds and ulcers as well as fevers caused by the derangement of the three dosas—*vāta, pitta* and *kapha.*

Bhṛṅgarājaḥ is acrid, bitter, hot and dry, reduces ***kapha*** and ***vāta*** and is a good rejuvenator. It is good for the hair and skin, expels intestinal worms, cures cough and asthma and strengthens body. It is considered a specific in nightblindness, eye diseases, headache and diseases pertaining to hair and its growth. Traditionally, the drug is extensively used against jaundice (Aiyer & Kolammal, 1962. 5: 119; Kurup *et al.*, 1979: 35). The whole plant enters into the composition of preparations like *Kayyanyādi tailaṃ, Nīlībhṛṅgādi tailaṃ, Nārasiṁharasāyanaṃ, Mahātraiphalaghṛtaṃ*, etc.

The synonyms indicate only the properties of the drug namely promoting growth of hair (*kundaḷavardhanaḥ*), giving black colour to the hair (*kēśarañjanaḥ*) etc.

Three varieties of this drug are mentioned in the texts, viz. the white flowered *śvētapuṣpī*, the blue-flowered *nīlapuṣpī* and yellow flowered *pītapuṣpī*. In practice, no distinction is made between the white and blue flowered varieties and *Eclipta prostrata* (Linn.) Linn. (= *E. alba* (Linn.) Hassk.) of Asteraceae, locally called ***kayyuṇṇi*** or ***kaññuṇṇi*** is used as the drug sorce (see Rheede, Hort. Malab. 10. 81–82, t. 41. 1690, *Canjennaeum*). These two, which may roughly correspond to the blue and white flowered varieties of the drug, were treated as two distinct species formerly, but they have been united subsequently. The yellow-flowered variety which is considered a different drug, is equated with *Wedelia chinensis* (Asteraceae), known as *maññakayyuṇṇi* in vernacular (Hort. Malab. 10. 83, t. 42. 1690, *Pee-canjennaeum*). The two plants can be identified as follows.

Eclipta prostrata (*Linn.*) *Linn.* **(Asteraceae)** (Fig. 41)
E. alba (Linn.) Hassk.

Erect or prostrate, strigosely hairy herbs; leaves acute, to 10.5 × 2.5 cms, serrulate on margins; flowers small, white, in axillary, peduncled rayed heads; involucre campanulate, bracts biseriate, the outer broader; receptacle flat with slender plumose paleae. Ray florets pistillate, disc florets bisexual; pappus of two minute, connate scales; corolla of pistillate flowers ligulate, 2-fid and those of bisexual flowers tubular with 4–5 lobes; stamens 5, epipetalous, syngenesious; ovary inferior, unilocular, 1-ovuled; achenes of ray florets triquetrous, warted, those of disc florets compressed.

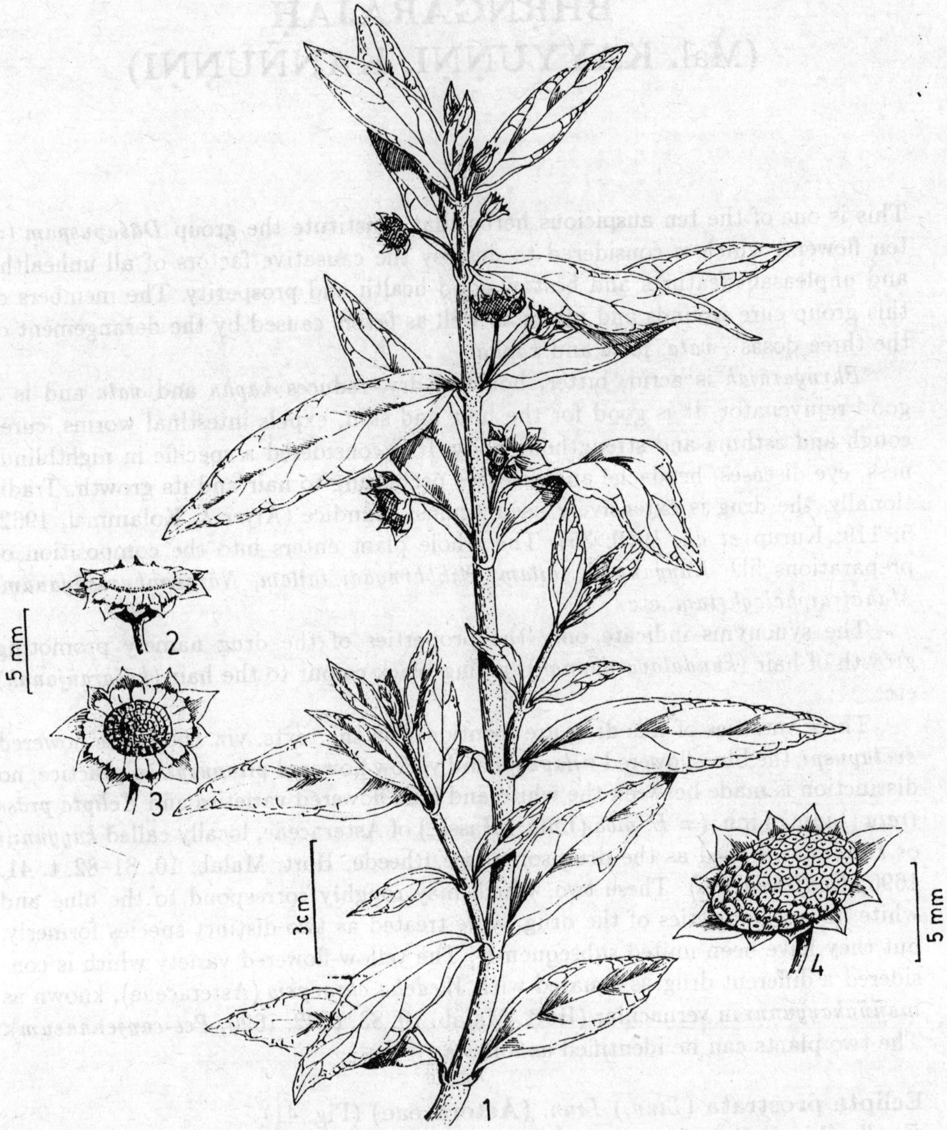

Figure 41: Eclipta prostrata (L.) L. 1, Habit; 2–3, Inflorescence; 4, Head in fruits.

Distribution: A pantropical weed, distributed throughout India in wet or moist waste lands and cultivated fields.

Note: *Eclipta prostrata* has been found to possess myocardial depressant and hypotensive effect (Gupta *et al.*, 1976). It is also found to be effective in the treatment of infective hepatitis (Dixit & Achar, 1979; Dube *et al.*, 1982). Chandra *et al.* (1987) found that *Eclipha alba* is effective against liver injury and inflammation.

Wedelia chinensis (*Osbeck*) *Merr.* **(Asteraceae)** (Fig. 42)
Wedelia calendulacea (Linn.) Less.

A scabrous procumbent perennial herb, stem terete, appressed hairy; leaves simple, opposite, short-petioled, linear to oblanceolate, acute, upto 9 × 2.5 cms, entire or crenate-serrate, scabrous above; heads axillary, solitary, peduncled, yellow, rayed, ray florets pistillate, disc florets bisexual; involucre campanulate, bracts biseriate, receptacle flat; corolla of ray florets ligulate, entire or 2–3 toothed, spreading, those of disc florets tubular, 5-lobed; stamens 5, epipetalous, anthers syngenesious; pistil bicarpellary, ovary inferior, unilocular, 1-ovuled; ray achenes triquetrous, pubescent and disc achenes compressed, tuberculate.

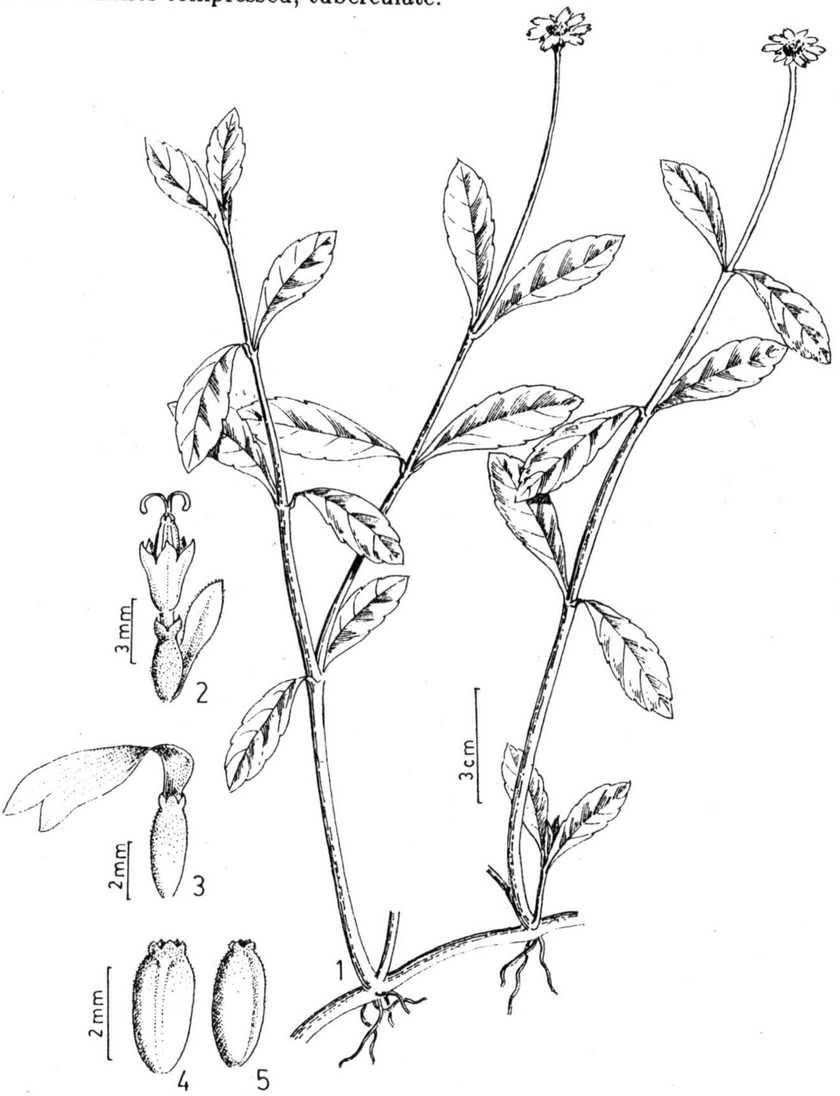

Figure 42: Wedelia chinensis (Osbeck.) Merr. 1, Habit; 2, Disc floret; 3, Ray floret; 4–5, Achenes.

Distribution: The plant is distributed in all plains districts of India, especially along E. and W. Coast, in wet places, also in Malaya and China.

Note: Yang *et al.* (1986) studied the antihepatotoxic effect of *Wedelia chinensis*. The isolated constituents of this plant exhibited strong activity against liver damage induced by chemicals.

BIṀBĪ (Mal. KŌVA)

In Indian medicine, *biṁbī* is highly valued for its antidiabetic potential. It is carminative, antipyretic, viriligenic, galactagogue and roborant. *Biṁbī* overcomes diseases due to vitiated *kapha*, cough, dyspnoea and other respiratory diseases, clarifies *pitta* and *rakta*, cures emaciation, fever with burning sensation, diabetes, ulcers and skin diseases. Juice of the plant is given in intermittent glycosuria and enlarged glands. Leaves are applied externally to sores, skin eruptions and bites of animals. Tender fruit is chewed to cure sores on the tongue. The whole plant is used medicinally (Nadkarni, 1954: 301; Mooss, 1976: 51; Kurup *et al.*, 1979: 43). In Siddha system of medicine, this drug is used against infective hepatitis (Rajasekharan *et al.*, 1984). *Vidāryādi ghṛtaṃ*, *Vidāryādi kaṣāyaṃ*, *Amṛtaprāśaghṛtaṃ*, *Vastyāmayāntaka ghṛtaṃ* etc. are some of the preparations using the drug.

Coccinia grandis (Linn.) Voigt. of Cucurbitaceae, locally called *kōva* is the accepted source of the drug. Rheede (Hort. Malab. 8: 27–28, t. 14. 1688) has described this under the name *Covel.*

Two varieties of *biṁbī* are recognised-a bitter variety and a sweet variety. The former grows wild and is preferred in medicine whereas the cultivated sweet variety is used as a vegetable (Sharma, 1983: 688).

Coccinia grandis (*Linn.*) *Voigt.* **(Cucurbitaceae)** (Fig. 43)
Coccinia indica Wt. & Arn.

Slender dioecious climber with tuberous roots; leaves simple, alternate, orbicular-cordate, 3–5 lobed, glabrous, 5 to 10 cm across; flowers unisexual, white, solitary, axillary. Male: calyx campanulate, glabrous, lobes 5, subulate; corolla campanulate, 5-lobed; stamens 3, inserted at the base of the calyx tube, filaments connate into a column, glabrous, anthers connate, triplicate, flexuous. Female: calyx and corolla as in male; stamens 0; ovary glandular-pubescent, ovules many, stigma 3-partite, fimbriate; staminodes 3, subulate; fruit ovoid or oblong, green with white stripes when young blood-red when ripe; seeds oblong-ovoid, compressed, glandular.

Distribution: The plant is distributed throughout India, common in most plains districts. It has also been reported from tropical parts of Asia, Africa and Australia.

Note: The pharmacognosy of *Coccinia grandis* has been discussed by Satyavati *et al.*, (1976: 262).

The drug has been found to be effective in the treatment of diabetes mellitus, due to its hypoglycaemic activity (Khan *et al.*, 1980; Pillai, N. R. *et al.*, 1980; Kuppurajan *et al.*, 1986; Choudhury & Misra, 1987). Rajasekharan *et al.* (1984) found that *Coccinia grandis* is very effective in the treatment of infective hepatitis (*maññakkāmila*).

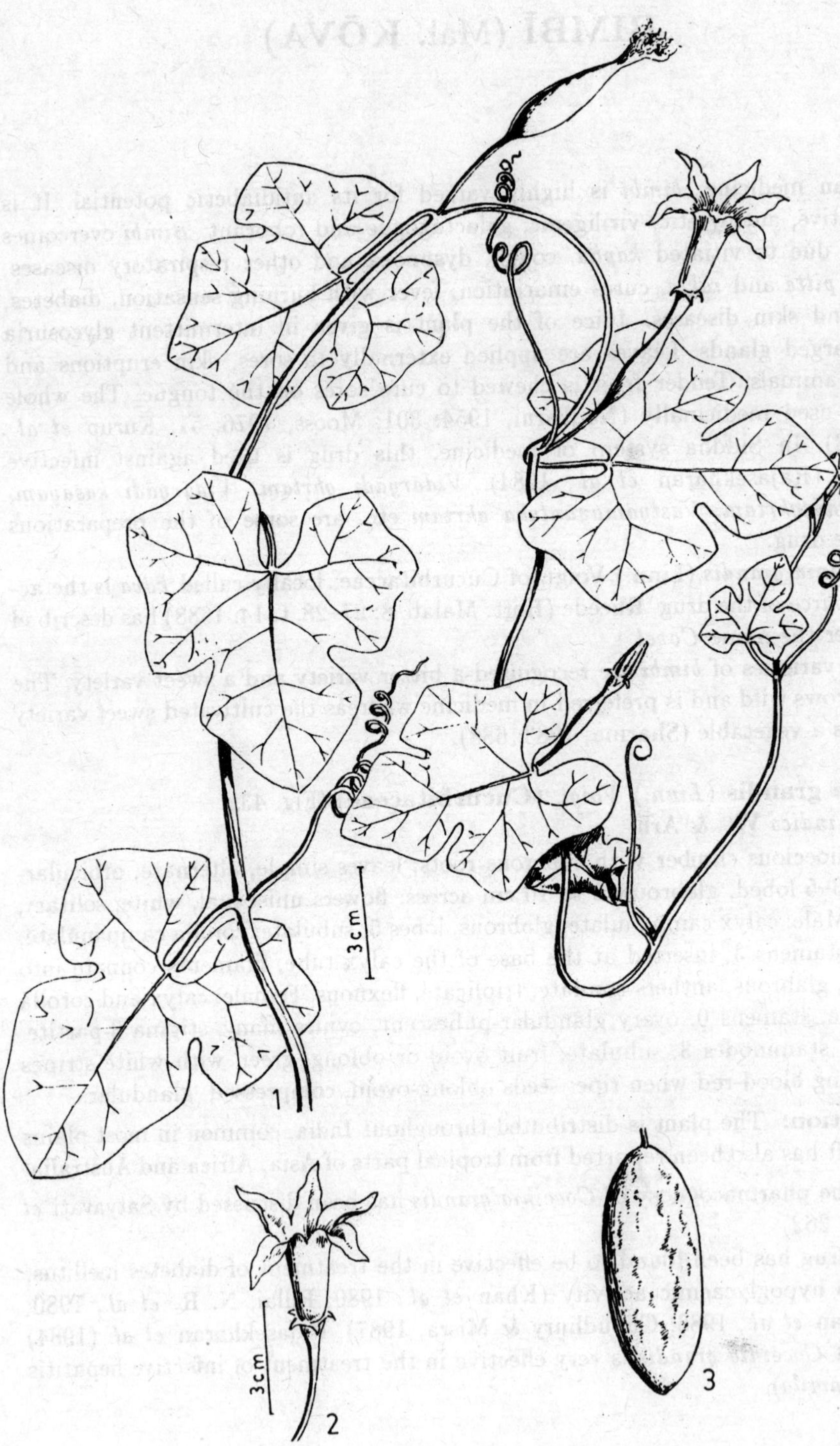

Figure 43: Coccinia grandis (L.) Voigt. 1, Vine with female flowers; 2, Male flower; 3, Fruit.

BRĀHMĪ (Mal. BRAHMI)

Brāhmī is an important *mēdhya* drug in Āyurvēda for improvement of intelligence and memory and revitalisation of sense organs. It is also capable of imparting youthful vitality and longevity. It clears voice and improves digestion. The drug is reported to be cold, sweet, astringent, diuretic, laxative and a tonic for heart and nerves. It is indicated against dermatosis, anaemia, diabetes, cough, dropsy, fever, arthritis, anorexia, dyspepsia, emaciation and insanity. It dispels poisonous affections, splenic disorders and impurity of blood (Aiyer & Kolammal, 1964. 8: 26). The whole plant is used in a variety of preparations like *Brāhmīghṛtaṃ, Sārasvatāriṣṭaṃ, Brāhmītailaṃ, Miśrakasnēhaṃ*, etc.

Resemblence of the leaves or flowers of this plant to the eye of fish (*matsyākṣī*) is the only indication given in the texts regarding the description of the drug. Most other synonyms like *vayasthā, kapōtavaṅgā, sōmavallī* and *sarasvatī* refer to its therapeutic properties and are not helpful in discerning the identity of the plant.

Abhidhānamañjari mentions four different types of *brāhmī* viz. *sātalabrahmī, mēdhābrahmī, munibrahmī* and *maṇḍūkaparṇī* (cf. Aiyer & Kolammal, 1964. 8: 20). But this is neither seen in other classical literature nor is it in vogue in practice. *Rājanighaṇṭu* has, however, equated *brāhmī* and *maṇḍūkaparṇī* as one and the same. This is being followed by some north Indian physicians also. (cf. Usman Ali *et al.*, 1981). But in the three great Āyurvēdic classics of Caraka, Suśrutha and Vāgbhaṭa, *brāhmī* and *maṇḍūkaparṇī* are spoken of as two distinct drugs. They are mentioned separately in the *Aṣṭāṅgaghṛta yōga* of *Aṣṭāṅgahṛdaya*. The fact that they have never been included in the same yōga by Caraka and Suśrutha also tend to show that they are distinct.

A critical study of the comparative phytochemistry, pharmacology and therapeutic properties of these two drugs also support the view that they are distinct. Caraka considers both of them as promoters of general mental ability (*mēdhya*) but suggests that *brāhmī* is superior to *maṇḍūkaparṇī*, in that the former is specified in mental diseases like *unmāda* (insanity), *apasmāra* (epilepsy) etc., whereas the latter helps regain general mental health through its *rasāyana* effect. This apart, they are found to have opposite effect on uterus, *brāhmī* promotes fertility and sustains implantation and pregnancy while *maṇḍūkaparṇī* tends to eject them. They also have different effect on *kāṇḍu*, a type of skin disease (Usman Ali *et al.*, 1981).

Moreover, they are found to differ in their *rasa*—*Bhāvaprakāśa* records that *brāhmī* is of *tikta rasa* (bitter) whereas *maṇḍūkaparṇī* is of *kaṣāya rasa* (astringent) as recorded by Suśruta (cf. Usman Ali *et al.*, 1981).

In Kerala, these two drugs have never been accepted as the same. The accepted source of *brāhmī* has always been *Bacopa monnieri* of Scrophulariaceae. This is a weak, creeping, herbaceous plant common in marshes and along backwaters and is called *brahmi* or *nīṛbrahmi* in vernacular. *Centella asiatica* (Apiaceae) known by the vernacular names *muttiḷ, koṭaṅṅal*, etc. is being used as the source of *maṇḍūkaparṇi* which is discussed elsewhere in the text. That this has been the practice since at least the 17th century is testified by Rheede's treatment of these two under *brāhmī* (Hort. Maḷab. 10: t. 14, 1690) and *codagen* (Hort. Malab. 10. t. 46, 1690) respectively.

Bacopa monnieri (*Linn.*) *Pennell* **(Scrophulariaceae)** (Fig. 44)
Lysimachia monnieri Linn.
Herpestris monnieria (Linn.) Kunth.
Creeping, glabrous, somewhat succulent herb; rooting at nodes; leaves simple, opposite, obovate-oblong, obtuse, entire, to 2×1 cm; flowers pale violet, axillary, solitary on long pedicels; calyx 5-partite, lobes unequal; corolla gamopetalous, funnel-like, white or pinkish with purple blotches; stamens 4, didynamous, included; ovary 2-chambered; ovules many on swollen axile placenta; capsules ovoid, included in the persistent calyx.

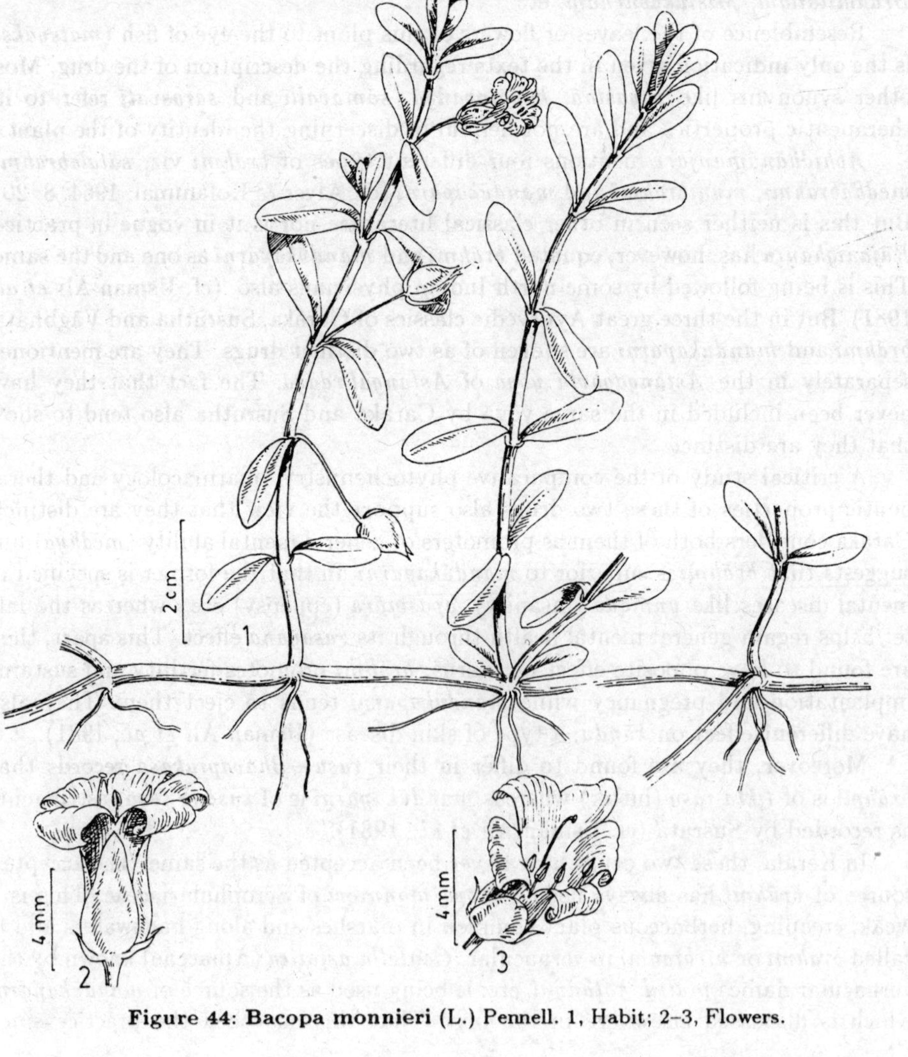

Figure 44: Bacopa monnieri (L.) Pennell. 1, Habit; 2–3, Flowers.

Distribution: This paleotropical weedy species is common in wet or marshy lowlands in all plains districts throughout India.

Note: *Bacopa monnieri* has been found to be very effective in cases of anxiety neurosis (Singh *et al.*, 1979) and in revitalising intellectual faculty (Sharma R. *et al.*, 1987a).

BṚHATĪ (Mal. VAḶUTINA)

An important constituent of *laghupañcamūla, bṛhatī* is reported to be constipating, digestive, acrid and bitter. It helps overcome vitiated *tridōṣās* and cures dyspepsia, fever, respiratory and cardiac disorders, skin ailments, vomiting, ulcers, and poisonous affections (Aiyer & Kolammal, 1960. 4: 81). Root is the major officinal part, but fruits and leaves are also used occasionally. *Bṛhatyādikaṣāyaṃ, Daśamūlariṣṭaṃ, Indukānta ghṛtaṃ*, etc. are the important preparations in which *bṛhatī* joins as an important drug.

From the texts, one can only infer that it is a prickly plant (*kaṇṭakārī, dusparśā, kaṇṭala*) with yellow fruits (*pītaphalā*). These synonyms are applicable to many species of *Solanum* and hence different authors have equated the drug with different species of the genus. Moreover, texts speak of a pair of *bṛhatī*, i.e. *bṛhatīdvayaṃ*. In Kerala these have been equated with a small fruited variety called *ceṛuvaḷutina* and a white fruited variety called *veḷ-vaḷutina*, also called *kaṛuttacuṇḍa* and *veḷutiacuṇḍa* respectively (cf. Mooss, 1980: 13).

Most of the authors have equated the former with *Solanum indicum* (now *S. violaceum*) of Solanaceae (see Kirtikar & Basu, 1918: 894; Vaidya, K.M. 1936. 397; Nadkarni, 1954: 1149, Singh & Chunekar, 1972: 277; Anonymous, 1978a: 252; Kurup *et al.*, 1979: 47; Dey, 1980: 32; Chunekar, 1982: 288; Sharma, 1983: 282) and the latter with *kaṇṭakāri* (*Solanum virginianum*). In Kerala, however, these two species are considered to be sources of different drugs (discussed elsewhere in the text) and are not eqated with *bṛhatīdvayaṃ*. Kerala physicians have, by and large, adopted the wild and cultivated varieties of *Solanum melongena* as the source of these two.

Solanum melongena *Linn.* **(Solanaceae)** (Fig. 45)

Erect, perennial, sparsely prickly shrub; leaves simple, alternate, or in sub-opposite unequal pairs, obliquely ovate, entire or angularly sinuated to shallowly or deeply pinnately lobed, acute, unequal-sided at base, stellate-pubescent; flowers blue, regular, in a few-flowered lateral or supra-axillary corymbose cymes; calyx gamosepalous, campanulate, 5-lobed, lobes linear-oblong or lanceolate, prickly; corolla rotate, 5–9 cleft or lobed; stamens 5; free, epipetalous; ovary globular; fruit a smooth, shiny, ovate-oblong, ellipsoid or globular berry.

Distribution: Widely cultivated throughout tropical India and the warmer parts of the world.

Solanum melongena *Linn. var.* **insanum** (*Linn.*) *Prain* **(Solanaceae)** (Fig. 46)
S. insanum Linn.

Very prickly, grey-pubescent, undershrub; leaves simple, alternate, ovate or elliptic-ovate, acute, 7–12 × 6–8 cm, oblique at base, irregularly lobed, stellate-pubescent, prickly along the nerves; flowers purple, 1–4, extra-axillary; calyx lobes 5, lanceolate, thick, stellate-pubescent; corolla rotate, deeply five-cleft, lobes 5, triangular;

stamens 5, free, epipetalous; ovary villous; berry oblong-globose, 3 cm across, fruiting calyx enlarging.

Distribution: Distributed throughout the tropical regions of India in the plains districts.

Note: Deb (1989) has now conducted extensive field studies on the morphological variability in *Solanum melongena* and has concluded that it is highly variable and the varieties recognised under it (var. *insanum* and var. *incanum*) do not hold good any more.

Solanum violaceum *Ortega* **(Solanaceae)** (Fig. 47)
Solanum angui Sensu Matthew & Rani
S. indicum sensu auctt., non Linn.

Armed shrub; leaves simple, alternate, or sub-opposite in unequal pairs, greyish green, ovate or oblong, sinuately lobed, 9–13 × 6–9 cm, base oblique or unequal-sided, stellately woolly or downy beneath, prickly along the midnerve; flowers pale purple, regular in 8–10 flowered, extra-axillary racemes; calyx cupular, lobes 5, triangular, thick, prickly; corolla rotate, deeply 5-cleft; stamens 5, free, filaments very short, anthers oblong-lanceolate; ovary glabrous, style stellately pubescent; berry globose, smooth, light green, variegated with dark green when young and orange-yellow when ripe.

Distribution: Sri Lanka and India. In India it is found all over the tropical parts in waste lands, roadsides etc. from sea level to about 2,000 ft.

S. virginianum *Linn.* **(Solanaceae)**
S. surattense Burm.f.
S. xanthocarpum Schrad. & Wendl.

(For descriptions and figure see under *Kaṇṭakārī*.)

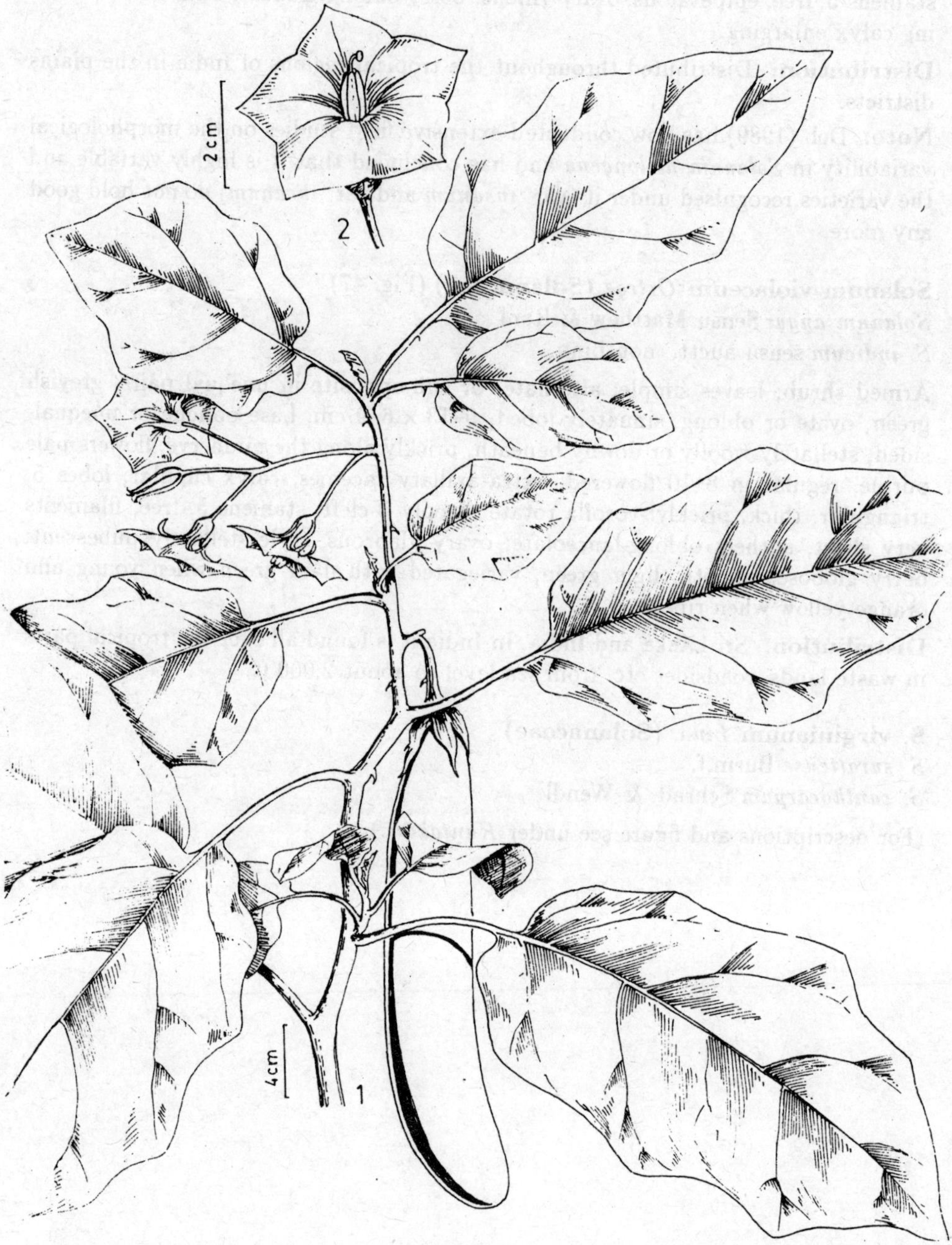

Figure 45: Solanum melongena L. 1, Twig with flowers and Fruits; 2, Flower.

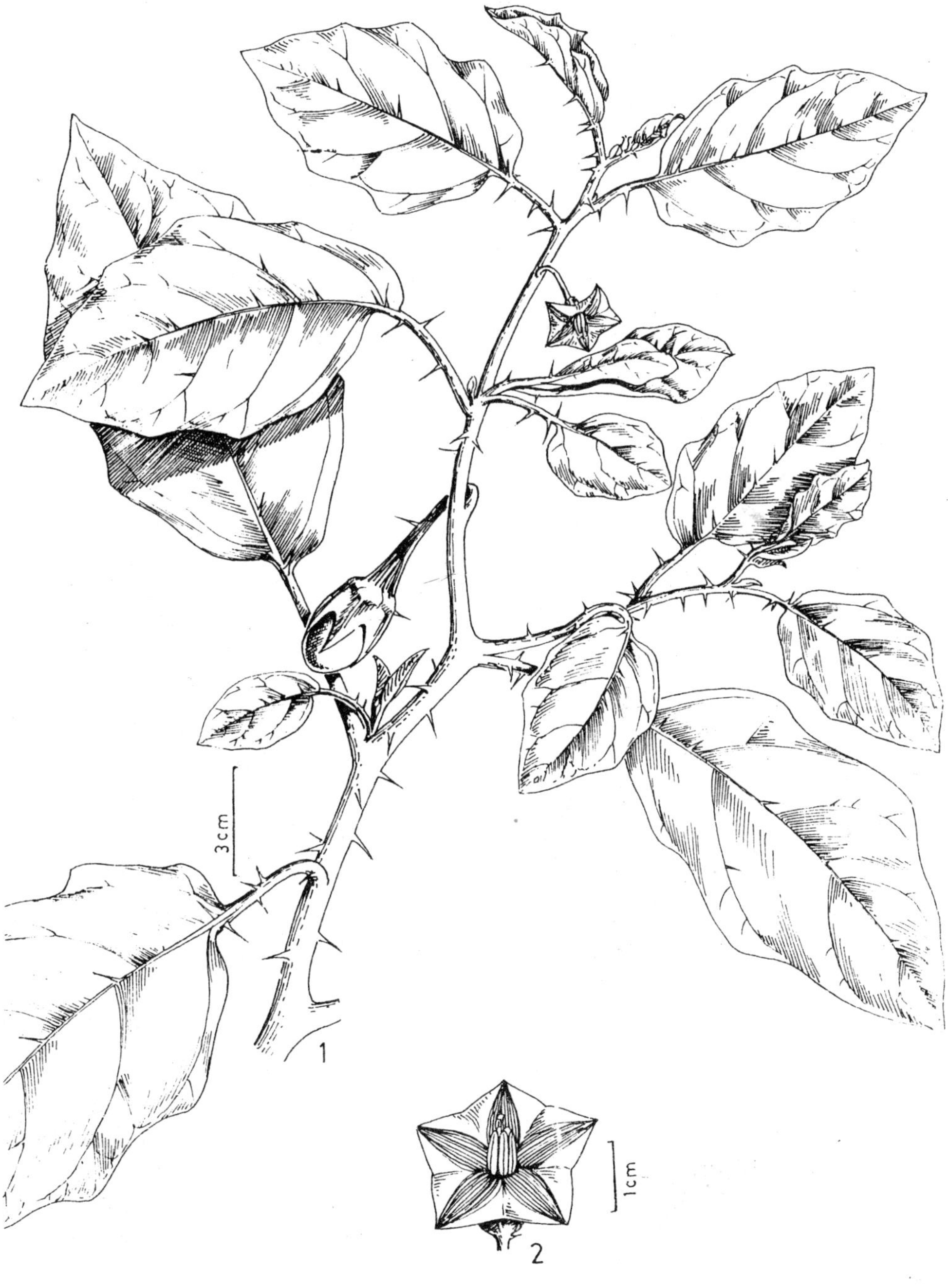

Figure 46: **Solanum melongena** L. var. **insanum** (L.) Prain. 1, Twig with flower and fruit; 2, Flower.

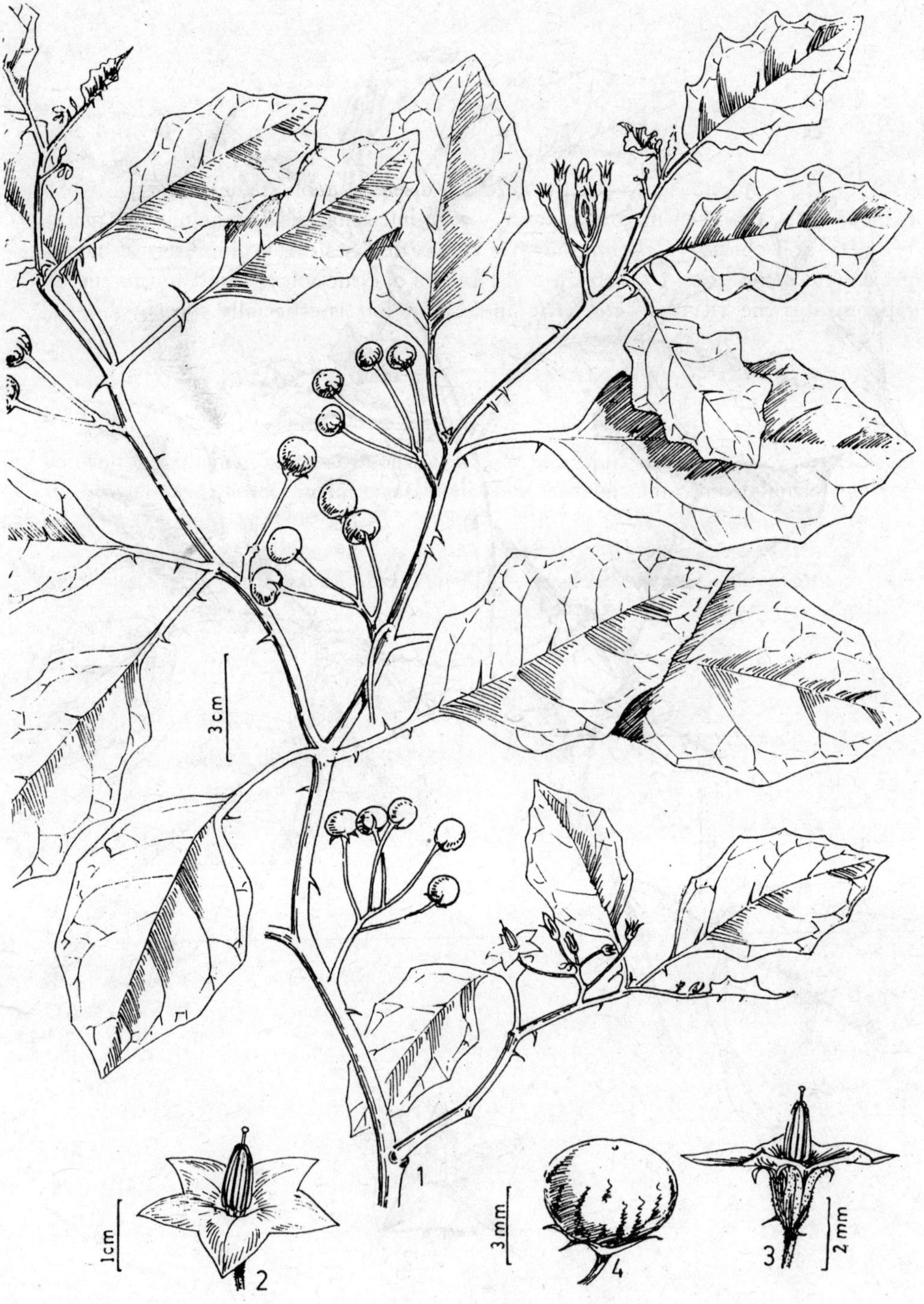

Figure 47: Solanum violaceum Ortega. 1, Twig; 2–3, Flowers; 4, Fruit.

CAKṚAMAṚDAḤ (Mal. TAKARA)

Cakṛamaṛdaḥ is considered a specific for all types of skin diseases. It is sweet, bitter, acrid, carminative, laxative and vermifuge and cures eczema, dermatosis, itching, ulcers, cough, dyspnoea and other respiratory diseases, anorexia, fever and phantom tumour. It is also used in constipation, gastro-intestinal disease, helminthic manifestation and obesity. *Cakṛamaṛdaḥ* overcomes diseases due to impurity of blood, gives good complexion to the skin and removes obstruction of urine and faecus. It rehabilitates the vitiated *vāta, pitta* and *kapha*, but is especially effective for deranged *vāta* and *kapha*. Seeds are recommended for arthritis, poisonous affections and hemicrania. Root paste with lime juice is specific for ringworm. Leaves used as poultice hasten suppuration and also forms a remedy in gout, sciatica and pains in the joints (Nadkarni, 1954: 292; Aiyer & Kolammal, 1964: 8. 74; Kurup *et al.*, 1979: 49). Leaves, seeds and sometimes the plant as a whole, are used in medicine. The important formulations using the drug are *Mahārājapṛasāriṇī tailaṃ, Yaṣṭimadhukādi tailaṃ, Surasādi tailaṃ*, etc.

From the synonyms given in ancient texts, one can infer that this plant with round foliage grows profusely (*cakṛī, cakṛaḥ, āvaṛtakaḥ*) and that it is relished by goats (*ēḍagajaḥ, ēḷagajaḥ.*) It cures eczema (*cakṛamaṛdaḥ, dadrughnaḥ, khaṛjughnaḥ*) but can cause impotence (*pṛapunnāṭaḥ, punnāṭaḥ, śukṛanāśanaḥ*) (cf. Aiyer & Kolammal, 1964: 8. 74).

Cassia tora *Linn.* **(Caesalpiniaceae)** (Fig. 48)

Weedy annuals; branchlets glabrous, leaves 6-foliolate, leaflets in three opposite pairs, obovate-obtuse, cuneate below, to 4 × 2.5 cms, thinly coriaceous, glabrous above, fine-pubescent below; flowers bright yellow in axillary, few-flowered clusters; calyx 5-partite; petals yellow, sub-equal; stamens 10, unequal, upper 3 reduced to staminodes; ovary sessile, linear, style incurved, stigma terminal; pods long, narrowly cylindrical, upto 15 cms, long; seeds oblong, many.

Distribution: The plant is a very common weed in waste places, fallow ground and as forest undergrowth during the rainy season. It is found throughout India and also in adjoining areas.

Note: Prakash & Prasad (1971) have made pharmacognostic studies on *Cassia tora*. Ethnobotanical study conducted by Khan and Chaghtai (1982) reveals that this species is used by the tribals of the suburbs of Bhopal for curing skin affections.

Taxonomic Note: *C. tora* can easily be distinguished from the closely similar *C. obtusifolia* Linn. by the presence of a gland between each pair of leaflets in the former while the latter having it only between one of the pairs of leaflets (See Brenan, 1958).

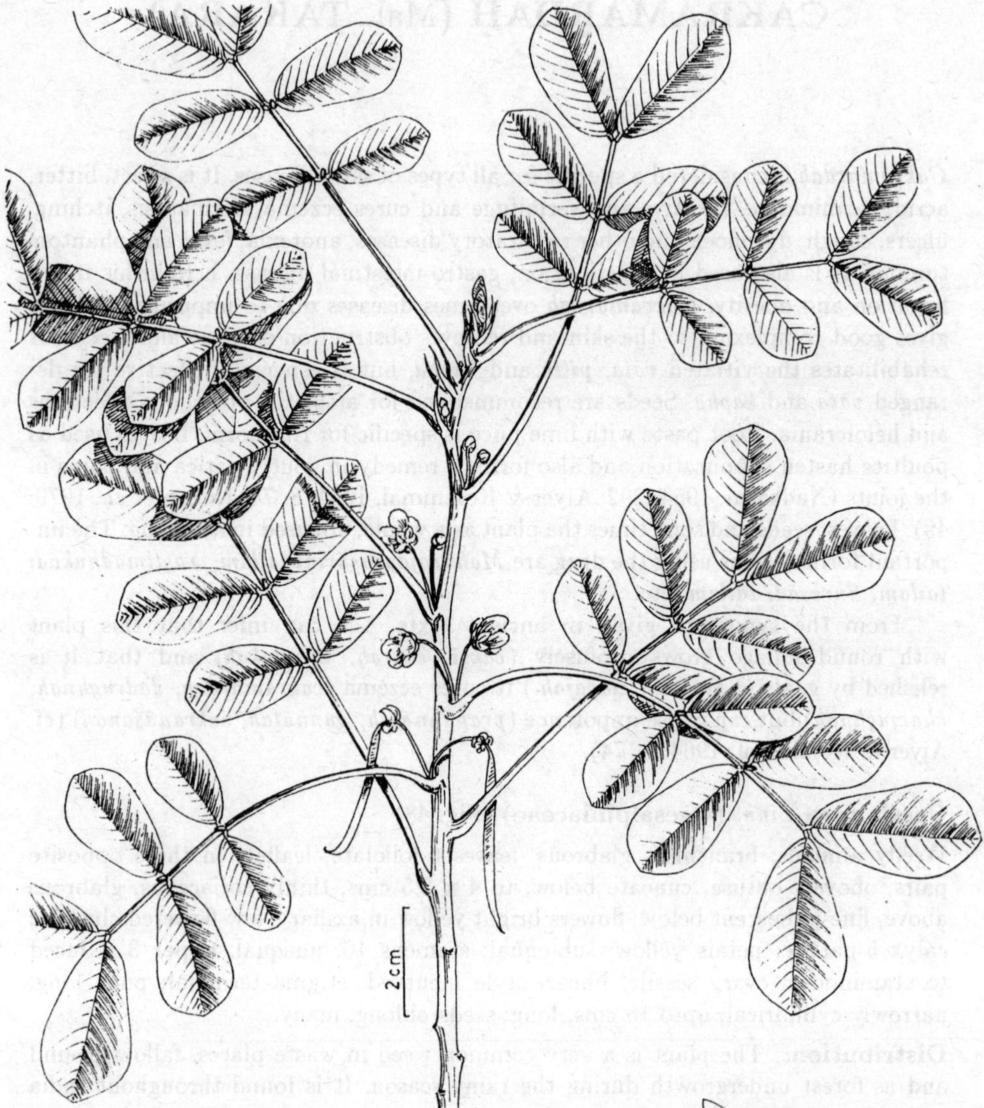

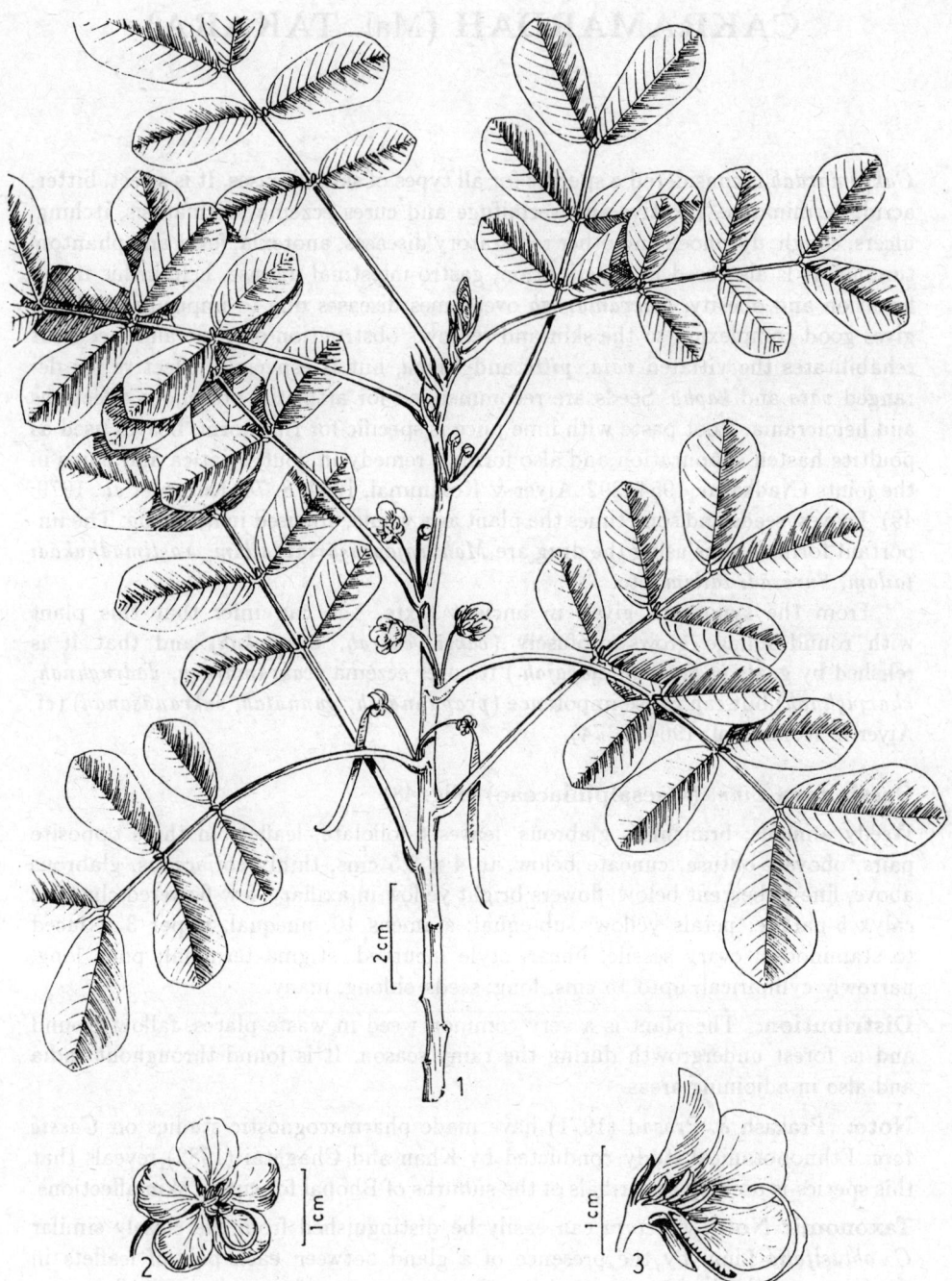

Figure 48: Cassia tora L. 1, Twig; 2, Flower; 3, Flower L.S.

CAṀPACA (Mal. CEṀPAKAṂ)

Caṁpaca flowers are considered to be bitter, cooling, stomachic, carminative and antispasmodic and are used in dyspepsia, nausea, fever and renal diseases. Oil from the flowers is an excellent application in ophthalmia, cephalalgia and gout. Bark is bitter, astringent, anthelmintic, diuretic and is useful in ulcers, skin eruptions, leprosy, intermittent fevers, oedema and menstrual disorders (Chopra *et al.*, 1956: 166; Sharma, 1983: 722).

Michelia champaca Linn. (Magnoliaceae) is the accepted source of the drug throughout the country (see also Rheede, 1: t. 19. 1678).

Michelia champaca *Linn.* (Magnoliaceae)

Tall, evergreen tree; leaves simple, alternate, ovate-lanceolate, acuminate, entire, base cuneate, upto 30 x 10 cms, glabrescent; flowers yellow, axillary, solitary, pedicel jointed, to 2.5 cm; perianth segments 9, in 3 series, outer ones oblong or ovate, inner ones linear; stamens many, anthers linear, apiculate; carpels many, free, ovoid, striate; follicles ovoid, warty, 2.3 cm across.

Distribution: South and S.E. Asia.

CAṆḌĀ (Mal. CAṆṆAKKŪVA)

Caṇḍā is one of the twenty eight drugs that constitute the *Ēladi gaṇa* of Vāgbhaṭa which subdues *vāta* and *kapha*, the effects of poison and promotes complexion. The tuberous root-stock is the officinal part. It is bitter, astringent, cooling, digestive stimulant and good for the heart. It cures *kapha* and *pitta* disorders, dyspepsia, fever, cough and other respiratory diseases, diabetes, oedema, blood diseases, leprosy and other skin ailments (Chunekar, 1982: 700; Sharma, 1983: 605). *Ēladi* oil, *Mañjiṣṭhādi tailaṃ, Asana mañjiṣṭhādi tailaṃ, Mañjiṣṭhādi cūrṇaṃ, Balādhātryādi tailaṃ*, etc. are some of the preparations using the drug.

The source-plant is reported to have conch-shell shaped flowers (*śaṅkhinī*) which opens during night (*cōrapuṣpī*) (Moosad, 1983: 361) *Costus speciosus* of Zingiberaceae, locally called *caṇṇakkūva* is being used as the drug source throughout Kerala. Rheede's illustration of the plant under the same vernacular name (Hort. Malab. 11: 15–16, t. 8. 1962, *Tsjana kua*) also supports the fact that this has long been accepted as the source of *caṇṇa* by Kerala physicians.

Some of the later authors have equated this plant with *kēbuka* or *kēmuka* (Kirtikar & Basu, 1918: 1260; Nadkarni, 1954; 385, Chunekar, 1982: 70; Sharma, 1983: 605). But *kēbuka* has been mentioned among the bitter vegetable group in the classical literature and so is treated as a different drug (Mooss, 1984: 57), equated with *Brassica oleracea* Linn. var *capitata* (Brassicaceae), the common Cabbage by many (Vaidya, K.M. 1936: 158; Menon, V.M.K., 1976: 456).

Bhiṣagārya has mentioned two varieties of *caṇḍā* namely a white variety and a yellow one which may be equated with *caṇṇa* and *naṟuṃ caṇṇa* of the people of Malabar. The former is undoubtedly identified as *Costus speciosus.* Mooss (1984) has opined that the second variety, *pīta-caṇḍā* of Bhiṣagārya, may be the *Mañjakua* figured and described by Rheede in his Hortus Malabaricus (11: 19, t. 10. 1690) which has been identified as *Boesenbergia rotunda* (Linn.) Mansf. (= *Kaempferia pandurata* Roxb.) of Zingiberaceae (see Nicols, *et al.*, 1988: 315).

This varietal distinction is not in vogue in Kerala practice and *Costus speciosus* is considered as the exclusive source of the drug *caṇḍā*.

Costus speciosus (*Koenig*) *Smith* (Zingiberaceae) (Fig. 49)

Succulent herb with tuberous rhizomes, stem spirally twisted; leaves spiral, oblong to oblanceolate, caudate-acuminate, 20 × 8 cms, glabrous above, silky pubescent beneath; flowers large, white in dense terminal spikes; bracts ovate, reddish brown; calyx tubular, base puberulous, 3-lobed; corolla white, labellum white with a yellow centre, broadly obovate with incurved margins; staminodes 0; stamen median, on an oblong petaloid process; ovary globose, 3-lobed, 3-celled, ovules many per cell; fruit an ovoid, 3-valved capsule.

Distribution: The plant is seen in all districts in moist localities, from sea level to 3,000 ft. Also found in Sri Lanka, Indo-China, Malesia to New Guinea, Taiwan.

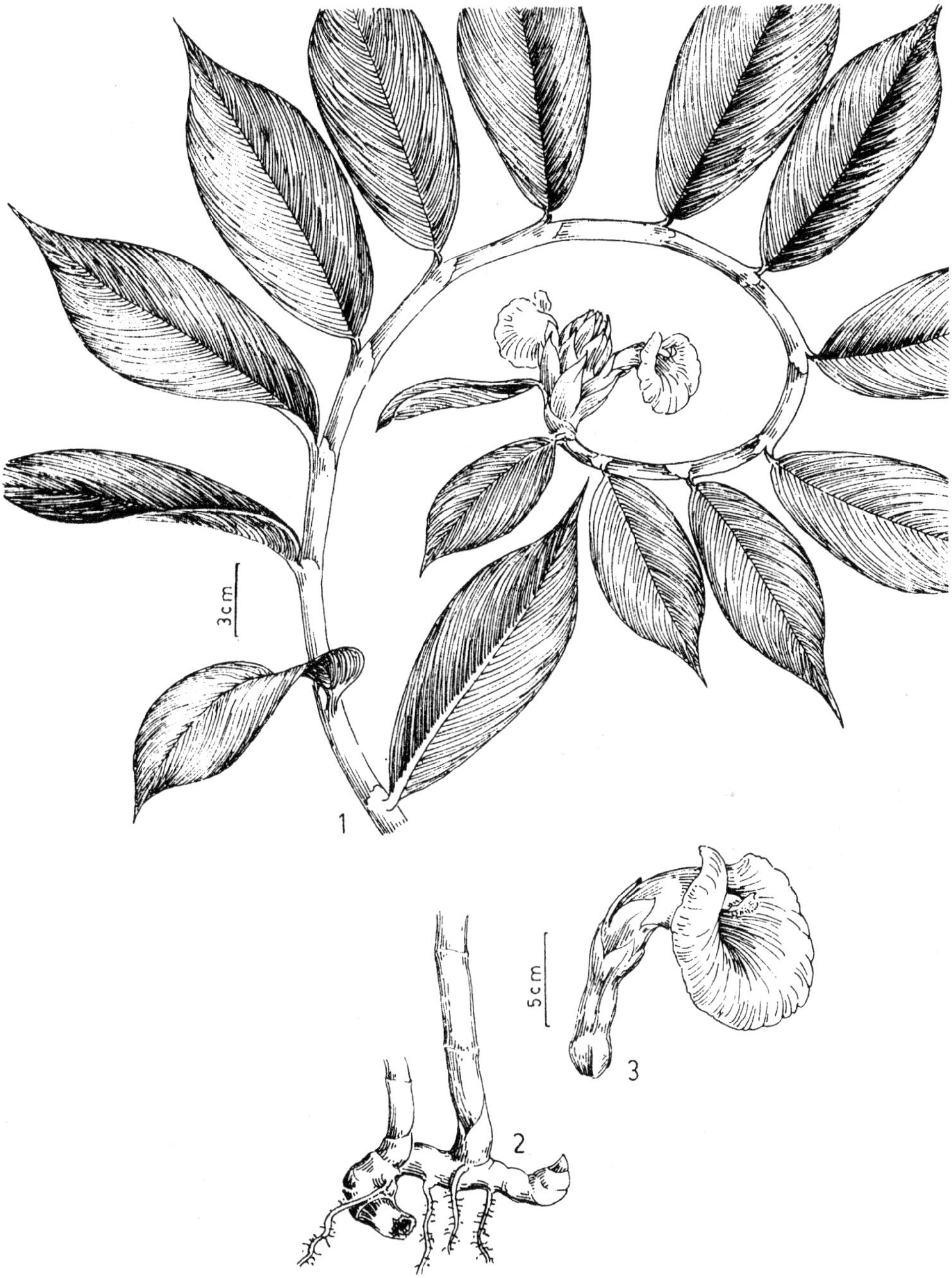

Figure 49: Costus speciosus (Koenig) Smith. 1, Aerial flowering shoot; 2, Rhizome; 3, Flower.

Note: Pharmacological studies conducted by Bhattacharya *et al.*, (1973) show that the rhizomes of *Costus speciosus* possess cardiotonic, hydrocholeric, diuretic and CNS depressent activity. Singh and Srivastava (1980) have studied the pharmacognosy of *Costus speciosus* (Koen.) Sm.

CANDANAṂ (Mal. CANDANAṂ)

Candanaṃ is considered sacred by the Hindus. The sweet-scented heart wood (*gandhasārah*) is valuable in religious rites and in medicine. It is reported to be cooling, bitter, cardiac, disinfectant, diuretic, sedative, resolvent and tonic and is useful in bronchitis, biliousness, fever, thirst, cystitis, dysentery, gonorrhoea, leucorrhoea, ulcers, dysuria, genito-urinary and bronchial tract troubles, gastric irritability and mental troubles. The wood paste is applied externally to inflammed swellings, ulcers, skin eruptions, the temples in headache, fevers and hemicrania and to other cutaneous affections to allay inflammation and pruritus. The heartwood and the essential oil extracted from it are used medicinally (Nadkarni, 1954: 1100; Dey, 1980; 35). The important formulations are *Aśokāriṣṭaṃ, Candanāsavaṃ, Aṇutailaṃ, Dhānvantaraṃ kaṣāyaṃ, Kalyāṇaka ghṛtaṃ*, etc.

Dhanvantarinighaṇṭu mentions five types of *candanaṃ* namely *candanaṃ, raktacandanaṃ, kucandanaṃ, kālīyakaṃ* and *barbarikaṃ* whereas *Rājanighaṇṭu* describes seven types. According to *Bhāvaprakāśa*, there are four types of *candana* i.e. *candanaṃ, raktacandanaṃ, kālīyakaṃ* or *pītacandanaṃ* and *kucandanaṃ* (Chunekar, 1982: 188). In practice, however, only two types are recognised viz. *candanaṃ* and *raktacandanaṃ*. *Santalam album* of Santalaceae, locally called *candanaṃ* is the accepted source of the former and *Pterocarpus santalinus* (Papilionaceae), known as the red sandal wood or *raktacandanaṃ* is the source of the latter throughout the country. These two together constitute the *Śiśiradvayaṃ* of *Śāribādi gaṇa* of Vāgbhaṭa.

Rheede has illustrated *Santalam album* in Hortus Malabaricus (4: 17–18, t. 8. 1683), but under a different vernacular name *Malla-Katoutsjambou*, which is not currently in use.

Santalum album *Linn.* **(Santalaceae)** (Fig. 50)

Small, semiparasitic tree; leaves simple, opposite, elliptic-ovate to lanceolate-acute, penninerved, glabrous above, glaucous beneath, upto 9.5 × 4.4 cm; flowers greenish yellow, turning brownish purple, in terminal paniculate cymes; perianth campanulate, lobes 4, ovate acute; stamens 4, disc lobes prominent, brown, fleshy, rounded; ovary semi-inferior, style elongate, stigma 2–3 fid; fruit an ovoid drupe, black when ripe.

Distribution: Common in Peninsular India, especially in dry, deciduous forests.

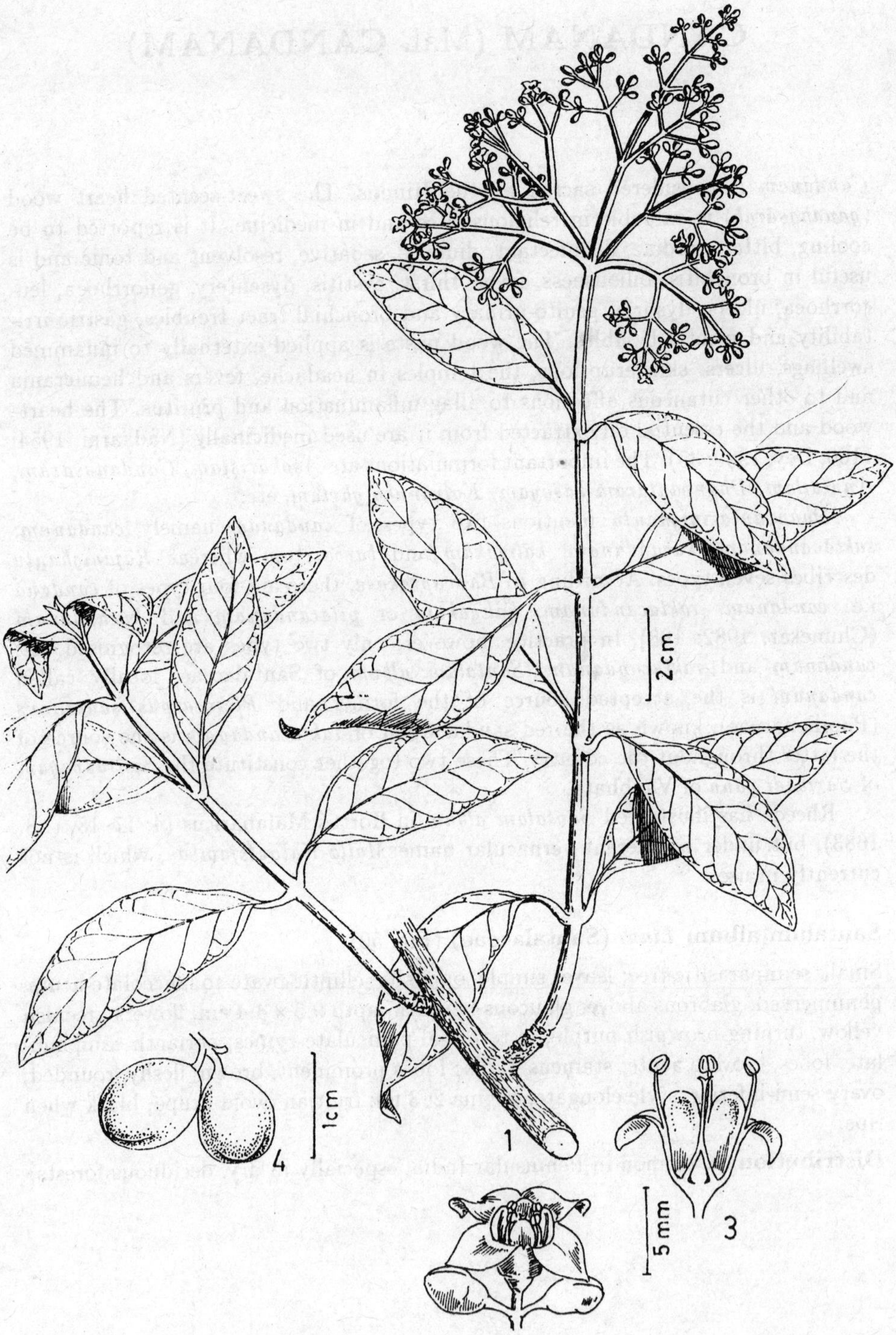

Figure 50: Santalum album L. 1, Twig; 2, Flower; 3, Flower L.S.; 4, Fruits.

CĀṄGĒRĪ (Mal. PUḶIYĀRAL)

The drug, boiled with buttermilk, is a reputed home remedy for indigestion and diarrhoea in children. The whole plant is medicinal. It is sour in taste, astringent, hot in action, digestive stimulant, alleviative of *vāta* and *kapha* and is beneficial in indigestion, dyspepsia, dysentery, piles, fever and biliousness. Leaves are used externally to remove corns, warts and other excrescences on the skin. It relieves pain and other inflammatory symptoms when applied as poultice to inflamed parts (Nadkarni, 1954: 890; Mooss, 1976; 94). The important preparations using the drug are *Cāṅgēryādi ghṛtaṃ*, *Pāṭhādi guḷika*, *Sūraṇādi ghṛtaṃ*, *Abhraṃ* (101) etc.

All the synonyms (*cāṅgērī*, *cukṛikā*, *aṁḷalōṇikā*, *aṁḷapatṛakaḥ*, etc.) indicate the sour taste of the leaves. It agrees well with the accepted source of the drug throughout the country, viz. *Oxalis corniculata* Linn. of Oxalidaceae, locally called *puḷiyāral*.

Oxalis corniculata *Linn.* **(Oxalidaceae)** (Fig. 51)

Diffuse herb; stem creeping, rooting at nodes, softly pilose; leaves digitately 3-foliolate; leaflets subsessile, obcordate, emarginate at apex, base cuneate, margin entire, 1.5 x 1.8 cm; flowers small, yellow, in umbellate clusters on slender axillary peduncles; sepals 5, ovate; petals oblanceolate, 6-nerved; stamens 10, staminal tube to 1.5 mm; ovary 5-celled, ovules many; capsule linear, 5-angled, puberulous, upto 2.25 cm; seeds many, bed-bug shaped.

Distribution: The plant is cosmopolitan. It is common on the banks of ponds and fields throughout the warmer parts of India upto 7,000 ft.

Note: The studies made by Gaitonde *et al.*, (1977) show that *Oxalis corniculata* exhibits significant anti-inflammatory, analgesic and antipyretic activities.

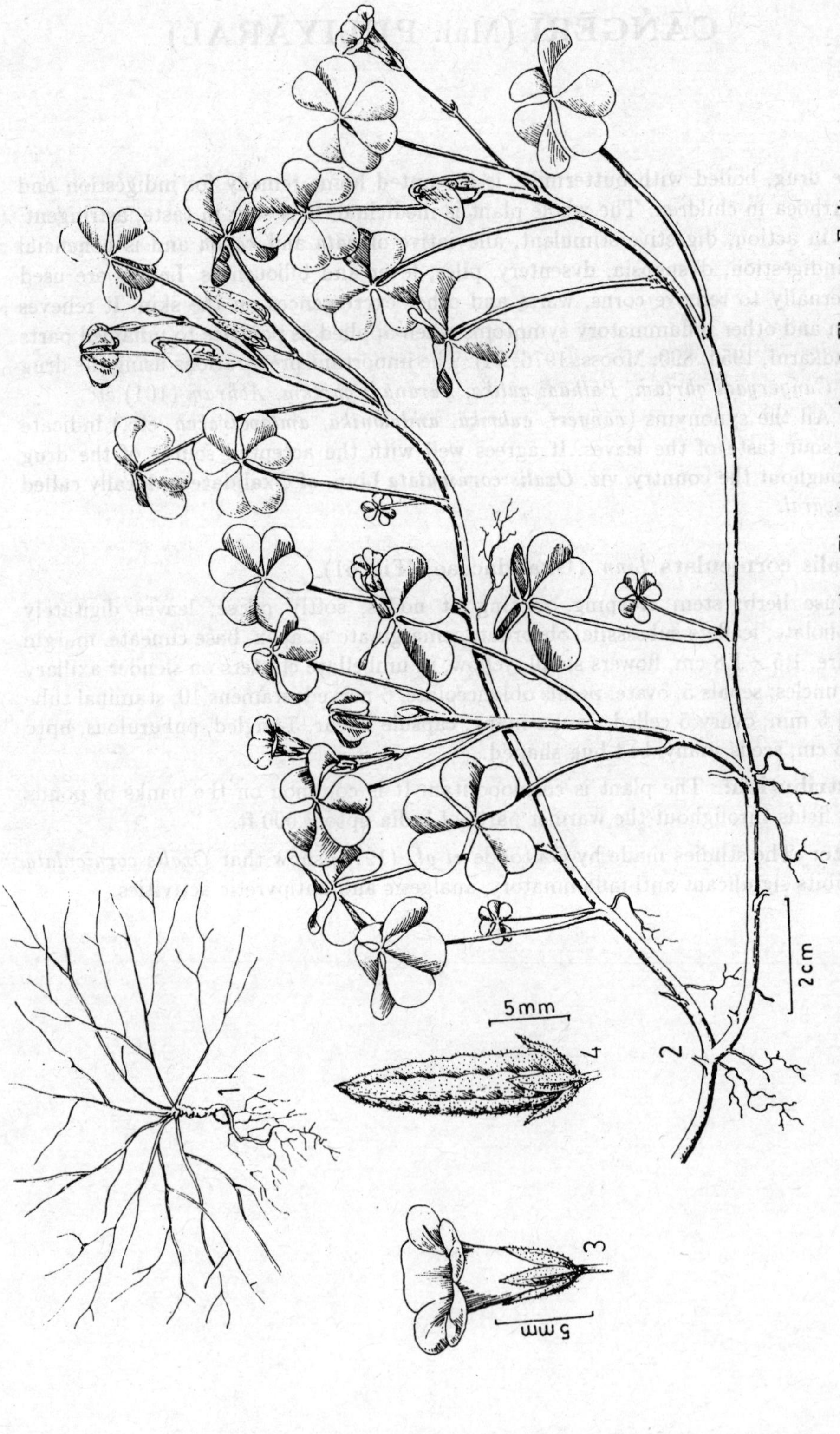

Figure 51: Oxalis corniculata L. 1, Habit (Diagrammatic); 2, Flowering branches; 3, Flower; 4, Fruit.

CIÑCĀ (Mal. PUḶI, VĀḶAṀPUḶI)

The pulp of the fruit is an important ingredient of Indian cuisine. It is sweet or sour, cooling, carminative, digestive, laxative, antiscorbutic and antibilious. Bark, leaves and seeds are astringent. Tender leaves and flowers are cooling and antibilious. All these parts are used medicinally. It is used in constipation, colic, cough, dyspepsia, fever, flatulence, gastro-intestinal diseases and urinary infection. Pulp of the fruit as well as a poultice of the leaves are recommended for external applications to inflammatory swellings to relieve pain. The ripe pulp of the fruit is considered as an effective laxative in habitual constipation and enters into many Āyurvēdic preparations. An infusion of the leaves is used as a gargle for aphthous sores and sorethroat and for washing indolent ulcers. Poultice of flowers is useful in inflammatory affections in conjunctiva (Nadkarni, 1954: 1192; Kurup *et al.*, 1979: 51). The important preparations using the drug are *Ciñcādi lēhaṃ, Pañcāmḷa tailaṃ, Hiṅguvacādi cūrṇaṃ, Koṭṭaṁcukkādi tailaṃ,* etc.

Tamarindus indica Linn. of Caesalpiniaceae, locally called *puḷimaraṃ* or *vāḷaṁpuḷi* is the plant used throughout the country. Rheede also describes and portrays this under the same name *Balam-pulli* (Hort. Malab. 1: 39–40, t. 23. 1678).

Tamarindus indica *Linn.* **(Caesalpiniaceae)** (Fig. 52)

Tree; leaves even-pinnate, leaflets 15–17 pairs, narrowly oblong-obtuse, entire, 1.5 × 0.7 cm, glabrous; flowers creamy yellow in axillary racemes; calyx tube narrowly turbinate, lobes 4, subequal, oblong; petals 3, yellow, outer one reflexed, pink-dotted, laterals clawed, subequal, oblong-oblanceolate; stamens 3, monadelphous, filaments pubescent at base, staminodes 2, bristly; ovary stipitate, style attenuate, stigma globose; pod oblong, thick, torulose, subcompressed; seeds obovoid or orbicular, compressed, brown.

Distribution: A native of tropical Africa, this is now naturalised and widely cultivated throughout India.

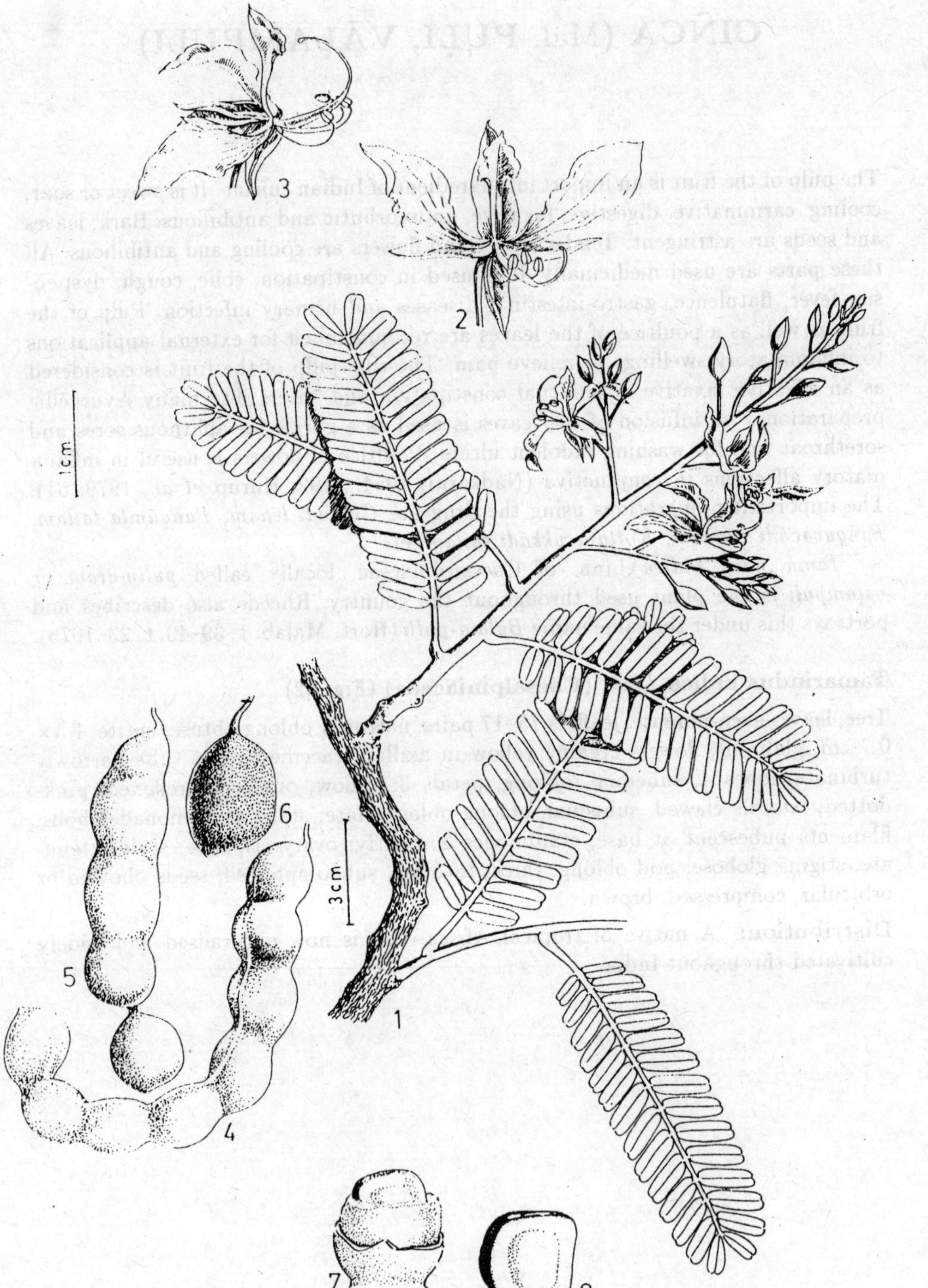

Figure 52: Tamarindus indica L. 1, Flowering twig; 2–3, Flowers; 4–6, Fruits; 7, Fruit C.S. showing seed embeded in the pulp; 8, Seed.

CIRABILVAḤ, PŪTĪKARAÑJAḤ (Mal. ÑEṬṬĀVAL)

In Kerala, the drug is commonly used in combination with *karañjaḥ* and they together form *karañjadvayaṃ*, an ingredient of different groups of Vāgbhaṭa namely *Āragvadhādi gaṇa, Varaṇādi gaṇa, Aṛkādi gaṇa*, etc. (cf. Mooss, 1980: 47, 56, 74). *Cirabilvaḥ* is reported to be bitter, astringent, hot, digestive, laxative and anthelmintic. It dispels diseases due to the morbidity of ***kapha*** and ***pitta***, oedema, diabetes, leprosy and other skin diseases. It purifies blood and overcomes dyspepsia, vomiting, intestinal disorders, piles, flatulence and sprue. A paste of the bark is applied externally on swellings (Sharma, 1983: 817). Bark and tender leaves are the officinal parts. The drug is used to prepare *Cirivilvādi kaṣāyaṃ, Ayaskṛti, Indukāntaghṛtaṃ, Valiya Pañcagavyaghṛtaṃ*, etc.

Holoptelia integrifolia (Roxb.) Planchon belonging to Ulmaceae, locally called *āvil* or *ñeṭṭāval* is the plant used as the drug source. (Chopra *et al.*, 1956: 135; Singh & Chunekar, 1972: 353; Mooss, 1980: 46; Sharma, 1983: 816; Nesamony 1985: 46). Due to the offensive smell of the bark of this tree, the synonyms *pūtikaḥ, pūtikarajaḥ*, etc. suit it well.

Holoptelia integrifolia (*Roxb.*) *Planchon* **(Ulmaceae)** (Fig. 53)
Ulmus integrifolia Roxb.

Large, deciduous tree; tender parts pubescent; leaves ovate-elliptic, acute, base rounded or subcordate, 8–14 x 4–9 cm, penninerved, pubescent below; flowers small, polygamous, in fascicles in the axils of fallen leaves; perianth simple, calycine; stamens 7–9, biseriate; fruit a dry, compressed, winged samara, 1 x 0.7 cm, wings membraneous; seeds flat, exalbuminous.

Distribution: The tree is common in N. Circars, in deciduous forests. Occasionally found in the hills of Deccan, E. Slopes of W. Ghats and in Travancore. Also distributed in Sri Lanka, Himalaya, Burma and Indo-China.

Note: Clinical studies conducted by Bambhole *et al.*, (1985) in rats show that the drug significantly reduces the body weight thereby proving its antiobesity properties.

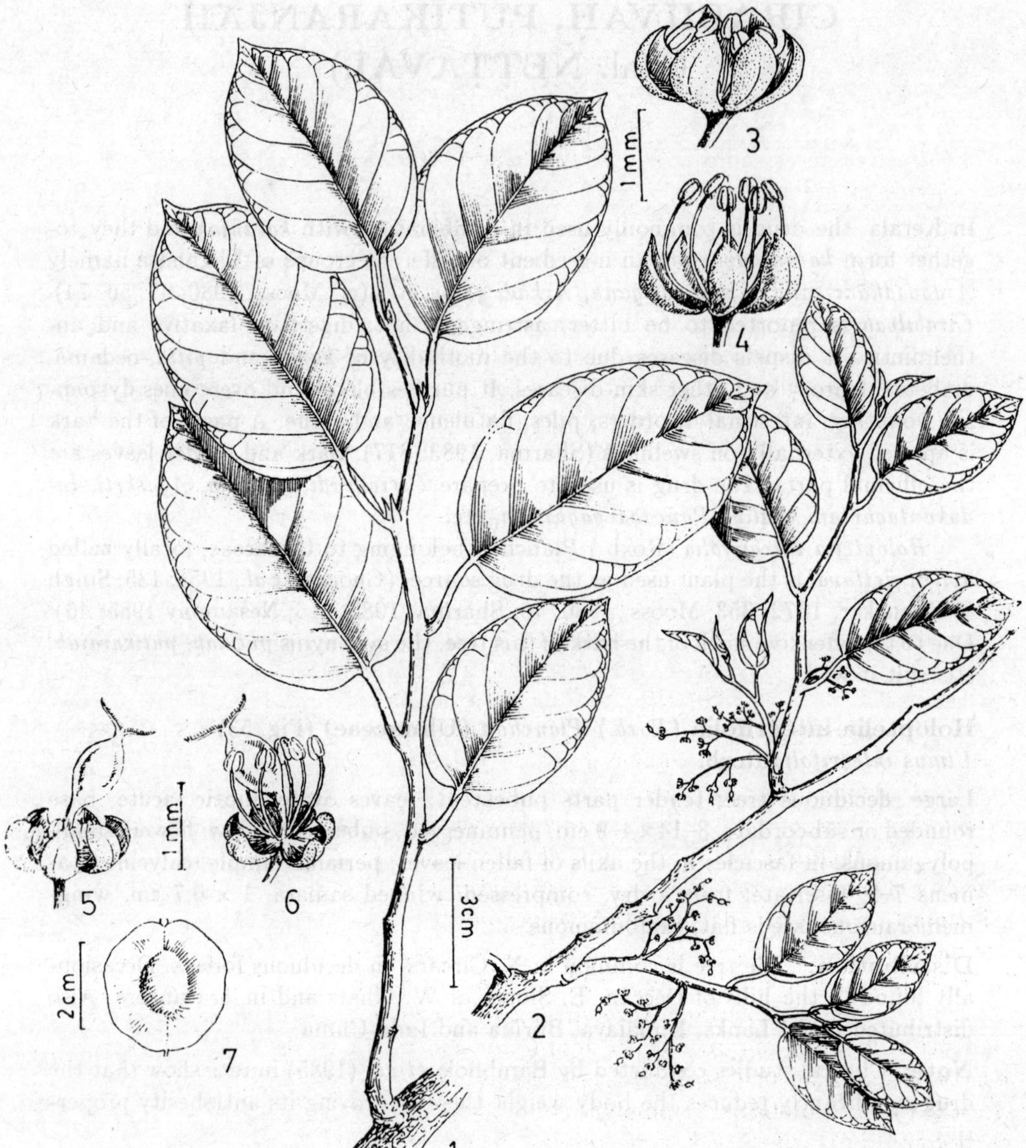

Figure 53: Holoptelia integrifolia (Roxb.) Planchon. 1, Vegetative branch; 2, Flowering twig; 3–4, Male flowers; 5, Female flower; 6, Bisexual flower; 7, Fruit.

CITṚAKAḤ (Mal. KOṬUVĒLI)

Citṛaka is an esteemed remedy for leucoderma and other skin diseases. The synonyms of fire like *agniḥ, vahniḥ, dahanaḥ, analaḥ,* etc. attributed to this drug, indicate the very caustic (burning) action of the root, causing blisters on the skin (*dāraṇaḥ, dāruṇaḥ*). The drug is used only after adequate curing and purification. The roots are digestive stimulants and aid digestion. It is pungent, astringent, diuretic, germicidal, vescicant and abortifacient. It overcomes flatulence, oedema, piles, cough, worms, diseases due to *vāta* and *kapha* predominance and haemorrhoidal anal inflammation and colic. The drug also cures enlargement of the abdomen, anaemia, diabetes, leucoderma, leprosy, diarrhoea, dyspepsia, anasarca and elephantiasis (cf. Aiyer & Kolammal, 1960. 4: 37; Mooss, 1976: 109; Kurup *et al.*, 1979: 52). Root is the officinal part and it enters into the composition of preparations like *Citṛakāsavaṃ, Daśamūlāriṣṭaṃ, Gulgulutiktakaṃ kaṣāyaṃ, Yōgarājacūrṇaṃ,* etc.

Caraka has mentioned three varieties of *citṛaka*, differentiated by the colour of flowers, viz. red, white and black (it may be noted that reference to black colour in ancient texts, often refers to blue). Vāgbhaṭa mentions a yellow flowered variety instead of the red flowered variety, the identity of which is not known (Mooss, 1976: 108).

Two varieties of *citṛaka* are recognised by men of Āyurvēda in Kerala and elsewhere, viz. the white flowered and the red flowered. Among these, the white flowered variety, which is equated with *Plumbago zeylanica* Linn. (Plumbaginaceae), is used in medicine in the northern parts of India. This plant, locally called *tumba codiveli* (See also Rheede, Hort. Malab. 10: 15, t. 8. 1690) or *veḷḷakoṭuvēli* is the source of *citṛaka* according to many authors (Kurup, *et al.*, 1979: 52; Kapoor & Mitra, 1979: 61; Dey, 1980: 37; Sharma, 1983: 359). However, the red-flowered variety, *Plumbago indica* Linn., is the accepted source of the drug in Kerala. This is known by the vernacular name *cettikoṭuvēli* (also see Rheede, Hort. Malab. 10: 17–18, t. 9. 1690 *Schetti-codiveli*) and is considered to be therapeutically more active. The black variety mentioned in the texts, may be the blue-flowered *Plumbago auriculata* Lam. (= *Plumbago capensis* Thumb.) which is often grown in gardens throughout India (Mooss, 1976: 106; Chunekar, 1982: 24, Sharma, 1983: 259). But this is not known to be used as the source of the drug anywhere.

Plumbago indica *Linn.* **(Plumbaginaceae)** (Fig. 54)
Plumbago rosea Linn.

Erect, rambling shrub with long tuberous roots; stem terete and striate; leaves simple, alternate, short-petioled, ovate-oblong, obtuse, 13 × 7 cms, glabrous; flowers bright red in long terminal spikes; calyx reddish, cylindric, 5 toothed, 5-ribbed, glandular-hairy outside; corolla tube slender, long, limb rotate, 5-lobed; stamens 5, filaments inserted on nectariferous disc; ovary oblong, style filiform, with 5 stigmatic branches; fruit a membraneous capsule enclosed within the persistent calyx.

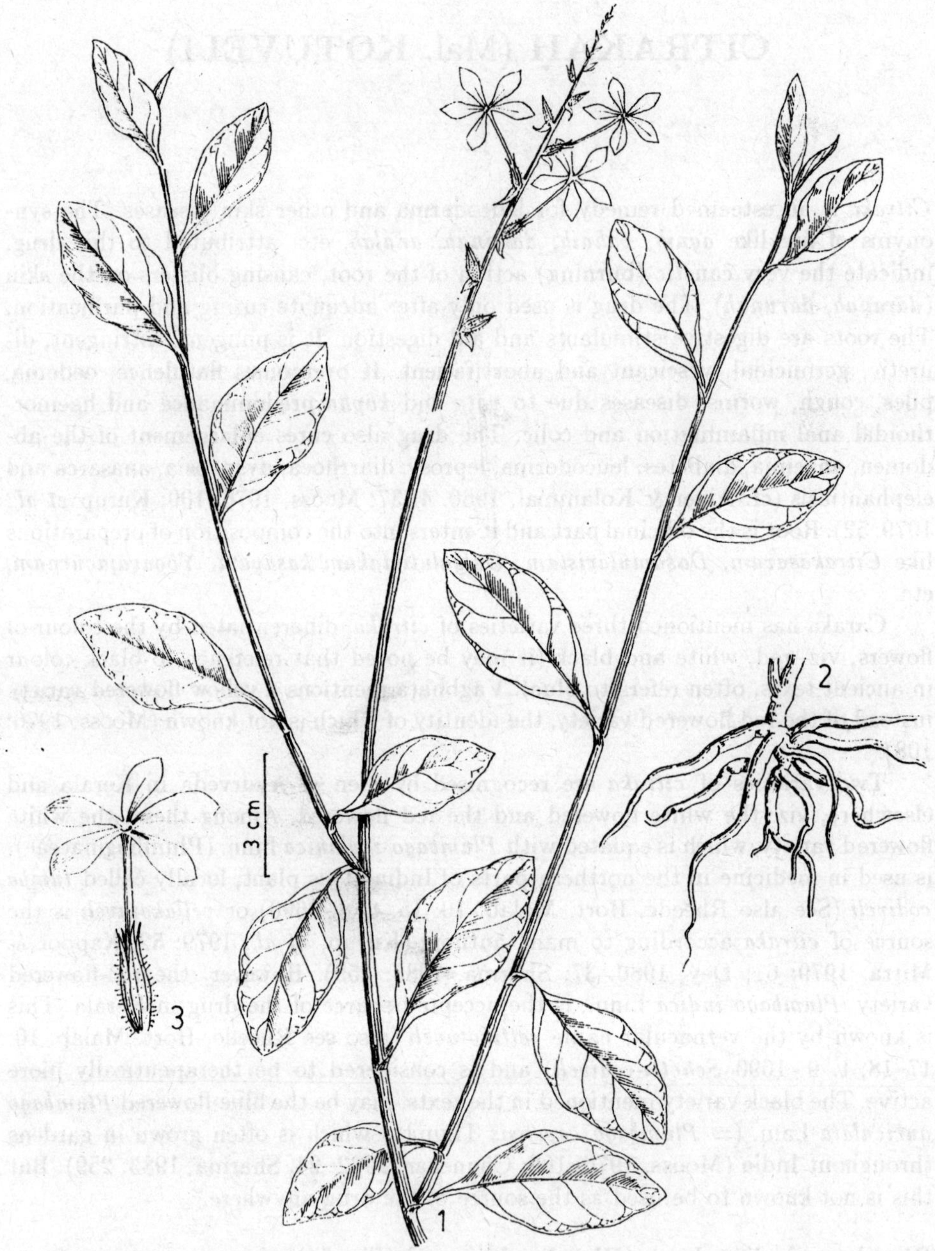

Figure 54: Plumbago indica L. 1, **Flowering branch; 2, Roots; 3, Flower.**

Distribution: A native of Coromandel Coast, this is found cultivated in several parts of India.

Plumgabo zeylanica *Linn.* **(Plumbaginaceae)** (Fig. 55)

Branched undershrub; roots long, tuberous; stem striate; leaves simple, alternate,

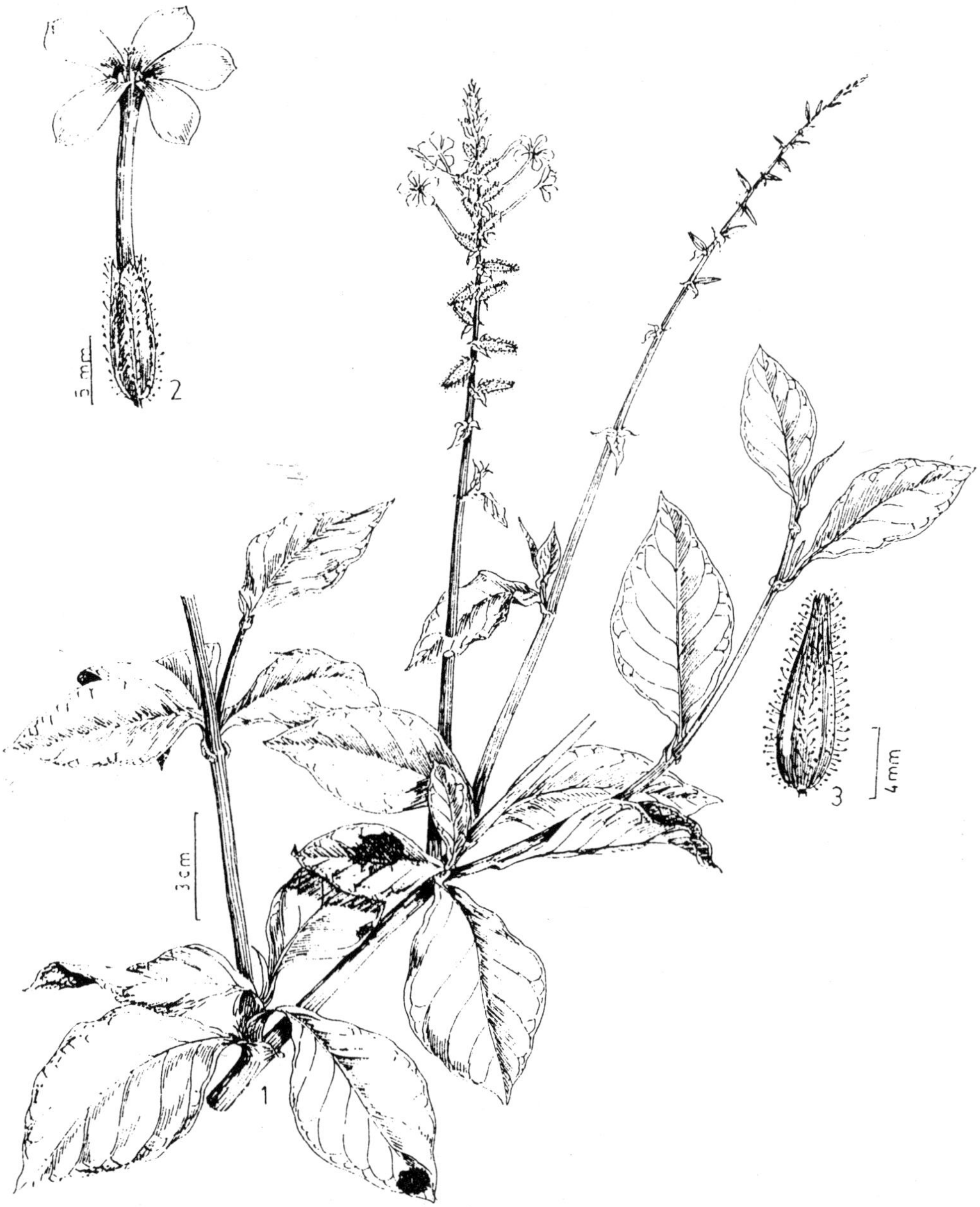

Figure 55: Plumbago zeylanica L. 1, Flowering shoot; 2, Flower; 3, Fruits.

short-petioled, ovate or ovate-oblong, acute with entire or wavy margin, 7 × 3.8 cms, glabrous; flowers white in terminal spikes; calyx tubular, glandular-hairy; corolla tube slender, limb rotate, 5 lobed; stamens 5 on a disc; style slender, stigmatic branches 5; fruit a membraneous capsule enclosed within the persistent calyx.

Distribution: Throughout the tropics and subtropics. In India, this runs wild.

Note: The pharmacognosy of the roots of both *P. zeylanica* and *P. indica* has been discussed by Satyavati *et al.* (1987). Clinical trials have demonstrated that plumbagin, isolated from *P. zeylanica*, has considerable antifertility potential (Bhargava & Dixit, 1985b) and that plumbagin oil from *P. indica* is useful in common wart (Pillai *et al.*, 1981).

DĀḌIMAḤ (Mal. UṞUMĀṀPAḶAṂ, MĀTAḶANĀRAKAṂ)

Dāḍimaḥ has long been esteemed as food and medicine and as a diet in convalescence after diarrhoea. The officinal part, rind of fruit, is astringent, digestive, cardiotonic, stomachic and is highly effective in chronic diarrhoea and dysentery, dyspepsia, colitis, piles and uterine disorders. The powdered drug boiled with buttermilk is an efficaceous remedy for infantile diarrhoea. The root bark is a vermicide and is found to be very useful in expelling tape worms. The fruit juice is costive, refrigerant, tonic and good for diarrhoea, dyspepsia, fever, biliousness and excessive thirst. Seed is nutritious (Nadkarni 1954: 1034; Mooss, 1978: 148). The important preparations using the drug are *Dāḍimādighṛtaṃ, Dāḍimāṣṭaka cūrṇaṃ, Hiṅguvacādi cūrṇaṃ, Hiṅgvādi guḷika*, etc.

Except for the term *lōhitapuṣpakaḥ* (having red flowers) the texts do not give any description about the plant.

Dhanvantarinighaṇṭu and *Rājanighaṇṭu* mention two varieties of *dāḍimaḥ* viz. *svādudāḍimaḥ* and *aṁḷadāḍimaḥ*. In addition to these two, *Bhāvaprakāśa* recognises a third variety called *svādvaṁḷadāḍimaṃ* (cf. Mooss, 1978: 146). The varietal difference is not in vogue, in practice and *Punica granatum* (Punicaceae), locally known as *uṟumāṁpaḷaṃ* or *mātaḷanārakaṃ* is being used as the drug source throughout India.

Punica granatum *Linn.* **(Punicaceae)** (Fig. 56)

Glabrous Shrub or a small tree; branchlets often spinescent; leaves simple, opposite, short-petioled, narrowly elliptic or lanceolate, obtuse, entire, glabrous, to 8 × 2.3 cms; flowers bright red, solitary, axillary, short-pedicelled; calyx tube funnel-shaped, thick, coriaceous, orange-coloured, adnate to the ovary below, lobes 5–7, triangular, persistent on the fruit; petals 5–7; stamens numerous; ovary inferior, style long, stigma capitate; fruit a large globose berry, yellowish red when ripe, upto 10 cm across, with a thick, coriaceous rind crowned with the persistent calyx lobes; seeds many, surrounded by a succulent pinkish white pulp.

Distribution: The plant is widely cultivated throughout India. Also reported in C & W. Asia and southern Europe.

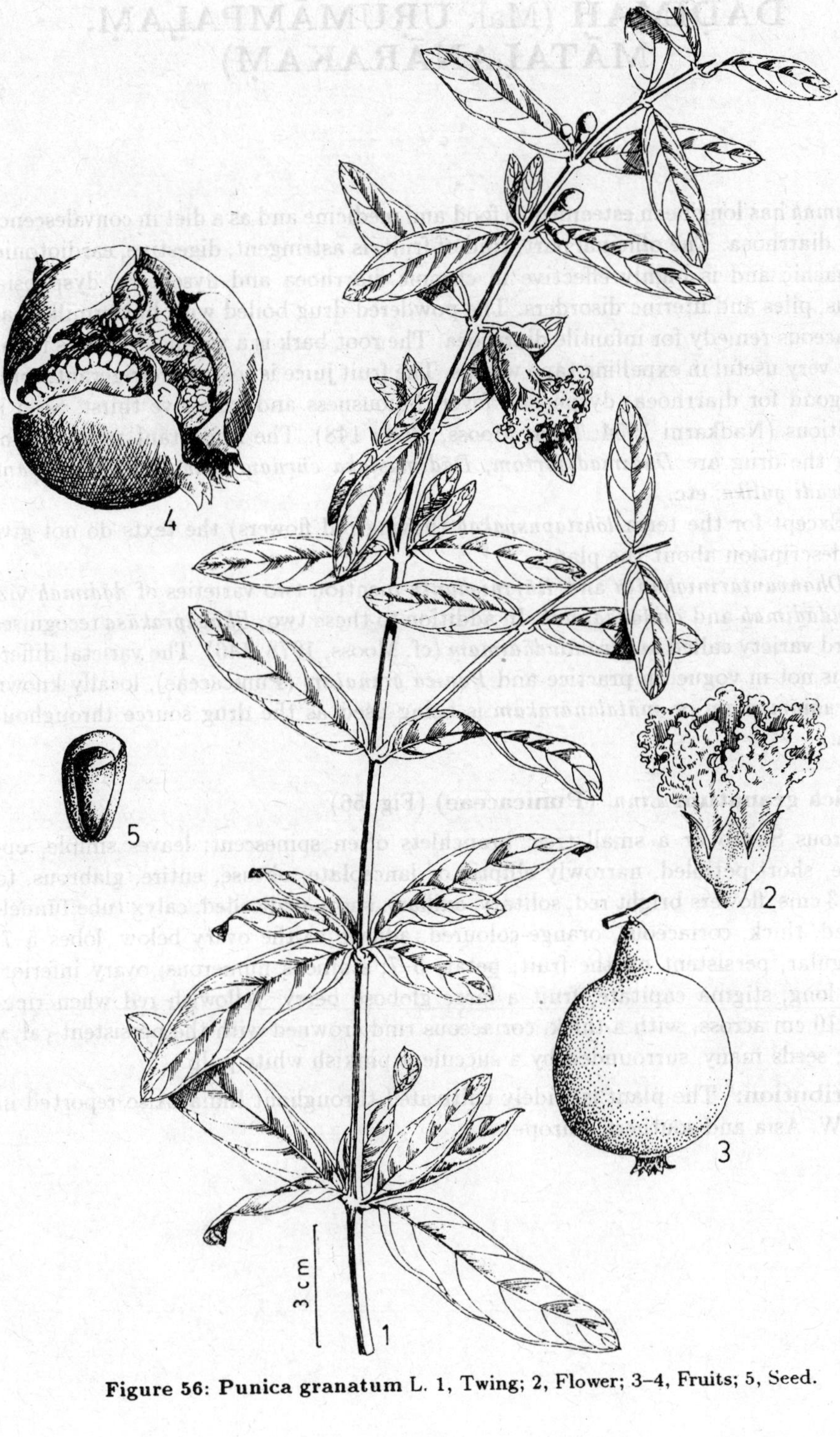

Figure 56: Punica granatum L. 1, Twing; 2, Flower; 3–4, Fruits; 5, Seed.

DANTĪ (Mal. NĀGADANTI)

The drug forms an important constituent of preparations like *Dantyariṣṭaṃ*, *Dantīharītakilēhaṃ*, *Kaiśōraguggulu guḷika*, etc. Root, which is the officinal part, is purgative, anthelmintic, carminative, rubefacient and anodyne. It is used in abdominal pain, constipation, calculus, general anasarca, piles, helminthic manifestations, scabies, skin disorders, suppurative ulcers and diseases caused by the morbidity of *kapha* and *pitta*. Root paste is applied to painful swellings and piles. Leaves cure asthma and seeds are used in snake-bite (Kurup *et al.*, 1979: 55, Sharma, 1983: 427).

Bhāvaprakāśa has mentioned two varieties of this drug, viz. *dantī* or *laghudantī*, the smaller variety and *bṛhatdantī*, also called *dravantī*, the larger variety. Caraka has recognised a third variety, *nāgadantī* also (cf. Chunekar, 1982: 399), but this distinction is not in vogue today. *Dantī* and *nāgadantī* are considered to be the same, at least in Kerala and is equated with *Baliospermum solanifolium* (= *B. montanum*) of Euphorbiaceae (see also Rheede, Hort. Malab. 10: 151, t. 76. 1690). However, the plant source of *bṛhaddantī*, has been in some confusion. Some people have equated this with *Croton tiglium*, while others have considered various species of *Jatropha* as the botanical source of this drug (for details see under *Dravantī*).

Baliospermum solanifolium (*J. Burm.*) *Suresh* **(Euphorbiaceae)** (Fig. 57)
Croton solanifolius J. Burm.
Baliospermum montanum (Willd.) Muell.-Arg.

Stout shrubs; leaves simple, alternate, with two glands at the base, variable in size and shape, lower ones long-petioled, petiole upto 17–18 cms, blade 3–5 lobed, or coarsely toothed, to 23 x 20 cms, upper ones smaller, ovate or lanceolate, acuminate, subentire, scabrous; flowers unisexual, small, greenish, in axillary monoecious fascicles; male flowers: perianth of 5 orbicular-concave lobes; stamens numerous on a central receptacle. Female flowers: calyx lobes 5, lanceolate, accrescent in fruit; ovary hairy outside, 3-celled, 3-ovuled, styles 3, each 2-fid; fruit a capsule separating into 3 cocci.

Distribution: Peninsular India.

Note: Pharacognosy and pharmacology of the plant have been discussed by Raghunathan & Mitra (1982: 238–249).

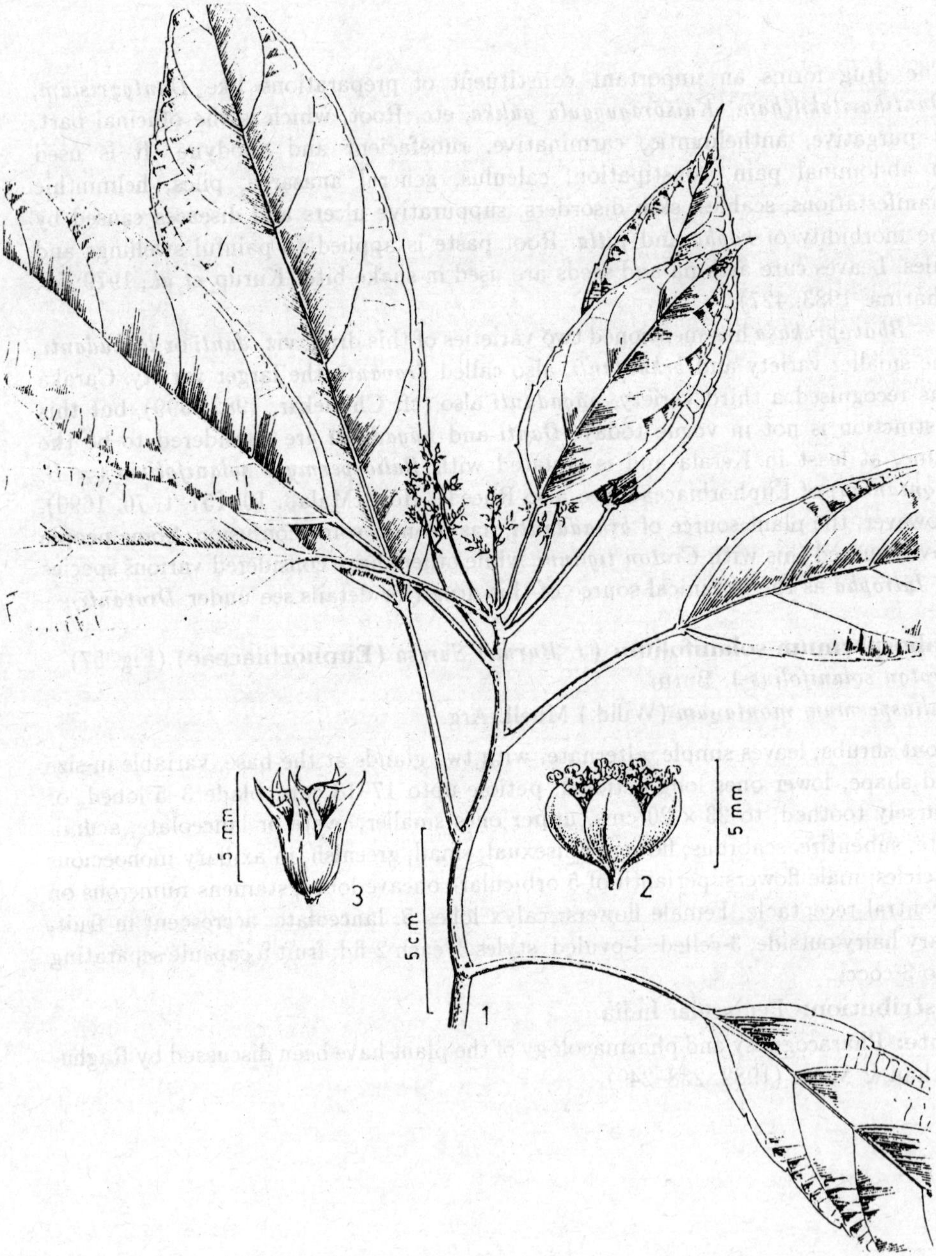

Figure 57: Baliospermum solanifolium (J. Burm.) Suresh. 1, Twig; 2, Male flower; 3, Female flower.

DAṚBHAḤ (Mal. DAṚBHA, DAṚBHAPPULLU)

This is called the 'sacrificial grass' or sacred grass as it is being used in 'Yagnas' and religious rites. Root is used in medicine. It is reportedly cooling, sweet, astringent, diuretic and galactagogue. It rehabilitates morbid *vāta, pitta* and *kapha*, dysentery, diarrhoea, thirst, urinary calculi, dysuria and other diseases of the bladder, *raktapitta* and skin diseases. (Chunekar, 1982: 382; Sharma, 1983: 635) *Varaṇādi kaṣāyaṃ, Valiya Candanāditailaṃ, Sukumāraghṛtaṃ*, etc. are some of the preparations using the drug.

Desmostachya bipinnata (Linn.) Stapf of Poaceae, locally called *daṛbha* or *daṛbhappullu* is the accepted source of the drug (see also Vaidya K. M., 1936: 285; Chunekar, 1982: 382; Sharma, 1983: 634). But, *Imperata cylindrica* is also used.

Desmostachya bipinnata (*Linn.*) *Stapf* **(Poaceae)**
Eragrostis cynosuroides (Retz.) Beauv.

Tufted perennial grass with a thick root-stock; leaves many, basal, linear-lanceolate, to 50 x 1 cm, with filiform tips and hispid margins, sheaths glabrous; panicles erect, narrowly pyramidal, clothed from base with sessile imbricating spikelets; spikelets many flowered, linear oblong, laterally compressed; glumes unequal, lanceolate, 1-nerved; lemma lanceolate, rigid, 3-nerved, keeled; palea slightly shorter, 2-keeled; stamens 3; grains obliquely ovoid, 0.5–0.6 mm, trigonous and laterally compressed.

Distribution: Throughout the Middle East to Indo-China, North and tropical Africa, India.

Imperata cylindrica (*Linn.*) *P. Beauv.* **(Poaceae)**
I. arundinacea Cyr.

Perennial grass; root-stock stoloniferous; culms erect, to 1 m tall; leaves lanceolate; panicles up to 20 cm long; spikelets 4–5 mm long, 2-nate, one short and the other long-pedicelled; glumes 3–5 nerved, densely hairy below; stamens 1–2; styles 2.

Distribution: Palaeotropical.

DHANAVALLĪ
(Mal. POITALACCI, VĀTAKKOṬI)

Dhanavallī seems to be another drug, exclusively used by Kerala physicians, which does not find mention in any of the Āyurvēdic classics. In Kerala, it is a constituent of *Kaccōrādi tailaṃ* and *Kaccōrādi cūrṇaṃ*. The whole plant is used medicinally. It is astringent, bitter, sweet, anthelmintic, depurative, anti-inflammatory and vulnerary and is useful in vitiated conditions of *pitta*, intestinal worms, skin diseases, leprosy, rheumatic pain, toothache, headache, colic, inflammations, wounds and ulcers (Anonymous, 1966. 7: 2). The roots and stems have a strong smell and are used by the tribals against headache.

In Kerala, *Naravelia zeylanica* (Ranunculaceae) is used as the source of the drug.

Naravelia zeylanica (*Linn.*) *DC.* **(Ranunculaceae)** (Fig. 58)
Atragene zeylanica Linn.
Climbing shrub; branches tomentose; leaves 3-foliolate, the terminal leaflet transformed into a tendril, lateral leaflets ovate-acuminate, to 11 × 9.5 cms, 5-nerved, margin serrate, pubescent above, woolly below; flowers greenish-yellow in axillary or terminal panicle; sepals 4 or 5, ovate, tomentose; petals 10–12, greenish yellow, linear to spathulate, glabrous; stamens many, filaments ligulate, connectives produced above; carpels 15–20, 1-ovuled, free; style short, stigma clavate; achenes tailed with the persistent, spirally twisted, feathery styles.

Distribution: Common on hedges and thickets in almost all districts, especially at higher elevations.

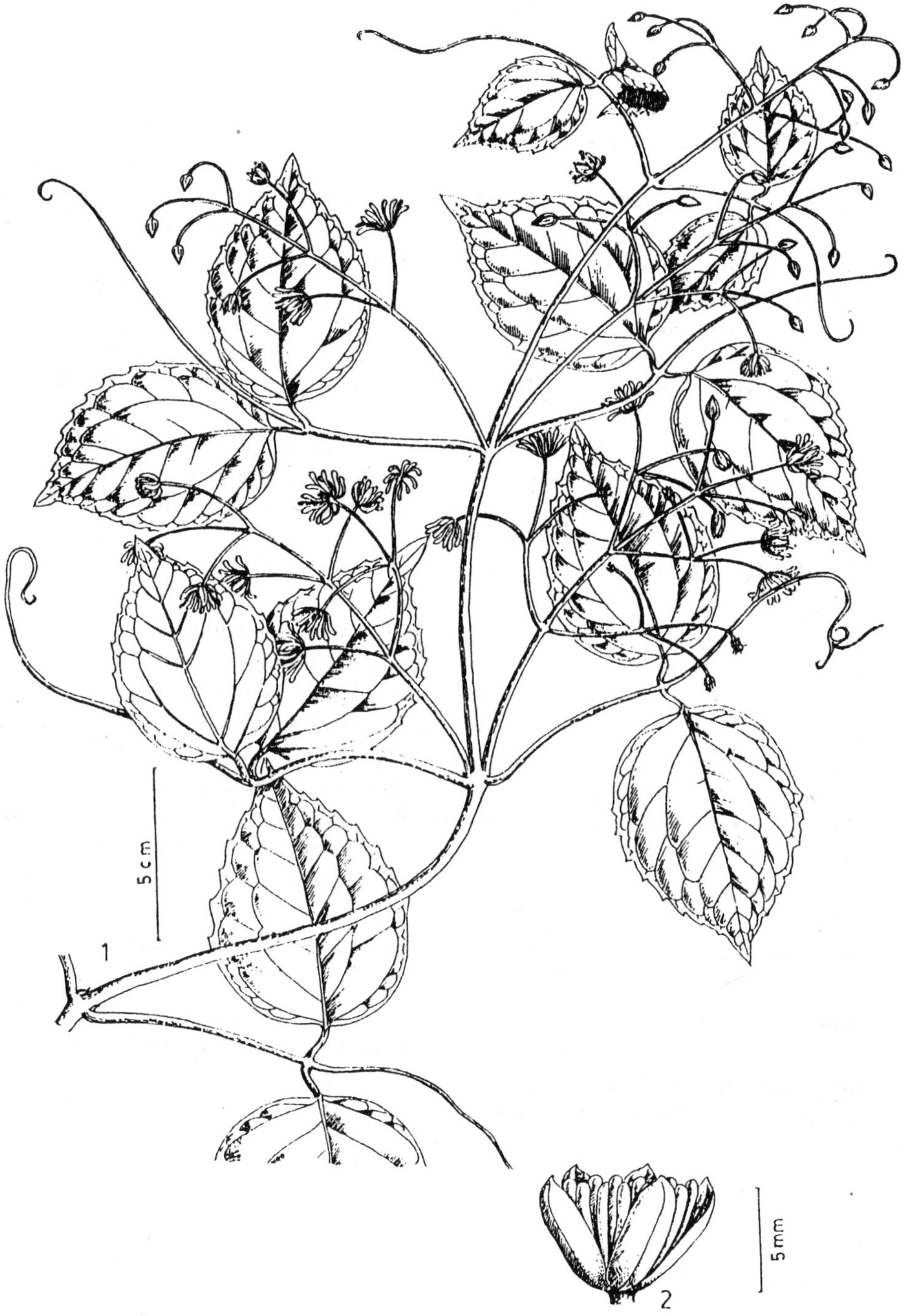

Figure 58: **Naravelia zeylanica** (L.) DC. 1, Habit; 2, Young flower.

DHĀTAKĪ (Mal. TĀTIRI)

The dried flowers of *dhātakī* are used in the preparation of *ariṣṭās* and *āsavās*, as it helps fermentation. *Dhātakī* is acrid, bitter, astringent, cold, light and intoxicant. It kills germs, purifies blood, allays thirst, heals ulcers, averts abortion, and cures heaemetemesis, erysipelas, dysentery, diarrhoea and uterine diseases, especially menorrhagia and leucorrhoea (Aiyer & Kolammal, 1966. 9: 5; Kurup *et al.*, 1979: 60). *Abhayāriṣṭaṃ, Kuṭajāriṣṭaṃ, Khadiraguḷika, Ceriya Arimēdastailaṃ* etc. are some of the preparations using the drug.

According to the texts, the plant bears attractive flowers in bunches (*dhātakī dhatṛupuṣpikā, gucchapuṣpā, saṅghapuṣpā*) which are red as the flames or fire (*agnijvālā, tāmṛapuṣpī, vahnipuṣpī, vahniśikhā*). Other synonyms like *madyasakhī, madyavāsinī, madanīyā, kuñjarikā*, etc. indicate the intoxicating properties of the flowers (Aiyer & Kolammal, 1966. 9: 4). *Woodfordia floribunda* of Lythraceae, locally called *tātiri* is the accepted source of the drug throughout India.

Woodfordia floribunda *Salisb.* **(Lythraceae)** (Fig. 59)
Woodfordia fruticosa Kurz.

Straggling woody shrub, young branches clothed with fine white pubescence; leaves simple, opposite, short-petioled, ovate-lanceolate acuminate, entire, to 11 × 3 cms, subcoriaceous, green glabrescent above, pale, hoary beneath; flowers numerous, short-pedicelled, deep orange-red, borne in cymose fascicles or panicled cymes arising from the older leafless portions of the branches in the axils of the leafscars; calyx 1.5 cm long, orange-red, slightly curved and striate, ending in a 6-toothed oblique mouth; petals small, narrowly linear, alternating with calyx teeth; stamens 12, filaments free, exserted; ovary sessile, cylindric, 2-celled, many ovuled, style long, ending in a punctiform stigma; fruit an ellipsoid capsule enclosed within the calyx tube; seeds minute, smooth.

Distribution: The plant is found distributed in most parts of India growing on rocky places.

Note: Atal *et al.* (1982) isolated a yeast strain (*Saccharomyces cerevisiae*) from *dhātaki* flowers which were found capable of producing alcoholic fermentation. The antipyretic activity of the alcoholic extract of *W. floribunda* flowers has been studied by Alam *et al.* (1986) in albino rats.

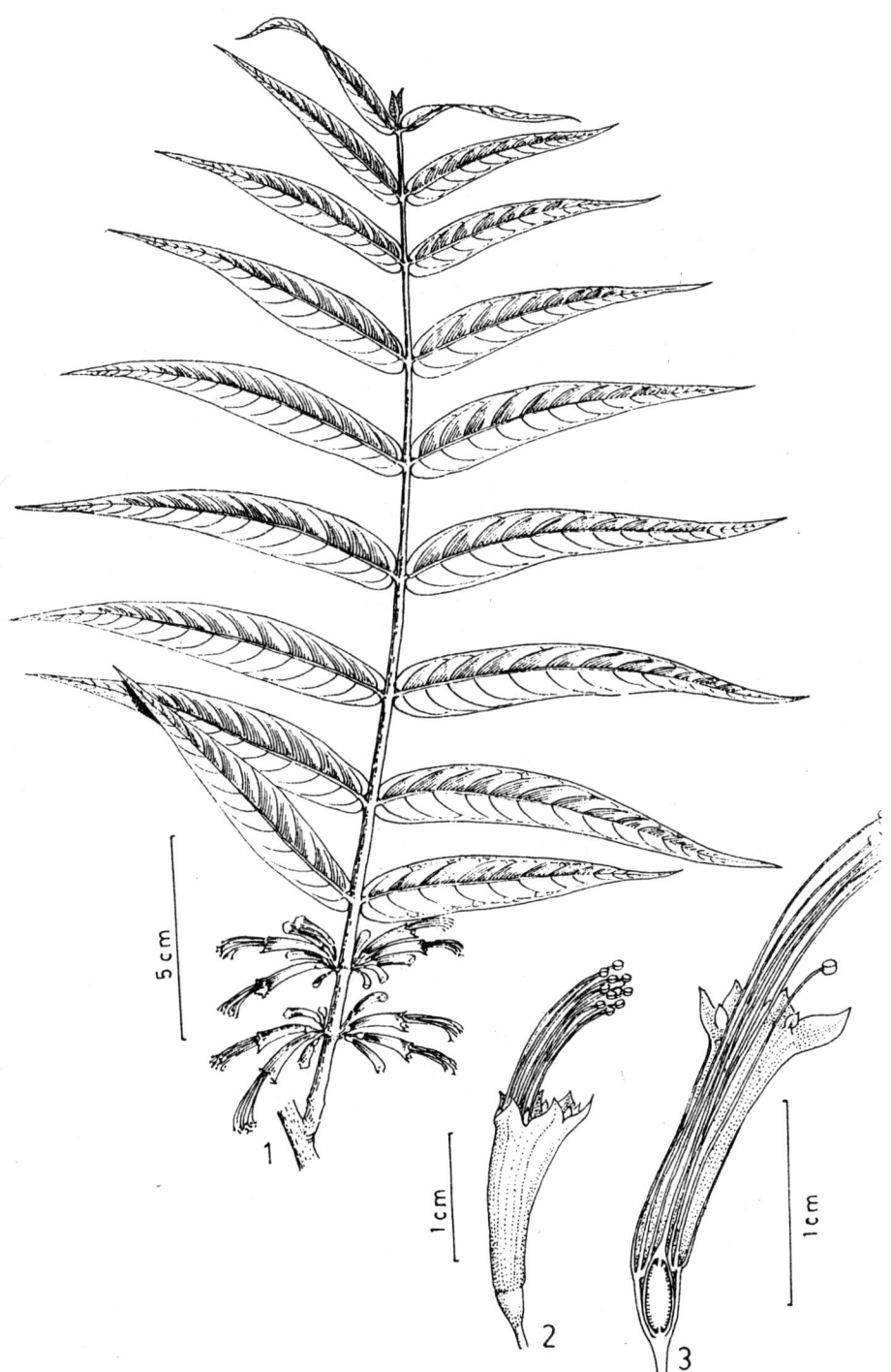

Figure 59: **Woodfordia floribunda** Salisb. 1, Flowering twig; 2, Flower; 3, Flower L.S.

DHATTŪRAḤ (Mal. UṀMAṂ)

In traditional medicine, this is a reputed drug in the treatment of rabid dog-bites and poisonous insect bites. It is reported to be bitter, acrid, astringent, germicidal, anodyne, antiseptic, antiphlogistic, narcotic and sedative. The drug gives good complexion, improves digestion and cures skin diseases such as itching, scabies, ulcers and leprosy, dandruff, fever, dysuria, piles, anaemia and inflammatory swellings. It is also useful in respiratory ailments, ear ache, eye diseases, insanity, rheumatism and elephantiasis (Kolammal, 1979. 10: 29; Kurup *et al.*, 1979; 61). Root, leaf and flower are used in medicine. The important formulations using the drug are *Kanakāsavaṃ, Dhuṛdhūradi tailaṃ, Dhuṛdhūrapatṛādi* coconut oil, *Mṛtasañjīvini*, etc.

Except the terms *kālapuṣpaḥ* and *syāmā* which indicate the blackish or dark colour of the flower, all other terms denote the qualities of the drug. Four varieties based on the colour of flowers, viz. white, blue, red and yellow are mentioned in the texts. In Kerala, two varieties namely the blue flowered and white flowered are generally met with. Those with blue flowers are considered to be the best for medicinal use, though all the varieties are reported to have similar properties (Kolammal, 1979. 10: 29).

Datura metel L. of Solanaceae, known as *uṁmaṃ* or *uṁmattu* in vernacular, is the source of the drug throughout the country (The blue flowered variety of this plant is locally called *nila-uṁmattu* (see also Rheede, Hort. Malab. 2: 49–50, 6. 29. 1679).

Datura metel *Linn.* **(Solanaceae)** (Fig. 60)
D. alba Nees
D. fastuosa var. *alba* (Nees.) C. B. Clarke
D. fastuosa auct. non L.

Erect subshrub; leaves simple, alternate, elliptic to angulate acute or acuminate, 10–18 × 7–15 cm, base unequally truncate, margin entire or sinuate or repand-dentate, often glabrous; flowers large, terminal, solitary; calyx gamosepalous, finely pubescent, long tubular, 5-toothed at apex; corolla gamopetalous, regular, long tubular, funnel-shaped with a spreading 5-angled plaited limb, white or purplish blue; stamens 5, filaments free, filiform, attached near the base of the corolla; ovary superior, clothed with soft prickles, 4-chambered and many ovuled, style filiform, stigma two-lobed; fruit a subglobose, greenish, fleshy capsule, 3 to 4 cm in diam., covered with short, blunt spines; seeds many, compressed.

Distribution: The plant is found in almost all districts of the hotter parts of India, as a weed in waste places, by roadsides and in garden land. It is also reported from tropical and subtropical Asia and Africa, now widely cultivated throughout the warmer regions of both hemispheres.

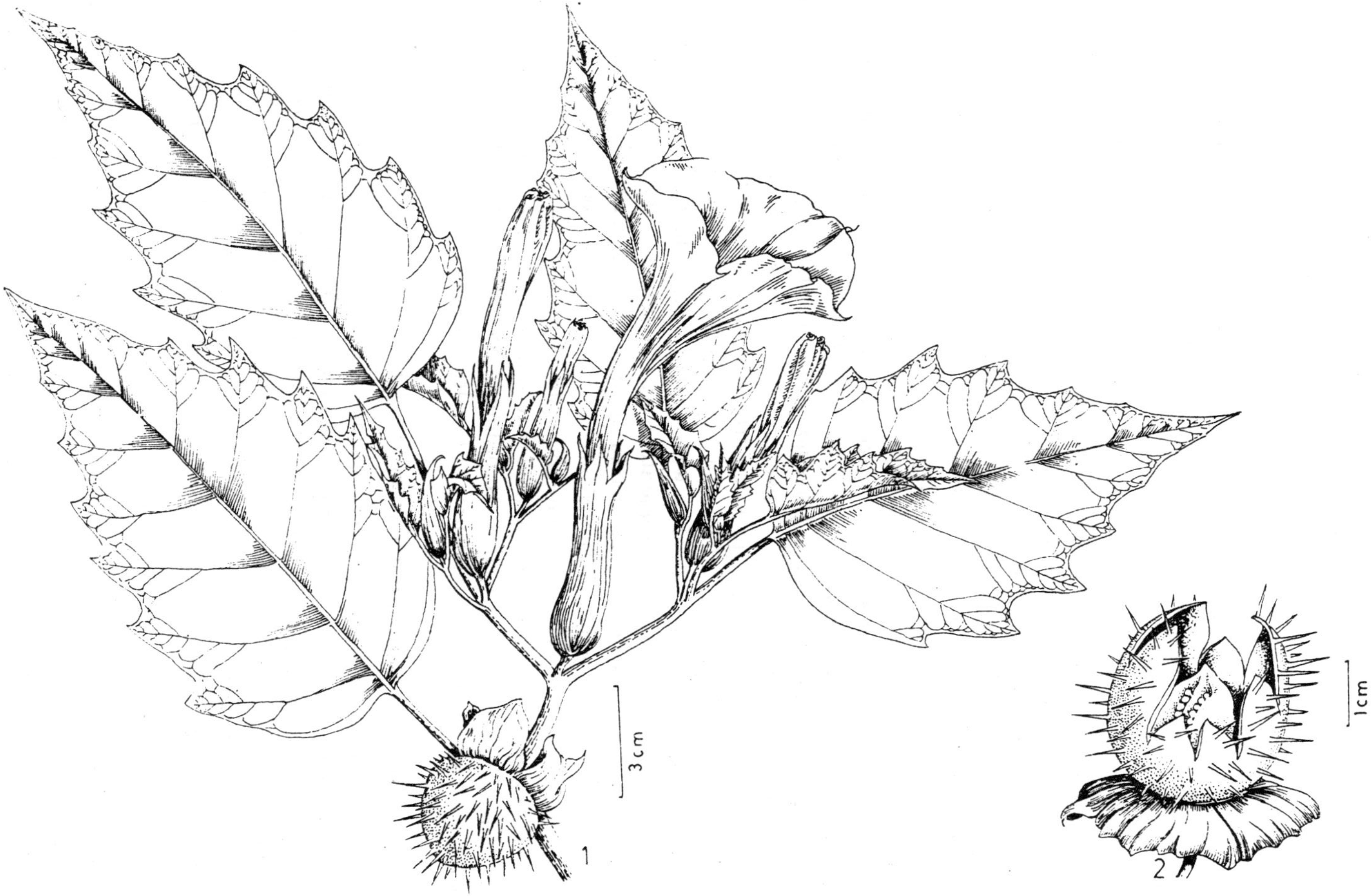

Figure 60: Datura metel L. 1, Branch with flowers and fruits; 2, Ruptured fruit.

DRAVANTĪ (Mal. KAṬALĀVAṆAKKU)

Dravanti, is reported to be bitter, acrid, astringent and anthelmintic. It serves to cleanse the entire system through its purgative property. It is useful in chronic dysentery, thirst, abdominal complaints, biliousness, anaemia, fistula, ulcer, diseases of the heart and skin. Root, leaf and fruit are used in medicine. The leaves are reported to be galactagogue, rubefacient, suppurative, insecticidal and are used in foul ulcers, tumours, and scabies. Fresh juice from the stem arrests bleeding from wounds, ulcers, cuts and abrasions. The seeds are powerful purgative, acrid, sweet, aphrodisiac, digestive, anthelmintic and are useful in piles, wounds, enlarged spleen and skin diseases. Seed oil is used as a cleansing application for wounds, sores, ulcers and rheumatism. It is an esteemed remedy for itch, herpes and eczema (Nadkarni, 1954: 705; Raghunathan & Mitra, 1982: 264).

The identity of *dravantī* is somewhat controversial. According to *Bhāvaprakāśa*, *dravantī*, also called *bṛhaddantī* is the bigger variety of *dantī*, the smaller variety being known as *laghudantī* or *dantī* which is *Baliospermum montanum* of Euphorbiaceae. Some people equate *bṛhaddantī* with a variety of *ēraṇḍa*, called *vyāghṛairaṇḍa* and identify it with *Jatropha curcas L.* of *Euphorbiaceae*. Some consider *dravantī* and *jayapāla* to be the same drug and *Croton tiglium* L. (Euphorbiaceae) as the source plant. (cf. Chunekar, 1982: 399). Mooss (1980: 114) and Sharma (1983: 428) also equate *dravanti* with *Croton tiglium*. In Kerala, however, *dravanti* and *jayapāla* are treated as separate drugs, the former being equated with *Jatropha curcas*, locally called *kaṭalāvaṇakku* or *kāṭṭāvaṇakku* and the latter with *Croton tiglium*, both belonging to Euphorbiaceae. People like Nadkarni (1954: 705) and Chopra *et al.* (1956: 145) also equate *Jatropha curcas* with this drug.

Our field studies have however, revealed that *Jatropha gossypifolia* Linn. is also used in some places as the drug source. According to Ayurvedic Formulary of India, *Jatropha glandulifera* is the actual source of the drug (Anonymous, 1978a: 249).

Jatropha curcas *Linn.* **(Euphorbiaceae)** (Fig. 61)

Glabrous shrub with an acrid latex; leaves simple, alternate, long-petioled, petiole upto 20 cms; lamina orbicular, subcordate, shallowly 3–5 lobed, 16 × 16 cms, 5-nerved; flowers yellowish green in axillary cymes; bracts lanceolate; sepals equal in male, unequal in female, ovate-obovate, sericeous at base within; petals obovate, villous within; stamens 10, 5 + 5, biseriate; capsule ellipsoid, obtuse.

Distribution: The plant is common in waste places throughout India and in the New World tropics.

Jatropha gossypifolia *Linn.* **(Euphorbiaceae)** (Fig. 62)

Tall shrub; branchlets glandular-hairy; leaves simple, long-petioled; petiole upto 17 cm, glandular, lamina deeply 3–5 lobed, 13 × 18 cms, lobes obovate, margin, entire, glandular-hairy, apex acute; flowers unisexual, reddish in terminal cymes;

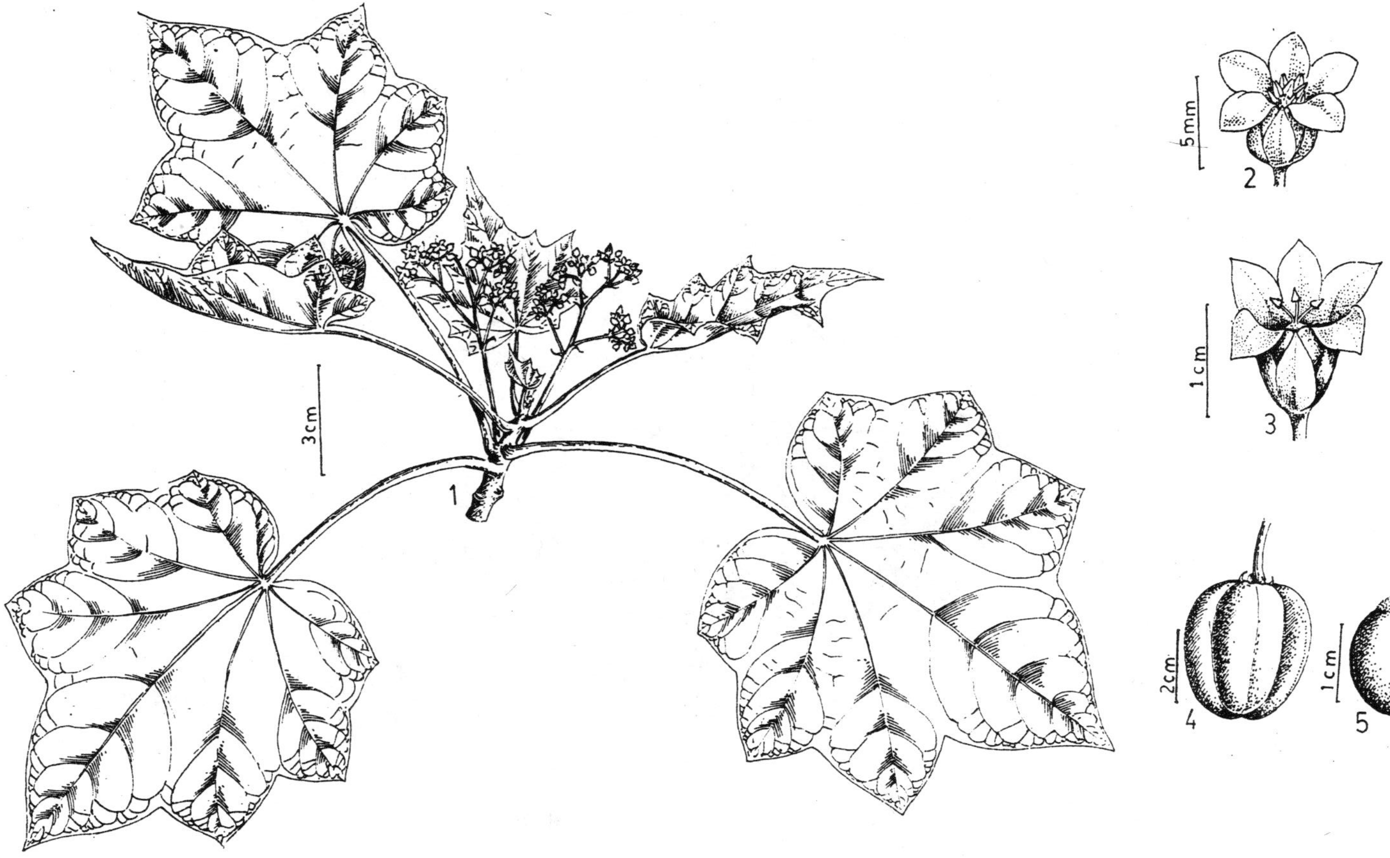

Figure 61: **Jatropha curcas** L. 1, Flowering twig; 2, Male flower; 3, Female flower; 4, Fruit; 5, Seed.

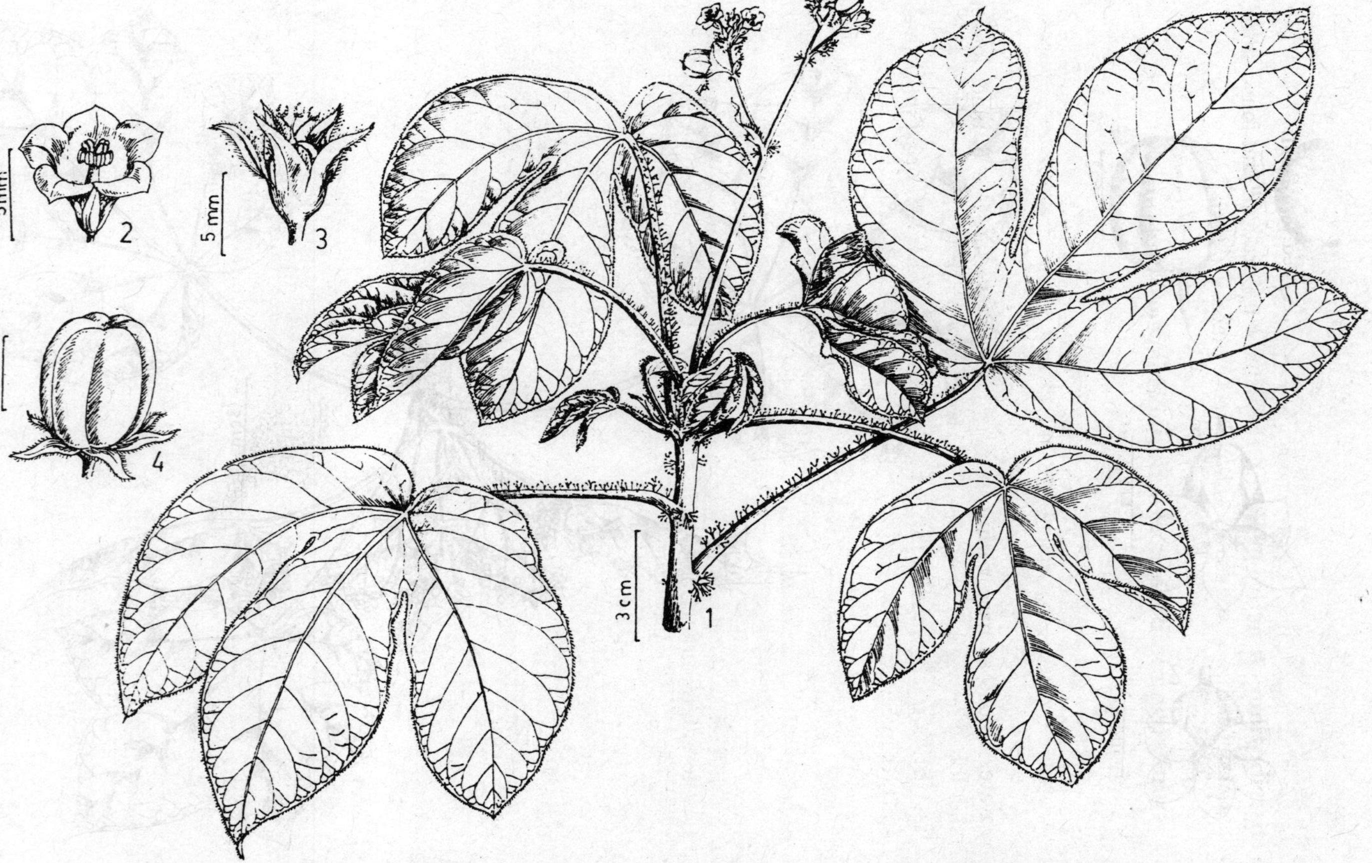

Figure 62: **Jatropha gossypifolia** L. 1, Flowering twig; 2, Male flower; 3, Female flower; 4, Fruit.

bracts lanceolate, glandular; outer sepals glandular-hairy, acuminate; inner ones reddish, campanulate, lobes ovate, ciliate, obtuse; stamens 8, 5 + 3 biseriate, filaments basally connate, inner 3 longer; capsule 3-lobed, ellipsoid.

Distribution: A native of Brazil, this is now naturalized and found in all plains districts of India on roadsides and in waste places.

Jatropha glandulifera *Roxb.* (Euphorbiaceae)

Shrub; leaves deeply 3–5 lobed, 6–9 × 6.5–8 cm, base (sub.) cordate, margin serrate, serratures gland-tipped, apex shortly accuminate; petiole 6–12 cm; stipules branched, filiform, to 1.5 cm, gland-tipped; flowers unisexual in terminal cymes; bracts linear-lanceolate, glandular-hairy; tepals free, outer lanceolate, inner ones obovate, villous at base within; stamens 8, diadelphous, 5 + 3, inner longer; capsule 3-lobed.

Distribution: It is found in Deccan and Carnatic. Also reported in Peninsula, Sri Lanka, tropical Africa.

Note: Jobert *et al.* (1984) and Aguye *et al.* (1985) have found the seeds of *J. curcas* to be highly toxic to children, producing a clinical syndrome of restlessness, severe vomiting and dehydration.

Pharmacognostic characters of *J. curcas* have been discussed by Gupta (1985) and a comparison with that of *J. gossypifolia* has been made with a view to check probable adulterants (Datta and Datta, 1983).

DRŌṆAPUṢPĪ (Mal. TUṀPA)

This is a reputed home remedy for worms, fever and intestinal catarrh in children. The whole plant is used medicinally. It is antihistaminic, antipyretic, antiseptic, carminative, febrifuge and wormifuge. It is used in anorexia, cough, dyspepsia, fever, helminthic manifestation, jaundice, psoriasis, respiratory diseases and skin diseases. Fresh juice of the plant is extensively used in jaundice and skin diseases (cf. Kurup, *et al.*, 1979: 64) *Kaccōrādi* oil, *Laśunaghṛtaṃ, Pāṭhādigulika, Kompañcādi guḷika,* etc. are some of the preparations using the drug.

The synonyms are not helpful in identifying the plant conclusively. Most of the authors equate the drug with different species of *Leucas* belonging to Lamiaceae. Some consider *Leucas cephalotes* as the drug source (Nadkarni, 1954: 739; Chopra *et al.*, 1956: 153; Chunekar, 1982: 463; Sharma, 1983: 707), while others accept *Leucas linifolia* (now *L. indica* (Linn.) R. Br. ex Vatke) as *drōṇapuṣpī* (Kirtikar & Basu, 1918: 1046; Vaidya, 1936: 296; Nadkarni, 1954: 740; Chopra *et al.*, 1956: 153). *Leucas aspera* (Willd.) Spr. is also equated with the drug by still others (Kurup *et al.*, 1979: 64; Mooss, 1980: 78; Nesamony, 1985: 274). This plant, locally called *tuṁpa* is the accepted source of the drug in Kerala. Rheede's illustration of the plant with the same vernacular name *Tumba* (Hort. Malab. 10: 181, t. 91. 1690) substantiates this fact.

Our field studies reveal that another species closely related to *L. aspera*, namely *L. stricta*, known by the same vernacular name, is also used as the drug source along with *L. aspera.* These two plants can be distinguished as follows.

Leucas aspera (*Willd.*) *Spr.* **(Lamiaceae)** (Fig. 63)
Phlomis aspera Willd.

Erect scabrid herb; leaves simple, opposite, linear-lanceolate, acute, to 7 × 1 cms, entire or dentate, puberulous; flowers small, white, in axillary, many-flowered verticels; calyx tube 6 mm, ribbed, mouth obliquely curved, teeth small, triangular; corolla 2-lipped, upper lip short and hairy, lower lip twice as long as upper, 3-lobed; stamens 4, didynamous, enclosed within the upper lip; nutlets oblong, angled on the inner face, smooth.

Distribution: India, Bangladesh, Indo China, Malesia and Mauritius. It is found in most plains districts of India upto 3,000 ft., as a weed in cultivated fields, waste lands and roadsides.

Leucas stricta *Benth.* **(Lamiaceae)** (Fig. 64)

Erect, densely hispid herb; leaves narrowly elliptic-lanceolate, acute, densely hairy on both surfaces; flowers white in axillary clusters in whorls; calyx pubescent, tube slightly curved and ribbed, mouth not oblique, teeth subequal, triangular. Other details similar to the previous species.

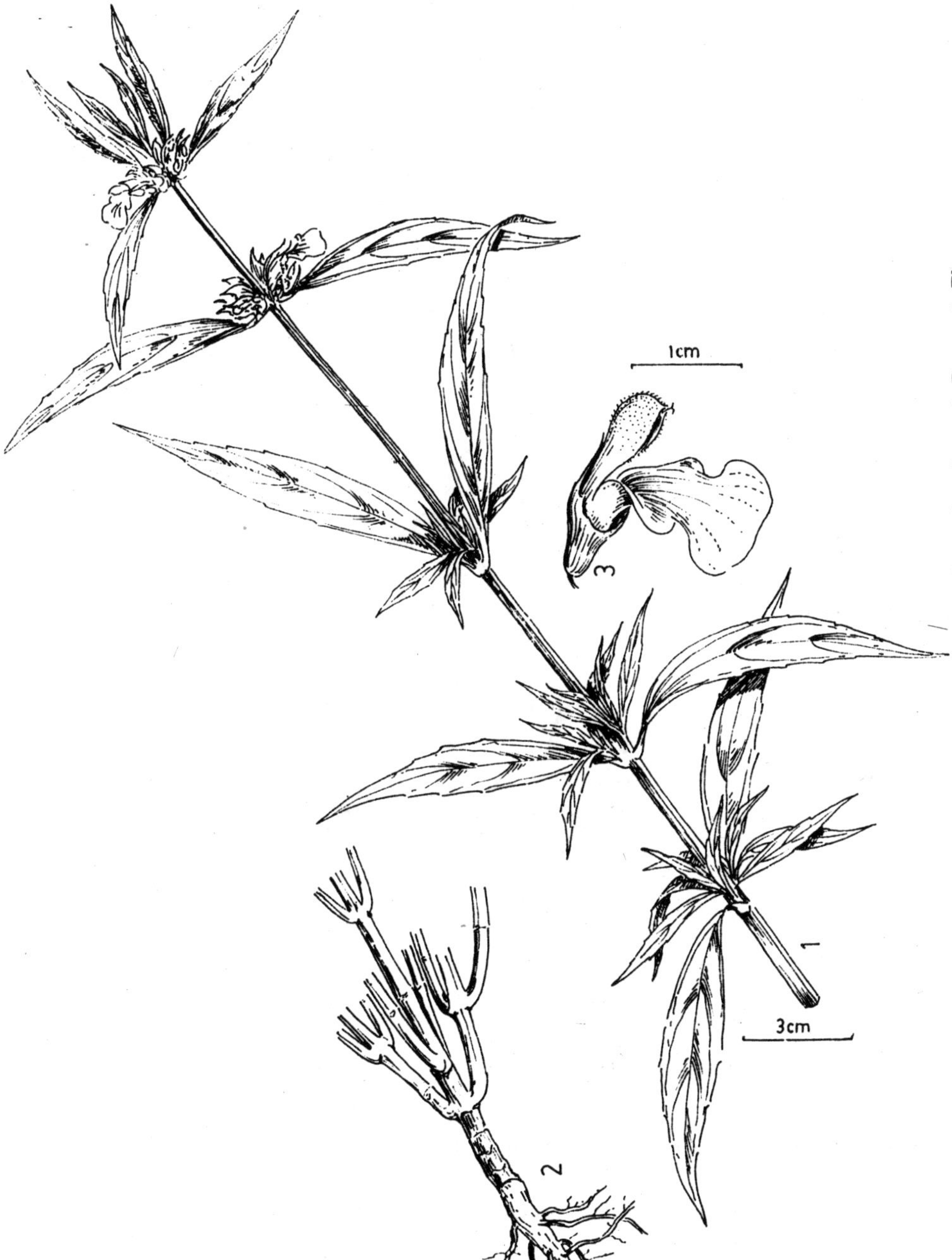

Figure 63: **Leucas aspera** (Willd.) Spr. 1, Flowering shoot; 2, Roots; 3, Flower.

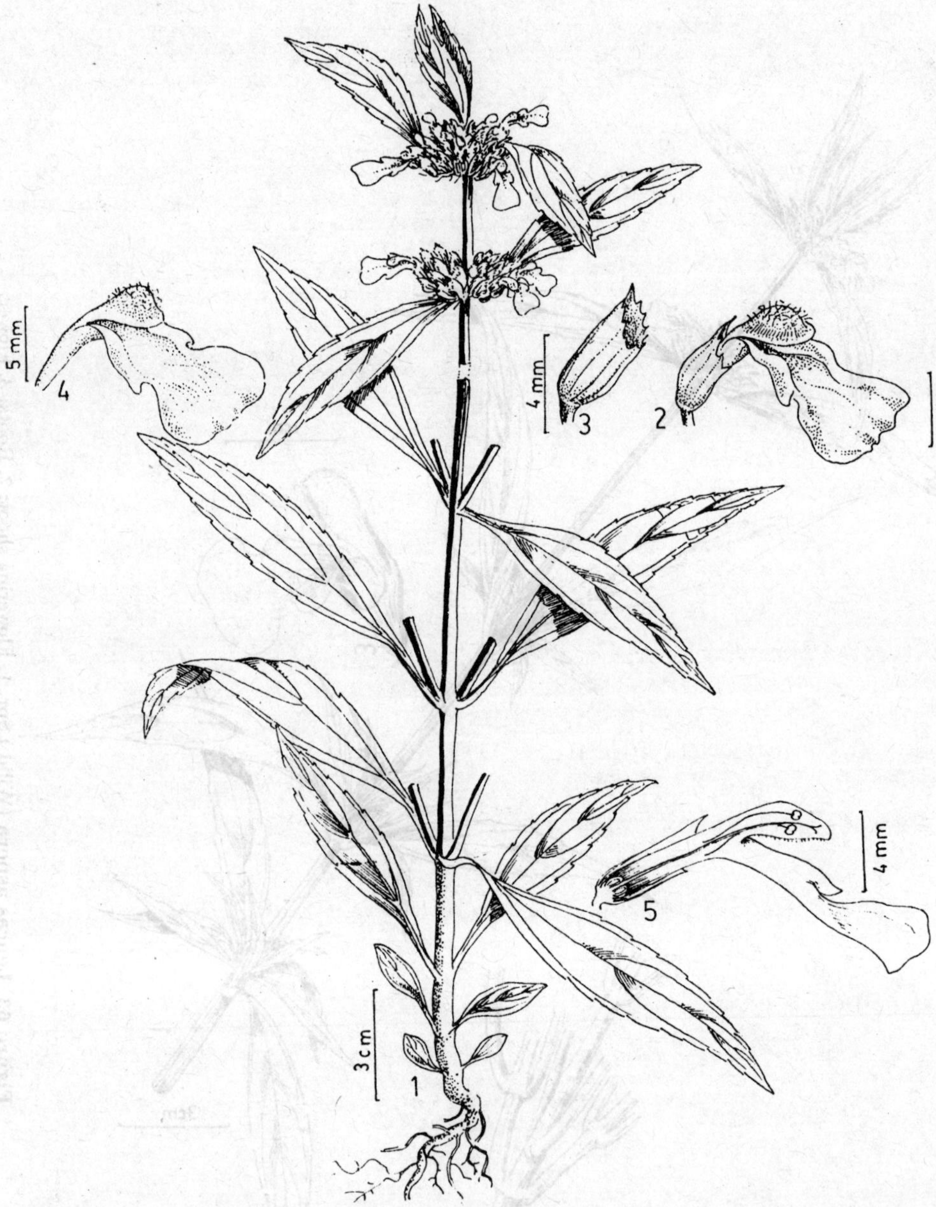

Figure 64: **Leucas stricta** Benth. 1, Habit; 2, Flower; 3, Calyx; 4, Corolla; 5, Flower L.S.

Distribution: A common weed in agricultural lands, sandy sea coast, and waste places throughout southern India.

Note: The antifungal activity of *L. aspera* has been studied by Thakur *et al.* (1982). Kannappareddy *et al.* (1986) found that the extract of the plant exhibits significant anti-inflammatory action on acute and chronic inflammation.

DUGDHIKĀ (Mal. NILAPPĀLA)

The plant *dugdhikā*, also called *kṣīrā, vikṣīriṇī*, etc. (all indicating the presence of milky latex in the plant body) is acrid, bitter, hot in action, diuretic and aphrodisiac. It overcomes diseases due to the morbidity of ***kapha*** and *vāta*, purifies blood and cures skin diseases, poisonous affections, cough, asthma and other respiratory disorders. Leaves and seeds are given in bowel complaints of children and worms. The plant juice is a good galactagogue (Nadkarni, 1954: 529; Chunekar, 1982: 459; Sharma, 1983: 302). The whole plant is medicinal.

Many authors recognise two different varieties of the drug, namely a bigger and a smaller variety, the former being equated with *Euphorbia hirta* Linn. and the latter with *Euphorbia thymifolia* Linn. of Euphorbiaceae (Chunekar, 1982: 458; Sharma, 1983: 300, 301). *Euphorbia microphylla* and *E. hypericifolia* are also considered as the smaller variety or *laghudugdhikā* by some (Vaidya Bapalal, 1982: 188; Chunekar, 1982: 459). But these are not known to be used in Kerala. In practice, in Kerala, *Euphorbia thymifolia*, locally called ***nilappāla***, is the one widely used as the source of *dugdhikā*. According to Ayurvedic formulary of India also, this is the accepted source (Anonymous, 1978a: 249). Rheede describes it under the name *Caicotti-n-pala* (Hort. Malab. 10: 65, t. 33. 1690). Our field studies reveal that *Euphorbia hirta* is also used in some parts of Kerala as ***nilappāla***. The two plants can be identified as follows.

Euphorbia thymifolia *Linn.* **(Euphorbiaceae)** (Fig. 65)
Chamaesyce thymifolia (Linn.) Millsp.

Softly hispid prostrate herb; leaves very small, bifarious, obliquely oblong-obtuse, finely serrate, to 1 x 0.5 cm; cyathia minute in axillary clusters; involucre campanulate, 0.8 x 0.7 mm; glands 4, equal, male: florets 1–4, ebracteolate, anthers 0.2 mm; female: laterally pendulous, ovary tomentose, styles 3, forked from base, erect; capsule 3-valved, appressed hairy; 1.5 mm across; seeds triangular, minutely tuberculate.

Distribution: The plant is found in all plains districts and on hills in Deccan and Carnatic at low elevations. Also distributed in tropical Asia.

Note: The antispasmodic and bronchodilating activity of *E. thymifolia* have been clinically proved on guinea pigs by Sharma and Sharma (1972), thus proving its efficacy in the treatment of *tamakaśvāsa* (Sharma *et al.*, 1982). Sinha *et al.* (1984) have studied the pharmacognosy of *E. thymifolia* Linn.

Euphorbia hitra *Linn.* **(Euphorbiaceae)** (Fig. 66)
Chamaesyce hirta (Linn.) Millsp.
Euphorbia pilulifera auct. non Linn.

Erect, hispid herb; leaves simple, opposite, broadly oblong to elliptic-oblong, acute, 4.3 x 1.8 cms, glaucous beneath, 3-nerved, base obliquely truncate, margin serrulate;

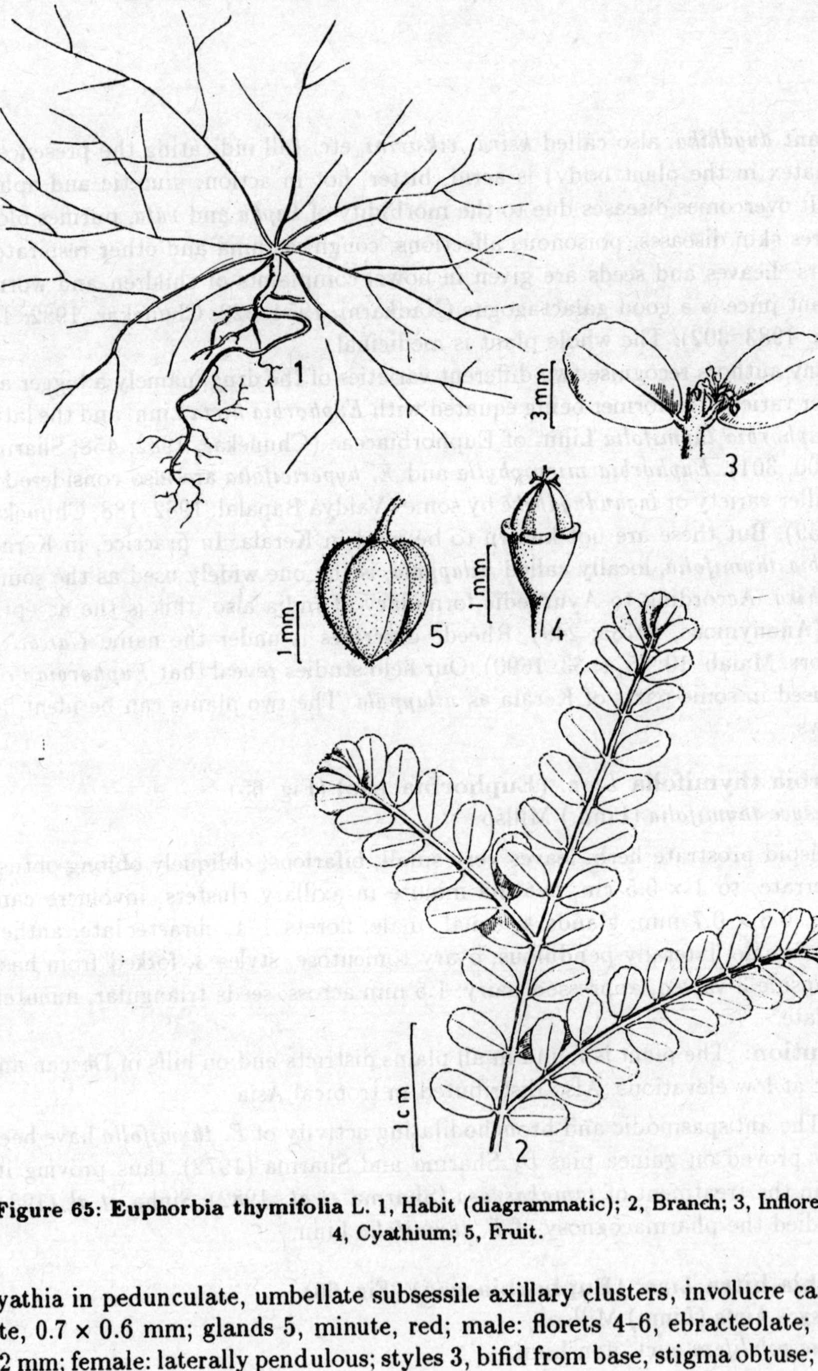

Figure 65: Euphorbia thymifolia L. 1, Habit (diagrammatic); 2, Branch; 3, Inflorescence; 4, Cyathium; 5, Fruit.

Cyathia in pedunculate, umbellate subsessile axillary clusters, involucre campanulate, 0.7 × 0.6 mm; glands 5, minute, red; male: florets 4–6, ebracteolate; anthers 0.2 mm; female: laterally pendulous; styles 3, bifid from base, stigma obtuse; capsule pubescent, 2 mm across; seeds 4-angled, minutely furrowed.

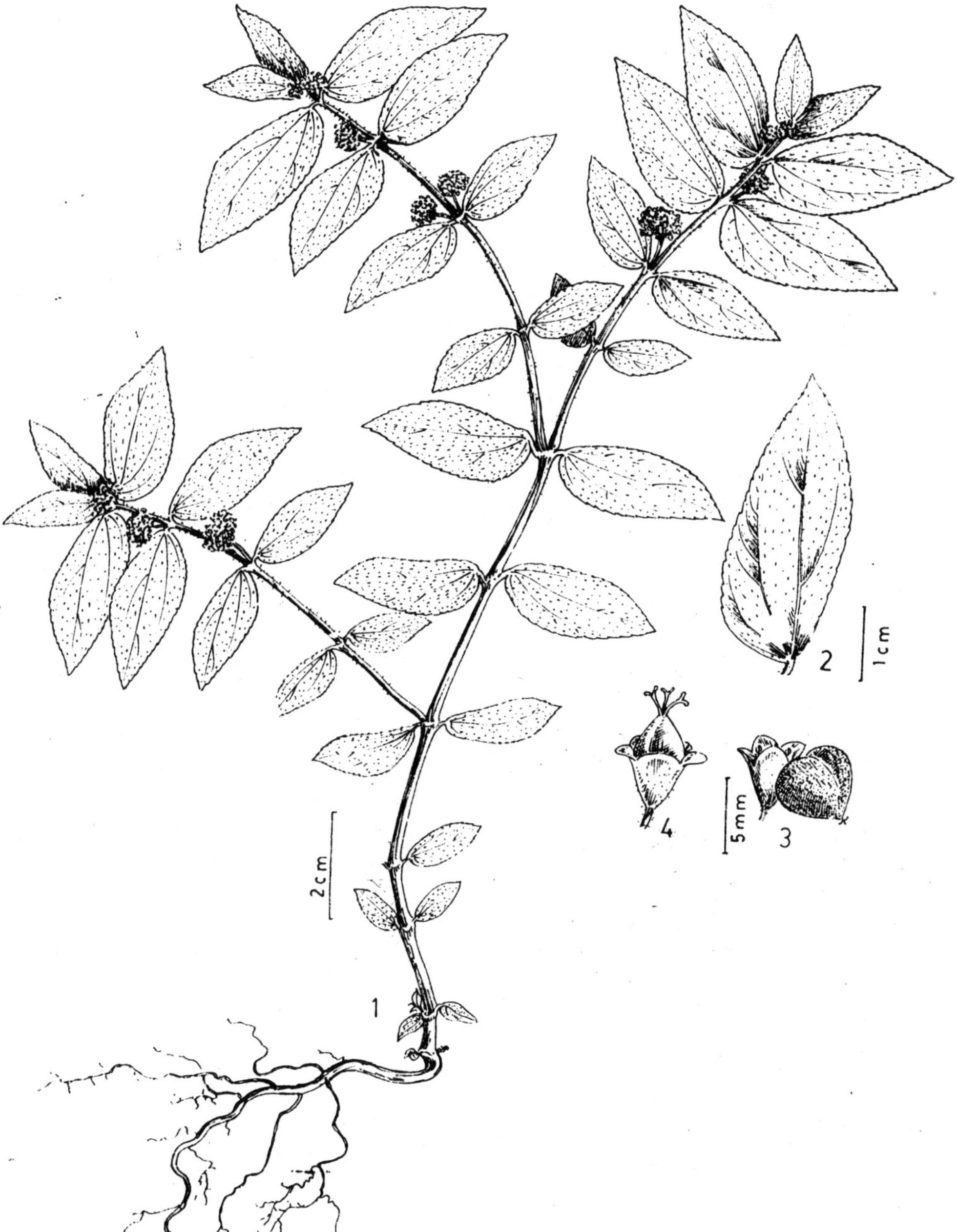

Figure 66: Euphorbia hirta L. 1, Habit; 2, Single leaf; 3–4, Cyathia.

Distribution: The plant is a pantropical weed seen in all plains districts especially on roadsides and waste land.

DURĀLABHĀ (Mal. KOṬITTŪVA)

The names *durālabhā, dusparśā, durālambhā, durabhigrahā*, etc. mean that which is difficult to handle, due to the presence of sharp thorns or stinging hairs (*kachura*) on the plant body. Āyurvēdic texts describe it as an inhabitant of dry, arid regions (*dhanvayāsaḥ, marutbhavaḥ*) with an extensive root system (*anantā, samudrāntā, dīrghamūlā*). It spreads over the ground (*yavāsaḥ*) and make the place unapproachable (*kunāśakaḥ*) (cf. Aiyer & Kolammal, 1963. 6: 103).

According to the texts, *durālabhā* is astringent, acrid and sweet. It purifies blood, cures asthma, toxicosis, all kinds of fevers, diarrhoea, phantom tumour, excessive urinary secretion, thirst, vomiting and dermatosis. It cures diseases caused by the discordance of *vāta, pitta* and *kapha* (Aiyer & Kolammal, 1963. 6: 104). The root system forms the officinal part. The important formulations using the drug are *Durālabhāriṣṭaṃ, Daśamūlāriṣṭaṃ, Rāsnādikaṣāyaṃ*, etc.

According to *Nighaṇṭuratnākara* and *Bhāvaprakāśa*, there are two kinds of *durālabhā* which are called *durālabha* and *yavāsa* or *yāsa* respectively. Both are considered to possess similar properties. Many others treat them as two different drugs. *Yāsa* or *yavāsa* is equated with *Alhagi maurorum* Baker (Papilionaceae) and *durālabhā* or *dhanvayāsa* with *Fagonia arabica* Linn. of Zygophyllaceae (see Singh & Chunekar, 1972: 328, 211: Mooss, 1980: 23; Chunekar, 1982: 411, 412; Vaidya Bapalal, 1982: 301; Sharma, 1983: 316, 319). Ayurvedic formulary of India accepts *Fagonia arabica* as the correct source and suggests *Alhagi maurorum* as substitute (Anonymous, 1978a: 250). In Kerala, however, *Tragia involucrata* (Euphorbiaceae) is being used for both *yavāsa* and *dhanvayāsa*. This plant is locally called *koṭittūva* or *coriyaṇaṃ* due to its stinging hairs that cause itching. (See also Rheede, Hort. Malab. 2: 73–74, f.39. 1679 *Schorigenam*). This plant is equated with the Sanskrit term *vṛścikāḷi* by some (Kirtikar & Basu, 1918: 1173; Nadkarni, 1954: 1226; Chopra *et al.* 1956: 246). But this term does not occur in the Sanskrit verses pertaining to *durālabhā* and so Kerala physicians consider *vṛścikāḷī* as a separate drug and use *Heliotropium indicum* (Boraginaceae) as the source plant.

The various plant sources can be identified as follows:

Tragia involucrata *Linn.* **(Euphorbiaceae)** (Fig. 67)

Slender, twining herb with stinging hairs all over; leaves simple, alternate, stipulate, 5–10 × 2–5 cms, very variable in form, from linear-oblong to ovate-lanceolate acuminate, coarsely serrate, hispid on both surfaces; flowers small, greenish in monoecious, terminal, leaf-opposed or axillary racemes. Pistillate flowers: calyx gamosepalous, 6-lobed, persistent, becoming rigid and enlarged in fruit; ovary superior, 3-lobed, 3-chambered with one ovule in each, styles 3, united below into a stout cylindric column; capsules of 3, 2-valved cocci; seeds globose. Staminate flowers: pale yellowish; calyx globose, 3-partite; stamens 3, filaments free.

Distribution: The plant is found distributed throughout India from Punjab, Ben-

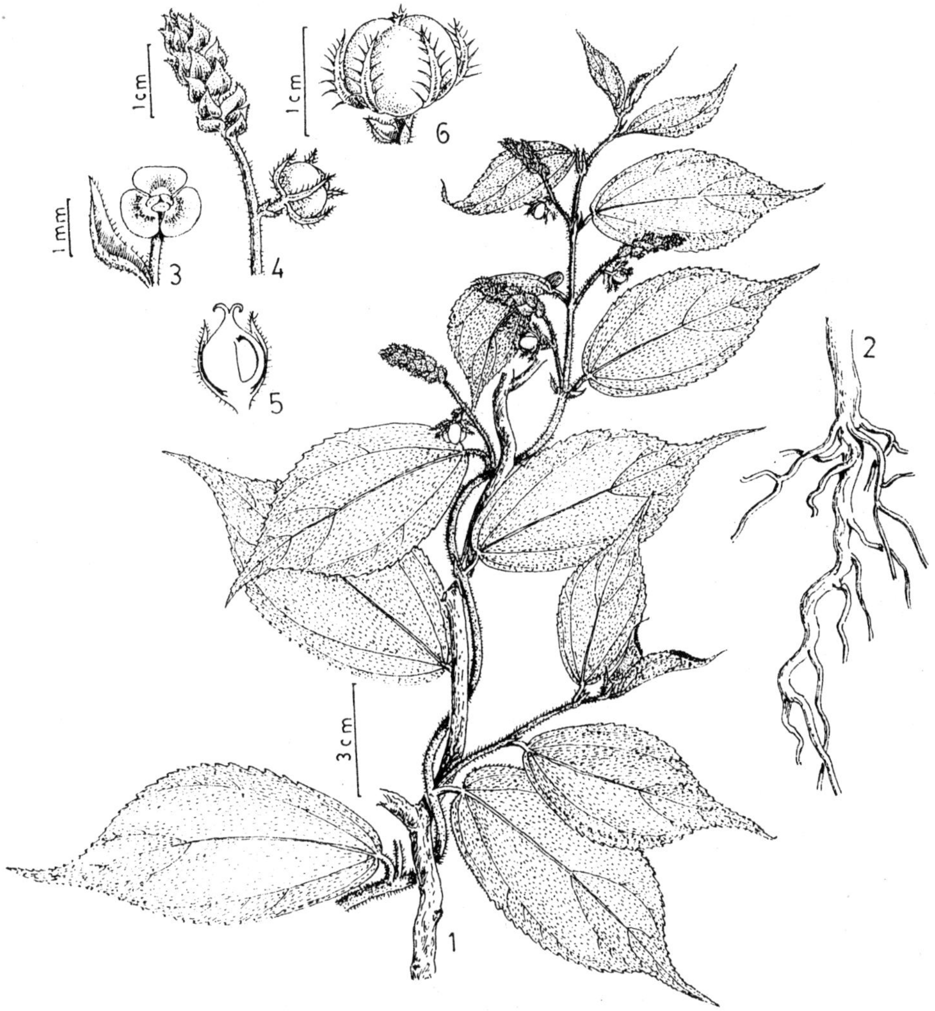

Figure 67: **Tragia involucrata** L. 1, Vine; 2, Roots; 3, Male flower; 4, Inflorescence; 5, Female flower L.S.; 6, Fruit.

gal, Assam, N. Circars, Deccan, Carnatic, the Western Ghats and Kerala. Also reported from Sri Lanka, Burma and China.

Fagonia arabica *Linn.* (Zygophyllaceae)

Fagonia cretica var. *arabica* Linn.

Small, much branched, thorny, undershrub, covered with glandular hairs; leaves opposite, 1-3 foliolate, stipulate, the stipules subulate and spiny appearing in whorls of 4 at a node, longer than the leaves; leaflets small, entire, elliptic-oblong or linear acute; flowers small, pale rose, solitary, pseudoaxillary; sepals 5, oblong or lanceolate, deciduous; petals 5, spathulate, clawed or unguiculate, caducous; stamens 10, inserted on the disc, filaments free, filiform; ovary sessile, hairy, 5-angled tapering into a subulate or 5 angled persistent style ending in stigma; fruit a five-cornered schizocarp of five, 2-valved, one seeded cocci; seeds compressed.

Distribution: The plant is recorded as occuring throughout Northwest India, W. Rajputana, Sindh, Punjab and Kutch, the upper Gangetic plain, Deccan, Kurnool and Ananthapur. It is an inhabitant of dry localities.

Alhagi pseudalhagi (Bieb.) Desv. **(Papilionaceae)**
Alhagi maurorum Baker
Alhagi camelorum Fisch.

Erect, thorny shrub; leaves simple, alternate, stipulate, the stipules minute and ensiform, very short-petioled, oblong or obovate-oblong, obtuse, apiculate or mucronate at tip, cuneate at base, glabrous or puberulous; flowers small, purplish on short racemes that end in bristly points; calyx gamosepalous, campanulate, 5-teethed; corolla exserted, papilionaceous; stamens 10, diadelphous; pistil monocarpellary, style filiform, incurved ending in a terminal capitate stigma; fruit a linear falcate or straight, thick, indehiscent pod about 2.5 cms long; seeds kidney-shaped, blackish brown.

Distribution: The plant is found in the deserts of the N.E. Region of India, Upper Gangetic Plain, Delhi, Sind, Gujarat, Konkan, United Provinces, etc.

DŪṚVĀ (Mal. KAṚUKA)

Dūṛvā is considered as a sacred herb by the Hindus and is used in religious rites. The whole herb is reputed as a remedy in epitaxis (*nāsāgadaraktapittaṃ*), haematuria (*adhōgaraktapittaṃ*) and scabies (*vicaṛcikā*). It is cooling, astringent, demulcent, diuretic, ophthalmic, haemostatic and suppurative. It checks bleeding from cut and wounds and is useful in fever, burning sensation, chronic diarrhoea, dysentery, anasarca, dropsy, catarrhal ophthalmia, dysuria, bleeding piles, eye affections, epilepsy, hysteria and insanity. The drug is used with benefit to remedy defects of *kapha, pitta* and *rakta*. (Nadkarni, 1954: 425; Aiyer & Kolammal, 1963. 6: 17; Dey. 1980: 46). The important preparations using the drug are *Dūṛvāditailaṃ, Gandhatailaṃ, Mānasamitṛavaṭakaṃ, Jātyāditailaṃ*, etc.

According to the synonymy, the plant is drought-resistant (*ruhā*), it grows extensively (*dūṛvā, anantā*) and it has numerous thin, wiry branches (*śatavallī*) with numerous joints or nodes (*śatapaṛvikā*). The many potent virtues of the plant are indicated by the term *sahasṛavīryā* (Aiyer & Kolammal, 1963. 6: 16).

Three varieties (*dūṛvātṛayaṃ*) namely *nīladūṛvā* with bluish or greenish stem, *śvētadūṛvā* with whitish stem and branches and *gaṇḍadūṛvā* with nodulose stem are mentioned in the *Bhāvaprakāśa nighaṇṭu*, giving separate synonyms and attributing different virtues to each (cf. Chunekar, 1982: 384–386). But such a varietal distinction is not in vogue in practice and *Cynodon dactylon* (Linn.) Pers. (Poaceae), locally called *kaṛuka* or *kaṛukappullu* is the accepted source of the drug.

The plant is also known by the name *Belicaraga* (See Rheede Hort. Malab. 12: 87, t. 47. 1693) because it is being used in the sacrificial ceremonies for the dead (called *Beli* in vernacular).

Cynodon dactylon (*Linn.*) *Pers.* **(Poaceae)** (Fig. 68)
Panicum dactylon Linn.

Perennial herb; stem slender, creeping, rooting at all nodes; branches erect; leaves narrowly linear, flat, upto 8×0.3 cm; spikes 3–7, umbellate; spikelets sessile, laterally compressed, arranged in two alternating series on the rachis, each spikelet one-flowered; glumes 3, 1 and 2 empty, keeled, glume 3 or lemma larger, boat-shaped, membraneous, 3-nerved, palea 2-nerved, both enclosing a bisexual flower; lodicules 2, short, glabrous; stamens 3; ovary glabrous; fruit oblong, laterally compressed grain.

Distribution: The plant is a very common weed throughout India and also in the tropical and warm temperate regions throughout the world.

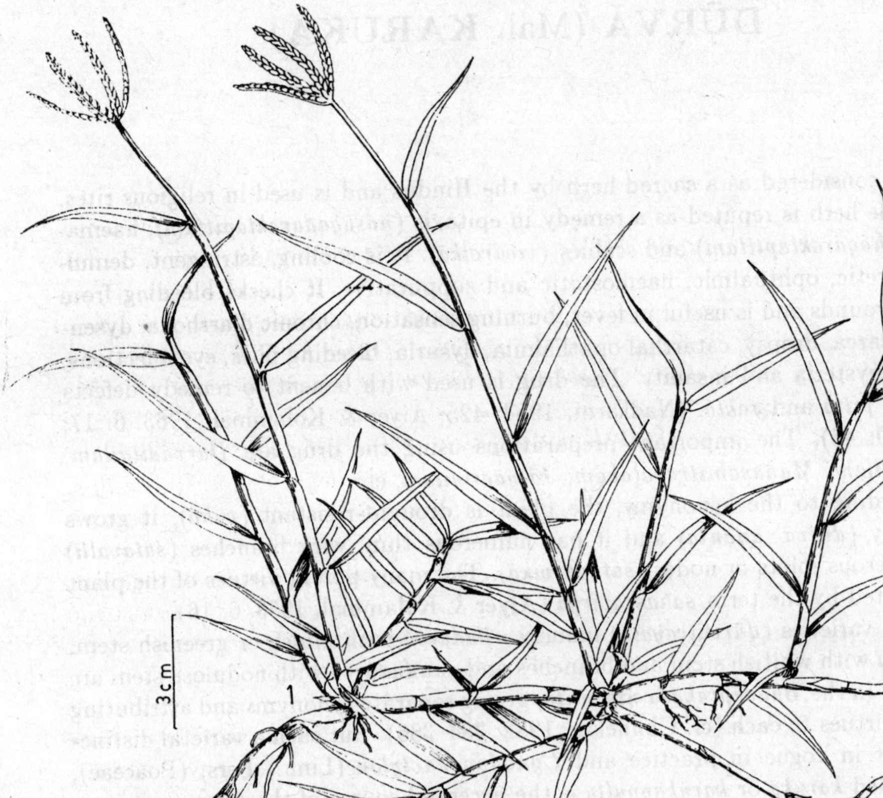

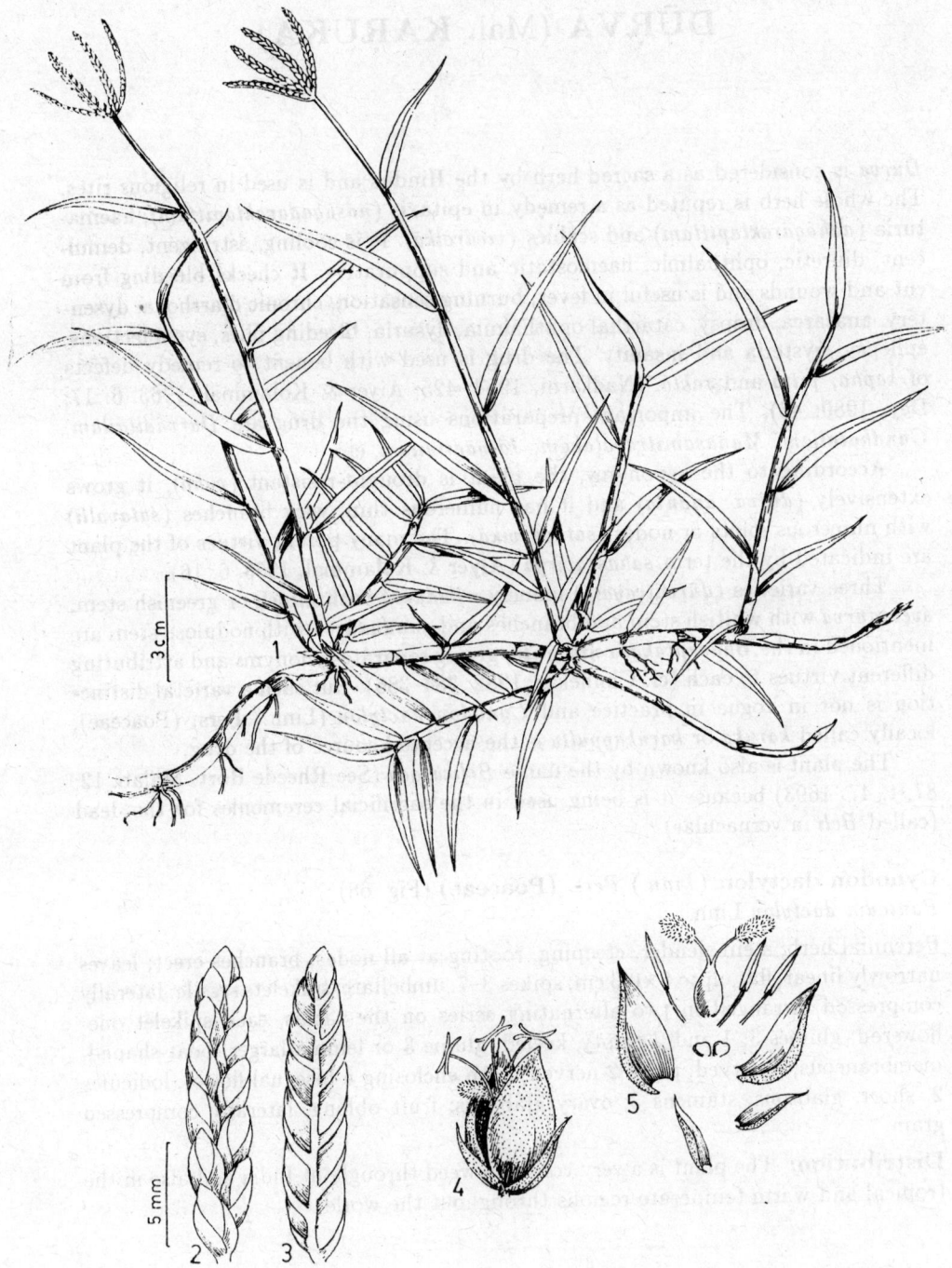

Figure 68: Cynodon dactylon (L.) Pers. 1, Habit; 2–3, inflorescence branch; 4, Floret; 5, Floral dissection.

ĒRAṆḌAḤ (Mal. ĀVAṆAKKU)

The name *ēraṇḍaḥ* indicates the property of the drug to dispel diseases. It is considered as a reputed remedy for all kinds of rheumatic affections (*vātāri, śūlaśatruḥ*). *Ēraṇḍa* is sweet, light, bitter, purgative and hot and cures dyspnoea, hydrocele, flatulence, dysentery, ascites, piles, cough, lumbago, headache, leprosy, arthritis, calculus and dysuria. It alleviates phantom tumour, splenic disorders, impurity of blood, dyspepsia and worm troubles. Root, leaves, seed and seed oil are used medicinally. Tender leaves cure pain in the bladder. Oil from seeds is sweet, hot in action, purgative and is a good remedy for all kinds of diseases due to morbid *vāta* and *kapha*, fever, scrotal enlargement, inflammation of the intestine and colic (Aiyer & Kolammal, 1966. 9: 18; Mooss, 1978: 153). The drug forms an ingredient of preparations like *Balāriṣṭaṃ, Aṣṭavargaṃ kaṣāyaṃ, Vidāryādi ghṛtaṃ* and *Vidāryādi lēhaṃ*.

According to the texts, the plant grows in any kind of soil (*vardhamānaḥ*) and has long slender stem (*dīrghadaṇḍakaḥ, cañcukaḥ*), large leaves resembling the ear of elephant (*hastikarṇakaḥ, gajakarṇaḥ, mahāpatraḥ*) with five protrusions or lobes resembling a human hand (*pancāṅgulaḥ, gandharvahastaḥ*) and 3-lobed fruits (*triputīphalaḥ*) having three seeds (*tribījaḥ*) which are mottled (*citraḥ, citrakaḥ*) (Aiyer & Kolammal, 1966. 9: 18).

In the ancient works on Āyurvēda, two varieties of *ēraṇḍaḥ* viz. a white variety and a red variety are mentioned. Among these, the white variety is preferred in medicine. *Ricinus communis* Linn. (Euphorbiaceae) is the plant used as the source of *ēraṇḍaḥ* throughout India. The two varieties are, differentiated by the colour of the young shoots, viz. 1) the white variety with greyish stems and leaves and 2) the red variety with reddish shoots and leaves. These two varieties of *ēraṇḍaḥ* are recognised by the physicians of Malabar, and the white variety is called *āvaṇakku* or *ciṭṭāvaṇakku* while the red variety *cuvanna āvaṇakku* in the vernacular (Mooss, 1978: 150). But, these are taxonomically not distinct. Rheede has described *Ricinus communis* under the names *Āvaṇacu, Citāvaṇacu, Pāndi-āvaṇacu* (Hort. Malab. 2: 57–60, t. 32. 1679).

Ricinus communis *Linn.* **(Euphorbiaceae)** (Fig. 69)

Tall glabrous shrub; stem grey or reddish, glaucous; leaves simple, alternate, long-petioled, stipulate, lamina peltate, nearly orbicular, digitately. 7–9 lobed, lobes acuminate, serrate; flowers small, unisexual, pale yellow in terminal monoecious panicles, the staminate flowers usually located in the distal part of the inflorescence and the pistillate flowers at the basal part. Male: perianth calycine, membraneous, splitting into 3–5 segments; stamens numerous, filaments branched; female: perianth spathaceous, caducuous; ovary superior, 3-chambered with 1 ovule in each, styles three, often large and brightly coloured, stigmas feathery; capsule 3-lobed, 3-valued and 3-seeded, spinous; seeds caruncalate and mottled.

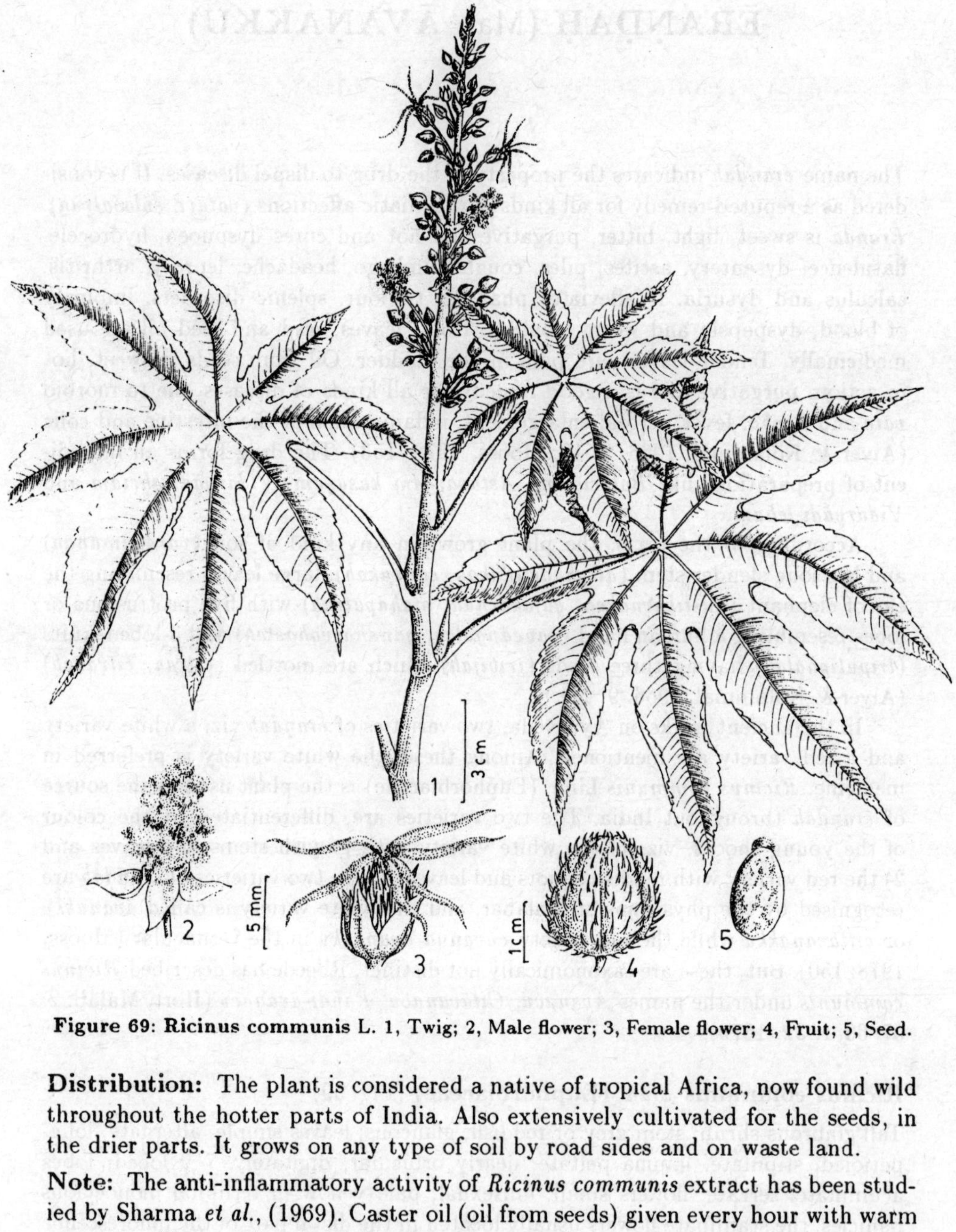

Figure 69: Ricinus communis L. 1, Twig; 2, Male flower; 3, Female flower; 4, Fruit; 5, Seed.

Distribution: The plant is considered a native of tropical Africa, now found wild throughout the hotter parts of India. Also extensively cultivated for the seeds, in the drier parts. It grows on any type of soil by road sides and on waste land.

Note: The anti-inflammatory activity of *Ricinus communis* extract has been studied by Sharma *et al.*, (1969). Caster oil (oil from seeds) given every hour with warm water or milk to patients suffering from *āmavāta*, has shown promising results without any toxic effect (Shastri, 1981). The macro and microscopical characters of the various parts of the plant, their cell contents, fluorescence analysis and phytochemistry have been discussed by Raghunathan and Mitra (1982: 312–319).

GŌDHĀPADĪ
(Mal. AMAṞCCAKKOṬI, COṞIVAḶḶI)

This is used as an ingredient of *Ayaskṛti* of the Kerala physicians. But there is little mention about this drug in ancient Āyurvēdic texts. It is reported that the leaves are astringent and refrigerant and are used to cure ulcers. Decoction of leaves checks uterine and other fluxes. The whole plant is acrid, refrigerant, costive and beneficial in hysteria, burning of the skin and diarrhoea (cf. Nadkarni, 1954: 1284; Chopra *et al.*, 1956: 56).

In their commentary on *Bṛhatṛayi*, Singh and Chunekar (1972: 97) equate *gōdhāpadī* with *kāṣṭhagōdha* which is considered to be one of the divine drugs used for *rasāyana* treatment. *Godhāpadī* is identified as *Cayratia pedata* of Vitaceae. Rheede has described two different varieties of this drug, viz. *Tsjorivalli* (Hort. Malab. 7. 17. t. 9. 1688) and *Belutta-tjori-valli* (Hort. Malab. 17: 19, t. 10. 1688) and has portrayed *Cayratia trifolia* and *C. pedata* as their respective source plants. In the current practice, the former is being used as the source of the drug *aṁḷavētasa* in some parts of Kerala, (described elsewhere) while the latter is invariably taken for *gōdhāpadī.*

Cayratia pedata (*Lam.*) *Juss. ex Gagnep.* **(Vitaceae)** (Fig. 70)
Cissus pedata Lam.
Vitis pedata (Lam.) Wall. ex Wt.

Liane; branchlets densely pubescent; leaves pedately 5–7 foliolate, leaflets 7–12 × 3–6 cm, terminal one elliptic-oblong or ovate-lanceolate acuminate, laterals inequilateral, pubescent; flowers greenish in axillary corymbose panicles; calyx 4-lobed, lobes rotund; petals 4, green, ovate; disc 4-lobed, crenulate at the rim; stamens 4; ovary 2-celled, ovules 2-per cell; berry depressed globose, 2–4 seeded.

Distribution: Common in western Peninsular India, in waste lands and scrub jungles. Also reported from Sri Lanka and Malaya.

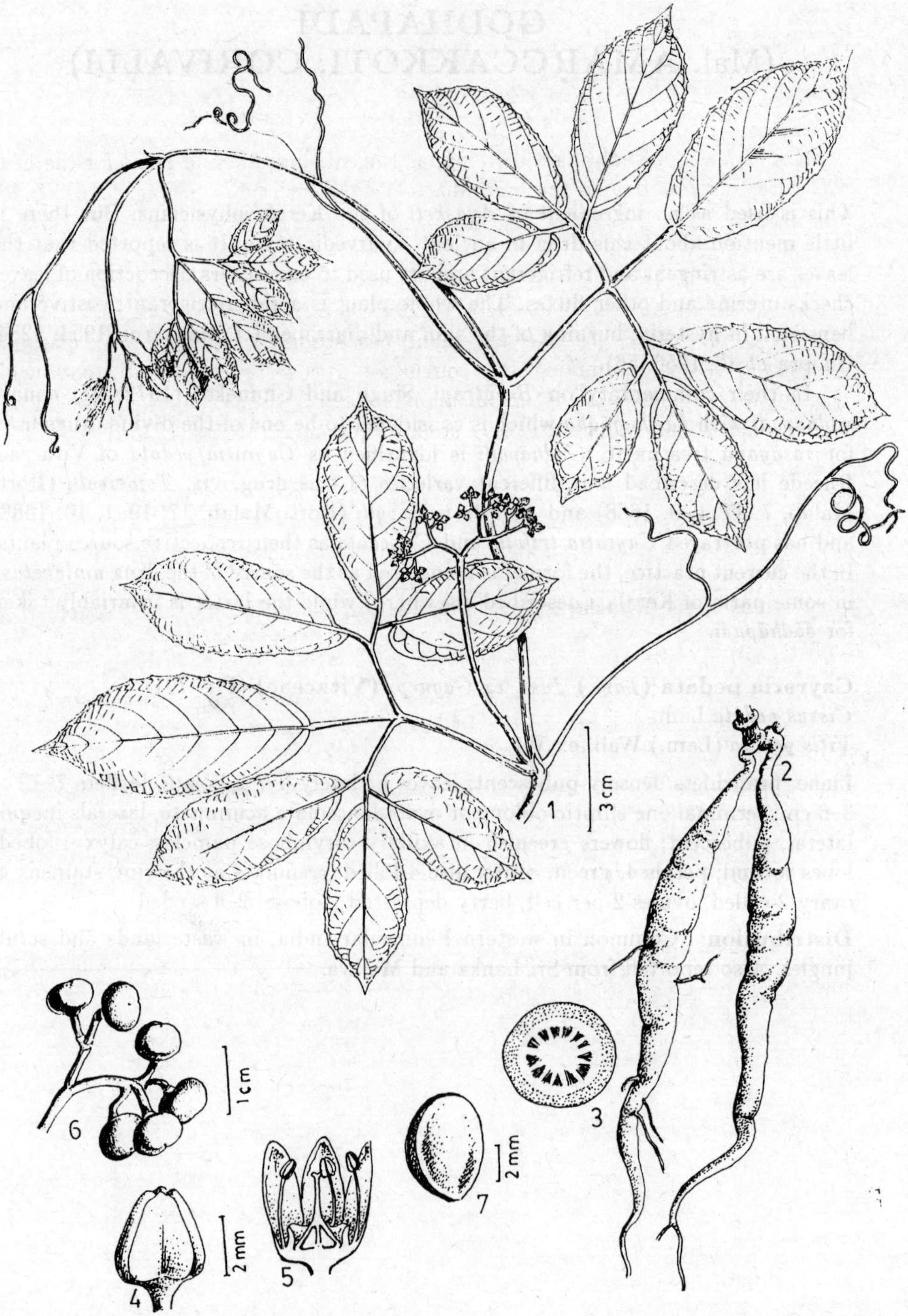

Figure 70: Cayratia pedata (Lam.) Gagnep. 1, Vine; 2, Roots; 3, Root, T.S.; 4, Flower bud; 5, Flower L.S.; 6, Fruits; 7, Seed.

GŌJIHVĀ (Mal. ĀNACCUVAṬI)

The drug is reportedly light, cooling, astringent, diuretic and good for the heart. It cures diseases due to the morbidity of *kapha* and *pitta*, cold, cough and other bronchial troubles, diabetes, hemopathy, ulcers and fever. It is also used in insomnia, mental weakness, constipation, jaundice, misperistalsis, dysuria, urethral discharges and general debility (Chunekar, 1982: 471; Sharma, 1983: 257). Root is the officinal part.

According to the texts, the plant has scabrid (*kharaparṇinī*), spathulate (*dārvikā*) leaves resembling the tongue of a cow (*gōjihvā*) and roots which resemble the tail of a jackal (*krōṣṭukamūla, sṛgālinī*). It has copper-coloured flowers (*tāmrāṁśuḥ*) and fruits borne on a stalk (*vṛntaphalā*) (Mooss, 1952: 1–6).

Ayurvedic formulary of India (Anonymous, 1978a: 247) has equated this drug with *Onosma bracteatum* Wall (Boraginaceae) and this has been supported by many (See Kapoor & Mitra, 1979: 62; Dey, 1980: 51; Vaidya Bapalal, 1982: 80; Sharma, 1983: 256). This is a well-known herb in unani medicine, where it is called *gowjaban*, also meaning the same as *gōjihva*. However, this plant restricted to the higher elevations of the Himalayas, has never been in use in Kerala as the source of the drug.

In the *Vākya-pradīpika* commentary on *Aṣṭāṅgahṛdaya* (ed. Mooss, 1950: 119–120), Parameswara has equated *gōjihvā* with the Malayalam name *ponnaṅṅāṇi*. In Kerala, *ponnaṅṅāṇi* is a synonym of *koḷuppa* (Mooss, 1952: 2) (Sans. *Lōṇikā*), the plant sources of which are discussed elsewhere in the text. None of these plants, however, compares well with the attributes provided for *gōjihvā* in the texts and hence Kerala physicians consider the two to be different drugs. The latter is equated with *Elephantopus scaber* of Asteraceae (See also Rheede, Hort. Malab. 10: 13–14. t. 7. 1690 *'Ana-schovadi'*). That this is the accepted source of the drug in most parts of India is evident from the fact that most authors on Āyurvēdic Materia Medica have equated this plant as the source of the drug (cf. Kirtikar & Basu, 1918: 672; Vaidya, K.M. 1936: 198; Nadkarni; 1954: 474; Chopra *et al.*, 1956: 105; Chunekar, 1982: 471; Vaidya Bapalal, 1982: 80).

Elephantopus scaber *Linn.* **(Asteraceae)** (Fig. 71)

Scapigerous, hirsute herb; leaves radical, oblanceolate-spathulate, 10–14 × 3.5–5 cm, scabrid-hairy on both surfaces, leaves on the scapes small, bract-like; heads compound, few-flowered, homogamous, sessile, enclosed in an involucre of 3 leafy bracts; pappus bristles long, 4–6; corolla violet, tubular, deeply 5-cleft; stamens 5, exserted, filaments filiform, anthers oblong-linear; ovary oblong; faintly ribbed, hairy, style hairy above, shortly 2-fid, recurved; achenes 10-ribbed.

Distribution: Forest undergrowth in all districts, also as a weed in waste lands in plains in India. Also reported from Sri Lanka, Burma, Indo China, Malay Peninsula, Malesia, Australia, tropical Africa.

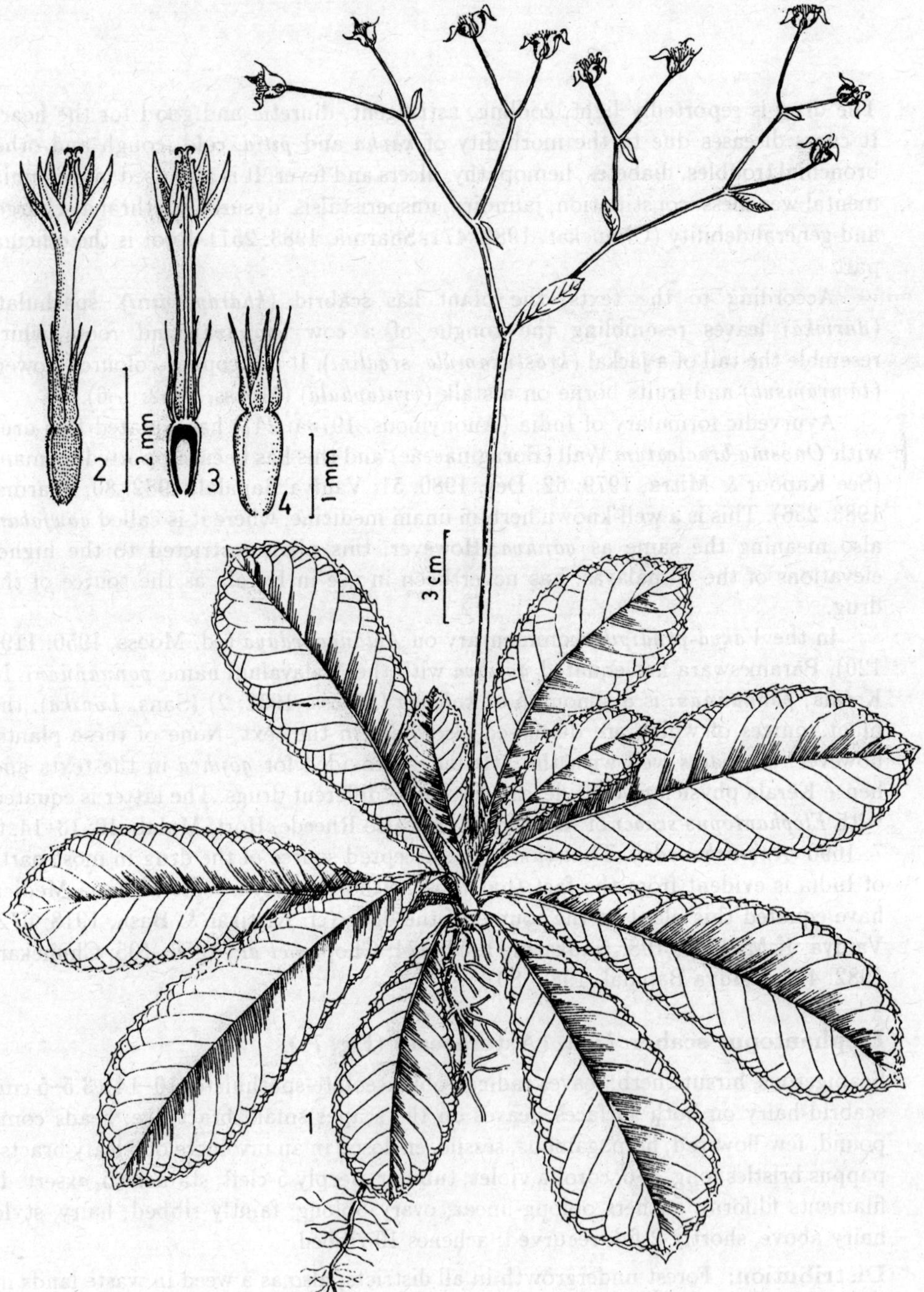

Figure 71: Elephantopus scaber L. 1, Habit; 2, Floret; 3, Floret L.S.; 4, Achene.

GŌKṢURAḤ (Mal. ÑERIÑÑIL)

This is one of the ten drugs that constitute the group *daśamūla* (ten roots). Due to the diuretic action of the fruits, it is found to be highly beneficial in renal calculus, difficult micturition, chronic cystitis and other genito-urinary disorders. It is also cooling, demulcent, tonic and aphrodisiac, promotes strength and digestive power and is useful in cough, difficult breathing, diabetes, piles, rheumatism, dropsy, burning sensation, impotence and diseases of the heart (Nadkarni, 1954: 1230; Kolammal, 1978. 2: 57). Fruit, which is the officinal part, enters into the composition of preparations like *Daśamūlāriṣṭaṃ, Bṛhatyādi kaṣāyaṃ, Himasāgaratailaṃ, Vastyāmayāntakaghṛtaṃ*, etc.

According to the description in the texts, the plant which grows wild (*vanaśṛṅgāṭaḥ*), has the smell of sugarcane (*ikṣugandhikā*) and it has spiny fruits (*gōkṣuraḥ, tṛikaṇṭaḥ, svādukaṇṭakaḥ*) resembling that of *śṛṅgāṭaka* (*Trapa bispinosa*). Two varieties are seen mentioned in the *Śāligrāma nighaṇṭu*, viz. the wild and the country type. The former is described as more erect, having yellow or white flowers, and fruits with four thorns, one at each conical portion and the latter as more prostrate with yellow flowers and fruits, having three pairs of thorns, one at each corner. (Kolammal, 1978. 2: 57). The wild form, locally called *kāṭṭu-ñeriññil*, also recognised as the large variety in *Bhāvaprakāśa nighaṇṭu*, is equated with *Pedalium murex* L. (Pedaliaceae) and the smaller variety with *Tribulus terrestris* L. (Zygophyllaceae) (Chunekar, 1982: 292, 293; Sharma, 1983: 632, 633). Though the large variety is also reported to have diuretic, tonic and aphrodisiac action, in practice, only *Tribulus terrestris* is used as the source of the drug.

The two plants can be identified as follows.

Tribulus terrestris *Linn.* **(Zygophyllaceae)** (Fig. 72)

Hirsute, prostrate herb; leaves opposite, pinnate, stipulate, leaflets 4–7 pairs, almost sessile or with very short petioles, oblong, entire, to 1.7 × 0.5 cms, villous; flowers yellow, solitary, extra axillary; sepals 5, free, linear-acute; petals 4, free, golden yellow, obovate, rounded at apex; stamens 10, inserted at the base of an annular lobed disc, filaments free; ovary sessile, hairy, 5-celled, style short, stigma 5-lobed; fruit a 5-angled, spinous, tuberulate, schizocarp, separating into 5 cocci, each with a pair of spines on them.

Distribution: The plant is distributed throughout India and also in the tropical and warm temperate regions of the world. It is a common weed of waste places and road sides, chiefly in hot, dry or sandy localities.

Note: The pharmacognosy of the roots of *T. terrestris* is studied by Ansari & Prasad (1970).

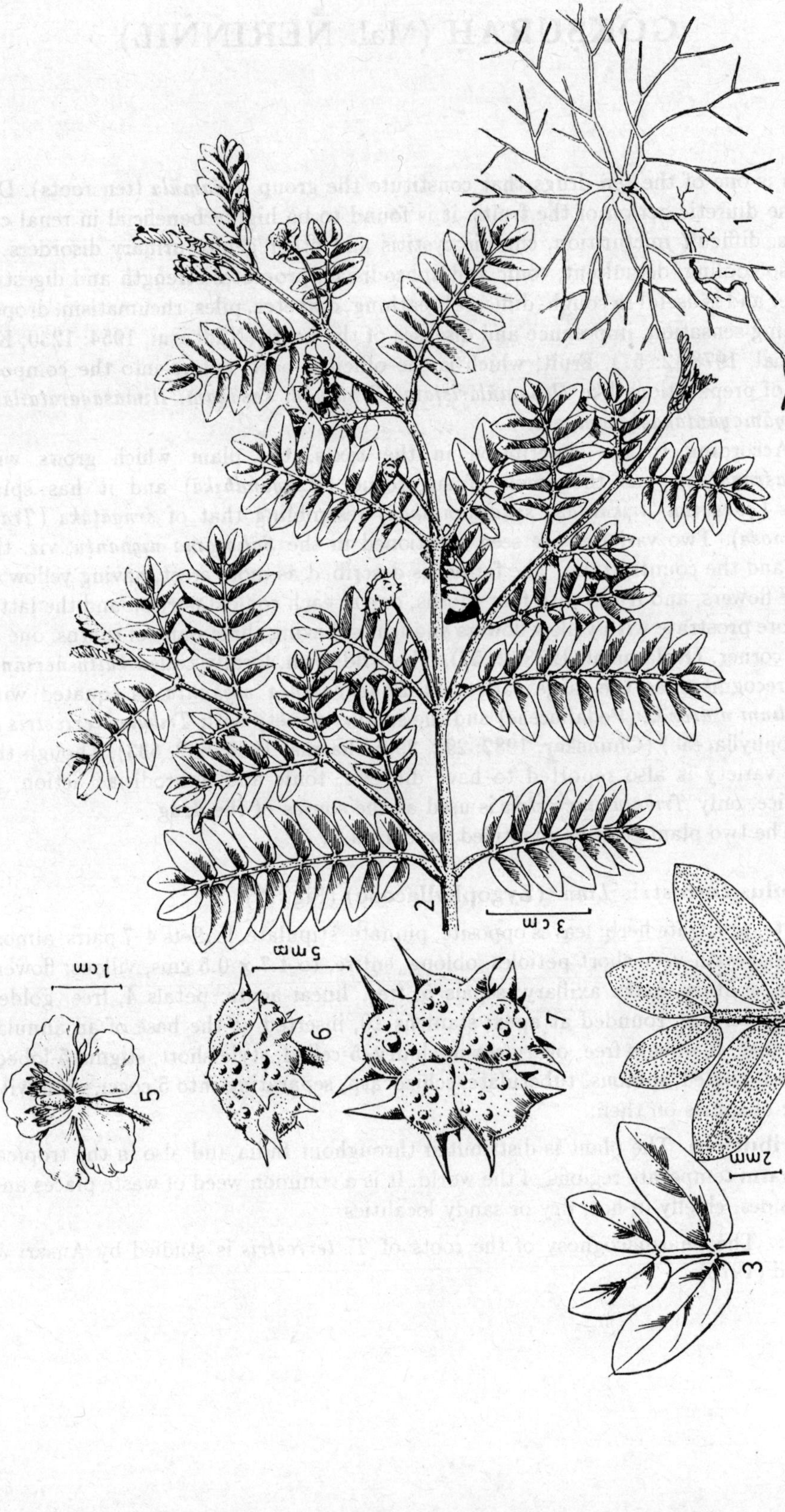

Figure 72: Tribulus terrestris L. 1, Growth habit (diagrammatic); 2, Twig; 3–4, Leaflets, front and back views; 5, Flower; 6–7, Fruits.

Pedalium murex *Linn.* **(Pedaliaceae)** (Fig. 73)

Glabrous, fleshy annuals; leaves simple, opposite, ovate-obtuse, coarsely toothed, with a pair of dark glands at the base; flowers yellow, solitary in the axils, 2.5 to 3 cms long, pedicel short; calyx 5-partite; corolla gamopetalous, lobes 5, round, spreading; stamens 4, didynamous; ovary 2-celled, style slender, stigma 2-lobed; fruits indehiscent, ovoid-obtuse, 4-sided at base with a sharp spine at each corner.

Distribution: Tropical Africa, Sri Lanka, India and Pakistan. In India it is found very commonly along the Western and Coromandel Coasts.

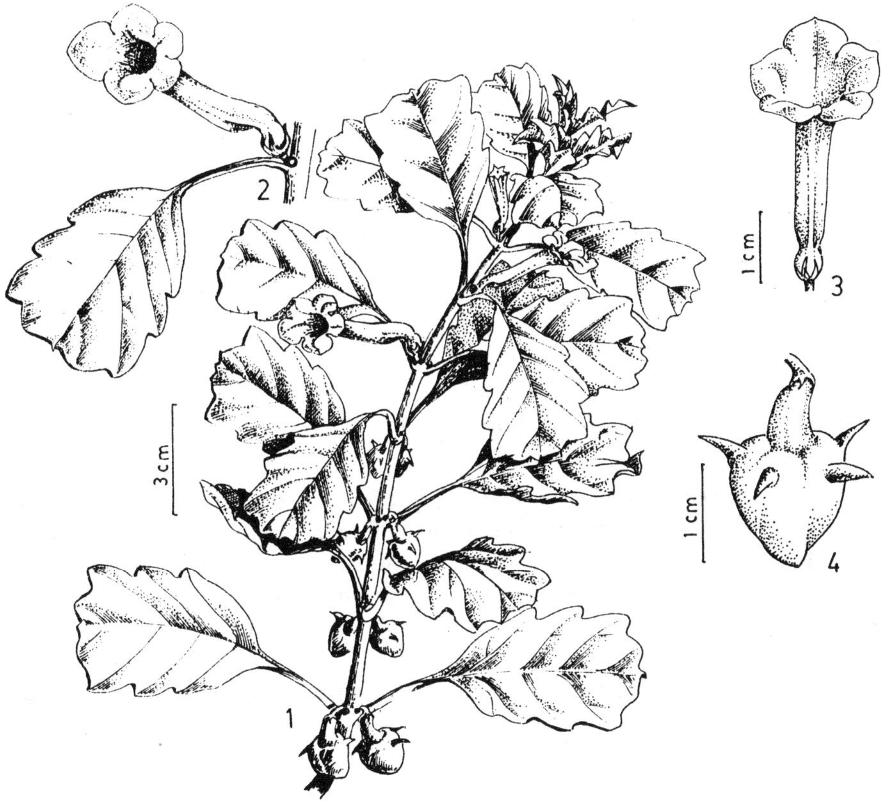

Figure 73: Pedalium murex L. 1, Twig; 2, Flower; 3, Flower, another view; 4, Fruit.

GUÑJĀ (Mal. KUNNI)

This drug seems to have been in use in Hindu medicine from very early times, as it is mentioned by Suśruta and other early Sanskrit writers. It is bitter, thermogenic, antihistaminic, antiseptic, aphrodisiac, emetic, tonic and vermifuge. *Guñjā* is beneficial for hair, cures diseases due to vitiation of *vāta* and *pitta*, fever, dryness of mouth, giddiness, difficult breathing, thirst and diseases of the eye. It improves sexual vigour and bodily strength and is useful in pruritus, ulcer, destruction of worms and similar parasites, alopacia and skin diseases (Aiyer, 1951: 35; Kurup *et al.*, 1979: 77). Roots, leaves and seeds are used medicinally. *Gōrōcanādi guḷika, Nīlībhṛṅgādi tailaṃ, Śvētaguñjādi guḷika, Abhraṃ* (101), etc. are some important preparations using the drug.

Two types of this drug are found mentioned in the texts, one with white seeds, locally called *veḷḷa-kunni* (*veḷḷa* = white) and the other with scarlet-red seeds with a black eye. Both are attributed the same properties but the latter, also called *raktaphalikā, kākaciñcī* and *kṛṣṇaraktikā* indicating the red and black colour of seeds, is considered more potent (Aiyer, 1951: 35). Both of them belong to *Abrus precatorius* of Papilionaceae, known as *kunni* in vernacular (See also Rheede, Hort. Malab. 8: 71–72. t. 39. 1688 *Konni*).

Abrus precatorius *Linn.* **(Papilionaceae)** (Fig. 74)

Perennial, wiry, twinning shrub; leaves pinnate, rachis ending in a bristle, leaflets 10–20 pairs, oblong-obtuse, mucronate, 1.5–2.5 × 0.6–0.8 cms, glabrous; flowers small, rose, clustered at the swollen nodes of rachis; calyx tube campanulate, pubescent; corolla papilionaceous, exserted; stamens 9, monadelphous; ovary subsessile, many-ovuled with short incurved style and capitate stigma; pod linear, more or less turgid, thinly septate, seeds subglobose, red with a black lateral blotch around the hilum or white.

Distribution: Throughout tropical India, Sri Lanka and Pakistan.

Note: The antifertility properties of the seeds of *Abrus precatorius* has been studied by Zia-Ul-Haque *et al.* (1983).

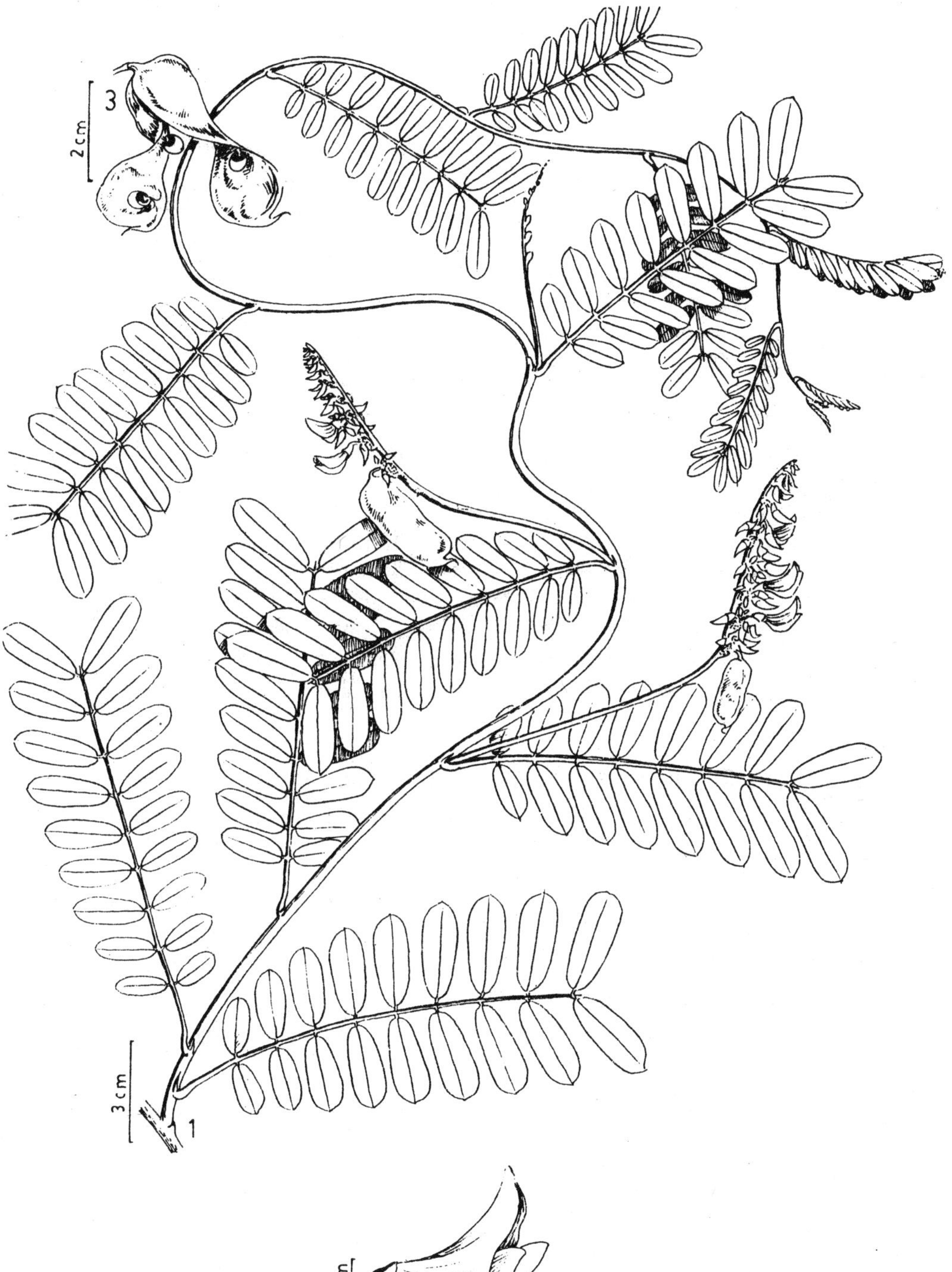

Figure 74: Abrus precatorius L. 1, Flowering branch; 2, Flower; 3, Fruit.

HALLAKAṂ (Mal. CEṄṄAḺINĪṚKIḺAṄṄU)

The drug is reportedly stomachic, anti-inflammatory and has been in popular use in the form of powder or as an ointment application to wounds and bruises to reduce swellings. A decoction of this drug is applied with much benefit to wounds with coagulated blood or purulent matter and also taken internally with the object of purifying the blood. It also improves complexion and cures burning sensation, mental disorders and insomnia (Nadkarni, 1954: 716). The officinal part is the root-tubers. *Aśōkāriṣṭaṃ, Cyavanaprāśaṃ, Kalyāṇakaghṛtaṃ, Balādhātryādi tailaṃ*, etc. are some of the preparations using the drug.

Amarakōśa attributes the synonyms ***saugandhikaṃ*** (aromatic), ***hallakaṃ*** (the flowers of which are visited by bees), ***ulpalaṃ*** and ***kalhāraṃ*** (water plant), while some others have given the names ***bhūmicaṁpaca*** and ***bhūcaṁpaca*** also to this drug. However, the names ***ulpalaṃ*** and ***kalhāraṃ*** are widely used for aquatic plants like lotus and water-lily. Moosad (1983: 233) in his commentary on *Amarakōśa*, has equated ***hallakaṃ*** with the *ceṅṅaḻinīṛkiḻaṅṅu* of Kerala physicians, which has been identified as *Kaempferia rotunda* of Zingiberaceae. This has been accepted by recent authors like Nadkarni (1954: 716) and Chopra *et al.* (1956: 147). However, Rheede (Hort. Malab. 11: 17–18. t. 9. 1692) has portrayed this species with the vernacular name *Malan-Kua* which is actually applied to *Zingiber zerumbet* of Zingiberaceae (See Nicolson *et al.*, 1988: 262). In practice, *Lagenandra toxicaria* (Araceae) is also found used as the drug source in some places.

Kaempferia rotunda *Linn.* **(Zingiberaceae)** (Fig. 75)

Herb with tuberous root-stock and several roots ending in ovoid tubers; leaves few, erect, oblong-acuminate upto 46 × 10 cms, variegated above, purplish below with white woolly hairs; flowers white with the lip purple or lilac, fragrant, on a short radical spike; bracts transparent, oblong-acute; calyx hyaline; the corolla tube 5–7 cms long, lobes 3, linear; staminodes oblong-acute, 6.5 cms long, lip 2-fid, segments suborbicular with deep purple patches; fertile stamen 1, with a 2-fid crest on the anther; ovary 3-celled, ovules many, axile.

Distribution: The plant grows wild in wet or humid shaded areas, especially in forests in southern India, also found cultivated.

Lagenandra toxicaria *Dalz.* **(Araceae)** (Fig. 76)

Marsh herb; root stock creeping; leaves long-petioled, coriaceous, oblong or elliptic-oblong obtuse or acute; spathe lanceolate, caudate-acuminate, slightly twisted, tube much shorter than the long-tailed limb; syncarp globose; carpels in many cycles; free; seeds several in each carpel, minute.

Distribution: The plant is seen in marshes in southern Concan to northern Kerala.

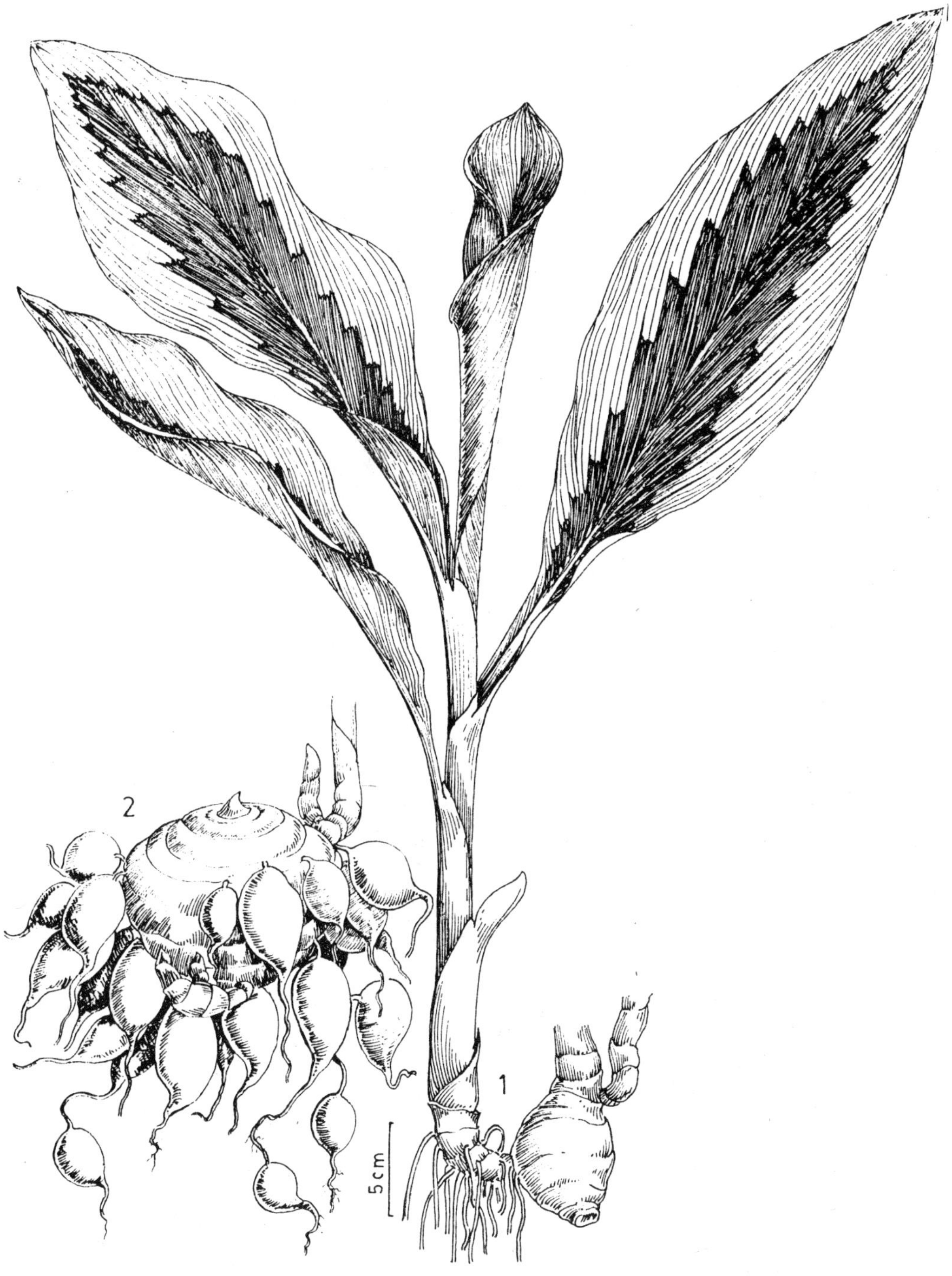

Figure 75: Kaempferia rotunda L. 1, Aerial shoot; 2, Rhizome.

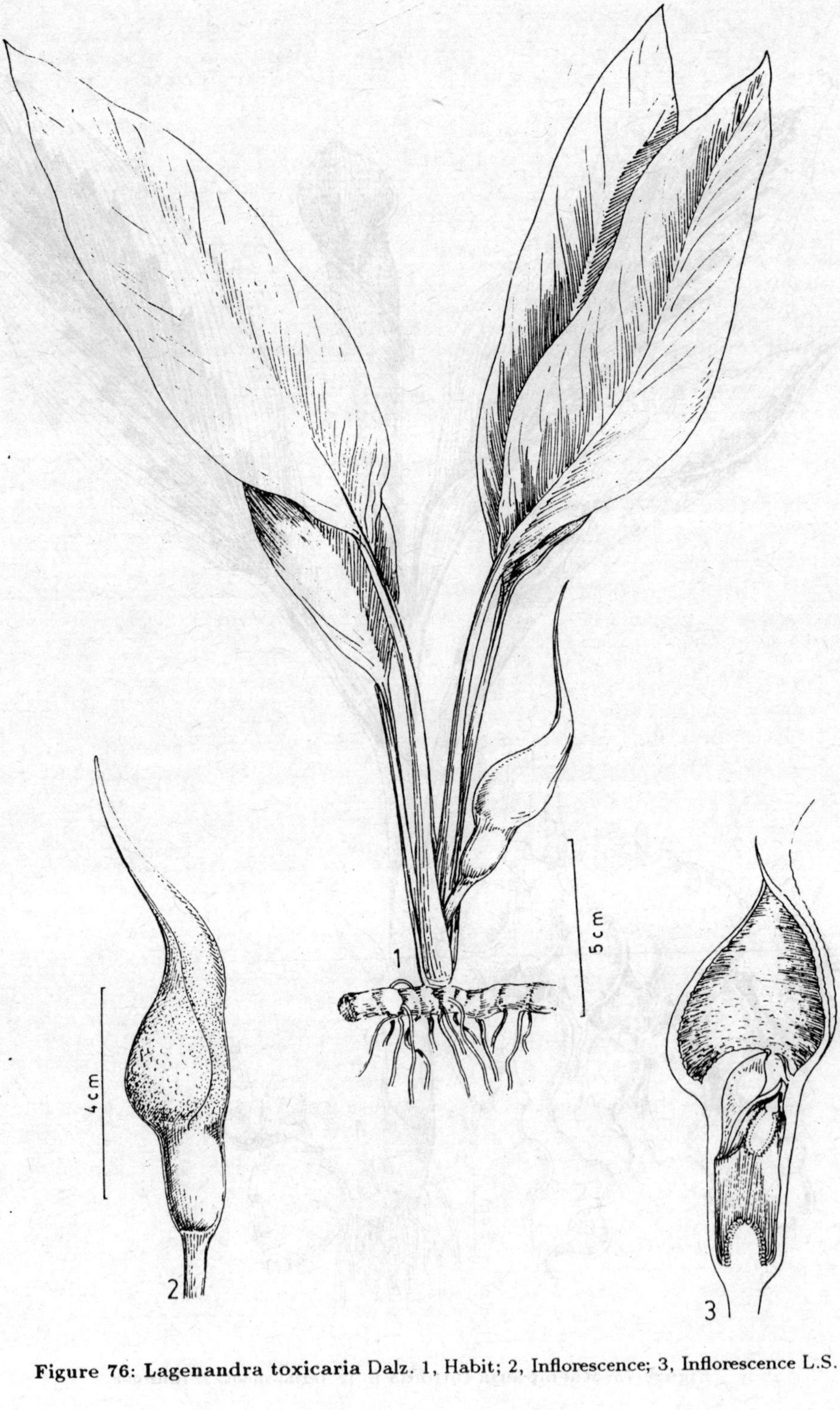

Figure 76: Lagenandra toxicaria Dalz. 1, Habit; 2, Inflorescence; 3, Inflorescence L.S.

HAṀSAPĀDĪ (Mal. NILAṀPARAṆṬA)

As the name indicates, the plant is described as one resembling the feet of swan. Vāgbhaṭa includes this drug in his *Vidāryādi gaṇa* along with 19 other drugs. The whole plant is applied externally to burns with great effect. It is also reported to be good for poisonous affections and skin diseases. Roots are considered carminative, tonic, diuretic and used in bilious complaints. Leaves, ground with cow's milk, are given to children for diarrhoea due to indigestion and also in convulsions. Juice of the fresh plant is applied to abscesses and wounds for quick healing (Nadkarni, 1954: 446; Chopra *et al.*, 1956: 94). The important preparations using the drug are *Vidāryādi ghṛtaṃ, Vidāryāsavaṃ, Mānasamitṛa vaṭakaṃ, Madhuyaṣṭyādi tailaṃ*, etc.

Most of the publications on Indian materia medica equate the drug with *Adiantum philippense* (= *Adiantum lunulatum*) of Polypodiaceae, commonly called 'maidenhair fern' (Vaidya 1936: 640; Singh & Chunekar, 1972: 463; Chunekar, 1982: 444; Sharma, 1983: 305). Rheede (Hort. Malab. 12: 72. t. 40. 1693) has portrayed this species but under a vernacular name *Avenka*. This name, however, has no currency at present and the plant is only known by the name *panna* in Kerala. Despite the fact that the pinnules (leaflets) have some resemblence to the webbed feet of swan, this common fern does not go well with its synonym '*tṛipādikā*' which probably means that the leaf is 3-segmented. In *A. philippense* leaves (fronds, as they are called in ferns) are pinnate.

The Malayalam equivalents given to this plant by Vaidya (1936: 640) are *ceṛuppuḷḷaṭi, paṇappuḷḷaṭi* and *nilaṁparaṇṭa*. Pāṭhya commentator also equates *tṛipādī* with *ceṛuppuḷḷaṭi* whereas Parameśwara considers *nilaṁparaṇṭa* as the Malayalam equivalent of *tṛipādī* (cf. Mooss, 1980: 32). In current practice, in Kerala, a small papilionaceous plant, *Desmodium triflorum* L. with trifoliate leaves (signifying the terms *tṛipādikā, haṁsapādī*, etc.) and which grows close to the ground (hence the name *nilaṁparaṇṭa*) is used as the source of the drug. The important characters of the plant are as follows.

Desmodium triflorum (*Linn.*) *DC.* **(Papilionaceae)** (Fig. 77)
Hedysarum triflorum Linn.

Prostrate or creeping slender herb; leaves alternate, trifoliate, leaflets obovate-retuse, base cuneate, margin entire, 4–8 × 4–7 mm, glabrous above, adpressed hairy beneath; flowers small, dark pink, 1–3 on axillary pedicels, calyx tube subequally 5-lobed; corolla papilionaceous; stamens diadelphous; lomentum 3–5 seeded, 1–1.5 cm long, straight on the dorsal suture, reticulate, glabrous.

Distribution: The plant is a common weed in all plains districts of India upto 3,000 ft. in hills. Also occurs in Sri Lanka, Burma, Indo-China, S. China, Hongkong, Formosa, throughout Malesia to N. Australia, New Caledonia and Polynesia.

Taxonomic Note: In the pharmacies, however, this species is often found mixed

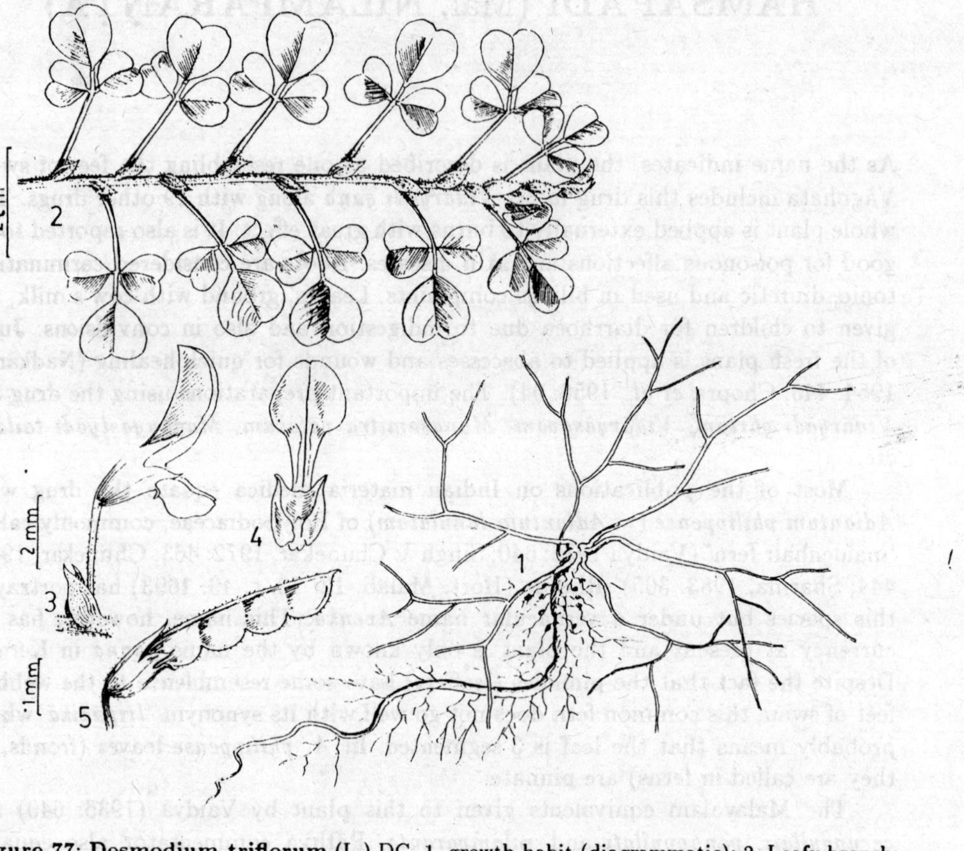

Figure 77: Desmodium triflorum (L.) DC. 1, growth habit (diagrammatic); 2, Leafy branch; 3, Flower; 4, Petal; 5, Fruit.

with another closely similar species, *Desmodium heterophyllum* which can easily be distinguished by its patently hairy stem and peduncles and much larger leaves rounded at apex.

Adiantum philippense *Linn.* **(Polypodiaceae)** (Fig. 78)
Adiantum lunulatum Burm. f.

A small, rhizomatous herb; rhizome covered with persistent leaf bases and scales; fronds simple pinnate, stipe glabrous, black, to 18 cm long; pinnae 10–15, stalked, ovate to lunate, minutely 5–8 lobed on the upper margin, each lobe bearing a transversely elongated sorus when fertile.

Commonly found in wet, shaded areas and on moist mud walls during monsoon.

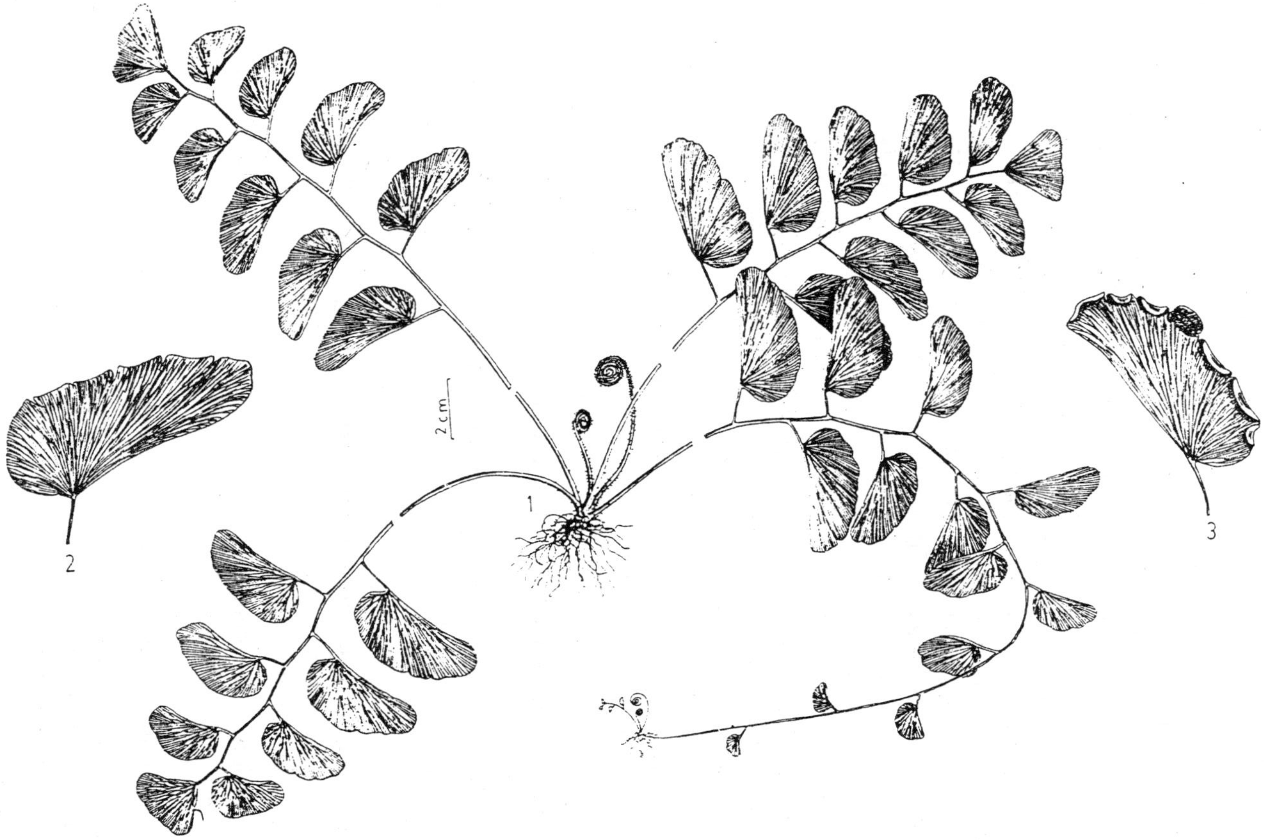

Figure 78: **Adiantum philippense** L. 1, Habit; 2, Fertile pinnule adaxial view; 3, Fertile pinnule abaxial view.

HAPUṢĀ (Mal. AṬAKKĀMAṆIYAN)

The drug is reported to be bitter, acrid, digestive, anthelmintic and alleviative of morbid *vāta* and *kapha*. It improves digestion, purifies blood and is useful in abdominal tumours, colic, indigestion, piles and hydrocele. It also cures cough, pectoral affections, diarrhoea, impotence, leucorrhoea and skin affections (Mooss, 1978; 165; Dey, 1980. 55). The whole plant forms an ingredient of preparations like *Kumāryāsavaṃ, Surasāditailaṃ, Dhānvantaraṃ ghṛtaṃ, Sukumāraṃ kaṣāyaṃ*, etc.

Most of the authors equate the drug with a gymnosperm, *Juniperus communis* L. of Pinaceae (Nadkarni, 1954: 710; Dey, 1980: 55; Chunekar, 1982: 50; Sharma, 1983: 644). But in Kerala, a different plant *Sphaeranthus indicus* L. (Asteraceae) locally known as *aṭakkāmaṇiyan* is being used as the drug source (see also Rheede, Hortus Malab, 10: 85–96, t. 43. 1690). But this plant is equated with the Sanskrit name *muṇḍī* or *muṇḍitiktā* by many of the writers (Kirtikar & Basu, 1918: 680; Nadkarni, 1954: 1162; Chopra *et al.*, 1956: 232; Chunekar, 1982: 413; Sharma, 1983: 804). Two types, *muṇḍī* and *mahāmuṇḍī* having similar properties, are described in the texts (Chunekar, 1982: 413). Mooss (1978: 160) mentions two varieties of *hapuṣā* viz. *rakta-hapuṣā* and *śvēta-hapuṣā* in his *Abhidhānamañjari*. These two are equated with the red-flowered *Sphaeranthus indicus*, and white flowered *S. africanus* by him (Mooss, 1978: 163, 160). Kerala physicians consider *hapuṣā* and *muṇḍī* to be synonymous and use *Sphaeranthus indicus* as the drug source.

Sphaeranthus indicus *Linn.* **(Asteraceae)** (Fig. 79)
S. hirtus Willd.

Much-branched, annual herb; stem winged, wings dentate; leaves alternate, subsessile, oblong-spathulate, obtuse, to 9 × 2.5 cms, lacerate or dentate, base decurrent, hirsute-pubescent, aromatic; heads globose, heterogamous, purplish pink, not rayed, outer florets female and inner bisexual. Bisexual: Corolla tubular-campanulate, 5-lobed; stamens 5, included; ovary angled, oblong. Female florets: corolla tube 2.5 mm long, minutely toothed above; ovary oblong, entire, densely hairy; achenes angular, glabrescent.

Distribution: The plant is distributed throughout the plains in India in wet places, Sri Lanka, Burma, Malesia and Australia.

Sphaeranthus africanus *Linn.* **(Asteraceae)** (Fig. 80)

Slender, glabrous, fragrant herb; branches ascending winged, wings entire; leaves obovate, denticulate, narrowed and decurrent at the bases; flowers white in globose heads; bracts rounded not imbricating; achenes small, angled, glandular.

Distribution: The plant is seen in swampy places in E. Coast, S. Canara and Malabar. Also distributed in Persia, Africa, Malay Islands, China, Philippines and Australia.

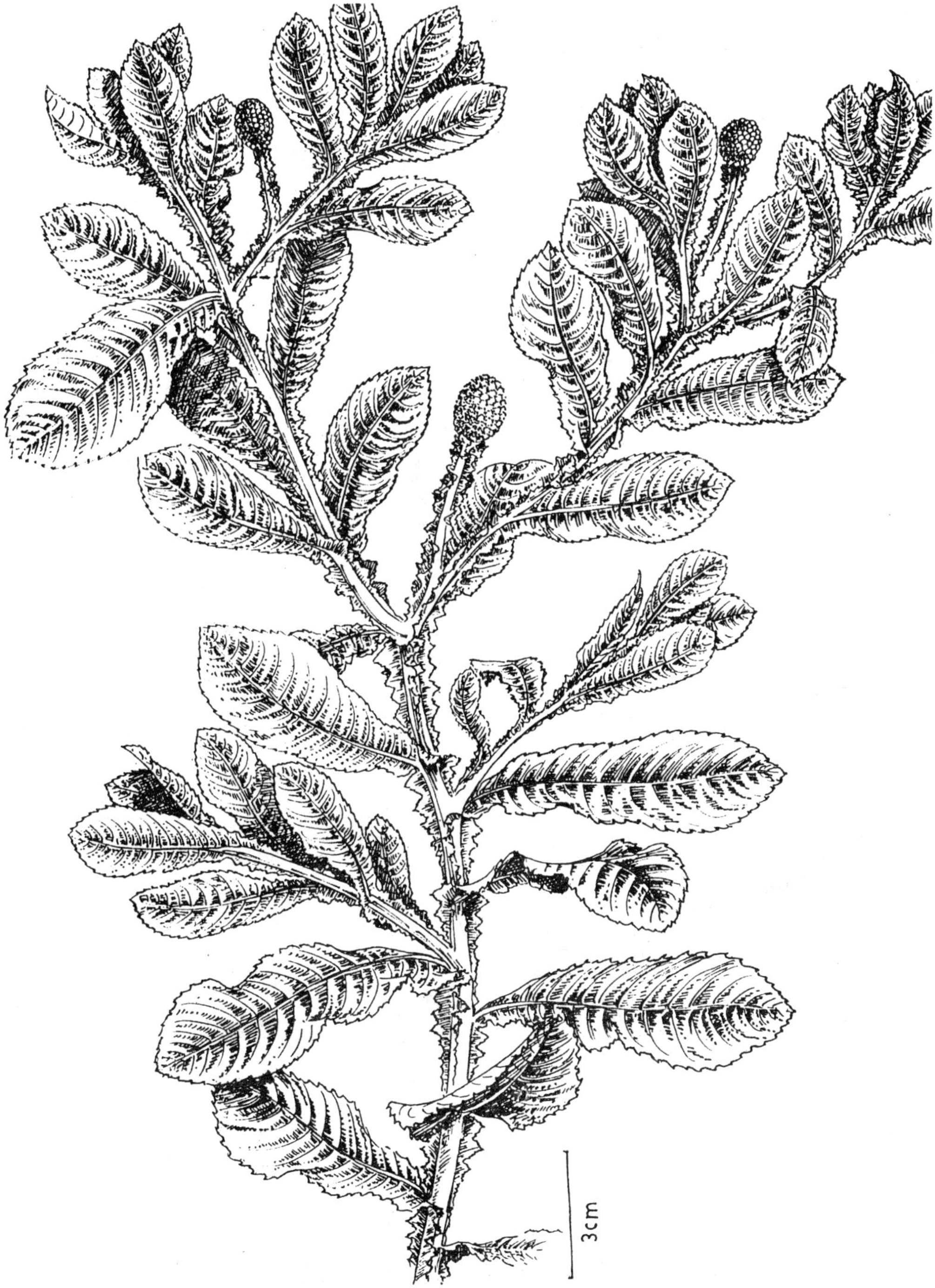

Figure 79: Sphaeranthus indicus L.

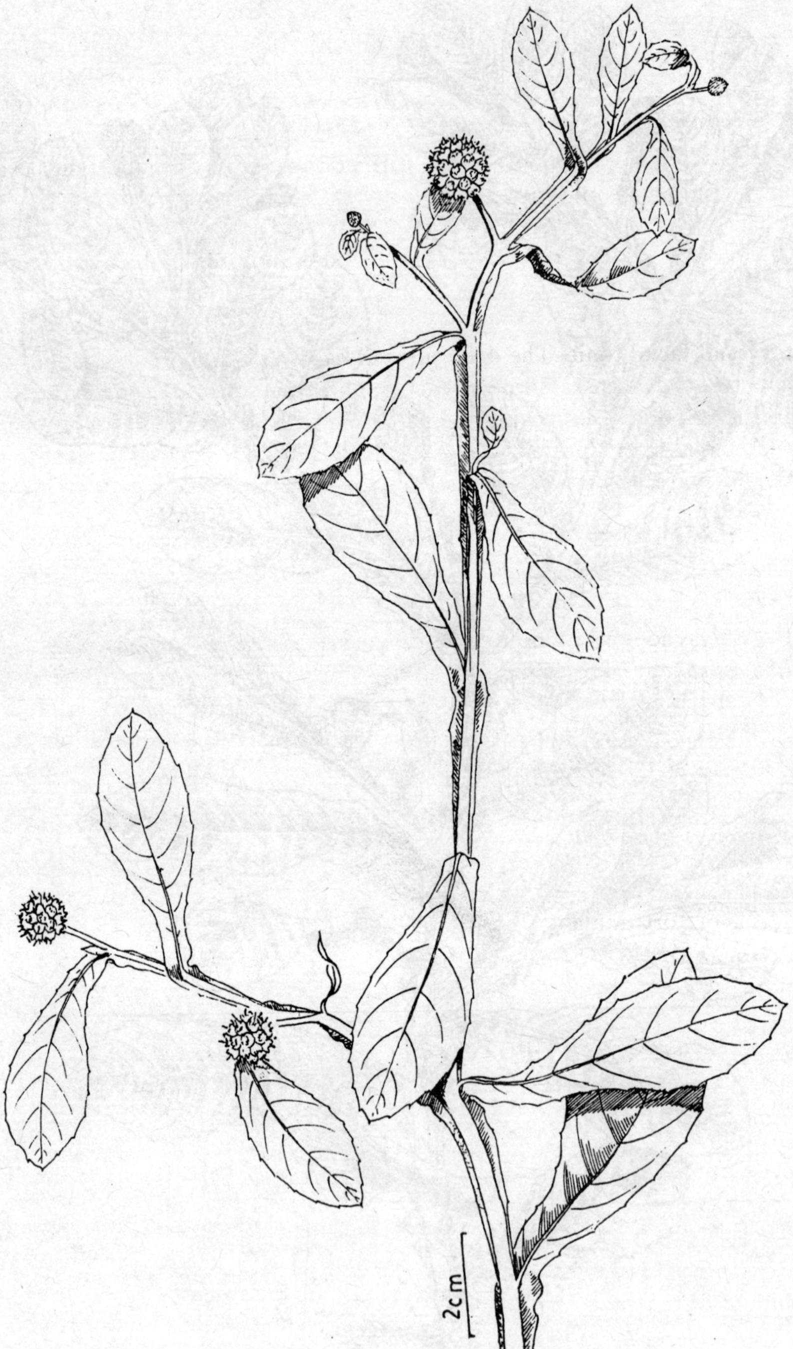

Figure 80: Sphaeranthus africanus L.

HARIDRĀ (Mal. MAÑÑAḶ)

Ethnologically *haridrā*, commonly called turmeric, occupies an important position in the life of Indian people in as much as that it foıms an integral part of the rituals, ceremonies and cuisine. Due to the strong antiseptic properties, *haridrā* has been used as a reputed remedy for all kinds of poisonous affections, ulcers and wounds. It is aromatic, alterative, antiperiodic, germicidal, carminative, stimulant, tonic and vermifuge. It gives good complexion to the skin and so applied to face as a depilatory and facial tonic. The drug cures diseases due to morbid *vāta, pitta* and *kapha*, diabetes, eye diseases, ulcers, oedema, anaemia, anorexia, leprosy and scrofula. It purifies blood by destroying the pathogenic organisms. A paste of turmeric alone, or combined with a paste of Neem (*Azadirachta indica*) leaves, is used to cure ringworm, obstinate itching, eczema and other parasitic skin diseases and also in chicken pox and small pox. The drug is also useful in cold, cough, bronchitis, conjuctivitis and liver affections (Nadkarni, 1954: 417; Kurup *et al.*, 1979: 78; Kolammal 1979: 10: 69). The rhizome is the officinal part and is an important ingredient of formulations like *Nālpāmarādi tailaṃ, Jātyādi tailaṃ, Nārāyaṇaguḷaṃ*, etc.

Most of the synonyms attributed to this drug refer to its golden yellow colour (*pītā, pītikā, suvarṇā, kāñcanī*) and its ability to impart this colour to other stuffs (*dīrgharāgā*). The names *varṇadātrī, varavarṇinī, śōbhanā, varṇavatī*, etc. indicate its ability to improve the complexion while *'kṛmighnā'* refers to its anthelmintic and antiseptic properties (of. Kolammal, 1979. 10: 68).

Two kinds of *haridrā* are mentioned in the texts. The ordinary *haridrā*, usually cultivated and the other growing wild in forests called *vanaharidrā*. In practice, however, only one *haridrā* is used which is *Curcuma longa* L. (Zingiberaceae).

Rheede has described two different plants with almost similar vernacular names, viz. *Manja-Kua* (Hort. Malab. 11. t. 10. 1692) and *Manjella Kua* (Hort. Malab. 11. t. 11. 1692). The terms *mañja* means yellow, while *mañjella* means turmeric. They are not to be confused as the former is *Beosenbergia rotunda* (Linn.) Mans. f. and the latter *Curcuma longa* Linn.

Curcuma longa *Linn.* **(Zingiberaceae)** (Fig. 81)
C. aromatica Salisb.

Aromatic, perennial, rhizomatous herb, rhizome bright yellow within, leaves oblong or oblong-lanceolate tapering to the base, caudate-acuminate at apex, 40–60 × 15–20 cms, glabrous, flowers pale yellow in bracteate, strobiliform spike arising from the centre of the leafy shoot; bracts rounded, pouched, pale green, upper ones (coma) sterile, larger and pinkish; calyx short, cylindric, corolla bright yellow; fertile stamen 1, staminodes 2, petaloid, labellum obovate, subentire, pale yellow with a deep yellow centre; ovary inferior, 3-celled, ovules many on axile placenta, style filiform, stigma two-lipped.

Distribution: The plant is found under cultivation in almost all states of India, especially in Punjab, Bengal, Bombay, Madras and Kerala.

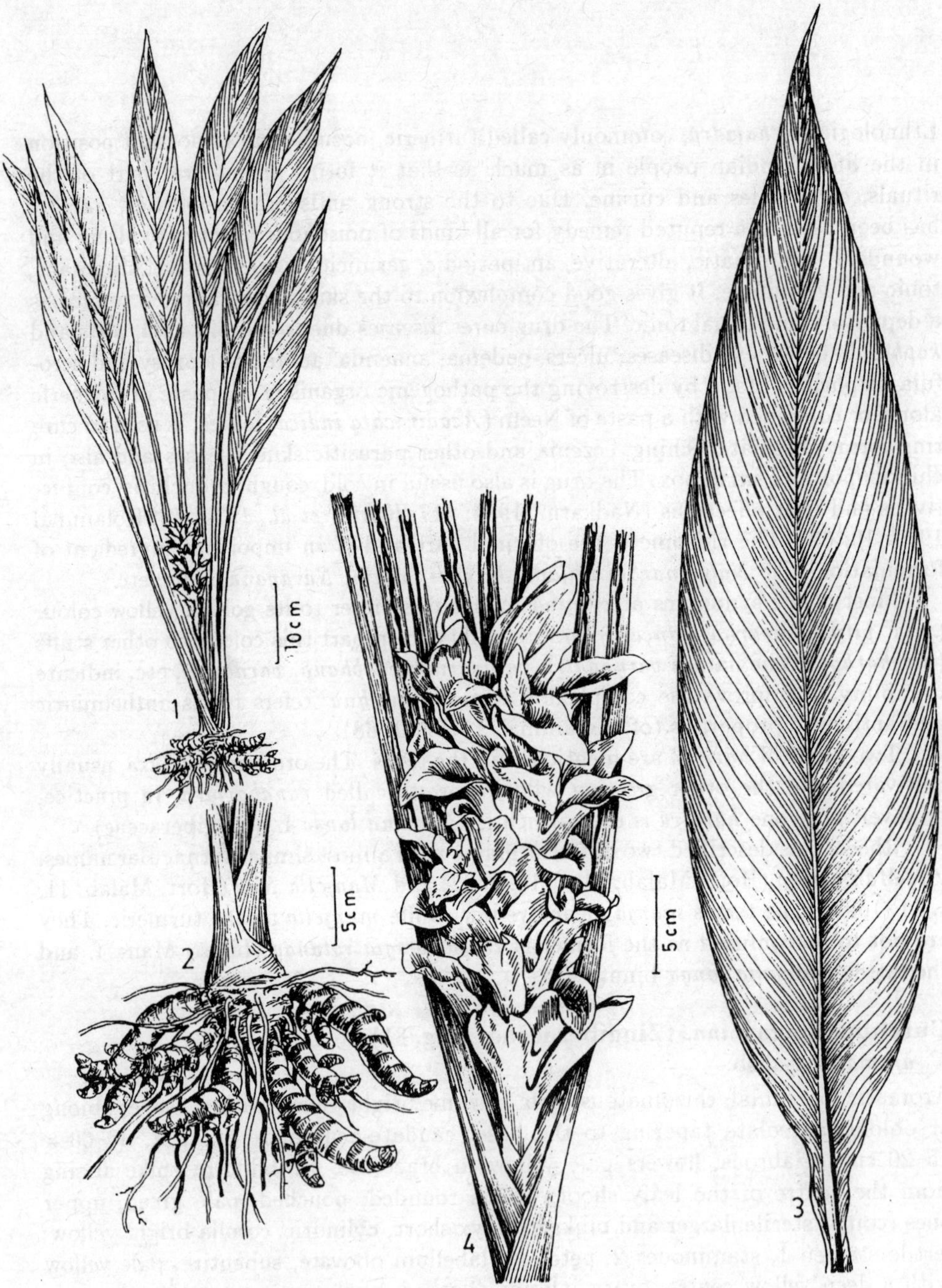

Figure 81: Curcuma longa L. 1, Habit; 2, Rhizomes; 3, Leaf; 4, Inflorescence.

Note: Oral administration of the powdered rhizomes of *Curcuma longa* had been found to produce significant relief in cases of *tamakśvāsa* (asthma) and *kāsa* (cough) (Jain *et al.*, 1979). The antirheumatic activity of curcumin, isolated from the rhizomes of *Curcuma longa*, has been clinically demonstrated in cases of rheumatoid arthritis by Deodhar *et al.* (1980). Due to the anti-inflammatory activity of curcumin, the powdered rhizomes of turmeric had been found to be effective in the treatment of sprain and inflammation (Mukhopadhyay *et al.*, 1982). Kiso *et al.* (1983) found that the rhizomes of *C. longa* exhibit intense antihepatotoxic action. Clinical and bactereological studies confirm that *C. longa* eye drops are efficacious in conjuctivitis (Srinivas & Prabhakaran 1987). Kuttan *et al.* (1987) found that an ethanol extract of turmeric and an ointment of curcumin produce remarkable relief in patients with external cancerous lesions. The pharmacognostical aspect of *C. longa* has been discussed in detail by Ahmad & Siddique (1987).

HARĪTAKĪ (Mal. KAṬUKKA)

Myrobalans, is an important group of three fruits (*triphalā*), which is widely used in Āyurvēdic medicine, since ancient times. Garcia da Orta (1563) has discussed the identity and application of this group of drugs in the ancient India, but has cautioned us that the "Mirobalanos" of the Europeans is different and it is an oil extracted from some sort of a fragrant, oily nut.

The Indian 'myrobalans' is constituted by the ripe fruits of *harītakī, vibhītakī* and *āmalakī* and is a *rasāyana* drug capable of imparting youthful vitality and receptivity of mind and sense organs.

Harītakī is astringent, light, easily assimilated, digestive, antiseptic, alterative, laxative, diuretic and carminative. It promotes digestive power, heals wounds and ulcers, cures local swellings, skin and eye diseases, diabetes, chronic and recurrent fever, anaemia, cardiac disorders, diarrhoea, dysentery, cough and dyspnoea. It dispels diseases caused by the vitiation of *vāta, pitta* and *kapha* and is useful in spleen enlargement, ascites, piles, hoarseness of voice, vomiting and blood pressure. *Harītakī* is one of the most coveted laxatives used by traditional practitioners. (Aiyer & Kolammal, 1963. 7: 99, 100; Kurup *et al.*, 1979: 80). The officinal part is the fruit-rind. The important preparations using the drug are *Abhayāriṣṭam, Triphalādi cūrṇam, Agastyarasāyanam, Daśamūlaharītakī*, etc.

While some authors are of opinion that *vijayā, rōhiṇī, pūtanā, amṛtā, abhayā, jīvantī* and *cētakī* represent seven different varieties of *harītakī*, an overwhelming number of them consider these names to be synonyms of the latter. Nor is this distinction in vogue in the current practice. All these names are indicative of the therapeutic value of the drug.

This drug, has universally been equated with *Terminalia chebula* Retz. of Combretaceae, known as *kaṭukka* in vernacular, and is widely used in Indian medicine. In Kerala, however, there are two varieties of the drug recognised, called *kaṭukka* and *kuruvillā kaṭukka* respectively in the vernacular, the latter being either tender or pathogenetic seedless fruits of the same species (see also Aiyer & Kolammal, 1963. 7: 98–99).

Terminalia chebula *Retz.* **(Combretaceae)** (Fig. 82)
Myrobalanus chebula (Retz.) Gaertner

Tree; branchlets rusty villous; leaves simple, opposite or sub-opposite, short-petioled, ovate-elliptic or obovate, acute or obtuse, entire, glabrous, 8–13 × 4–6.5 cm, thinly coriaceous; flowers small, cream-coloured in axillary spikes; calyx tube villous, lobes 5, petals absent; stamens 10, ovary 1-celled, fruit a glabrous obovoid or ellipsoidal drupe, 4 × 2.5 cm, faintly 5 angled.

Distribution: The plant is found throughout India chiefly in deciduous forests, on dry slopes upto 3,000 ft. The plant is also reported in Sri Lanka, Nepal and Burma.

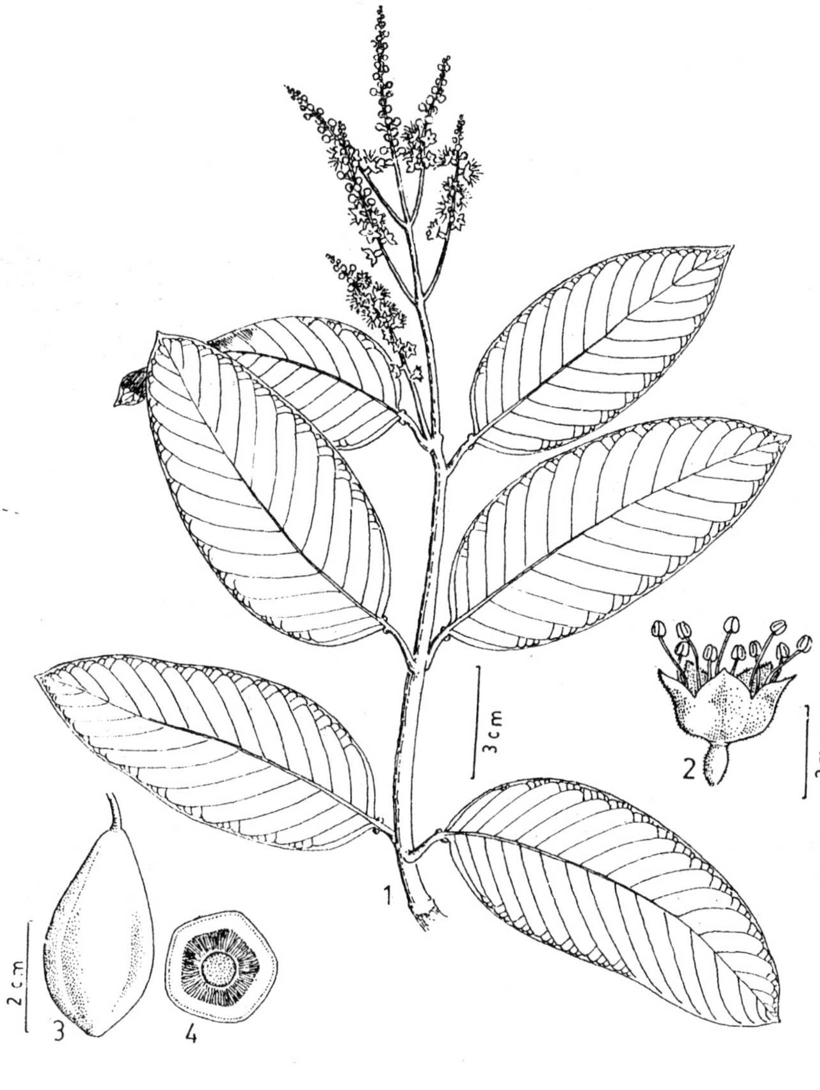

Figure 82: Terminalia chebula Retz. 1, Flowering twig; 2, Flower; 3, Fruit; 4, Fruit C.S.

Note: *Terminalia chebula* has been found to be effective in the treatment of simple constipation (Tripathi *et al.*, 1983).

IKṢUḤ (Mal. KARIṀPU)

This is one of the five ingredients of the group *tṛṇapañcamūla* i.e. roots of five grasses and it enters into the formulations like *Balātailaṃ, Dhātṛyādighṛtaṃ, Balājīrakādi kaṣāyaṃ, Amṛtaprāśaghṛtaṃ, Kūśmāṇḍakaghṛtaṃ*, etc. Along with other seventeen drugs, *ikṣuḥ* constitutes the *Śyāmādi gaṇa* of Vāgbhaṭa which cures *gulma*, effect of poison, anorexia, disorders of *kapha*, dysuria, etc. (Mooss, 1980: 114).

Ikṣuḥ is cooling, sweet, restorative, aphrodisiac, diuretic, laxative and is used in general debility, haemophilic conditions, impotence, jaundice and urinary diseases. It overcomes diseases due to the morbidity of *vāta* and *pitta*, cough, asthma, *raktapitta* and cardiac problems. Fresh juice and root are used in medicine. (Kurup *et al.*, 1979: 82; Sharma, 1983: 639). The source plant abounding in sweet juice (*rasālaḥ*) has been equated with *Saccharum officinarum* L., the common sugarcane, of Poaceae, throughout the country.

Saccharum officinarum *Linn.* **(Poaceae)** (Fig. 83)

Tall, stout perennial herb, culms jointed and leafy, upto 6 m high; leaves linear-lanceolate, acuminate, upto 1.5 m long and 5 cms wide, margins scabrid; flowers minute in large, white silky terminal panicles, spikelets surrounded by long silky hairs; florets 2; glumes 2, equal, often chartaceous below, membranous to hyaline upwards; lemma hyaline, the lower empty; lodicules 2; stamens 3; styles 2.

Distribution: Cultivated in the hotter parts of India.

Note: Takahashi *et al.* (1986) have proved that the six glycans A, B, C, D, E and F yielded from the non-sucrose portion of the stalks of *Saccharum officinarum* exert remarkable hypoglycaemic action in normal and alloxan-produced hyperglycaemic mice.

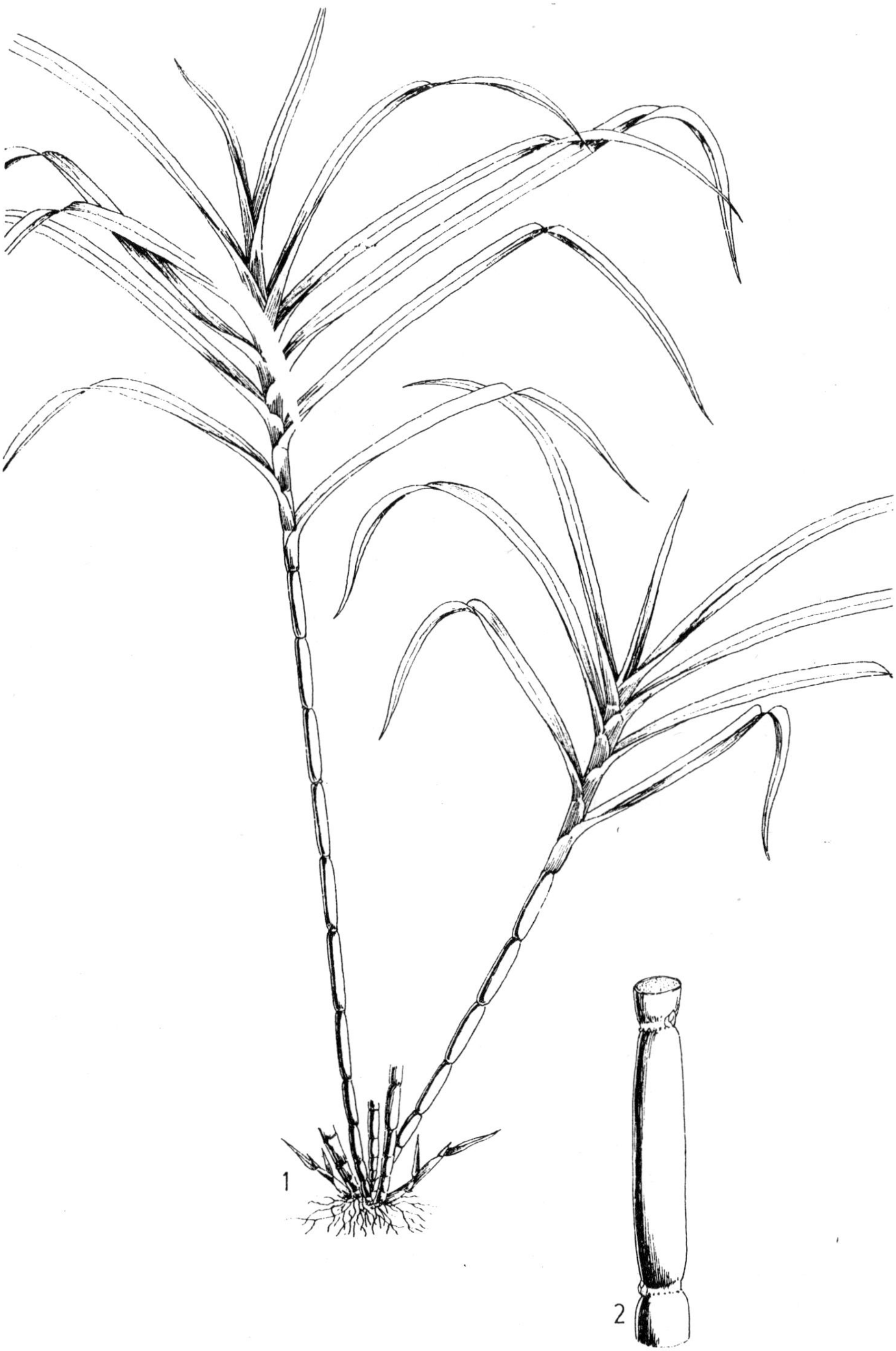

Figure 83: **Saccharum officinarum** L. 1, Habit; 2, Portion of stem.

IKṢVĀKUḤ (Mal. KAIPPANCURA)

This is one of the twenty-two emetic drugs which constitute the *Madanādi gaṇa* of Vāgbhaṭa. Due to the emetic property, the drug is particularly indicated in overcoming diseases caused by the morbidity of *kapha* and *pitta*. The fruit is bitter, hot, acrid, cooling, cardiotonic and emetic. It cures oedema, pain, ulcers, cough, asthma and other bronchial disorders, fever and poison. The roots and leaves are also emetic. Leaves are recommended for jaundice. Ashes of the bitter fruit mixed with honey, applied to eyes, cures nightblindness (Nadkarni, 1954: 722; Menon, 1976: 480–482) *Kaccōrādi tailaṃ* and *Pārantyādi* coconut oil are some of the important preparations using the drug.

Except for its extreme bitterness, which makes even sugarcane tasteless (hence the name, *ikṣuākuḥ, ikṣuḥ* = sugarcane), references in the texts, do not give us any other indication of the nature of the plant (cf. Moossad 1983: 384).

Two varieties of this drug, sweet and bitter, are mentioned in the texts, the former known by the Sanskrit synonyms *ālābu* and *tuṁbī* and the latter by names like *ikṣuāku, kaṭutuṁbī, mahāphalā*, etc. The sweet variety is generally used as a vegetable, while the bitter wild variety is preferred in medicine. *Lagenaria siceraria* belonging to Cucurbitaceae, known as bottle-gourd in English is the botanical source of the drug.

Lagenaria siceraria (*Molina*) *Standley* **(Cucurbitaceae)** (Fig. 84)
L. vulgaris Seringe

Large tendril-climber; branchlets densely hirsute, tendrils 2-fid; leaves large, orbicular, 3–5 angled or lobed, 7–10 × 10–12 cm, hirsute; flowers white, solitary, axillary, unisexual. Male flowers: calyx campanulate, tube narrow, lobes 5, linear; petals 5, free, white; stamens 3. Female flowers: calyx and corolla as in male; ovary densely villous, style thick, stigmas 3, bilobed; fruit bottle-shaped with a hard shell-like epicarp and numerous seeds.

Distribution: The plant is distributed in tropical Africa and Asia. This is widely cultivated in all warmer regions as a vegetable.

Rheede has portrayed two varieties of *cura* namely *Bela-Schora* (Hort. Malab. 8: 1–2 t. 1. 1688) and *Caipa-Schora* (Hort. Malab. 8: 9. t. 5. 1688). The former is the variety cultivated widely for its fruits and used as a vegetable. The latter is found wild in some areas of Kerala and has bitter fruits. Botanically both belong to the same species, but in medicine, it is the latter which is preferred. Nevertheless, because of the difficulty in procuring the wild variety, the edible variety is now being used in medicine as well.

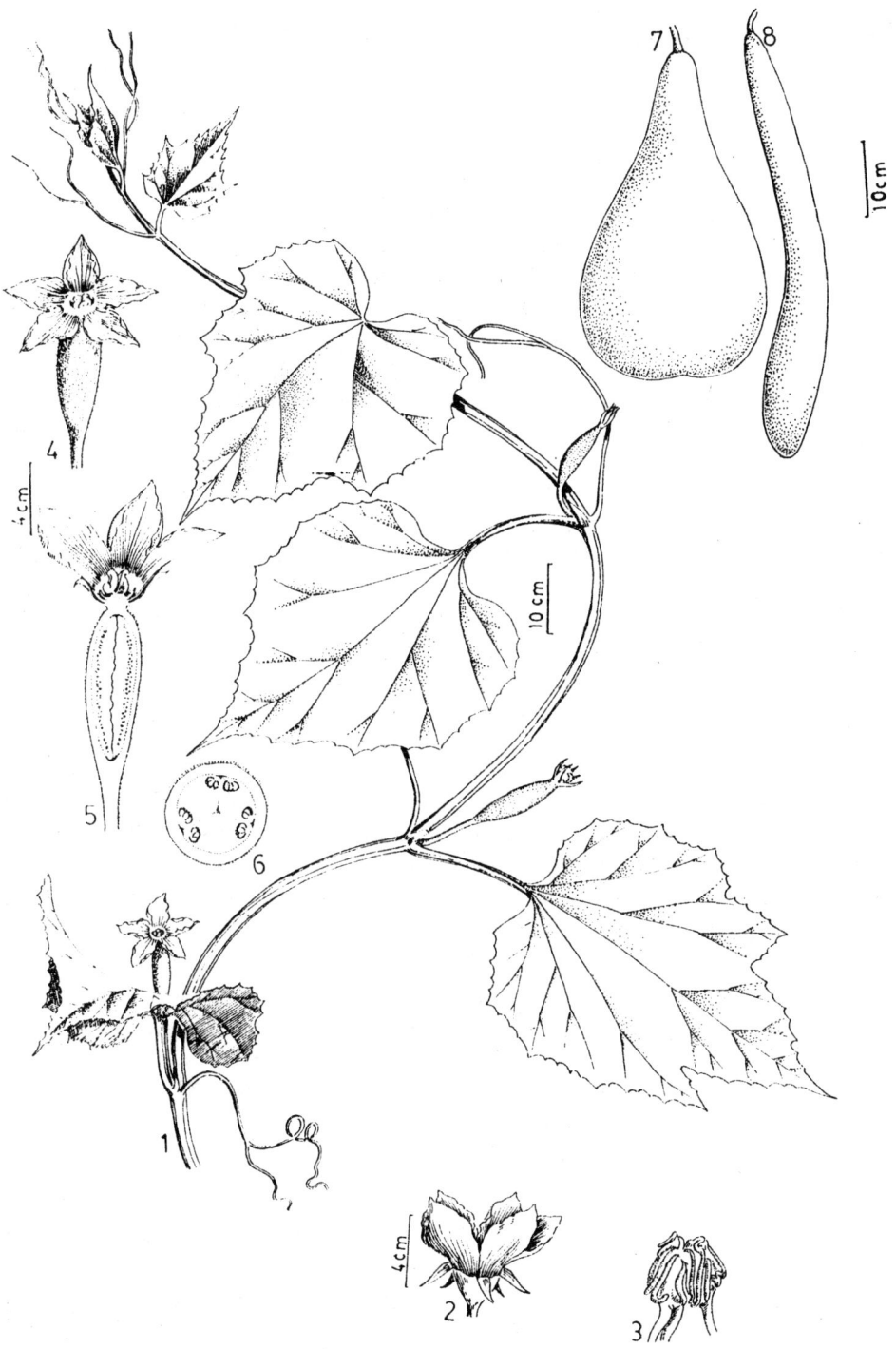

Figure 84: Lagenaria siceraria (Molina) Standley. 1, Habit; 2, Male flower; 3, Stamens; 4, Female flower; 5, Female flower L.S.; 6, Ovary, T.S.; 7–8, Fruits.

INDRAVALLĪ (Mal. UḶIÑÑA)

This is one of the ten auspicious herbs that constitute the group *Daśapuṣpaṃ*. The entire plant is used in medicine. Root and leaves are diuretic, laxative, stomachic and alterative. It is good for hair growth and is useful in rheumatism, nervous diseases, piles, chronic bronchitis, fevers, hydrocele, amenorrhoea, sprains and oedema. Juice of the plant is dropped into the ear in earache (Nadkarni, 1954: 272; Aiyer & Kolammal, 1963. 6: 21). *Nīlībhṛṅgādi tailaṃ, Āṛukālādi tailaṃ*, etc. are some of the preparations using the drug.

There is no mention about this drug in the classical Āyurvēdic texts. Kerala physicians however use this widely and this is equated with *Cardiospermum halicacabum* Linn. of Sapinadaceae, locally called *uḷiñña*, as the drug source (see Rheede, Hort. Malab. 8: 53–54, t. 28. 1688).

Cardiospermum halicacabum *Linn.* **(Sapindaceae)** (Fig. 85)

Annual scrambling shrubs climbing by means of tendrillar hooks; stem and branches wiry and furrowed; leaves alternate, exstipulate, biternate; leaflets deeply dentate or lobed, acute at tip upto 6 × 3 cms, glabrous; flowers small, white, polygamous on axillary long peduncles; sepals 4, greenish, rounded, the outer pair smaller, the inner larger; petals 4, free, rounded or oblong, slightly tapering towards the base, the upper pair partially adnate to the sepals and provided with an emarginate suprabasal scale, the lower pairs smaller, each furnished with a small glandular yellow scale; stamens 8, filaments unequal; pistil tricarpellary, syncarpous; ovary three angular, 3-chambered with one ovule in each, style very short, 3-fid; fruit an inflated trigonous 3-valved capsule; seeds globose, black.

Distribution: The plant is found throughout India, mainly in N. Çircars, Carnatic, the Coromandel and West Coast. It is a very common plant of waste places found scrambling over hedges etc.

Note: *Cardiospermum halicacabum* has been found to exhibit significant diuretic (Santhakumari *et al.*, 1981) and anti-inflammatory activity (Chandra and Sadique, 1984). The plant also shows sedative effect on central nervous system, significant analgesic, vaso depressant and anti-spasmodic effects (Pillai, NR & Vijayamma, 1985).

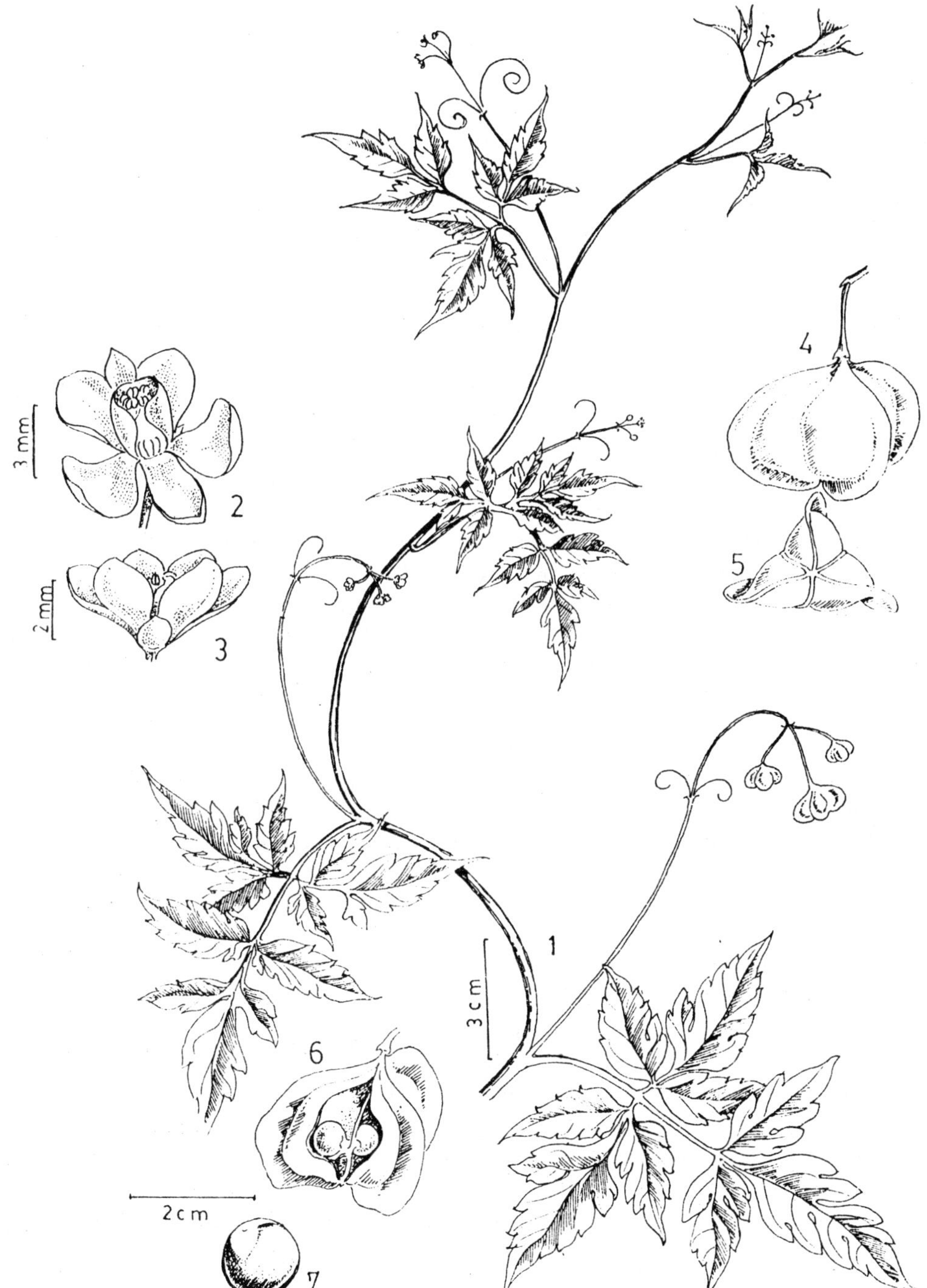

Figure 85: Cardiospermum halicacabum L. 1, Habit; 2–3, Flowers; 4–6, Fruits; 7, Seed.

INDRAVĀRUṆĪ (Mal. KĀṬṬUVEḶḶARI)

The drug *indravāruṇī* (the name signifying its efficacy against a wide variety of ailments) derived from a trailing plant (*gavākṣī, gōtuṁbā*) with fanciful multi-coloured fruits (*citṛā*), is reported to be light, bitter, hot, abortifacient, purgative, blood purifier and cathartic. The fruit is useful in ascites, biliousness, jaundice, cerebral conjestion, colic, constipation, dropsy, fever, worms and sciatica. Root is given in cases of abdominal enlargement, cough, asthma, inflammation of the breast, ulcers, urinary diseases and rheumatism. Oil from seeds is used for poisonous bites, bowel complaints, epilepsy and also for blackening the hair (Nadkarni, 1954: 337; Dey, 1980; 60). The important formulations using the root and fruit are *Abhayāriṣṭam, Mahātiktakaṃ kaṣāyaṃ, Mānasamitṛavaṭakaṃ, Cavikāsavaṃ, Madhuyaṣṭyādi tailaṃ*, etc.

There are two varieties of this drug mentioned in the texts, viz. a smaller variety called *indravāruṇī* with smaller fruits and a large variety (also called *viśālā*) with larger fruits (*mahāphalā*). The smaller variety has been unanimously identified as *Citrullus colocynthis* of Cucurbitaceae (see Kirtikar & Basu, 1918: 598; Vaidya, K.M. 1936; 59; Nadkarni, 1954; 335; Kapoor & Mitra, 1979: 63; Anonymous, 1978a; 243; Dey, 1980; 59; Chunekar, 1982: 403; Sharma, 1983: 436), known as *ceṛiya kāṭṭuveḷḷari* in vernacular. But, there is some confusion with regard to the identity of the latter. Some of the authors have identified it as *Cucumis trigonus* (See Kaitikar & Basu, 1918: 578; Nadkarni, 1954: 405; Chopra *et al.*, 1956: 83) while others have equated it with *Trichosanthes palmata* (now *T. tricuspidata*) (See Vaidya, K.M. 1936: 525; Chunekar, 1982; 405; Sharma, 1983: 436), both belonging to Cucurbitaceae.

In Kerala, however, *T. tricuspidata* is being used as the source of a different drug *kākatiktā*, locally called *kākkattoṇḍi*. Moreover, the varietal distinction is not in vogue here and both *Citrullus colocynthis* and *Cucumis callosus* are used as the drug source. The important characters of these plants are described below.

Citrullus colocynthis (*Linn.*) *Schrad.* **(Cucurbitaceae)** (Fig. 86)
Cucumis colocynthis Linn.

Trailing scabrid herb; branchlets hirsute; leaves ovate or narrowly triangular, 6–10 × 4–7 cm, deeply 3–5 lobed, lobes sometimes pinnatified, densely villous hirsute below; flowers yellow, axillary, solitary, unisexual. Male: Calyx campanulate, 5-lobed, hirsute without; petals ovate, hirsute; stamens 3. Female: Calyx and corolla as in male; fruit globose, 5–7 cm in diameter, striped green and white when young, yellow when ripe; seeds ovoid.

Distribution: Tropical and subtropical N. Africa and Asia. In India, the plant is seen in Deccan, on dry sandy or rocky lands.

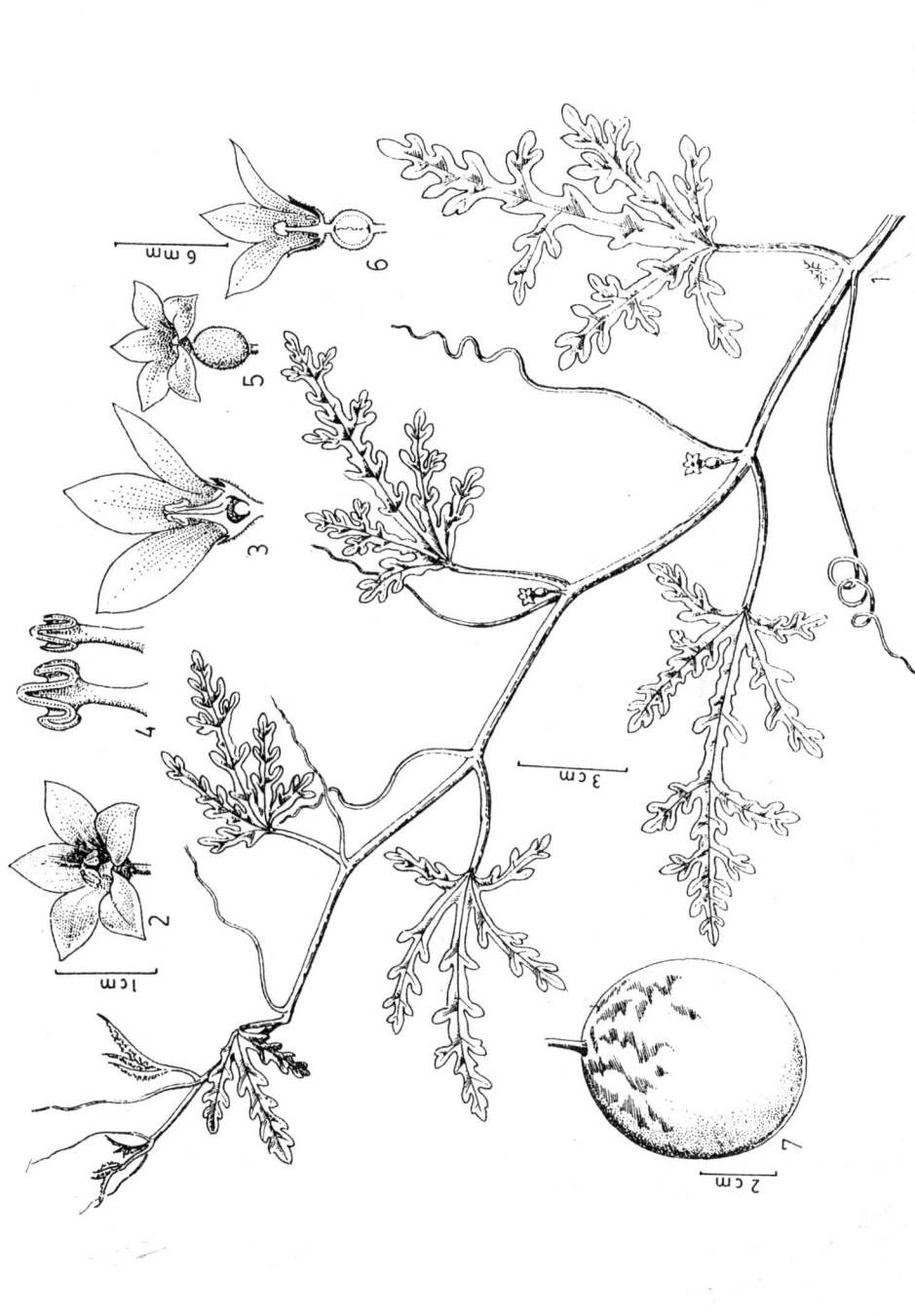

Figure 86: **Citrullus colocynthis** (L.) Schrad. 1, Habit; 2, Male flower; 3, Male flower L.S.; 4, Stamens; 5, Female flower; 6, Female flower L.S.; 7, Fruit.

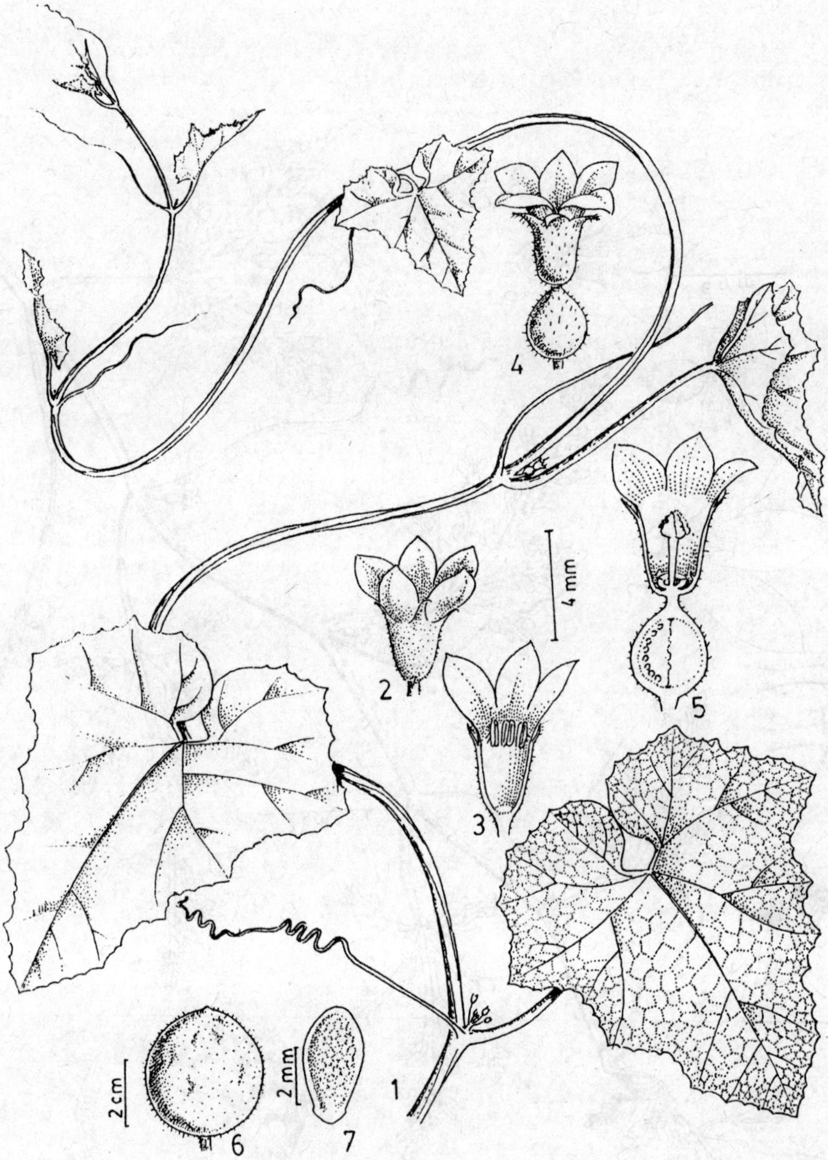

Figure 87: **Cucumis callosus** (Rottl.) Cogn. 1, Habit; 2, Male Flower; 3, Male flower L.S.; 4, Female flower; 5, Female flower L.S.; 6, Fruit; 7, Seed.

Cucumis callosus (*Rottl.*) *Cogn.* **(Cucurbitaceae)** (Fig. 87)
Cucuminus trigonus (Roxb.)

Trailing herbs; branchlets hispid; leaves suborbicular, deeply 5-lobed, 3–4.5 × 2.5–3.5 cm, chartaceous, hispid, obovate. Male flowers in axillary few-flowered clusters, yellow: calyx hirsute, lobes linear; petals obovate, hirsute without; stamens

3, anthers flexuous, connectives apically prolonged, pistillode globose, 3-fid. Female: Calyx and corolla as in male; fruit smooth, globose, to 5 cm in diam. with green and white streaks.

Distribution: Peninsular India. Seen in Deccan and Karnatic; in dry districts.

Trichosanthes tricuspidata *Lour.* **(Cucurbitaceae)** (Fig. 88)
T. bracteata (Lam.) J. Voight.
T. palmata Roxb.

Large climbers; leaves polymorphous, ovate or suborbicular, cordate, palmately lobed, lobes oblong or ovate-elliptic, 10–15 × 9.5–12 cm, scabrous. Male racemes with large laciniate bracts; calyx glabrous, lobes lanceolate; corolla white; petals ovate, ovate-lanceolate; stamens 3, anthers ciliate, connectives slightly produced at the apex. Female, solitary, ebracteate; calyx lobes lanceolate; petals laciniate, involute in bud; fruit globose, red when ripe.

Distribution: Peninsular India, China, Japan, Malesia and tropical Australia.

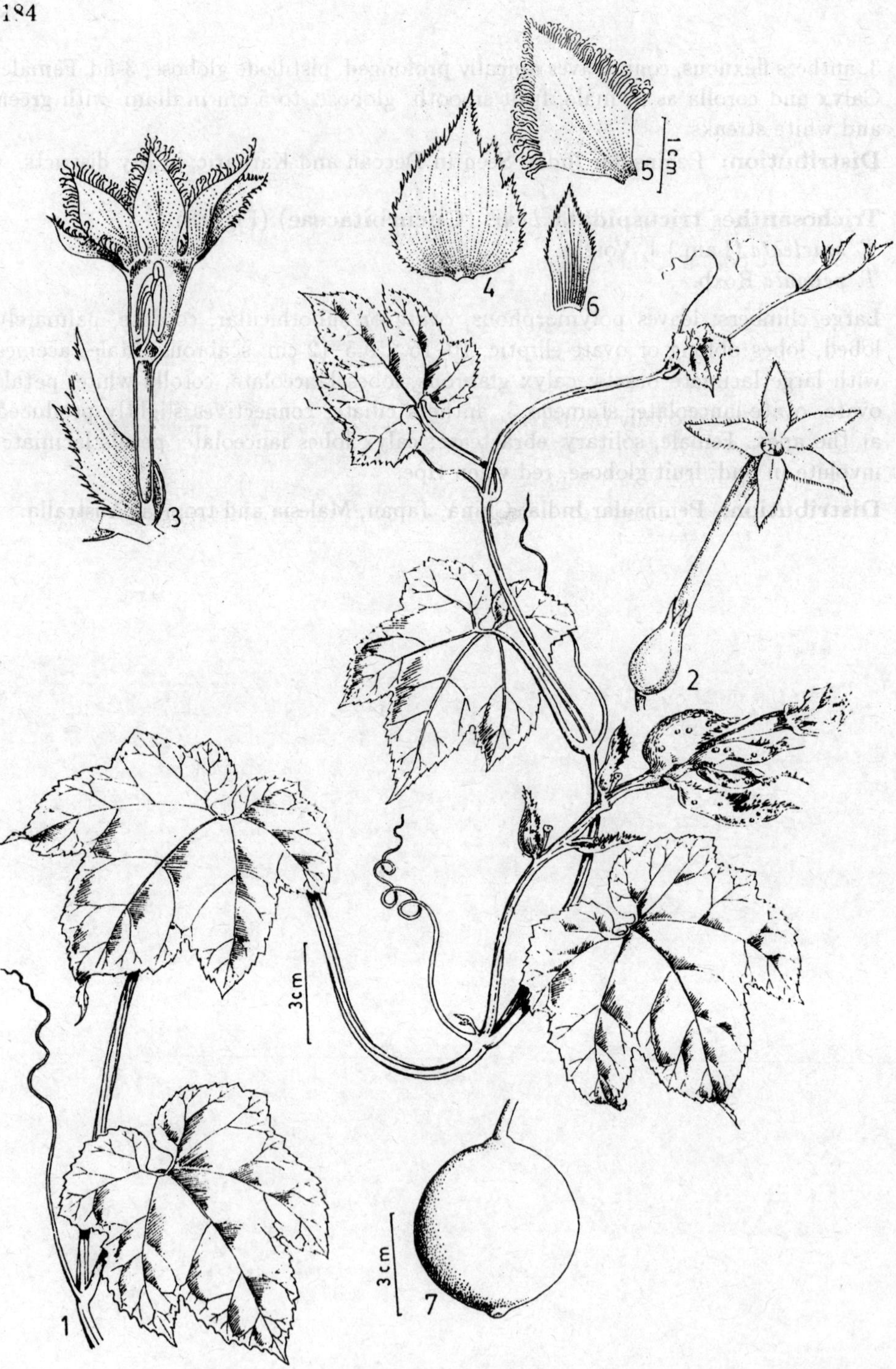

Figure 88: Trichosanthes tricuspidata Lour. 1, Habit; 2, Female flower; 3, Male flower L.S.; 4–6, Bracts; 7, Fruit.

ĪSWARĪ (Mal. KARAḶAYAṂ)

As the name *īswarī* indicates, the plant is believed to have the power to neutralise or resist snake poison. Other synonyms (*nākulī, gāruḍī, karaḷakaḥ, viṣaghnī, viṣavēga*) also imply its property of destroying the toxic effects of all poisons, especially snake poison. It is a purifier of blood (*asṛadōṣajit*) and hence useful in skin diseases. It heals wounds and dispels diseases due to the morbidity of *vāta, pitta* and *kapha*. It is an appetiser, aphrodisiac and anthelmintic and relieves burning sensation. Chiefly the root and occasionally the leaves are used in medicine. Fresh juice of the leaves is a favourite antidote to snake poison. Juice of the leaves and also of the bark is used in the bowel complaints of children, diarrhoea and in intermittent fevers. Roots are sometimes used for abortion by quacks (Nadkarni, 1954: 139; Aiyer & Kolammal, 1963. 6: 78) *Nīlīdaḷāditailaṃ, Pārantyāditailaṃ, Pāṭhādi guḷika*, etc. are some of the preparations using the drug.

According to the synonyms given in the texts, the plant has long roots (*mahāmūlaḥ*) and a long, twining stem (*dīṛghakāṇḍaḥ, dīṛghalatā*) which is very strong (*dṛḍhalatā*) (Aiyer & Kolammal, 1963. 6: 77).

There is mention of two kinds of *nākulī* known as *nākulī* and *gaṇdhanākuli* in the texts, distinguished from each other by the aroma of the latter. It is therefore suggested that *Rauvolfia serpentina* (Apocynaceae) and *Aristolochia indica* (Aristolochiaceae) may respectively be called *nākulī* and *gandhanākulī* (Vaidya, K.M., 1936: 313; Chunekar, 1972: 219) (See also notes under *Saṛpagandhā*).

In practice, *Aristolochia indica* Linn. of Aristolochiaceae, known as *karaḷayaṃ* or *īsvaramulla* in vernacular, which is widely used against snake bites, is the accepted source of the drug as has been mentioned by Kirtikar & Basu (1918: 1088), Nadkarni (1954: 139), Chopra *et al.* (156: 25) and Sharma (1983: 594). Rheede has described the plant under the name *Careloe-Vegon*, a decayed form of '*karaḷakaṃ*' or *karaḷayaṃ* as it is known widely in Kerala (Hort. Malab. 8: 49, t. 25. 1688).

Aristolochia indica *Linn.* **(Aristolochiaceae)** (Fig. 89)
A. lanceolata Wight

Perennial twiner with long, slightly tuberous roots; leaves simple, alternate, short-petioled, ovate-lanceolate, acute, entire, 10×4 cm; flowers greenish purple in axillary cymes; perianth monochlamydous and gamophyllous, pitcher-shaped, upto 3.8 cms long, basal part swollen or inflated, the middle part contracted to form a narrowly funnel-shaped tube and the distal part expanded into an obliquely two-lipped limb; stamens 6, adnate to the short stylar column; ovary inferior, elongate, grooved and six-celled with many ovules on parietal placentae; capsule 5 to 6 cm long, 6-valved, truncate below; seeds many with papery wings.

Distribution: The plant is distributed in all the provinces of India and in Sri Lanka, Nepal and Bangladesh. It is usually found scrambling over hedges and bushes.

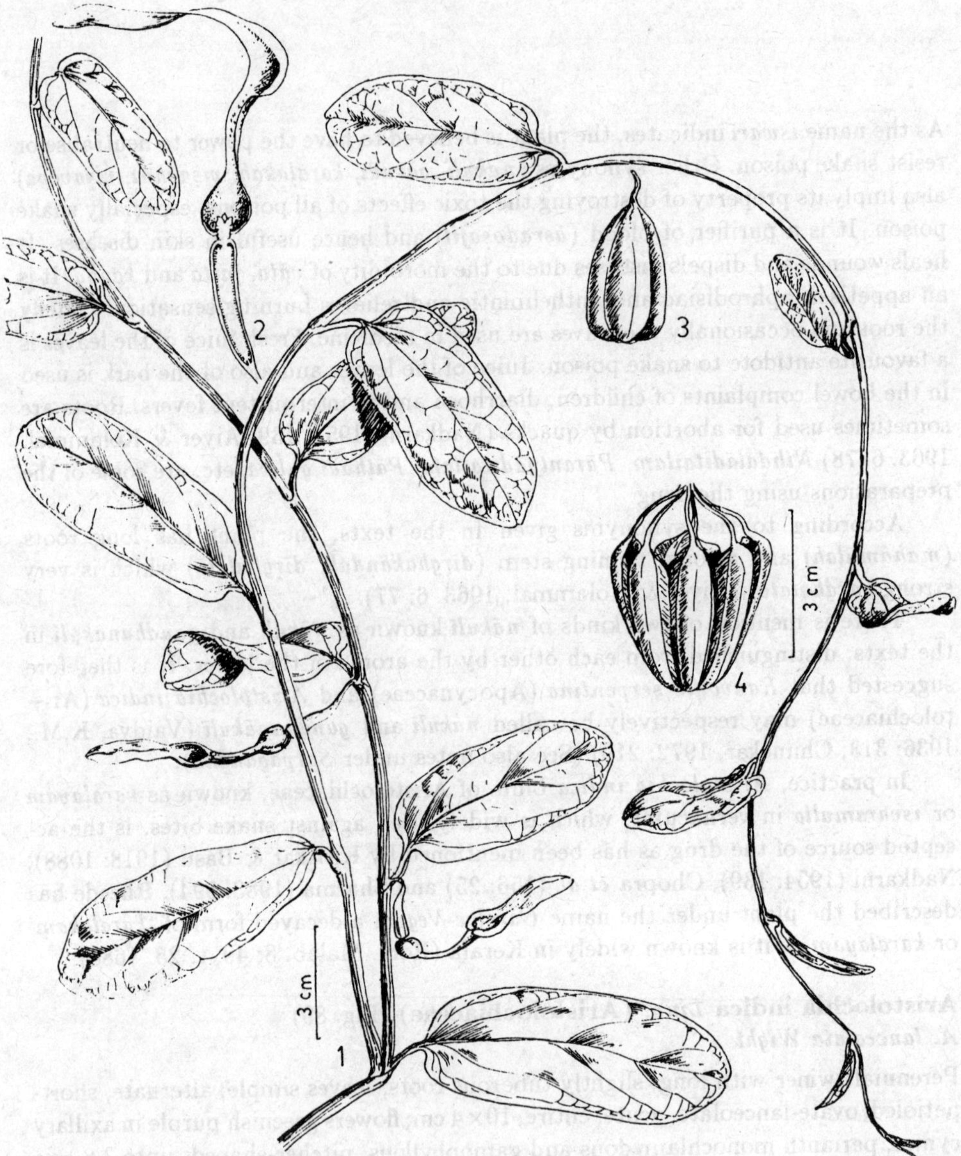

Figure 89: Aristolochia indica L. 1, Habit; 2, Flower L.S.; 3–4, Fruits.

Note: The antifertility effect of *Aristolochia indica* roots has been studied by Pakrashi and Shaha (1978).

We have three species of the genus in southern India viz. *A. indica*, *A. tagala* and *A. krisagathra*, of which only *A. indica* is currently used in medicine. Studies on the pharmacognosy and phytochemistry of this plant have been carried out by Nayar *et al.* (1976). Consequent to over-exploitation of this herb, its population has dwindled considerably. Yoganarasimhan *et al.* (1981) has suggested that *A. tagala* would prove to be a useful alternative for *A. indica.* The former can easily be distinguished from the latter by its much larger size, deeply cordate leaves, larger inflorescence, flowers and fruits.

JAṀBŪḤ (Mal. ÑĀVAL, ÑĀṚA)

In traditional medicine, this is extensively used against diabetes and sore throat. The bark and fruit are the officinal parts. The bark is considered a specific for dysentery. It is astringent to the bowels, unctuous, alleviative of *kapha* and *pitta*, cures haemorrhages, burning sensation, dysentery, diarrhoea, diabetes, excessive thirst, dyspepsia, cough, and asthma (Mooss, 1976: 142; Kurup *et al.*, 1979: 85). *Uśīrāsavaṃ, Vārāhyādighṛtaṃ, Lōhasindūraṃ*, etc. are some of the preparations using the drug.

According to the texts, *jaṁbūḥ*, which grows along river banks (*vētasī*) is an evergreen tree (*mēghamōdinī, ghanapriyā*) having stout stem and branches (*mahāskandā*), sweet smelling leaves (*surabhipatrā*) and large (*mahāphalā, bṛhatphalā*), blue black fruits (*kṛṣṇaphalā, kākanīlā, nīlaphalā, kāṣṭajaṁbū*) which attract cuckoos (*bhṛamēṣṭā*) and beetles (*bhṛamarēṣṭā, bhṛṅgavallabhā, bhṛṅgēṣṭā*) and are eaten by birds (*pikabhakṣyā, kākaphalā*) (Aiyer & Kolammal, 1962. 5: 52).

Āyurvēdic texts mention several types of this drug, namely *mahājaṁbūḥ, rājajaṁbūḥ, kākajaṁbūḥ, bhūmijaṁbūḥ* and *kṣudrajaṁbūḥ* (cf. Aiyer & Kolammal, 1962. 5: 53). But this is not observed in present day practice in Kerala. However, Kerala physicians recognise two varieties, locally called *ñāval* and *ñāṛa*, which together is believed to constitute what is called *jaṁbūdvayaṃ* (a pair of *Jambu*) (cf. Mooss, 1976: 140). *Ñāval* is usually equated with *Syzygium cumini* and *ñāṛa* with *S. caryophyllatum* of Myrtaceae. Rheede (Hort. Malab. 5: 57, 58, 29, 1685; 5: 53, t. 27, 1685) has illustrated these species under the vernacular names *Perin-njara* and *Njara* respectively.

Syzygium cumini (*Linn.*) *Skeels* **(Myrtaceae)** (Fig. 90)
Eugenia jambolana Lam.
Syzygium jambolanum (Lam.) DC.

Tree; branchlets glabrous; leaves simple, opposite, elliptic or ovate-lanceolate, acute or acuminate, entire, 5.5–11.5 × 2.5–6.5 cm, coriaceous, glabrous; flowers numerous, small, sweet-scented, dull white in axillary or terminal panicled cymes; calyx tube persistent, cup-shaped or shortly turbinate, glabrous, lobes 4; petals 4, orbicular; stamens numerous, free, anthers small; fruit an oblong, ellipsoid or globose berry, dark purplish black when ripe; seed roundish, smooth.

Distribution: The tree is found in moist localities in all forest districts of India and is often cultivated as an avenue tree. Also distributed in Sri Lanka, Malesia and Australia.

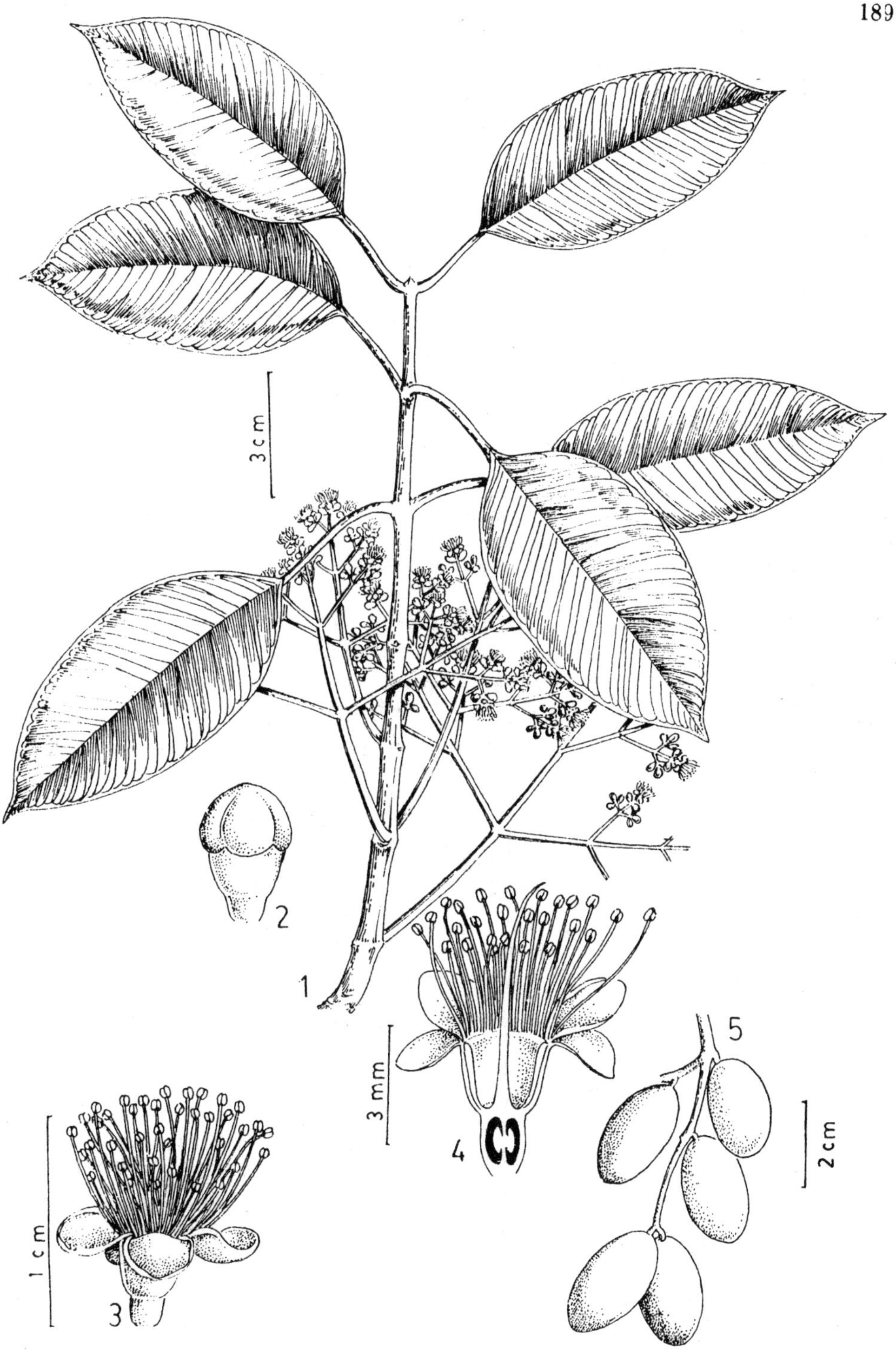

Figure 90: Syzygium cumini (L.) Skeels. 1, Flowering twig; 2, Flower bud; 3, Open flower 4, Flower L.S.; 5, Fruits.

Syzygium caryophyllatum (*Linn.*) *Alston* **(Myrtaceae)** (Fig. 91)
Myrtus caryophyllata Linn.
Syzygium caryophyllaeum Sensu auctt. non Gaertn.

Small tree; leaves simple, opposite, very short-petioled, elliptic to obovate, obtuse or emarginate, entire, 12.5 × 6–7 cms, sub coriaceous, dark green above, pale beneath; flowers small, white in lax terminal corymbose cymes; calyx shortly turbinate, 4 or 5 lobed; petals 4–5; stamens numerous, free; fruit a smooth, globose, berry, dark purplish or black when ripe; seeds globose.

Distribution: The tree is found near streams especially in W. Coast and W. Ghats from S. Canara southwards upto 5,000 ft.

Note: The hypoglycaemic activity of the seeds of *S. cumini* had been clinically studied by many. (Srivastava *et al.*, 1983; Nair & Santhakumari (1986) etc.) Sinha *et al.* (1986) found that its seed extract is a potential source for male contraception.

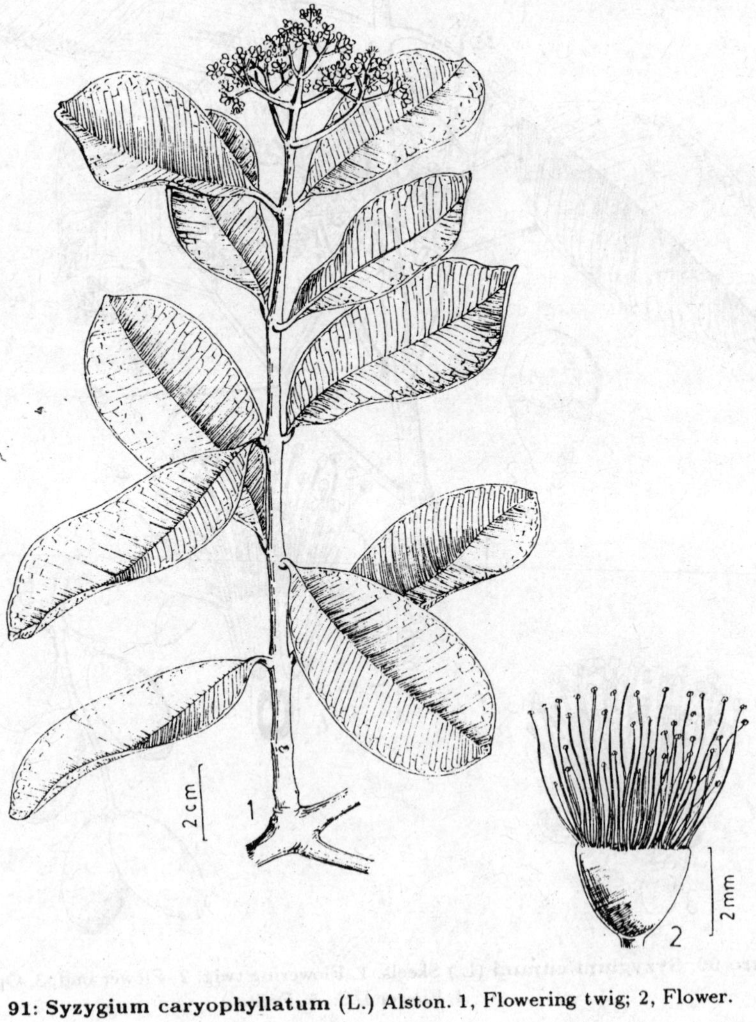

Figure 91: Syzygium caryophyllatum (L.) Alston. 1, Flowering twig; 2, Flower.

JAPĀ (Mal. CEṀPARUTTI)

In traditional medicine, *japā* is extensively used for blackening of hair. Flowers are reported to be astringent, constipating, hypoglycaemic, aphrodisiac and are used in treating alopacia, burning sensation in the body, diabetes, menstrual disorders and piles. It is also useful in fever, cough, menorrhagia, strangury, cystitis and other irritable conditions of the genito-urinary tract. Leaves and flowers are good for healing ulcers and for promoting the growth and colour of the hair (Nadkarni, 1954: 631; Kurup *et al.*, 1979: 86). The drug forms an important ingredient of *Ceṁparuttyādi* oil.

Except the name *japāpuṣpaṃ* which means flowers that lose its freshness quickly, the synonyms are not indicative of any particular feature of the plant. *Hibiscus rosa-sinensis* Linn. (Malvaceae), locally called *ceṁparutti* is the accepted source of this drug throughout the country. (See also, Rheede, Hort. Malab. 2: 25–26. t. 17. 1679. *Schem-Pariti*).

Hibiscus rosa-sinensis *Linn.* **(Malvaceae)** (Fig. 92)

Glabrous shrub; leaves simple, alternate, long-petioled, petiole upto 6–7 cms, lamina ovate, acuminate, crenate-serrate, 15 x 9 cms, basally three-veined; flowers large, axillary, solitary; bracteoles linear, free and form a whorl of epicalyx; calyx gamosepalous, petals 5; stamens numerous united to form a staminal tube bearing the anthers towards the top; ovary 5-celled, style long, slender, stigma 5, capitate, velvety.

Distribution: This species, now widely cultivated in the tropics as an ornamental, has several forms with varying colours of flowers. In medicine, however, the red-flowered variety is preferred.

Note: *Japā* flowers have been found to be effective in the treatment of arterial hypertension (Dwivedi *et al.*, 1977) and to have significant antifertility effect (Singh *et al.*, 1982; Sethi *et al.*, 1986). The pharmacognostic studies on *Hibiscus rosa-sinensis* have been conducted by Wahi *et al.* (1974).

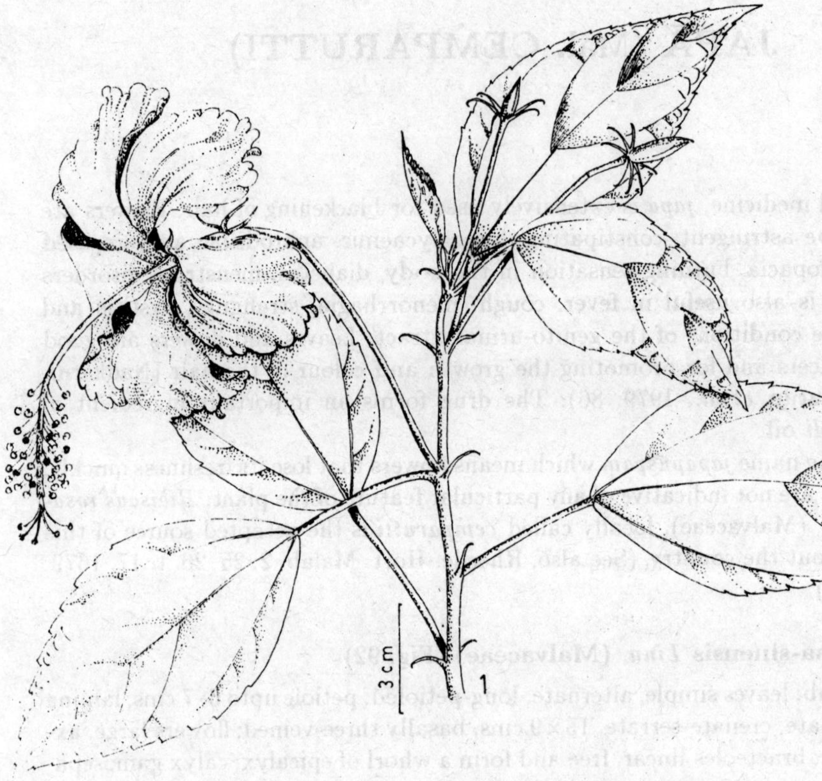

Figure 92: Hibiscus rosa-sinensis L.

JAYAPĀLAḤ (Mal. NĪṚVĀḶAṂ)

The drug is well known for its drastic purgative property. The seeds and seed oil are mainly used in Āyurvēda. The drug is also irritant, diaphoretic, rubefacient, vermifuge and vesicant. It is found very useful in ascites, anasarca, cold, cough, asthma, constipation, calculus, dropsy, fever and enlargement of the abdominal viscera. It is given only when a drastic purgation is required, as in dropsy and cerebral affections like convulsions, insanity and other fevers, attended with high blood pressure. The seed-paste is a good application for skin diseases, painful swellings and alopacia. The seed oil is useful in chronic bronchitis, laryngeal affections, arthritis and lock-jaw (Nadkarni, 1954: 397; Dey, 1980: 66; Sharma, 1983: 429). *Miśraka-snēhaṃ* is an important preparation using the drug.

Croton tiglium L. (Euphorbiaceae) is the source of the drug throughout the country. (Kirtikar & Basu, 1918: 1158; Nadkarni, 1954: 396; Chopra *et al.*, 1956: 82; Kapoor & Mitra, 1979: 75; Dey, 1980: 65; Chunekar, 1982: 401). A little confusion in the identity of the actual plant source stems from the fact that some authors consider *jayapālaḥ* and the larger variety of *dantī* (called *bṛhaddantī* or *dravantī* in Āyurvēdic parlance) to be the same (cf. Chunekar, 1982: 399). However, current practice in Kerala does not corroborate this. In Kerala, these two are considered different, *jayapālaḥ* being known as *nīṛvāḷaṃ* and *bṛhaddantī* as *kaṭalāvaṇakku* in the vernacular. The former is equated with *Croton tiglium* and the latter with some species of *Jatropha* (Euphorbiaceae). Rheede's portrayal of *Croton tiglium* under the vernacular name *Cadel-Avanacu* (Hort. Malab. 2: 61–62. t. 33. 1679), seems to be a mistake, because, nowhere in Kerala, this plant is known by this vernacular name.

Croton tiglium *Linn.* **(Euphorbiaceae)** (Fig. 93)

Shrubs; leaves simple, alternate, membraneous, elliptic to ovate, acuminate, upto 14 x 6 cm; flowers small, unisexual, greenish yellow in monoecious terminal raceme; sepals 5, ovate-obtuse; petals 5, linear with white hairs at the tip; stamens in male flowers many on a villous receptacle, filaments free, inflexed in bud; ovary in female tricarpellary, 3-celled with a single ovule in each, styles 3, long, slender, 2-cleft; capsule 3-lobed, obovoid, 3-valved.

Distribution: Almost throughout India.

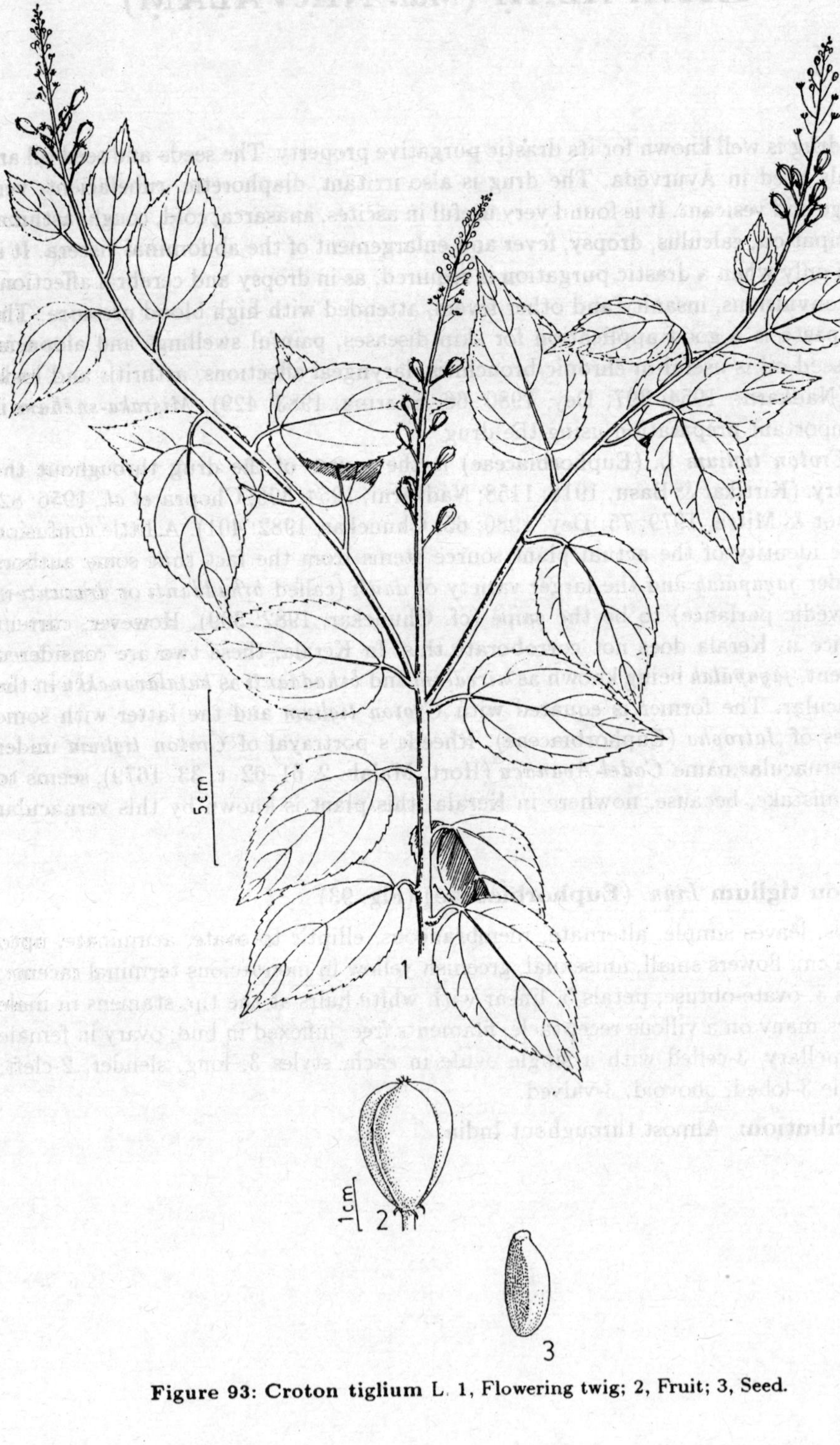

Figure 93: Croton tiglium L. 1, Flowering twig; 2, Fruit; 3, Seed.

JĪVANTĪ (Mal. AṬAKOḌIYAN, AṬAPATIYAN)

As the name *jīvantī* and other synonyms like *jīvanī, jīvā, jīvanīyā, jīvadā*, etc. indicate, the drug is considered to have the property to bestow health and liveliness to the consumer. Caraka treats it as an important *rasāyana* drug, capable of maintaining the youthful vigour and strength and Vāgbhaṭa includes it among the ten drugs that constitute the *Jīvanīya gaṇa* or the vitalising group.

Jīvantī is cold, sweet, aphrodisiac, rejuvenative and easy of digestion. It promotes health and vigour, improves voice, alleviates the three *dōṣās-vāta, pitta* and *kapha* and cures eye diseases, haemetemesis, emaciation, cough, dyspnoea, fever and burning sensation. Dysentery, nightblindness, poisonous affections and tuberculosis are also relieved by the use of the drug (Kolammal, 1979. 10: 20; Chunekar, 1982: 296). The root, which is the officinal part, enters into the composition of preparations like *Jīvantyādi ghṛtaṃ, Mānasamitravaṭakaṃ, Balāriṣṭaṃ, Aṇutailaṃ*, etc.

According to the description in the texts, the plant is a good vegetable (*śākaśrēṣṭhā*) having a copious exudation (*madhusṛavā, payasvinī*) which has a golden yellow colour (*suvarṇikā, svarṇavarṇinī, svarṇalatā*) and yellowish flowers (*hēmapuṣpī*) (Aiyer & Kolammal, 1979: 10: 19).

The most widely used name for this drug, *jīvantī*, is, however a homonym of several other drugs like *gudūcī, abhayā, mēdā, kākōḷī* and *vṛkṣādanī*, resulting in a lot of confusion in the identity of the drug source. Classical literature mention six different varieties of this drug viz. *śākapuṣpikā, kharakhōṭikā, śṛṅgarōtikā, tiktajīvantikā, arkapuṣpikā* and *bṛhajjīvantikā* which probably represent different plants (Aiyer & Kolammal, 1979. 10: 20) Mooss (1976: 77), however, recognises only two varieties, *jīvantī* and *bṛhatjīvantī*. In the actual practice, this discrimination is not recognised.

The botanical identity of the drug is highly disputed. Some of the authors from the north have equated it with *Flickingeria nodosa* (Dalz.) Seiden f. (= *Dendrobium macraei* auct.), an orchid (Nadkarni, 1954: 444; Chopra *et al.*, 1956: 95; Dey, 1980: 67; Chunekar, 1982: 296). The whole plant being golden yellow in colour, it is reportedly being used as *suvarṇajīvantī* in Bengal and some other parts of India (Vaidya Bapalal, 1982: 278). Yet others consider an Asclepiadaceae plant, *Leptadenia reticulata* W. & A. as the source of the drug (Singh & Chunekar, 1979: 62; Chunekar, 1982: 295; Sharma, 1983: 743). According to Caraka, *jīvantī* is the best among vegetables (*śākaśrēṣṭhā*). In Gujarat and Kathiawar people use *Leptadenia* as a pot herb and consider it to be a good cure for tuberculosis and eye diseases. So *Leptadenia reticulata* is treated as the real *jīvantī* by some (Vaidya Bapalal, 1982: 277). Ayurvedic formulary of India also accepts this plant as the true drug (Anonymous, 1978a: 248).

Jīvantī, according to Parameswara is the *Aṭapatiyan* or *Aṭakoḍiyan* of Kerala physicians, which has been identified as *Holostemma adakodien* Schult. (= *Holostemma annulare* (Roxb.) K. Schum.) belonging to Asclepiadeceae (cf. Mooss, 1980: 26). The fact that the roots of this plant are being used as *jīvantī* in Kerala from times immemorial, is substantiated by Rheede's description and illustration of the plant under the name *Adakodien* (Hort. Malab. 9: 9–10, t. 7. 1689). This may be the variety *arkapuṣpikā* mentioned in the texts since its flowers are very similar to that of *Calotropis gigantea.* The general colour of the roots, the presence of yellowish latex and other features tally with some of the synonyms attributed to this drug. This plant also satisfies the claims attributed to it, being found beneficial in the diseases for which it is prescribed (see Aiyer & Kolammal, 1979, 10: 20).

The various plants equated with the drug can be identified as follows:

Holostemma ada-kodien *Schult.* **(Asclepiadaceae)** (Fig. 94)
Holoslemma annulare (Roxb.) K. Schum.
Holostemma rheedii Wall.

Large, perennial, laticiferous climber; stem slightly reddish, glabrous; leaves simple, opposite, ovate or ovate-oblong, entire, acute, deeply cordate at base, 4–6 × 2–3.5 cms, chartaceous, puberulous below; flowers large, crimson-pink in axillary cymes; calyx deeply 5-partite, lobes broadly ovate-obtuse; corolla gamopetalous, deeply 5-lobed, subrotate, pinkish outside and purplish within; stamens 5, adnate to the base of the corolla tube, the filaments cohering in a ten-winged column; pistil bicarpellary, ovaries free, style slender, ending in an oblong 5-winged stigma; follicles lanceolate.

Distribution: The plant has been recorded as occuring in the tropical Himalayas, Dehradun, Konkan, Bombay, Deccan, N. Circars, Canara, Carnatic, Kerala and Kanyakumari district. It grows over hedges and in open forests especially on the lower slopes of the hills. Also distributed in Sri Lanka, Burma, W.China.

Leptadenia reticulata (*Retz.*) *Wt. & Arn.* **(Asclepiadaceae)** (Fig. 95)
Cynanchum reticulatum Retz.

A climbing shrub with milky latex; leaves pale, elliptic-oblong or lanceolate, acute, 4.7 × 1.5–3 cm, chartaceous, base truncate, obtuse or rounded; flowers yellowish in axillary or terminal umbellate cymes; calyx cupular, lobes subequal; corolla campanulate, lobes linear-lanceolate; corona double, outer corolline, alternating with corolla lobes, inner staminal, of 5 shallow annular lobes around staminal column; follicles paired, cylindric, bluntly acute to both ends; seeds winged.

Distribution: The plant is found in N. Circars, Deccan & Carnatic, west ward to the E. slopes of the Ghats, upto 3,000 ft chiefly in hedges. Distributed in Mauritius, Madagascar, Sri Lanka, tropical Himalaya, Burma.

Flickingeria nodosa (*Dalz.*) *Seiden f.* **(Orchidaceae)**
Desmotrichum fimbriatum Auct.
Dendrobium macraei auct. p.p. non Lindley

Epiphytic herb with annulate creeping rhizome; stem smooth, pendulous, nodose, pseudobulbs narrowly fusiform, uninodal, 2.5–6.5 cms long, shining; leaves linear-oblong, obtuse, 5–20 cms long; flowers white or pinkish speckled with red, the midlobe of the lip greenish yellow, 1–3 together from near the base of the leaf.

This plant is found in the Deccan plains.

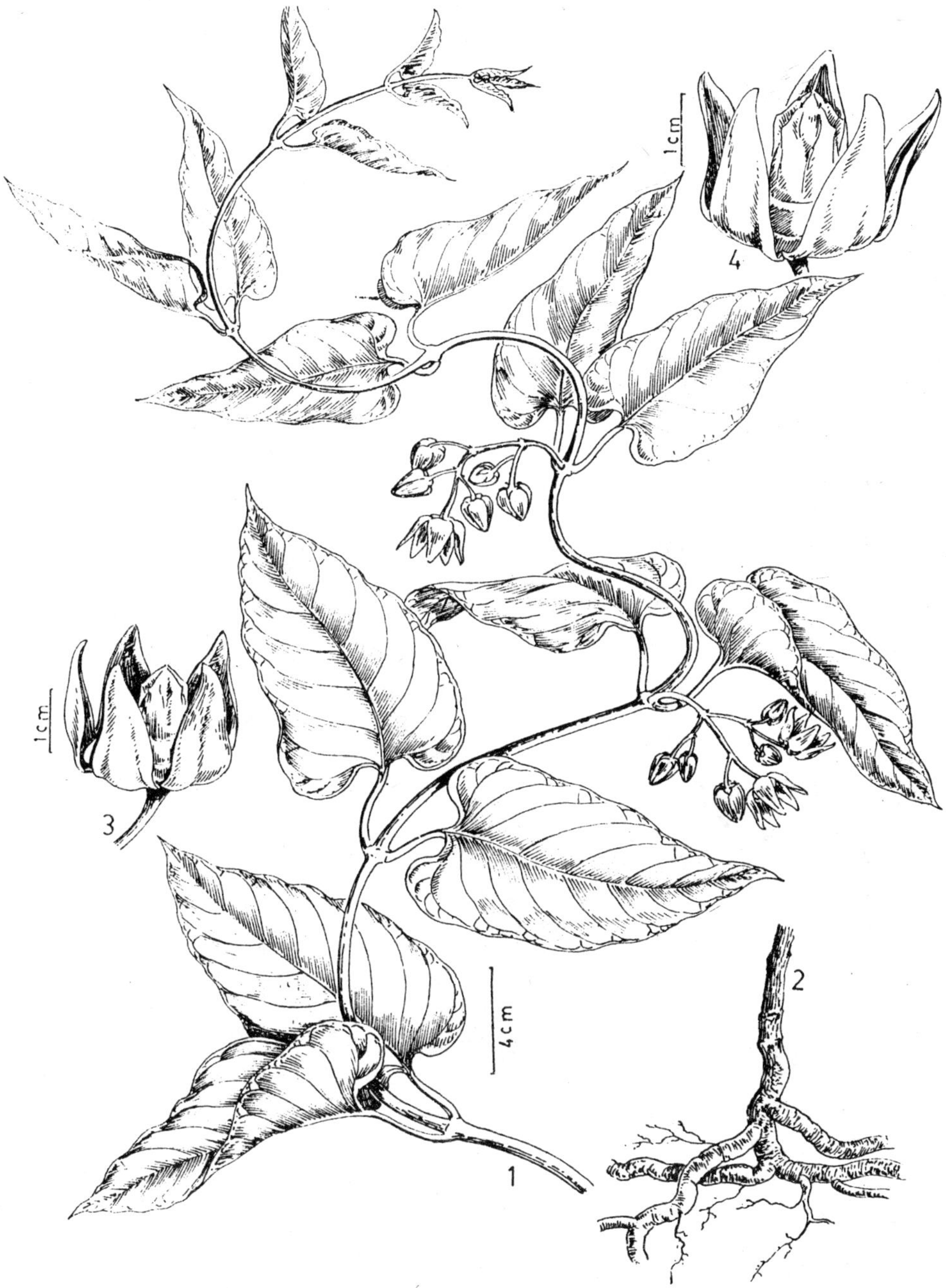

Figure 94: **Holostemma ada-kodien** Schult. 1, Flowering vine; 2, roots; 3–4, Flowers.

Note: The pharmacognosy, chemistry, pharmacology and clinical studies on *Leptadenia reticulata* have been discussed in detail by Satyavati *et al.* (1987: 152–158).

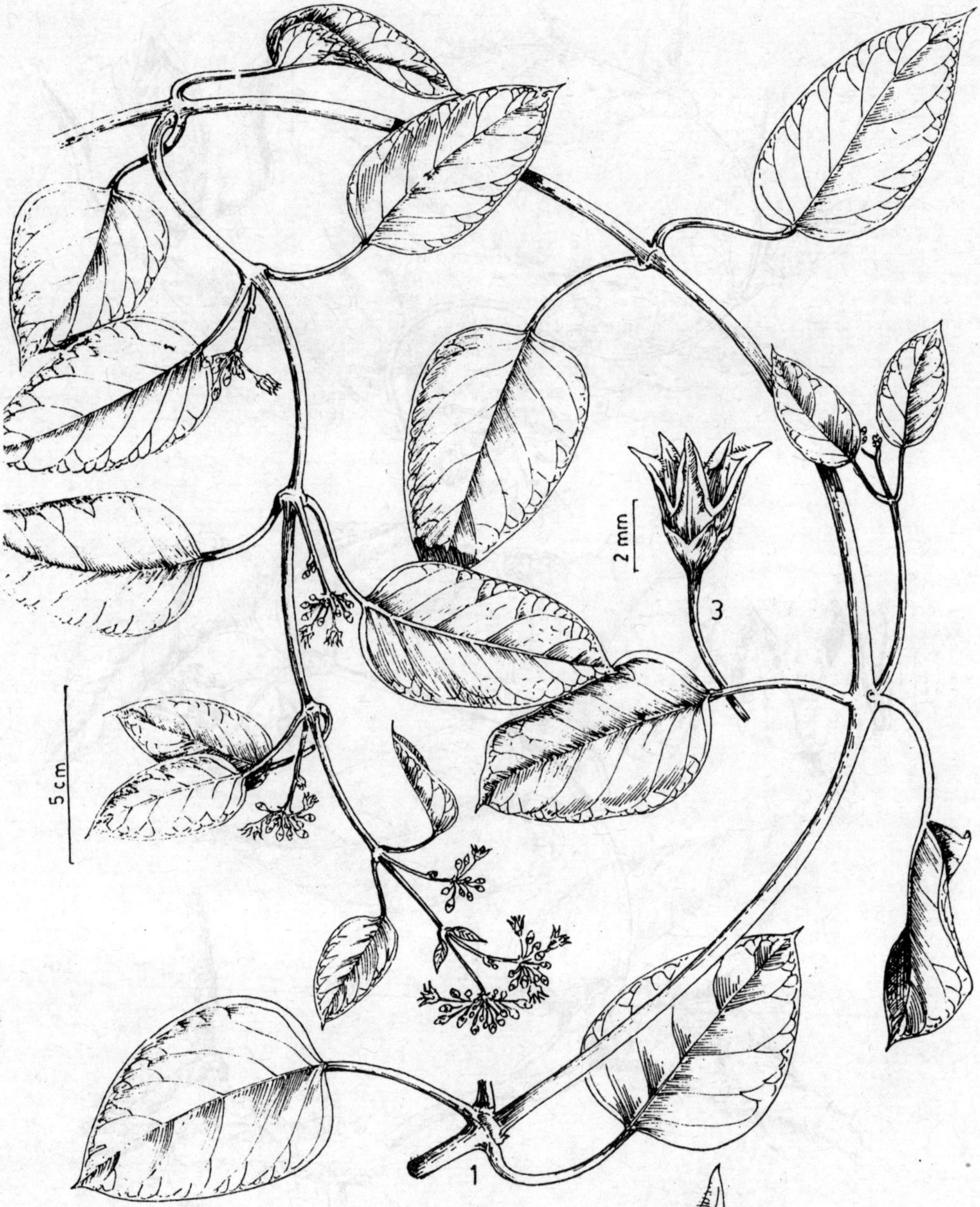

Figure 95: Leptadenia reticulata (Retz.) Wt. & Arn. 1, Flowering vine; 2–3, Flowers.

KAIḌARYAḤ (Mal. KARIVĒPPU)

The plant is highly esteemed for its leaves which promote appetite and digestion and destroy pathogenic organisms, and hence form an important ingredient in Indian cuisine. It is reported to be acrid, bitter, astringent, cool and light and is useful in emaciation or wasting conditions, skin diseases, hemopathy, worm troubles, neurosis and poisons. *Kaiḍaryaḥ* improves voice, stimulates digestion and destroys concocted poisons in the system. Leaves, bark and root are used in medicine. The important preparations using the drug are *Kāḷaśākādi kaṣāyaṃ, Pāmāntaka tailaṃ, Jātyādi tailaṃ, Jātyādi ghṛtaṃ*, etc.

The synonyms attributed to this drug provide us with some important indications about the plant. It resembles *niṁbaḥ* (Neem tree), but is darker in colour (*kṛṣṇaniṁbakaḥ*), with dark (*kāḷaśākaḥ*) and scented leaves (*surabhiḥ, surabhicchadaḥ*) and is white flowered (*kumudikā*) (Aiyer *et al.*, 1957.3: 33).

All these synonyms match well with the plant viz. *Murraya koenigii* (Rutaceae) that is being used as the source of the drug throughout Kerala (see also Rheede, Hort. Malab. 4: 109–110. t. 53. 1683 *'Karibepou'*).

The author of *Rājanighaṇṭu* considers *kaiḍaryaḥ* to be the same as *mahāniṁbaḥ* and some others equate it with *kaṭphalaḥ* or *pūtīkarañjaḥ* (cf. Aiyer *et al.*, 1957. 3: 32, Singh & Chunekar 1972: 118). But in Kerala, this is considered distinct from both.

Murraya koenigii (*Linn.*) *Spreng.* **(Rutaceae)** (Fig. 96)
Bergera koenigii Linn.

Small trees; leaves alternate, imparipinnate, pubescent when young, strongly aromatic; leaflets short-stalked, alternate, elliptic to ovate-lanceolate, 4.5 × 1.8 cms, gland-dotted, finely serrate, oblique at base; flowers white, fragrant in dense terminal corymbose panicles; calyx five-cleft, pubescent; petals 5, free, oblong-obtuse; stamens 10, attached around a disc; ovary superior, 2-celled; style cylindric, thick with a capitate stigma; berries small, ovoid or subglobose, green when young and black when ripe.

Distribution: The plant is largely cultivated for its fragrant leaves and is common in most parts of India. Also found in Sri Lanka, Burma, Indo-China, S. China, Hainan, elsewhere in cultivation.

Note: The hypoglycaemic potential of *Murraya koenigii* has been successfully tested by Santhakumari *et al.*, (1985) in animals and human beings.

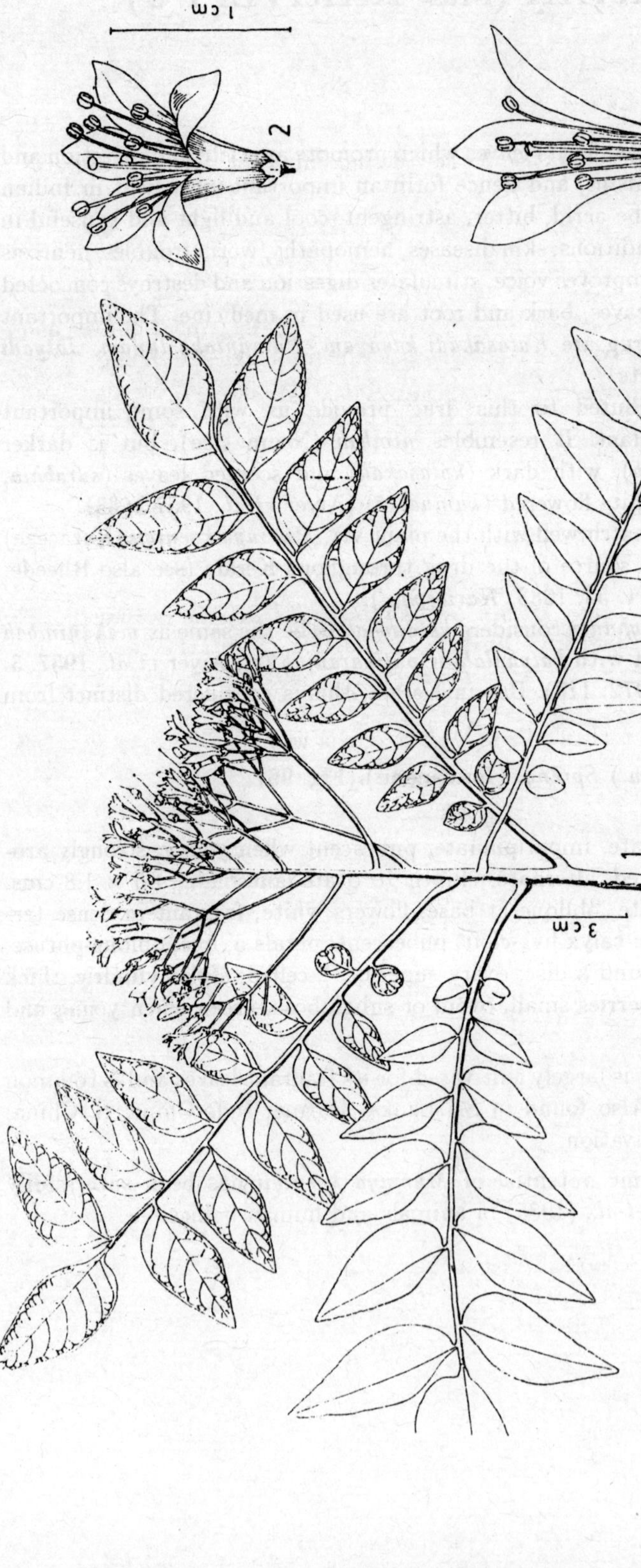

Figure 96: Murraya koenigii (L.) Spr. 1 Flowering twig; 2 Flower; 3 Flower LS.

KĀKAMĀCĪ (Mal. MAṆATAKKĀḶI)

According to *Bhāvaprakāśa*, *kākamācī* is demulcent, hot, bitter, diuretic, cardiotonic, antidiabetic, laxative and restorative and is useful in overcoming the vitiation of the three *dosas*. It promotes or improves voice and semen, cures oedema, leprosy, piles, fever, urinary diseases with increased urination, eye diseases, hiccough, vomiting and heart ailments. Fresh extract of the plant has been recommended in dropsy, inflammatory swellings and enlargement of liver and spleen. Decoction of the berries and flowers is useful in cough (Nadkarni, 1954: 1153; Aiyer and Kolammal, 1960: 4. 74; Kurup *et al.*, 1979: 96). Whole plant and fruits are used medicinally.

From the Sanskrit synonomy, one can only deduce that the whole plant is bitter (*varatiktā, sarvatiktā*) and that the fruits produced in bunches (*bahuphalā, gucchaphalā*) are acrid (*kaṭuphalā*) and are liked by crows (*kākamācī*) (cf. Aiyer & Kolammal, 1960. 4: 73).

Almost all the practitioners equate *kākamācī* with *Solanum americanum* (*S. nigrum* auct.) of Solanaceae locally known as *maṇatakkāḷi*. (Kirtikar & Basu 1918. 2: 889; Vaidya 1936: 117; Nadkarni, 1954: 1152; Kapoor & Mitra 1979: 64; Kurup *et al.*, 1979: 96; Chunekar 1982: 438; Sharma, 1983: 540). However, Pāṭyakāra, Paramesvara and Bhiṣagārya have treated *kākamācī* and *kariṁtakāḷi* as the same drug (cf. Mooss, 1980: 80). Mooss (1980: 80) has agreed with this and has equated this drug with *Geophila reniformis* (now *G. repens*) of Rubiaceae. In Kerala, however, these two are considered as different drugs. *Kākamācī*, locally called *maṇa* (*maṇi*) *takkāḷi*, has been equated with *Solanum americanum* and *kariṁtakkāḷi*, also called *karimuttiḷ*, with *Geophila repens*. Rheede (1690) has portrayed both under the respective local names (Hort. Malab. *Karimtakali* 10: 41. 6. 21 is *Geophila repens* and 10: 145. t. 73 *Nelemtsjunda* is *Solanum americanum*).

Solanum americanum *Mill.* **(Solanaceae)** (Fig. 97)
S. nigrum auct. non Linn.

Glabrous annual herb; leaves ovate or ovate-lanceolate, acute, entire or bluntly toothed, thin, membraneous, 8–14 × 4–7 cms; flowers small, white in lateral, umbellate cymes borne on slender drooping pedicels; calyx persistent; corolla rotate, 5-lobed, lobes spreading; stamens 5, epipetalous, filaments short, anthers yellow, oblong-obtuse; ovary globose; fruit a globose shiny berry, green when young and purplish black when mature, 0.5 cm across; seeds many, discoid.

Distribution: The plant is found throughout India as a weed in open waste lands, gardens, cultivated land and roadsides.

Detailed pharmacognosy of the plant has been studied by Brinda *et al.* (1982).

Taxonomic Note: This species is usually attributed the name *S. nigrum* L. A lot of biosystematic work on this complex group has been carried out in the recent past and the name *S. nigrum* is now reserved for the hexaploid group in this complex.

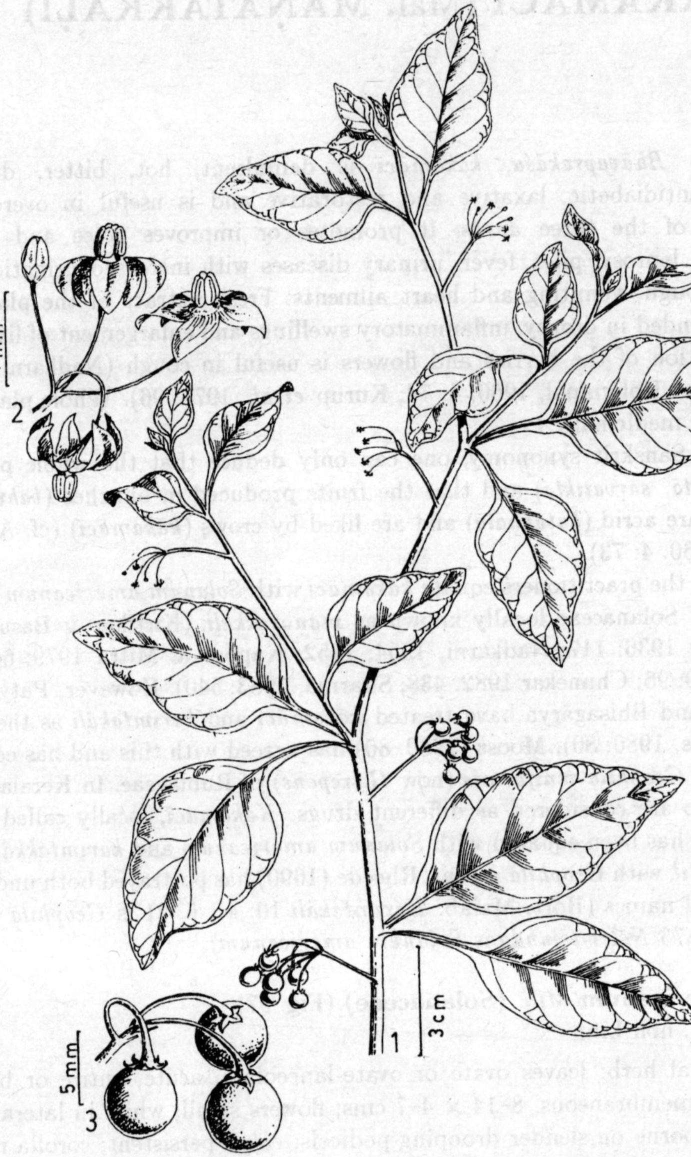

Figure 97: Solanum americanum Mill. 1, Flowering branch; 2, Inflorescence; 3, Fruits.

The diploid Indian materials are hence treated under the name *S. americanum* (See Symon, 1981 & Nicolson *et al.*, 1988).

Note: Afaq *et al.* (1985) found that the ripe fruit of this species are effective in treating the diseases of heart and eye, piles, leucoderma, asthma, jaundice, etc. due to the presence of the active principle solasodine which is in great demand in pharmaceutical industry.

KAṀPILLAKAḤ (Mal. KAṀPIPPĀLA)

Kaṁpillakaḥ is a drug well known for its anthelmintic property and is a reputed remedy against tape worms. With curd or milk, it expels worms from the intestine of children. Vāgbhaṭa includes it in his *Nikuṁbhādi gaṇa* (purgatives). The crimson-coloured powder consisting of glandular hairs on the fruit forms the officinal part. It is bitter, cathartic, anthelmintic, styptic, aphrodisiac and cures abdominal disorders, hemopathy, calculus, flatulence, leprosy and skin diseases and is applied externally as an ointment in cases of ringworm, syphylitic ulcers, freckles and pityriasis (Nadkarni, 1954: 762; Kurup *et al.*, 1979: 101). The drug forms an ingredient of *Jīvantyādi yamakaṃ, Vindūghṛtaṃ, abhraṃ* (101), etc.

Except for the mention of the red powder on the fruit (*raktāṅgaḥ, raktaphalaḥ*) the synonyms do not provide any clue which could have enabled us to determine the actual plant source of this drug.

Most authors have equated the drug with the crimson-red powder on the fruits of *Mallotus philippensis* of Euphorbiaceae (Kirtikar & Basu, 1918: 1165; Nadkarni, 1954: 760; Singh & Chunekar, 1972: 74; Kurup *et al.*, 1979: 101; Dey, 1980: 71; Mooss, 1980: 8; Sharma, 1983: 521). The synonyms *raktāṅgaḥ, raktaphalaḥ*, etc. which indicate the red powder on the fruit, also agree well with this plant. But in Kerala, the vernacular name *kaṁpippāla* is attributed to another laticiferous plant, *Tabernaemontana alternifolia* (Apocynaceae) which is accepted as the plant source of the drug. This equation may be due to the misinterpretation of the usage *"kaṁpillakaṃ payaḥ"*, mentioned in some of the formulations, to the milk (milky latex) of *kaṁpillakaṃ* (which actually means a combination of *kaṁpillakaṃ* and milk) or due to the similarity in the vernacular and Sanskrit names. Rheede describes this plant under the name *Curutu-pala* (Hort. Malab. 1: 83–84, t. 46. 1678).

This is an example in sight as to how different (mis) interpretation of the classical Sanskrit verses can cause confusion in the identification of the actual drug and its plant source. It is yet to be investigated whether *Tabernaemontana alternifolia* has the same properties attributed to the real drug i.e. *Mallotus philippensis*. The important features of the two plants are described below.

Mallotus philippensis (*Lam.*) *Muell-Arg.* **(Euphorbiaceae)** (Fig. 98)
Croton philippensis Lam.
Rottlera tinctoria Roxb.

Trees; branches rusty tomentose; leaves simple, alternate, ovate-lanceolate, acuminate, 20 × 10 cm, 3-veined from base, fulvous tomentose below; flowers small, unisexual in terminal panicles. Male: Tepals 4, free, obovate, acute, recurved; stamens many, anther cells unequal. Female: Tepals 3, lanceolate, bifid; ovary pubescent, 3-locular; capsule smooth, 3-valved, pubescent, red-glandular; seeds globose, black.

Distribution: The plant is found in all forest districts in N. Circars, Deccan, W. Ghats, also in hills of Carnatic; upto 5,000 ft. Also reported from Sri Lanka, Malesia, Australia and Melanesia.

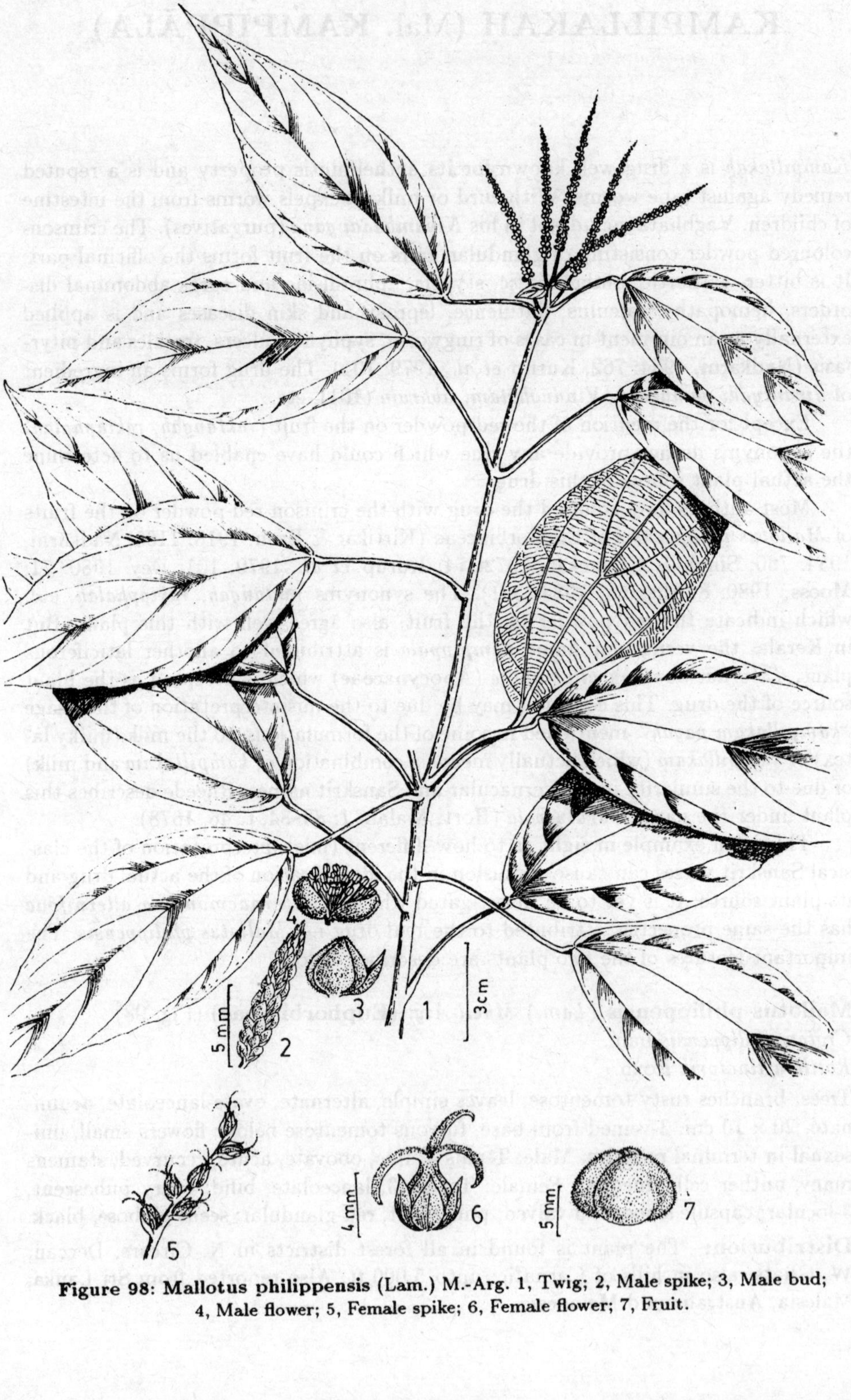

Figure 98: Mallotus philippensis (Lam.) M.-Arg. 1, Twig; 2, Male spike; 3, Male bud; 4, Male flower; 5, Female spike; 6, Female flower; 7, Fruit.

Tabernaemontana alternifolia *Linn.* **(Apocynaceae)** (Fig. 99)
T. heyneana Wall.
Ervatamia heyneana (Wall.) Cooke

Small trees; leaves simple, opposite, elliptic-oblong, acuminate, 23 × 6.5 cm, prominently nerved, glabrous above, glaucous beneath; flowers white in corymbose cymes; calyx lobes 5, thick, connate at base; corolla salver-shaped, tube cylindric, dilated at top, lobes 5; stamens 5, inserted within the dilated part of corolla tube, filaments very short, anthers linear-acute; ovary bicarpellary, syncarpous, style slender, stigma oblong with a bifid apiculus; fruit of 2 oblong, boat-shaped, orange-yellow follicles, upto 4 cm long, with recurved beaks.

Distribution: The plant is found in W. Ghats in Malabar and Travancore, in open forests upto 3,000 ft.

Taxonomic Note: Nicolson *et al.* (1988: 57) has discussed the nomenclature of this species in some detail.

Note: Coronaridine hydrochloride, an active principle from roots of *Tabernaemontana heyneana* was found to be an antifertility agent (Mehrotra and Kamboj, 1978). Rao and Singri (1979) found that mature leaves of *T. heyneana* indicated the presence of a rare alkaloid, isovoacristine, having anticholinergic and antihistaminic activities.

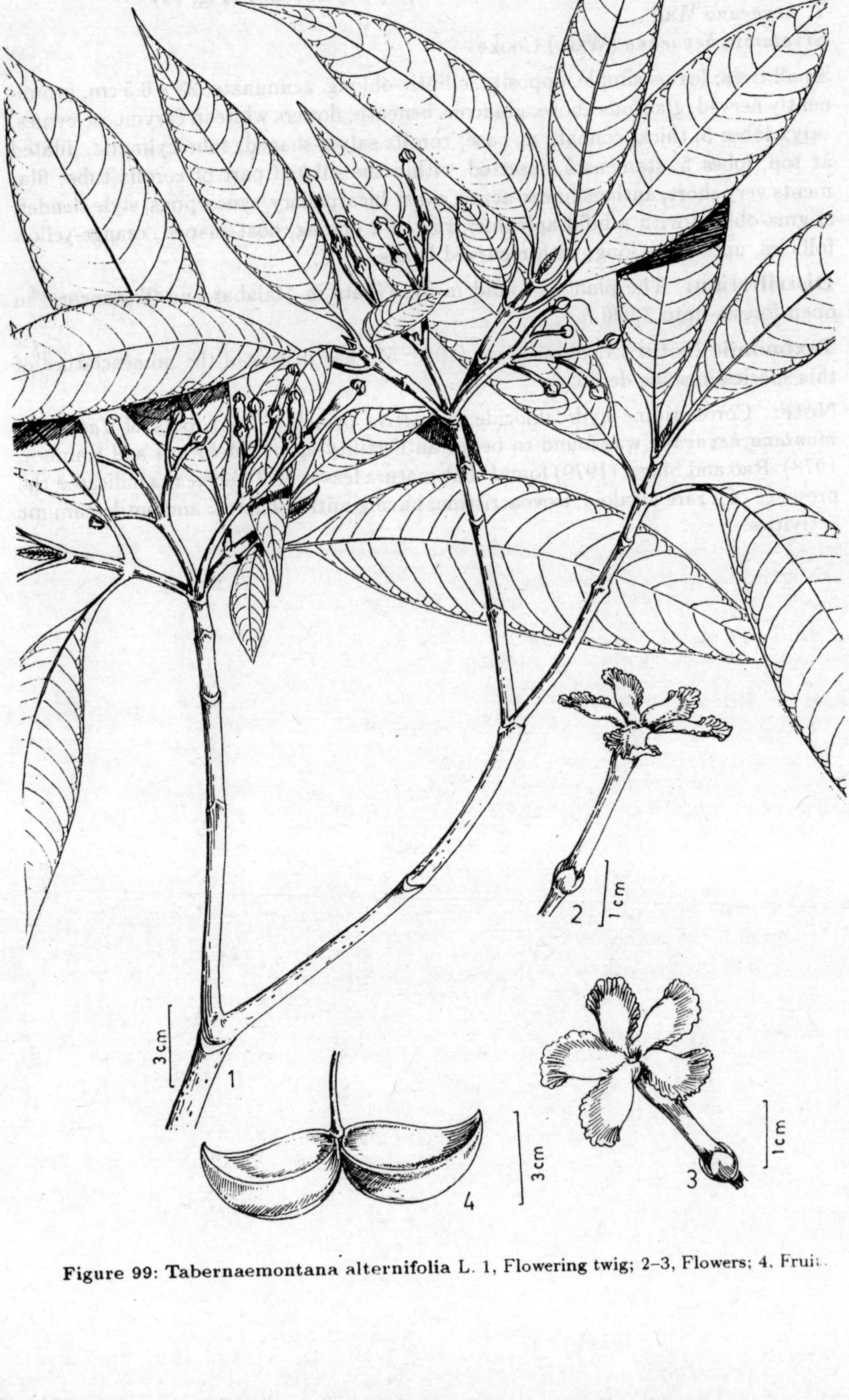

Figure 99: Tabernaemontana alternifolia L. 1, Flowering twig; 2–3, Flowers; 4, Fruit.

KĀÑCANĀRAḤ (Mal. MANDĀRAṂ)

In traditional medicine, this drug is extensively used in glandular diseases and as an antidote to poison. Bark is the officinal part. It is light, cool, astringent, anthelmintic, acrid and overcomes vitiated *pitta* and *kapha*. It cures ulcers, swellings, leprosy, cough, menstrual disorders, glandular diseases and prolapse of rectum. The drug is also reported to be useful in dysentery, diarrhoea, piles and worms (Kurup *et al.*, 1979: 102; Sharma, 1983: 235) *Uśīrāsavaṃ* and *Candanāsavaṃ* are some of the preparations using the drug.

Bhāvaprakāśa nighaṇṭu recognises two types of this drug namely *kāñcanāraḥ* and *kōvidāraḥ*, but attributes same properties to them. *Rājanighaṇṭu* and *Dhanvantarinighaṇṭu* also treat them as synonymous. *Nighaṇṭuratnākara*, however, recognises three types—red, white and yellow and attribute different properties to them. These three are well known locally also, as has been called by different local names viz. *cuvanna mandāraṃ*, *veḷutta mandāraṃ* and *mañña mandāraṃ*. *Cuvanna mandāraṃ* has been equated with two different species, *Bauhinia purpurea* and *B. variegata*, *veḷutta mandāraṃ* with *B. acuminata* and *mañña mandāraṃ* (also known as *Canschenapou* means golden flowered) with *B. tomentosa* (also see Rheede, Hort. Malab. 1. 57–64. tt. 32–35 1678). In practice, however, physicians prefer *B. variegata* and *B. tomentosa* as the source plants of this drug.
The various species can be identified as follows.

Bauhinia variegata *Linn.* **(Caesalpiniaceae)**

Tree; leaves ovate, 5–10 × 6–11 cm, leaflets connate for about two thirds, thin-coriaceous, 10–12 nerved, glabrous above, puberulous along nerves below, base deeply cordate, margin entire, apex obtuse, mucronate at the cleft; flowers light pink in terminal panicles; bracts ovate; buds ovoid, apex beaked; calyx tube irregularly lobed, 2.5 × 1.5 cm; petals light pink, odd one dark, variegated; stamens 3; pod oblong, 20 × 15 cm, distinctly reticulate, base and apex narrow, horned.

Distribution: Possibly a native of China, this is now found in dry deciduous forests, especially on rocky hills throughout India.

Note: Prakash *et al.* (1978) have carried out the pharmacognostical study of *Bauhinia variegata* Linn.

Bauhinia tomentosa *Linn.* **(Caesalpiniaceae)** (Fig. 100)

Small tree; leaves orbicular, 3.5–5.5 × 3.5–6.5 cm; leaflets connate for about half their length, chartaceous, 7-nerved, glabrous above, pubescent below, base truncate or subcordate, apex obtuse, margin entire; flowers yellow in 2–5 flowered terminal racemes; calyx spathaceous, lobes 5, oblong; petals 5, yellow, obovate, 6 × 3 cm; stamens 10, unequal; pod oblong to 10 × 1.5 cm, compressed, distinctly reticulate, downy puberulous, base subacute-cuneate, apex obtuse and horned; seeds ovoid.

Distribution: Africa and Asia. In India it is found wild in dry deciduous forests. Often cultivated.

Bauhinia purpurea *Linn.* **(Caesalpiniaceae)** (Fig. 101)

Tree; leaves oblong, 5.5–11.5 × 6–12 cm, leaflets connate about half way, 11–13 nerved, plaited below, base subcordate, apex obtuse, margin entire; flowers rose in terminal or axillary panicles or racemes; buds narrow, obovoid, obtuse; calyx 2-cleft above; petals 5, rose or pink, equal, obovate-obtuse, entire; stamens 3 (5); pod oblong, 30–40 × 1.5–2 cm, compressed, narrow at base, apex horned; seeds ovoid, flat, beaked.

Distribution: South and South East Asia. In India it is found in deciduous forests. Also grown as ornamental.

Bauhinia acuminata *Linn.* **(Caesalpiniaceae)**

Shrubs; leaves tomentose beneath, glabrous above, lobes subacute; flowers large, showy, white; pods oblanceolate, acuminate, ridged on both sutures, compressed; seeds few, compressed.

Often cultivated in gardens.

Note: The experimental studies conducted by Sijoria and Prasad (1979) on animals indicate that *Bauhinia purpurea* is very effective in normalising the thyroid gland.

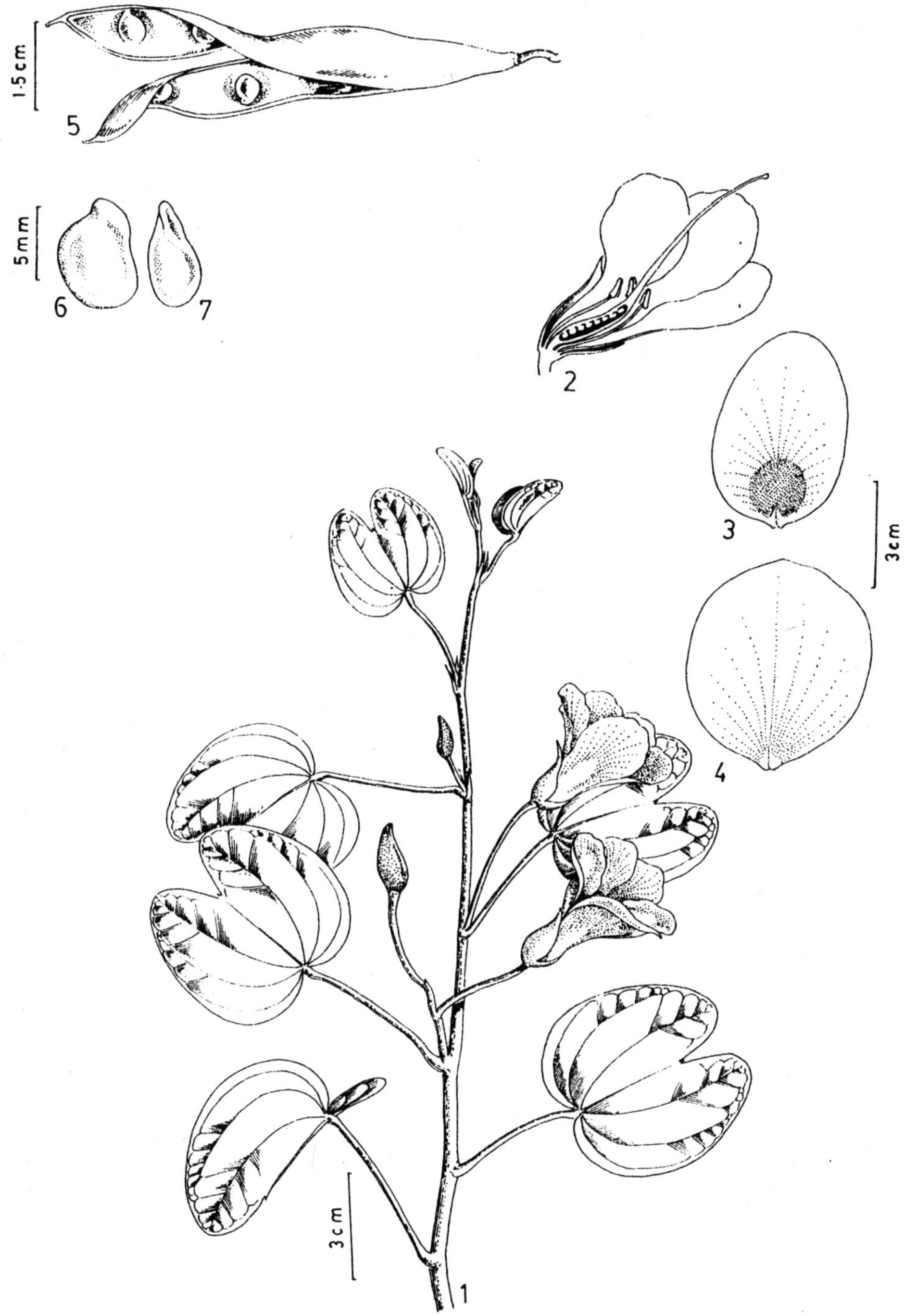

Figure 100: Bauhinia tomentosa L. 1, Flowering twig; 2, L.S. of flower; 3, Petal inside view; 4, Petal back view; 5, a dehisced pod; 6–7 Seeds.

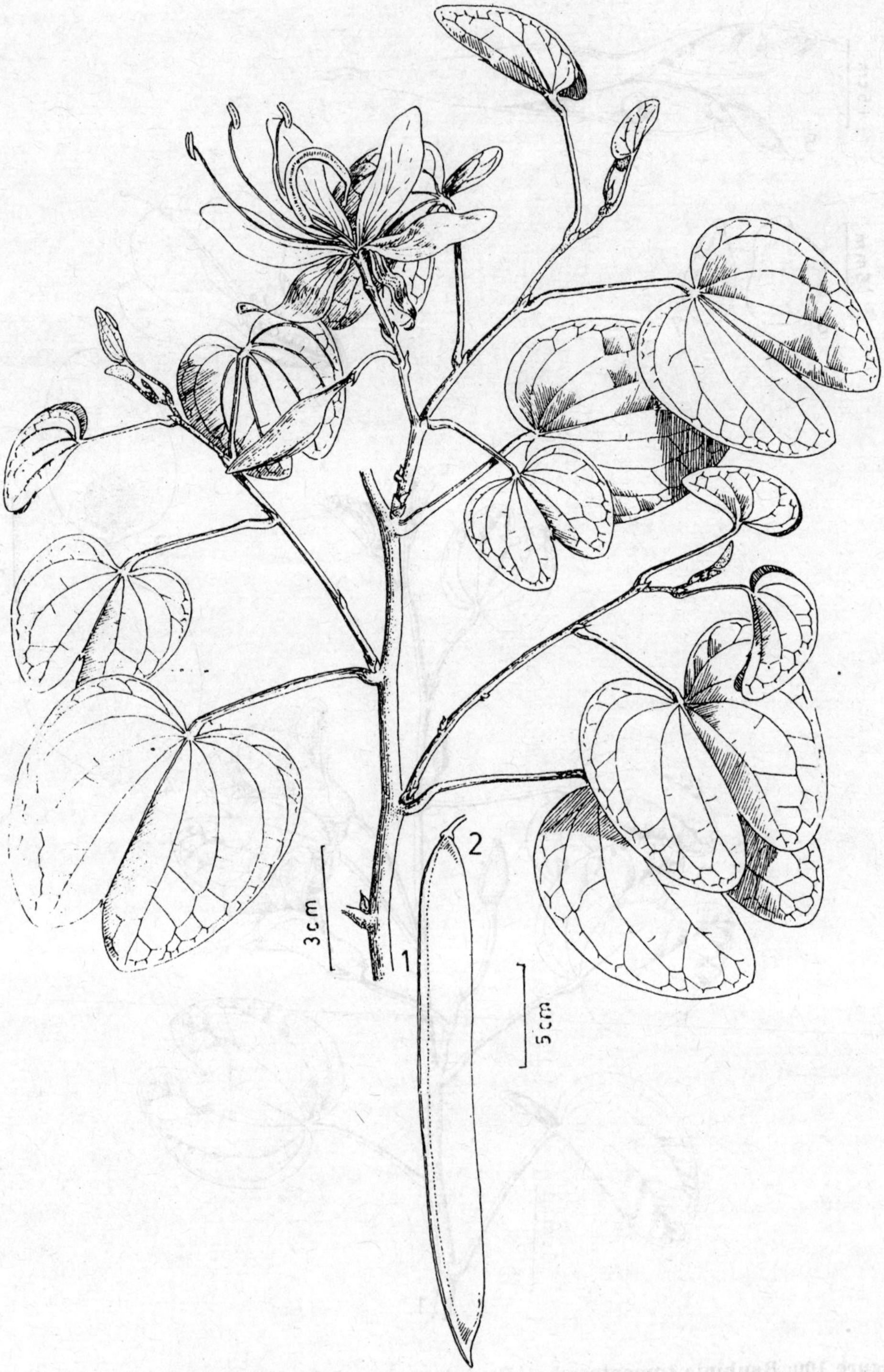

Figure 101: Bauhinia purpurea L. 1, Flowering twig; 2, Pod.

KAṆṬAKĀRĪ (Mal. KAṆṬAKĀRI VAḶUTINA)

Kaṇṭakārī is an important therapeutic agent for dislodging tenacious phlegm and is extensively used in the treatment of cough, bronchitis and asthma. It is also useful in cases of influenza, enteric fever and allied conditions. The drug is diuretic, expectorant, febrifuge, cardiotonic, laxative, stimulant and is also used against difficult urination, bladder stones, rheumatism, sore-throat, enlargement of liver and spleen, vomiting and skin diseases. Fumigation with the seeds is a reputed cure for toothache (Nadkarni 1954: 1157; Kurup *et al.*, 1979: 105; Dey 1980: 75). Roots, fruits and occasionally the whole plant are used in medicine. The important formulations using the drug are *Kaṇṭakāri ghṛthaṃ, Kanakāsavaṃ, Pūtīkarañjāsavaṃ, Sūraṇādi lēhaṃ*, etc.

Classical literature informs us only that the plant is difficult to touch (*dusparśā*) due to sharp spines all over the plant body (*kaṇṭakārī, kaṇṭakāriṇī, vyāghrī*) (Aiyer & Kolammal, 1960. 4: 79).

Two varieties of *kaṇṭakārī* are mentioned in the texts viz. the blue-flowered and the white-flowered ones, of which the blue-flowered is more common (Chunekar, 1982: 289; Sharma, 1983: 280). In practice, the blue flowered *Solanum surattense* Burm. f. (now *S. virginianum* Linn.) (Solanaceae) is being used as the drug source in Kerala. Our field studies have revealed that *Solanum aculeatissimum* (now *S. capsicoides*) is also used as the source of *kaṇṭakārī* in some parts of Kerala. Whether this can be equated with the white-flowered variety mentioned in the texts is not known.

There is a view point that *kaṇṭakārī* is a constituent of the reputed *bṛhatīdvayaṃ* (= pair of *Solanum*) of the *daśamūla group*. Pāthya commentator also has agreed with this idea (cf. Mooss, 1980: 13). However, according to Kerala physicians, this is constituted by what are known as *ceṛu-vaḷutina* and *veḷ-vaḷutina*, which have been equated with different varieties of *Solanum melongena*. *Kaṇṭakārī* is considered as a distinct drug. *Bṛhatīdvayaṃ* is discussed separately elsewhere in this treatise.

S. virginianum *Linn.* **(Solanaceae)** (Fig. 102)
Solanum surattense Burm.f.
S. xanthocarpum Sch. & Wendl.

Diffuse herbs, very prickly on stem, leaves and calyx; leaves ovate-oblong, acute, pinnately 7–11 lobed, sparsely stellate-pubescent, 3.5–8 × 1.5–5 cms; flowers purple in few-flowered axillary cymes; calyx 5-lobed, prickly, corolla rotate, shallowly 5-lobed, pubescent outside; stamens 5, filaments very short, anthers yellow, long, opening by apical pores; fruit a glabrous, globular berry variegated with green and white stripes when young, yellow when mature; seeds smooth, compressed, reniform.

Distribution: The plant is found in all districts in the plains and low hills throughout India. It grows as a weed along roadside and wastelands. Also distributed in S. E. Asia, Malesia, Australia and Polynesia.

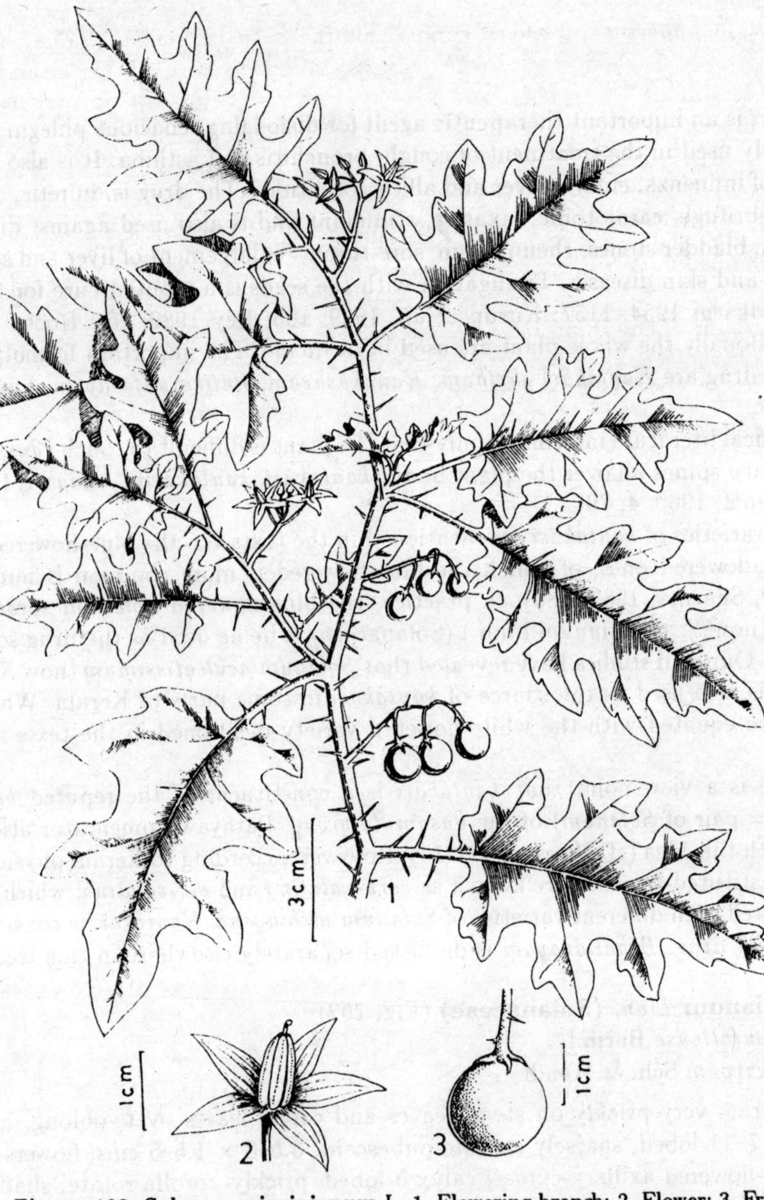

Figure 102: Solanum virginianum L. 1, Flowering branch; 2, Flower; 3, Fruit.

Note: The efficacy of *kantakārī* in the treatment of bronchial asthma (*shwās* & *kās*) and non-specific cough has been tried by Sharma K. *et al.* (1971) and Jain (1980) while Ansari *et al.* (1971) have studied the pharmacognosy of this species.

Solanum capsicoides *All.* **(Solanaceae)** (Fig. 103)
Solanum aculeatissimum Jacq.

Very prickly undershrub; leaves simple, alternate or in unequal pairs, broadly ovate, shallowly 5-lobed, dark green, sparsely hairy above, pale below and beset with prickles along the midrib and lateral veins on both sides; flowers white in few-flowered, supra axillary inflorescence; calyx gamosepalous, prickly outside, 5-lobed, persistent; corolla gamopetalous, regular, rotate, deeply 5-cleft; stamens 5, free, epipetalous, filaments short, anthers linear, 2-celled with apical pores; ovary 2-chambered, many ovuled, style short, stigma capitate; fruit smooth, globose berry, light green or variegated when young, orange-red when ripe; seeds many, slightly winged.

Distribution: Though an introduced one, the plant is found growing as a weed in waste places in Kerala and other states.

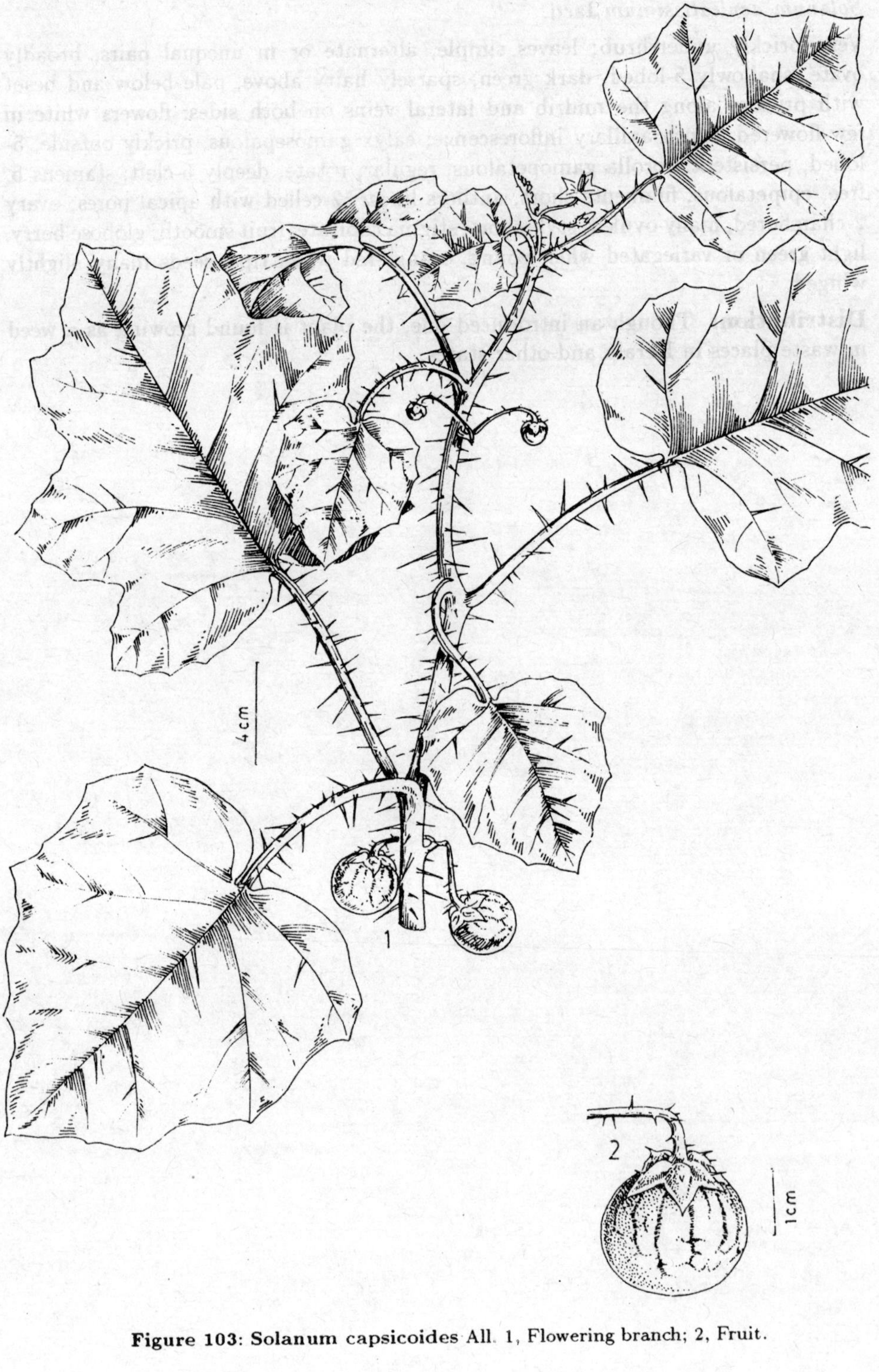

Figure 103: Solanum capsicoides All. 1, Flowering branch; 2, Fruit.

KARAÑJAḤ (Mal. UṄṄU, POṄṄAṂ)

This is reported to be an effective remedy for all skin diseases like scabies, eczema, leprosy and ulcers. According to *Bhāvaprakāśa*, *karañjaḥ* is acrid, active and hot and cures vaginal diseases, skin diseases, intestinal obstruction, *gulma* (phantom tumour), piles, ulcer, abdominal and splenic enlargement. Bark is the main part used. Leaves, root, fruit and oil from seeds are also medicinal. Leaves cure piles, parasites, oedema and morbid *kapha* and *vāta*. Fruit overcomes urinary diseases, piles and skin diseases. Oil from seeds is applied to scabies, sores, herpes and other skin diseases. (Aiyer & Kolammal, 1960, 4:11). The drug enters into the composition of preparations like *Nāgarādi tailaṃ*, *Varaṇādi kaṣāyaṃ*, *Varaṇādi ghṛtaṃ*, etc.

This plant, which is a reputed remedy for skin ailments (*kacchudāraḥ*), is described in the texts as foul-smelling (*pūtikaḥ*, *pūtiparṇaḥ*) with clustered flowers (*mañjarīpuṣpaḥ*, *lājapuṣpaḥ*, *gucchakaḥ*) and oiliferous seeds (*ghṛtapūrṇakarañjaḥ*) (cf. Aiyer & Kolammal, 1960. 4:9)

Bhāvaprakāśa mentions three varieties of *karañjaḥ* namely 1. *kaṇṭaka karañjaḥ* (syn: *karañjaḥ*, *naktamālaḥ*, *karajāḥ*, *cirivilvakaḥ*) 2. *ghṛtakarañjaḥ* (syn: *pūtikaḥ*, *pūtikarañjaḥ*, *sōmavalkaḥ*, *prakīryaḥ*) 3. *karañjī* (syn: *udakīryaḥ*, *hastivāruṇī*, *karabhañjikā*, *vāyasī*, *ṣaḍgrandhā*) (cf. Chunekar, 1982:350). Modern writers have also recognised three varieties of *karañjaḥ* namely, *vṛkṣa karañjaḥ*, *kaṇṭa karañjaḥ* and *cirivilvaḥ* and have equated them with *Pongamia pinnata* (Papilionaceae), *Caesalpinia bonduc* (Caesalpiniaceae) and *Holoptelia integrifolia* (Ulmaceae) respectively (cf. Sharma, 1983: 144, 706, 816).

Kerala physicians recognise two types of *karañja* and call it *karañjadvayaṃ* or *dvikarañjaṃ*. They are prescribed in formulations like *Āragvadhādi gaṇa*, *Varaṇādi gaṇa*, *Arkādi gaṇa*, etc. (cf. Mooss, 1980: 46, 56, 74). *Karañjaḥ* is equated with *Pongamia pinnata* (Papilionaceae), locally called *uṅṅu* or *poṅṅaṃ*. This has been described by Rheede (6: 5–6 t. 3. 1686) with the local name as *Poṅgam* and *pūtīkarañja* or *cirivilva* with *Holoptelia integrifolia* of Ulmaceae, locally called *āvil* or *ñeṭṭāval*. *Caesalpinia bonduc* is not considered as a variety of *karañjaḥ* by Kerala physicians, but is used as a separate drug under the name *kubērākṣī*, described elsewhere in the text.

Pongamia pinnata (*Linn.*) *Pierre* **(Papilionaceae)** (Fig. 104)
P. glabra Vent
Derris indica (Lam.) Bennet

Trees, leaves alternate, imparipinnate, 5–7 foliolate, leaflets elliptic-acuminate, 15 × 8 cms, glabrous; flowers small, pinkish white in axillary racemes; calyx cup-shaped, shortly 4–5 toothed; corolla papilionaceous, much exserted; stamens 10, monadelphous, anthers uniform; ovary subsessile, 2-ovuled, style incurved, glabrous, ending in a capitate stigma; pod woody, compressed, obliquely oblong; seed solitary.

Distribution: The plant is common throughout India. Often planted along roadsides as an avenue tree. Also distributed in Himalaya, Sri Lanka, Burma, Malaya, N. Australia and Polynesia.

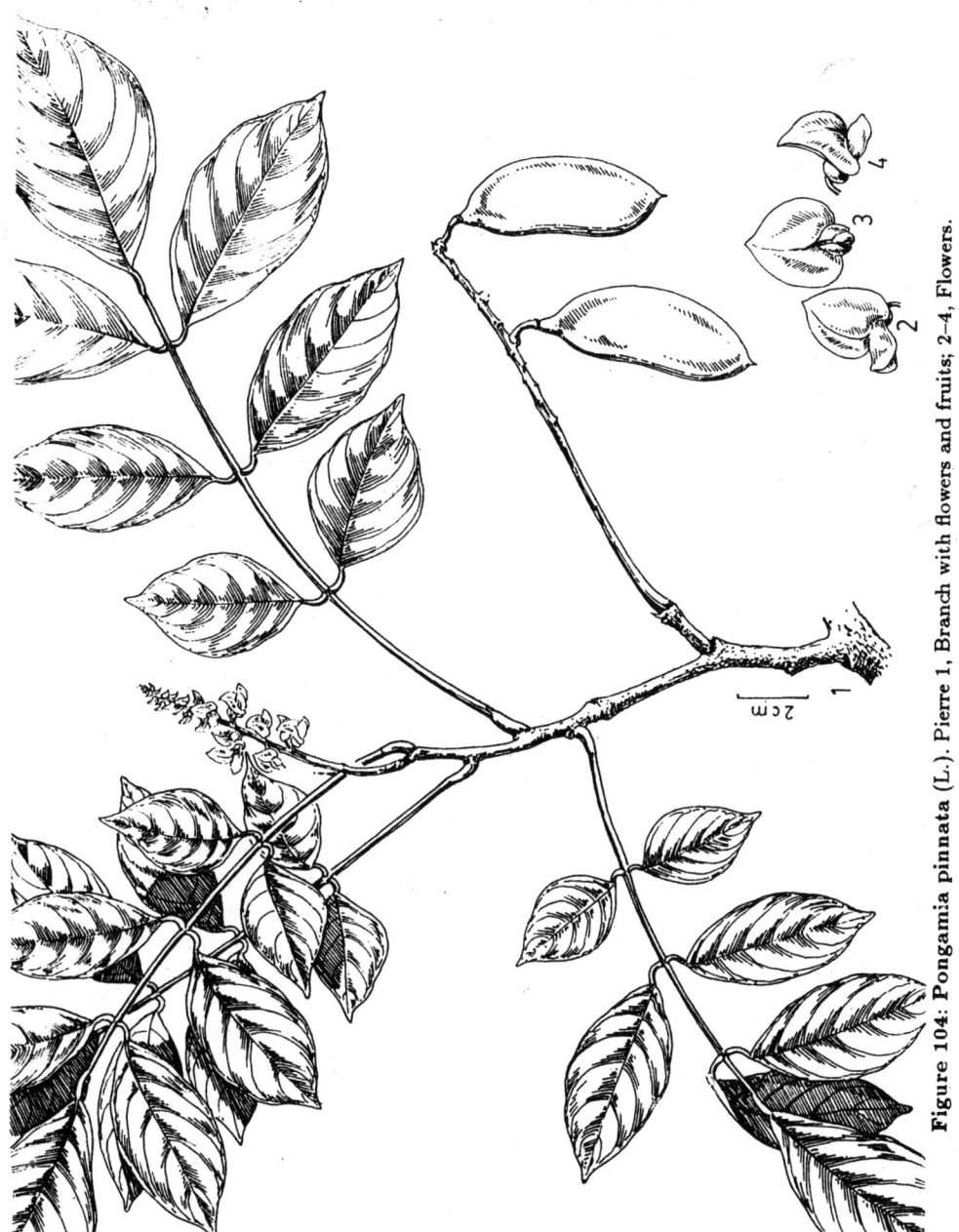

Figure 104: Pongamia pinnata (L.). Pierre 1, Branch with flowers and fruits; 2–4, Flowers.

KĀRASKARAḤ, KUPĪLUḤ (Mal. KĀÑÑIRAṂ)

The drug, commonly called 'nux vomica' is highly toxic to man and animals, producing stiffness of the muscles and convulsions, ultimately leading to death. But in small doses, it can also serve as efficacious cure for certain forms of paralysis and other nervous disorders. The seeds are bitter, nervine, stomachic, tonic, aphrodisiac, spinal, respiratory and cardiac stimulant. It is used as a remedy in intermittent fever, dyspepsia, chronic dysentery, paralytic and neuralgic affections, worms, epilepsy, chronic rheumatism, insomnia and colic. The drug is also useful in impotence, neuralgia of the face, heart disease, spermatorrhoea, skin diseases, toxins, wounds, emaciation, cough and cholera. Bark is employed as tonic and febrifuge. (Nadkarni, 1954: 1178, Kurup *et al.*, 1979: 127)

Strychnos nux-vomica Linn. (Loganiaceae), known as *kāññiraṃ* in Malayalam, is the plant used as the drug throughout the country. (See also Rheeds Hort. Malab. 1: 67–68, t.37.1678, *Canniram*).

Strychnos nux-vomica *Linn.* **(Loganiaceae)** (Fig. 105)

Trees; leaves simple, opposite, broadly ovate, acute, 7–12.5 × 5–8.5 cm, glabrous, 3–5 nerved; flowers greenish white in terminal many flowered cymes; calyx 5 lobed, pubescent, corolla tube cylindric, slightly hairy near the base within, 4–5 lobed; stamens 5; ovary pubescent; berries orange-red when ripe, thick-shelled, 5–6 cm across, seeds discoid.

Distribution: The plant is found in N. Circars, Deccan, Carnatic, also in W. Coast, in deciduous forest upto 4,000 ft. in hilly country. Also distributed in Sri Lanka, Siam, Indo China and Malesia.

Note: Nux-vomica and *Lignum colubrinum* were two drugs which had found their way to the European pharmacies from South India and Ceylon, since ancient times. Rheede has described three species of *Strychnos* which yield the drug, under the vernacular names *Caniram* (Hort. Malab: 1: 67 - 68, t. 37. 1678), *Modira-Caniram* (Hort. Malab. 8: 47 t. 24. 1688) and *Schem-Katu-valli-Kaniram* (Hort. Malab. 7: 9 t. 5. 1688) which have now been identified as *S. nux-vomica, S. colubrina* and *S. minor* respectively (Nicolson *et al.*, 1988. 163–164). The former is a tree while the other two are tendril-climbers. Bisset (1972) has made a comprehensive study of literature on the source and use of this drug. In Kerala, at present, only *S. nux-vomica* is used.

There is, however, another not-so-important drug, locally known as *vaḷḷikāññiraṃ*, the accepted source of which is *Tiliacora acuminata* (Menispermaceae), since at least Rheede's times (Hort. Malab. 7: 5–6. t. 3. 1688). Botanically speaking, except for some superficial similarity in the foliage, this has no what-so-ever relationship with the genus *Strychnos* (*kāññiraṃ*).

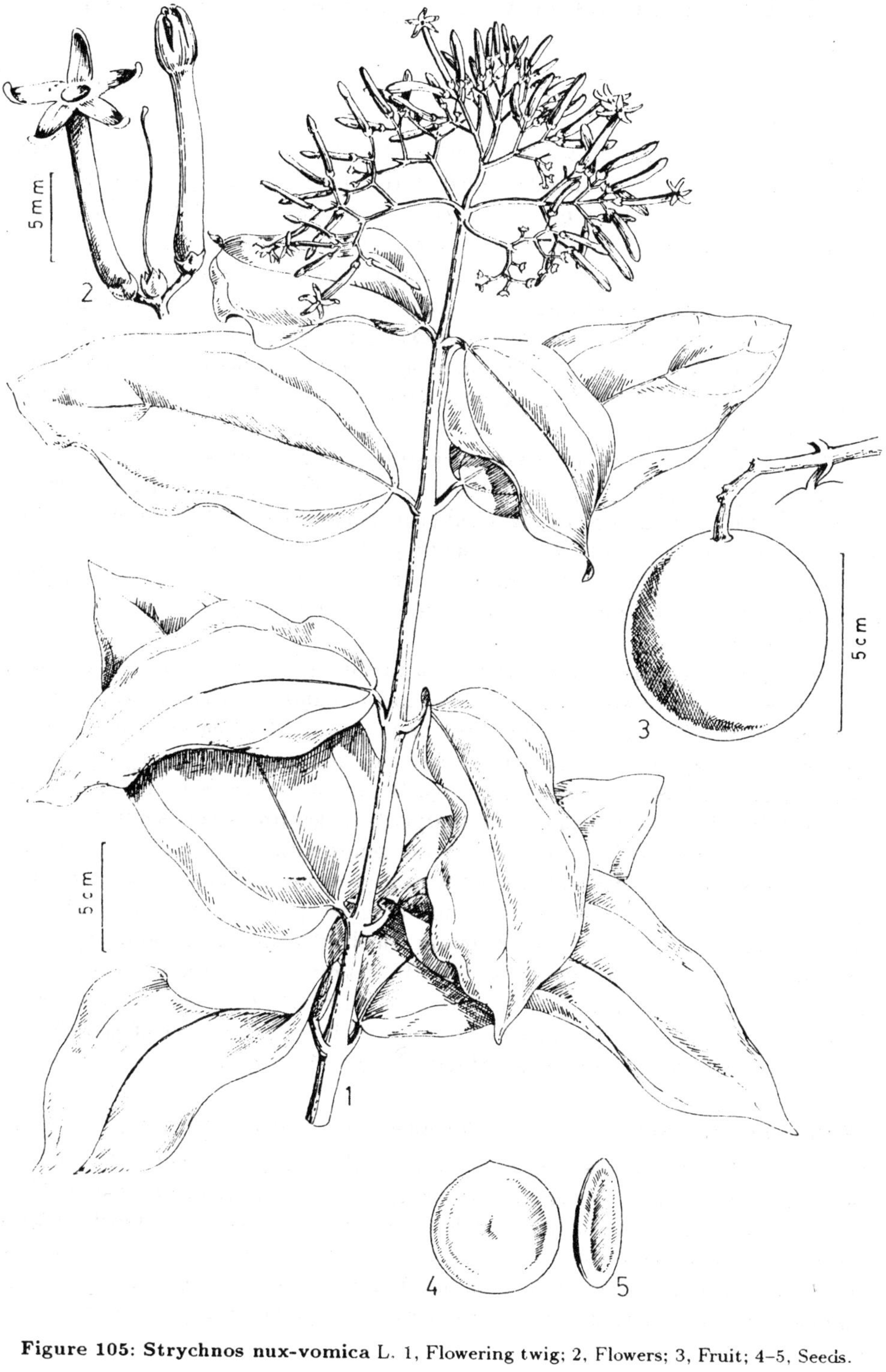

Figure 105: Strychnos nux-vomica L. 1, Flowering twig; 2, Flowers; 3, Fruit; 4–5, Seeds.

KĀRAVĒLLAṂ (Mal. PĀVAL, KAIPPA)

Kāravēllaṃ is a reputed medicine prescribed for diabetic patients by traditional physicians. The fruits, commonly called 'bitter-gourd' is a highly sought-after vegetable, while the whole plant is used in medicine. It is bitter (*kaṭhillaḥ*), anthelmintic, antidiabetic, cardiotonic, laxative and a digestive stimulant. It is used in cough, respiratory diseases, fever, intestinal worms, skin diseases and poisonous affections. The drug improves digestion, calms down sexual urge, quells diseases due to *pitta* and *kapha* and cures anaemia, anorexia, leprosy, ulcers, jaundice, flatulence and piles. Fruit is useful in gout, rheumatism and complaints of liver and spleen (Nadkarni, 1954; 806; Aiyer & Kolammal, 1966. 9: 86, 87; Mooss, 1976: 85; Kurup *et al.*, 1979: 107).

Kaccōrādi tailaṃ is an important prepartion using the drug.

According to the description in the texts, the plant gives forth pretty fruits (*suṣavī*) and it emits a penetrating smell (*ugragandhā*) (Aiyer & Kolammal, 1966. 9: 86). Other synonyms indicate only the properties of the drug.

The accepted source of this drug throughout the country is species of *Momordica* (Cucurbitaceae) and the synonyms *suṣavī* and *ugragandhā* seem to fit the genus very well.

Bhiṣagārya recognises three varieties of this drug, namely *kāravēlla, kāravallī* and *vanyakāravallī*. However, Kerala physicians recognise only two types, *kāravallī* and *vanyakāravallī* which are called *pāval* or *kaippa* and *kāṭṭupāval* respectively, in the vernacular. Mooss (1976. 83) has equated the former with *Momordica charantia* and the latter with *M. tuberosa* respectively. *M. tuberosa* Cogn. is a rather rare, wild species with tuberous roots and small, sharply 6-angled fruits, very similar to those of *Luffa* and hence has been removed to the genus with the name *Luffa tuberosa* Roxb. (Chakravarty, 1982). This species, has never been found in use in Kerala, probably because, it is difficult to procure it in adequate quantity. Instead, it is the two different varieties of *M. charantia* which is found most commonly used. The cultivated form with large fruits (viz. *M. charantia* var. *charantia*) is the one usually taken for *kāravallī* while the accepted source of *vanyakāravallī* is the wild variety (var. *muricata*) with small fruits. However, it is the latter which is preferred in medicine (also see Rheede, Hort. Malab. 8: 19, t. 10. 1688).

Momordica charantia *Linn. var.* **charantia (Cucurbitaceae)** (Fig. 106)

Slender climber; branchlets villous; tendrils simple, opposite to leaves; leaves simple, alternate, orbicular-cordate, 5–7 lobed, apex acuminate or mucronate, 4–8.5 × 3.5–8.5 cm; flowers yellow, solitary in the axils, on a long, slender peduncle, with a reniform bract towards base; calyx tube campanulate, greenish-pubescent, adnate to the ovary; corolla yellow; stamens 3, inserted at the mouth of the hypanthium in staminate flowers, filaments short; in pistillate flower pistil syncarpous; fruit oblong, echniate, 8–20 cm long, fusiform.

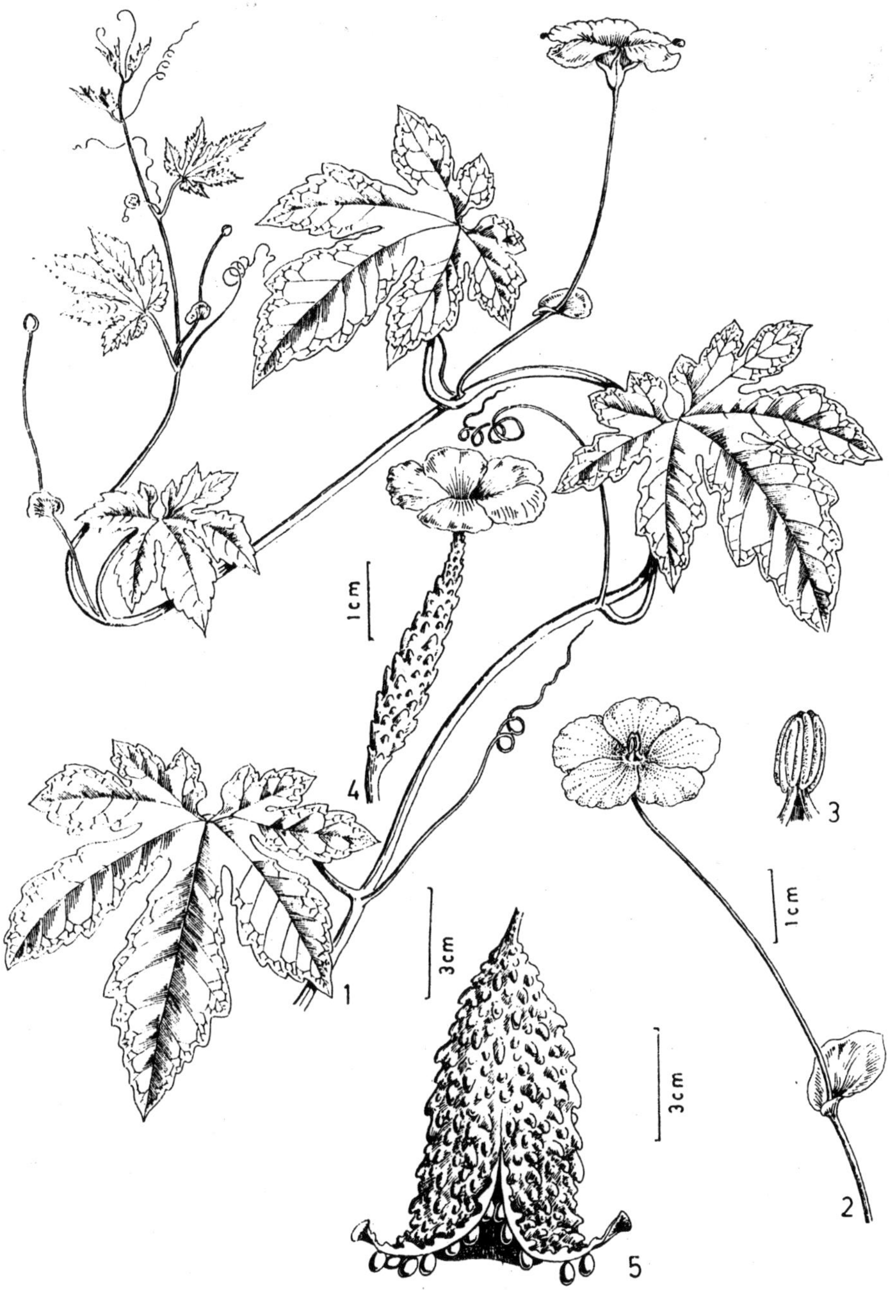

Figure 106: Momordica charantia L. var. **charantia.** 1, Vine; 2, Male flower; 3, Stamens; 4, Female flower; 5, Fruit.

Distribution: The plant is commonly cultivated as a vegetable in tropical and warm countries.

M. charantia *var.* **muricata** (*Willd.*) *Chakr.*
M. muricata Willd.
This variety can easily be distinguished from the var. *charantia* by its faintly nerved leaves and small fruits (5–7.5 cm long) tapering at both ends.

Occuring throughout the area of distribution of var. *charantia*, this is very common, but difficult to distinguish, unless we get mature fruits.

Note: The significant hypoglycaemic activity of the fruits of *M. charantia* has been clinically tested by many. Akhtar *et al.* (1981) and Karunanayake *et al.* (1984) found that oral administration of *M. charantia* fruit causes a decrease in blood sugar level of normal and alloxan diabetic rabbits and rats. The hypoglycaemic and hypocholesterolemic activity of the water and ether extracts of bitter gourd powder have been clinically proved by Upadhyaya *et al.* also (1986). The studies made by Meir & Yaniv (1985) prove that the fruit of this plant contains two inhibitory compounds, one against hexo kinese activity and the other against glucose uptake by rat intestinal fragments.

The chemical, pharmacological and clinical studies done on this plant have been discussed in detail by Satyavati *et al.* (1987: 262–268).

KARAVĪRAḤ (Mal. KAṆAVĪRAṂ)

The root of *karavīra* is one of the several vegetable root poisons, but if administered carefully, it is a powerful cardiac tonic. It is bitter, hot, astringent, anthelmintic, carminative, diaphoretic and is valuable for curing ulcers, leprosy and skin diseases. It overcomes morbid *kapha* and *vāta*, cures dyspepsia, intestinal disorders, cardiac asthma, fever, respiratory disorders and worm. A paste of the root is externally applied to ulcerations in leprosy, scorpion stings and snake bites. Paste of the root bark and leaves is used in ring worm and other skin complaints. Fresh juice of the leaves is dropped into the eyes in opthalmia and to improve eye sight (Nadkarni, 1954: 848; Chunekar, 1982: 314; Sharma, 1983; 212). The drug enters into the composition of preparations like *Mālatyādi tailaṃ* and *Mustāmṛtādi cūrṇaṃ*.

The poisonous nature of the plant is well indicated by the synonyms *aśvamārakaḥ, hayamārakaḥ*, etc. which mean that it is capable of killing horse. The plant is described to have two varieties viz. white-flowered (*śvētapuṣpaḥ*) and red flowered (*raktapuṣpaḥ*). But none of them gives any idea regarding the accurate identity of the plant.

Bhāvaprakāśanighaṇṭu and *Dhanvantarinighaṇṭu* mention two varieties of *karavīra* i.e. the white and red flowered ones, having identical properties. In *Rājanighaṇṭu*, four varieties with white, red, yellow and black (blue) flowers are described, while modern writers recognize only three varieties namely white, red and yellow. The first two are equated with the same plant *Nerium oleander* L. of Apocynaceae which is locally known as *kaṇavīraṃ* or *araḷi*. Rheede also describes and portrays the two varieties under the names *Tsjovanna-areli*, the red-flowered (Hort. Malab. 9: 1–2, t. 1. 1689) and *Belutta-areli*, the white-flowered (9: 3, t. 62. 1689) which have been identified as the same plant *Nerium oleander* (Nicolson *et al.*, 1988: 160). The yellow-flowered variety, called *pītakaravīra* is equated with *Cascabela thevetia* (= *Thevetia peruviana*) of the same family. Like *karavīr*, this is also considered to be a good cardiotonic, having the property to strengthen the functioning of heart and to cure cardiac asthma, oedema and skin diseases, despite its poisonous properties (Chunekar, 1982: 324–326; Sharma, 1983: 211–213).

Though the red and white flowered varieties are preferred in medicine, the yellow flowered *Cascabela* is also found used in some Āyurvēdic preparations. The two plant sources of the drug can be identified as follows.

Nerium oleander *Linn.* **(Apocynaceae)** (Fig. 107)
Nerium indicum Miller
Nerium odorum Soland.

Evergreen shrub; leaves in whorls of 4–6, linear-lanceolate, acuminate, 15 × 2.5 cms, thickly coriaceous, midrib stout, secondary veins numerous, close and parallel; flowers large, showy, sweet-scented, single or double in terminal cymes; sepals subulate-

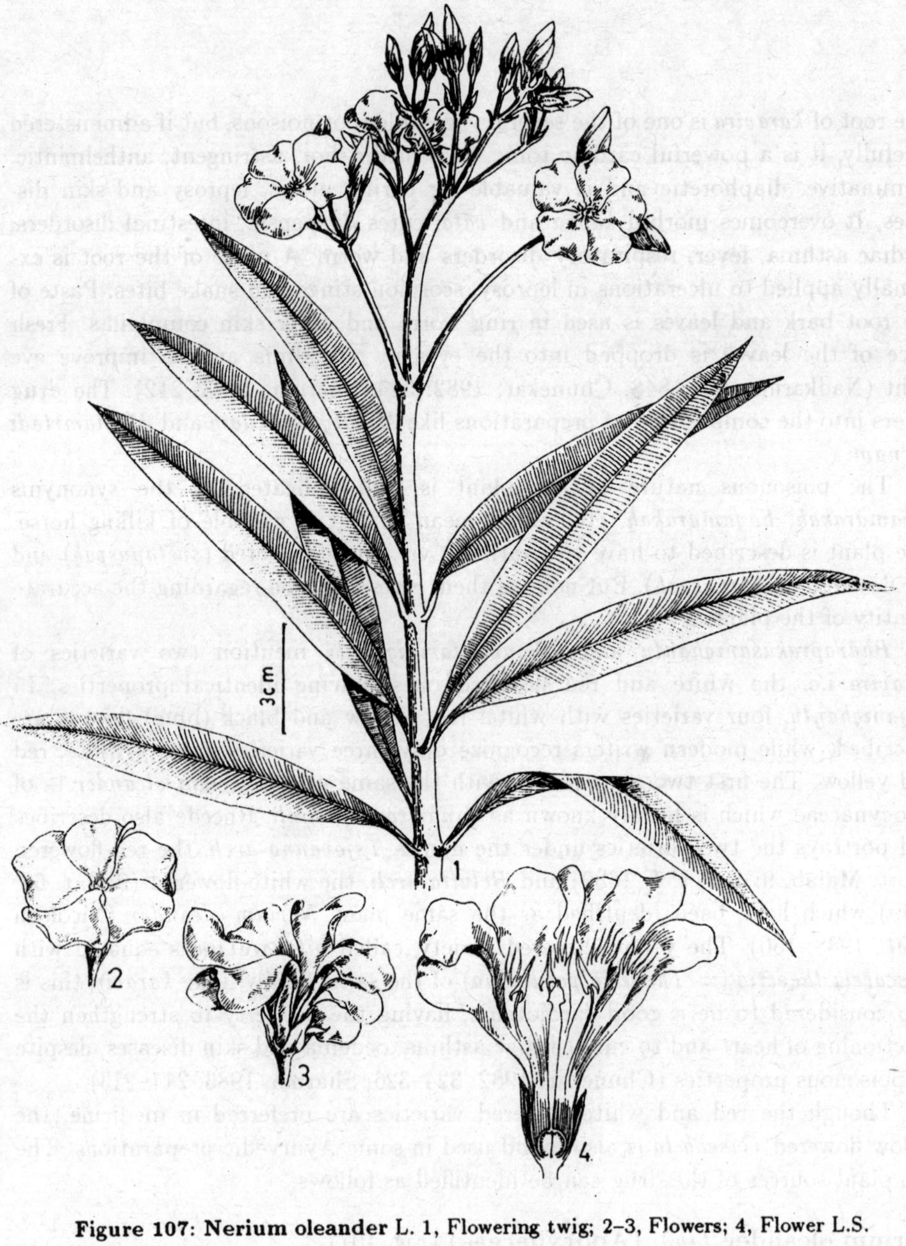

Figure 107: Nerium oleander L. 1, Flowering twig; 2–3, Flowers; 4, Flower L.S.

lanceolate; corolla funnel-shaped; follicles 2, cylindrical, 15–17.8 cm; seeds linear, ribbed, villous.

Distribution: Tropical and subtropical Asia, Europe and Africa. In southern India, this plant is found only under cultivation.

Note: Widely cultivated ornamental with white, pink, red and yellow, single and double flowers. This plant has been known as highly toxic for live-stock and human beings. Theophrastus has mentioned about the poisoning of military animals of Alexander, the Great, during his conquest (334. 323 B.C.). Dioscorides and Pliny also have mentioned that the leaves and flowers can kill animals. The toxicity is such that there are several mentions about this plant in ancient war chronicles. In 1796, some French soldiers in Corsica died immediately after eating meat skewered on an oleander branch and in Africa several soldiers who slept on pallets made of Olender branches either died or were seriously poisoned. In human beings the symptoms of Oleander poisoning are depression, dizziness, fever, nausea, diarrhoea, weak heart beat and pulse, paralysis, loss of consciousness and death through heart failure.

Despite this, the use of this plant in medicine has also been known since ancient times. Dioscorides, the personal physician of the Roman emperor Nero, has mentioned that the Oleander poison taken with wine and rue (*Ruta graveolens*) is antivenum for snake bites. This has also been found to have anticancerous properties in the recent times.

Cascabela thevetia (*Linn.*) *Lippold* (**Apocynaceae**) (Fig. 108)
Thevetia peruviana (Pers.) Merr.
Thevetia neriifolia Juss. ex Steudel.

Shrub or small tree; leaves alternate, linear-lanceolate acute, upto 19 × 2 cms, glabrous, midrib prominent, lateral nerves faint; flowers large, bright yellow in terminal, peduncled cymes; calyx lobes 5, unequal, shortly united, lanceolate; corolla yellow, funnel shaped, tube 4 cm narrowed from below the middle, throat villous, lobes 5, overlapping to left; stamens 5, included, anthers oblong-cordate, mucronate, ovary 2-locular, depressed-conic; drupe broadly turbinate, 3 cm across, compressed laterally; seeds few, flattened.

Distribution: A native of tropical America, this plant is widely naturalised elsewhere in tropics. Seen wild and also cultivated in gardens in India.

Note: The pharmacognosy of *Nerium oleander* has been worked out by Sharma and Kapoor (1970). Studies by Singh *et al.* (1970) and Trivedi *et al.* (1978) have proved the cardiotonic effect of this drug. Dev and Wasir (1985) have discussed in detail the pharmacology and clinical application of *Cascabela thevetia*.

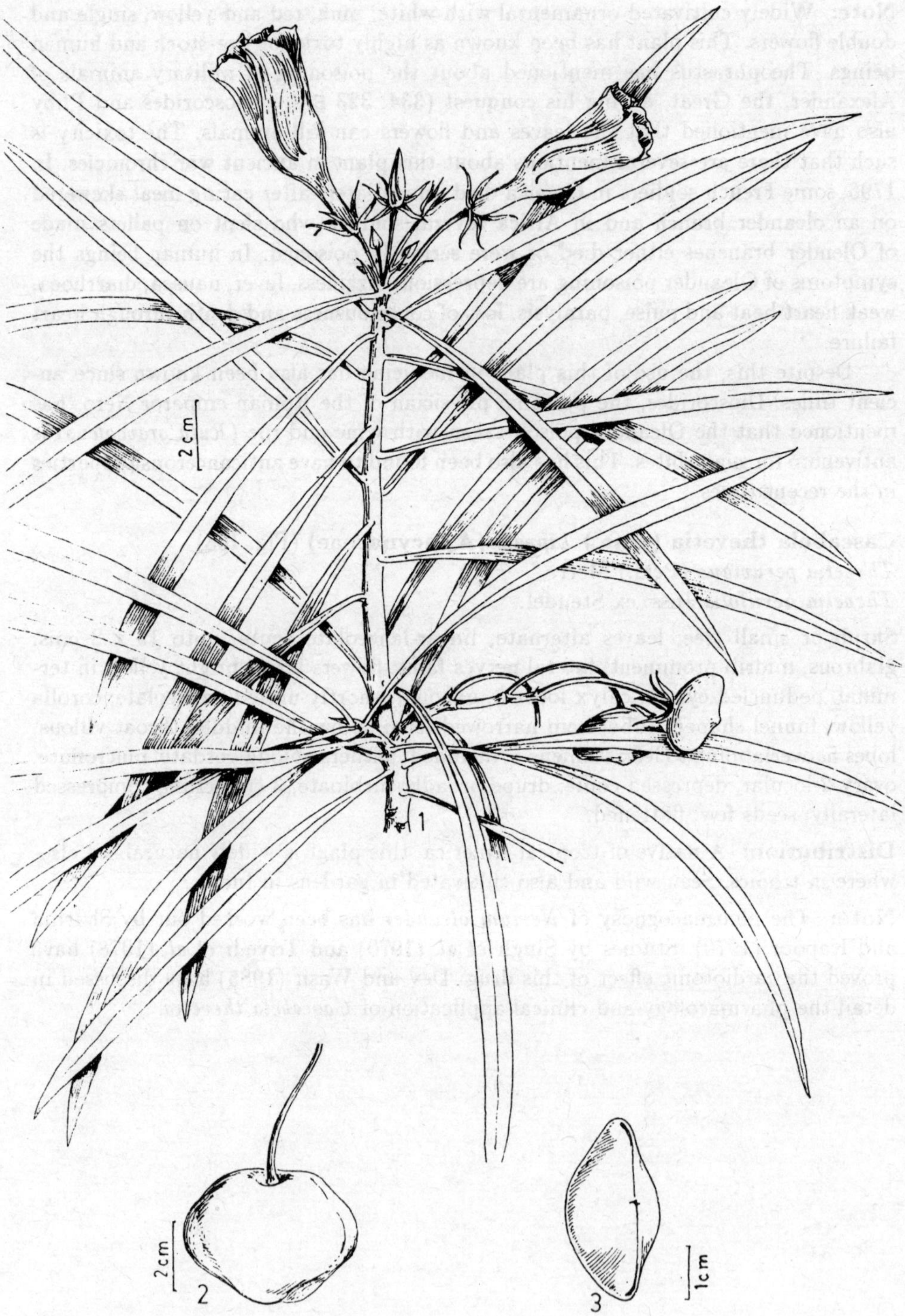

Figure 108: Cascabela thevetia (L.) Lippold. 1, Flowering twig; 2–3, Fruits.

KAṚCŪRAḤ (Mal. KACCŌLAṂ)

Karcūra is a reputed remedy for all diseases caused by the morbidity of *vāta* and *kapha* and is especially useful in respiratory ailments like cough, bronchitis and asthma. The drug is reported to be acrid, hot, bitter, aromatic and light. It cures skin diseases, wounds and splenic disorders. It promotes digestion, removes bad odour of the mouth and destroy pathogenic organisms (Aiyer & Kolammal, 1964. 8: 91). The officinal part is the rhizome and it is a constituent of a wide variety of Āyurvēdic preparations like *Daśamūlariṣṭaṃ, Valiya Rāsnādi kaṣāyaṃ, Kaccōrādi cūrṇaṃ, Asanaelāditailaṃ, Valiya Nārāyaṇa tailaṃ*, etc.

From the texts, one can infer that this drug is capable of alleviating a variety of ailments (*vēdhamukhyaḥ, śaṭi* etc.) it occurs mainly in the colder regions (*himōdbhavā*) and that it has several, strongly aromatic roots (*karcūraḥ, karbūrā, ṣaḍgrandhikā, gandhamūlī, sugandhamūlā*) (See Aiyer & Kolammal, 1964. 8: 91). Nevertheless, the identity of the plant source of this drug is a matter of debate.

Moreover, there is difference of opinion among men of Āyurvēda, as to whether *śaṭī* and *karcūra* are the same drug or different. Many authors consider them different and equate *śaṭī* with *Hedychium spicatum* Smith and *karcūra* with *Curcuma zedoaria*, both belonging to Zingiberaceae (Kurup *et al.*, 1979: 195, 109; Chunekar, 1982: 245, 247; Sharma, 1983: 292, 294). However, some others treat them to be the same and equate it with *Curcuma zedoaria* (Kirtikar & Basu, 1918: 1247; Vaidya, 1936: 544; Nadkarni, 1954: 408; Kapoor & Mitra, 1979: 64).

Hedychium spicatum is a plant found in the Himalayas with its spikes sometimes reaching a length of 35 cm. This is not available in the south, nor it has been the source of the drug in Kerala. *Curcuma zedoaria* is available in Kerala. With its yellowish white, fragrant rhizomes having a sharp pinching taste, it suits the synonymy rather well, but goes under the name *kua* in Malabar (See Rheede, Hort. Malab. 11: 13–14, t. 7. 1692, *Kua*). There is some evidence to believe that the tubers of *Curcuma zedoaria* have been the source of this drug in Kerala in the early times. Garcia da Orta (1563: 455) while describing the drug *'Zedoary'* says "... the Guzeratis and Deccanis (call it) *Cochora*, the people of Malabar *Cua*" (orthographic variants of *kaccōlaṃ* and *kua* respectively). "Most of it is in Malabar, namely Calicut and Cannanore. It grows in the woods, but is planted or sown and thrives in many parts". The description that "The leaf is like that of ginger" also suits *C. zedoaria* well.

However, the source of *karcūra* in Kerala in the recent times has been *Kaempferia galanga* of the same family. Rheede's description of this plant under the name *Katsjula Kelengu* (katsjula = kaccola, kilangu = tubers) (Hort. Malab. 11: 81, t. 41. 1692) proves that this has been the drug source, at least since the 17th century. The tubers of *K. galanga* compare well with the characters indicated in the synonymy. The objection of Duthie that it is not a native of India and hence cannot be considered as the source of this drug is not true (See Burtt in Dassan & Fosb., Rev. Handb. Fl. Ceylon 4: 509, 510, 1983, where it is described as a native of India).

Curcuma zedoaria (*Christm.*) *Roscoe* (Zingiberaceae) (Fig. 109)
Amomum zedoaria Christm.
Curcuma zerumbet Roxb.
Large perennial herb with yellowish-white rhizomes and fibrous roots; pseudostem about 40 cm tall; leaves large, elliptic to oblong-lanceolate, acuminate, to 45 × 30 cms, greenish and often blotched with purple down the middle on the upper side, glabrous, flowers yellow in the axils of pouched bracts in dense strobiliform spikes; calyx whitish, membraneous, irregularly 3-toothed; corolla funnel-shaped, limb 3-lobed, whitish, lateral staminodes petaloid and connate with the broad filament of the fertile stamen; lip orbicular, obscurely 3 lobed; ovary inferior, 3-chambered, hairy, style slender, stigma 2-lipped; capsules globose.
Distribution: Most parts of India and S.E. Asia

Kaempferia galanga *Linn.* (Zingiberaceae) (Fig. 110)
A geophilous perennial herb with very fragrant, white rhizomes and ovoid tubers at the tips of fibrous roots; leaves 2–3, radical, spread over the floor, broadly ovate or orbicular, 20 × 15 cms, glabrous, green above, tawny below; flowers rose-coloured with purple spots, 2–3 in a subsessile spike, lasting only for a day; calyx spathaceous, corolla tubular, 3-lobed; fertile stamen 1, staminodes petaloid, lip deeply 2-lobed; ovary inferior, 3-celled, style filiform ending in a turbinate, urceolate stigma; capsules oblong.
Distribution: A native of India; common in the plains, at low elevations, especially in shaded areas on the forest floor.

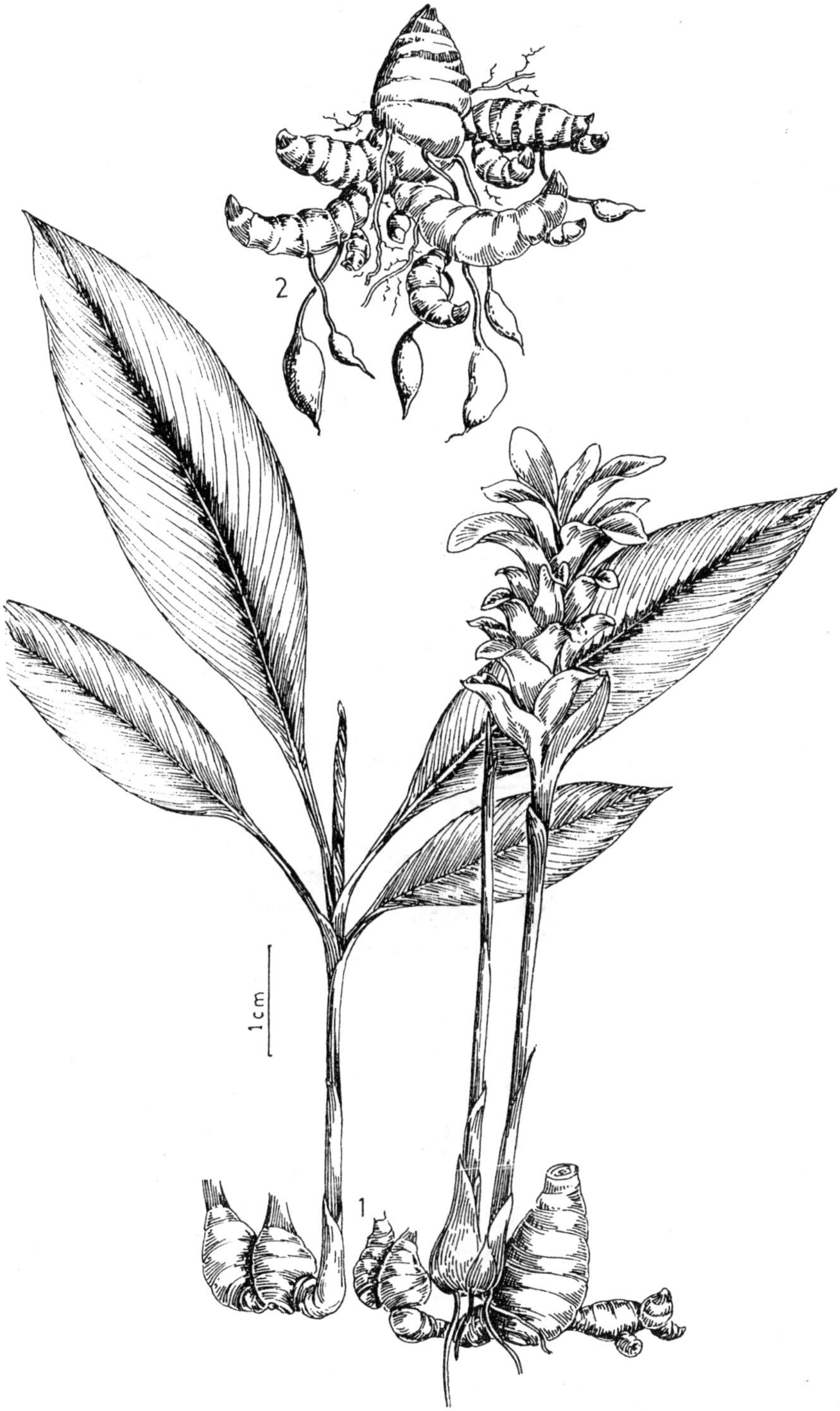

Figure 109: Curcuma zedoaria (Christm.) Rosc. 1, Habit; 2, Rhizome.

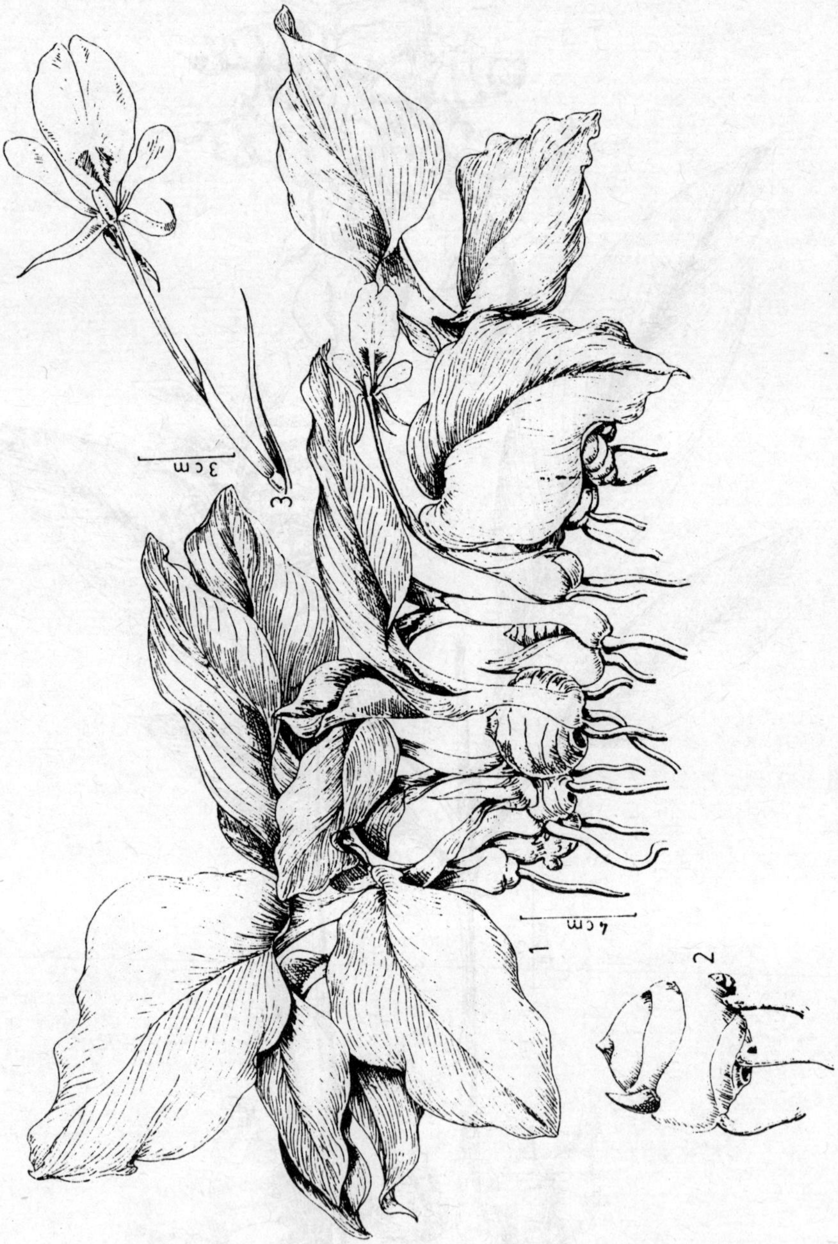

Figure 110: Kaempferia galanga L. 1, Habit; 2, Rhizome; 3, Flower.

KĀṚPĀSAḤ (Mal. PARUTTI)

In traditional medicine, this drug is considered to be an effective remedy against rheumatism. The officinal part is the seed. It is sweet, light, and galactagogue. It gives strength to the body, dispels diseases caused by the morbidity of *tridōṣās* and cures thirst, burning sensation, lysuria, oedema, uterine disorders, anaemia and genitourinary diseases. Leaves are diuretic and are beneficial in mental disorders. They repress boils and cure skin diseases and rat poison. The flowers are germicidal and they purify blood and heal ulcers due to leprosy. The seeds are aphrodisiac and unctuous and are recommended in scanty lactation and diarrhoea. (Kolammal, 1979. 10: 3, Kurup *et al.*, 1979: 110). The drug forms an ingredient of preparations like *Kāṛpāsāstyādi tailaṃ, Kāṛpāsāstyādi kuḷambu, Saṛvāmayāntaka ghṛtaṃ, Śvētaguñjādi guḷika*, etc.

Ancient texts have described it as a drug of manifold application (*kāṛpāsī, guṇāsū*), the seeds of which are capable of long-distance dispersal (*samudrāntā, vāmani, sāraṇī*) and the hair-like appendages of which are usually woven into cloth (*paṭaḥ, chādanaḥ, vāsasī, tūlā*) (cf. Kolammal, 1979. 10: 3).

There are two varieties of this drug, mentioned in the texts: *kāṛpāsa* and *vanakāṛpāsa* (the wild one). The plant source of the former is almost universally accepted to be species of *Gossypium*, the cotton plant of Malvaceae. The latter has been equated with *Thespesia lampas* of the same family, which runs wild throughout India. (Chunekar, 1982: 375; Sharma, 1983: 601). But this is not very much in use in medicine.

There are two different species of *Gossypium* used as the source of *kāṛpāsa*. Most of the North Indian physicians equate it with *Gossypium herbaceum* Linn. (Nadkarni, 1954: 587; Kurup *et al.*, 1979: 110; Kapoor & Mitra, 1979: 64; Chunekar, 1982: 374; Sharma, 1983: 600), while the southerners usually prefer *G. arboreum L.* (see also Rheede, Hort. Malab. 1: 55–56, t. 31. 1678, *Cudu-Paritti*). Nevertheless, consequent to the widespread cultivation of commercial cotton in various parts of India and with the resultant introduction of more species and varieties, the drug that now comes to the market is a mixture of seeds of all the available ones (see also Kolammal, 1979. 10: 4).

Gossypium arboreum *Linn.* **(Malvaceae)** (Fig. 111)

Erect shrub, leaves simple, alternate, long-petioled, broad ovate-cordate, deeply palmately 3–5 lobed, glabrescent; lobes linear oblong to oblong-lanceolate, mucronate, under surface punctate with black dots; flowers large, reddish with darker centre or rarely yellowish, axillary, solitary; bracteoles 3, large, foliaceous, ovate-cordate, laciniate, punctate; calyx truncate, punctate; corolla of five free spreading petals, adnate at base to the base of the staminal column; stamens many, monadelphous; ovary 3-celled; fruit a loculicidal capsule, seeds covered with white cotton fibres.

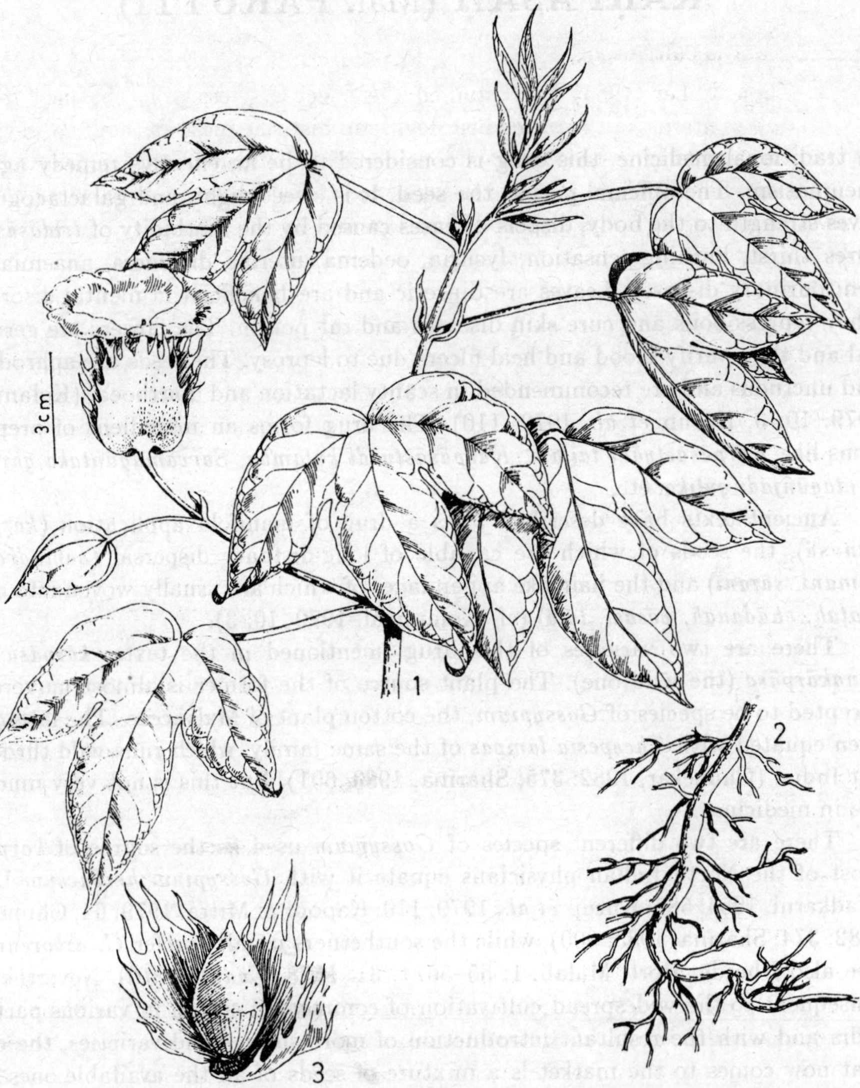

Figure 111: Gossypium arboreum L. 1, Twig; 2, Roots; 3, Fruit.

Distribution: The plant is found throughout the greater part of India in the plains districts. It is at times cultivated as an ornamental in gardens.

Gossypium herbareum *Linn.* **(Malvaceae)**

Erect, subglabrous shrub; leaves cordate, 3–5 lobed, lobes broadly ovate-acuminate; flowers axillary, solitary, yellow with a purple centre; involucral bracts 3, ovate-dentate; calyx truncate or obsoletely crenulate; petals spreading, obovate or cuneate; stamens many, filaments united to form the tube with the free ends bearing anthers; capsule ovate, globose, mucronate, 3–5 valved; seeds 5–7 in each cell, ovoid, with white or brownish adpressed fibres.

The plant is cultivated.

Note: Zhou & Lei (1984) have studied the effect of Gossypol (obtained from *Gossypium*) on uterus and ovary by histologic and histochemical methods. Gossypol has been employed in gynaecologic clinics for the treatment of endometriosis and functional uterine bleeding. It has been found to act on the uterus directly as well as indirectly by inhibiting ovarian secretions and antagonising the effect of oestrogen in the female.

KARPŪRAVALLĪ (Mal. KAÑÑIKKŪṚKA, PANIKKŪṚKA)

This aromatic plant (*karpūravallī*) with its distinctive smelling leaves (*gandhaparṇikā*) is a common home remedy for infantile cough, cold and fever. The drug is hot, digestive, carminative, diuretic, anthelmintic and constipating. It overcomes diseases due to *kapha* and *vāta*, cures poisonous affections and stimulates the function of liver. It is given in epilepsy and other convulsive affections, kidney and bladder stones, indigestion, diarrhoea, dysentery, cholera and bilious affections. Crushed leaves are used as a local application for headache and to relieve the pain and irritation caused by poisonous bites (Nadkarni, 1954: 371; Sharma, 1983: 462). Leaves form an ingredient of preparations like *Gōpīcandanādi guḷika, Abhraṃ* (101), *Puḷilēham*, etc.

The accepted source of this drug in Kerala is *Coleus ambonicus* Lour. of Lamiaceae. Many authors have equated this plant with *pāṣāṇabhēdaḥ* (Kirtikar & Basu, 1918: 1017; Vaidya K.M., 1936: 33; Nadkarni, 1954: 371; Chopra *et al.*, 1956: 74; Kapoor & Mitra, 1979: 74; Chunekar, 1982: 105; Vaidya Bapalal, 1982: 6), may be because of its reported property to have specific action on the bladder. However, Kerala physicians accept it as the source of the drug *karpūravallī*, though there is no mention of it in any of the Āyurvēdic texts.

Coleus ambonicus *Lour.* **(Lamiaceae)** (Fig. 112)
C. aromaticus Benth.
Plectranthus ambonicus (Lour.) Spreng.

Much branched, fleshy, highly aromatic pubescent herb; leaves simple, opposite, long-petioled, lamina broadly ovate or orbicular-obtuse, crenate-serrate on margin, to 9 cm across, fleshy, bullate above; flowers small, purple, in dense whorls at intervals on a terminal racemose axis; calyx 2-lipped, tube decurved; corolla 2-lipped; stamens 4, didynamous; fruit of 4 orbicular nutlets.

Distribution: The plant is a Malay species, cultivated and found run wild. It grows in Circars, Deccan and Carnatic.

Note: Rheede (9: 145–146 t. 74: 1689) has portrayed this species, but has wrongly attributed the name 'Iribeli'. These are two distinct drugs used in Indian medicine which are taken from closely related species of *Coleus*, viz. *C. ambonicus* and *C. zeylanicus* respectively. These two can be easily recognised by the flaccidness of leaves and by their distinctive odour.

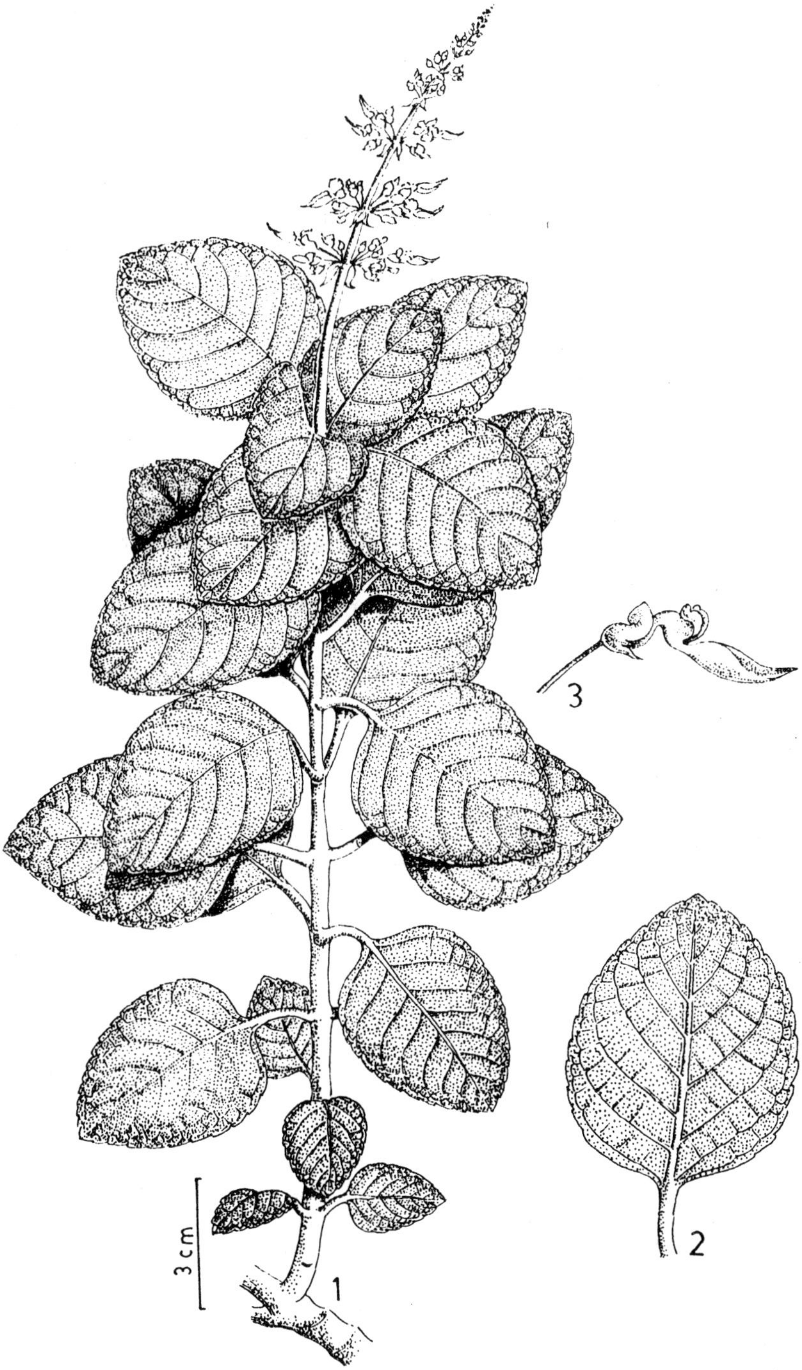

Figure 112: **Coleus ambonicus** Lour. 1, Flowering twig; 2, Leaf; 3, Flower.

KĀSAḤ (Mal. KUŚA)

This drug enters into the composition of preparations like *Valiya Candanāditailaṃ, Sukumāraṃ kaṣāyaṃ, Vīratarādi ghṛtaṃ, Sukumāraṃ lēhaṃ, Traikaṇṭaka ghṛtaṃ*, etc. It is reported to be sweet, cooling, astringent, diuretic, galactagogue and overcomes vitiated *vāta* and *pitta*, cures *raktapitta*, tuberculosis, dysentery, bleeding piles, kidney and bladder stones, dysuria, thirst and burning sensation (Chunekar, 1982: 380; Sharma, 1983: 637). Root is the officinal part.

Saccharum spontaneum L. (Poaceae), is the accepted source of the drug. (See Vaidya K.M. 1936: 132; Nadkarni, 1954: 1088; Anonymous, 1978a: 245; Mooss, 1980: 62; Dey, 1980: 80; Chunekar, 1982: 380; Sharma, 1983: 636).

Saccharum spontaneum *Linn.* **(Poaceae)**

Tall, erect, perennial grass; culms slender, 0.8–1 cm wide; leaf sheaths to 20 cm, glabrous; leaves narrowly linear, finely acuminate, rigid, coriaceous, ligule ovate, membraneous; panicles 20–50 cm, silky white, spikelets in pairs, one pedicelled and the other sessile; glumes 4, lanceolate, ciliate, lower glume glabrous, 2-dentate, 2-keeled, upper glume 1-keeled, shortly aristate; lower lemma sparsely ciliate, epaleate; grains oblong to subglobose.

Distribution: Distributed throughout India, Pakistan and the warmer regions of the Old World.

KĀSAMARḌAḤ (Mal. PONNĀVĪRAṂ)

Kāsa, in Sanskrit, means cough. As the synonyms *kāsamarḍaḥ* and *kāsārī* indicate, this is often recommended against cough, asthma and other respiratory ailments. It helps regain the balance of the three *dōṣās—vāta, pitta* and *kapha*, improves digestion, clears throat and purifies blood. A paste made out of roots is considered as a specific for ringworm, eczema and other skin ailments. (Aiyer & Kolammal, 1964. 8: 80). Bark, roots, leaves and seeds are used in medicine. The drug is an ingredient of *Surasādi tailaṃ*.

Many of the authors consider *Cassia occidentalis* Linn. (Caesalpiniaceae) as the plant source of this drug (Vaidya, 1936: 134; Singh & Chunekar, 1972: 677; Chunekar, 1982: 97; Sharma, 1983: 287). Some others equate *Cassia sophera* Linn. also with *kāsamarḍaḥ*, in addition to *C. occidentalis* (Kirtikar & Basu, 1918: 470, 472; Nadkarni, 1954: 280; 290; Chopra *et al.*, 1956: 54, 55) giving separate vernacular names viz. *ponnāṁtakara* and *ponnāvīraṃ* or *natraṃtakara* respectively. Mooss (1976: 36) is of opinion that *Cassia occidentalis*, being not truely indigenous to India, cannot be considered as the *kāsamarḍa* of the ancient Āyurvēdic works (However, this plant has been naturalised in India since very early periods and this seems to be an argument of doubtful merit. There are quite a few species of plants, introduced and naturalised in India which are now widely used in the system). Instead, he mentions two different varieties of *kāsamarḍa* in his *Abhidhānamañjarī* viz. *kāsamarḍa* and *sitakāsamarḍa*, known as *ponnāvīraṃ* and *veḷutta ponnāvīraṃ* (*veḷutta* = white) respectively in vernacular and considers *Cassia sophera* as the source of both. According to him the basis of recognising the two varieties is the colouration of the shoot of *C. sophera*, i.e. one with reddish purple stem and the other having greenish stem. However, this type of distinctive colouration of the shoot is met with in both *C. occidentalis* and *C. sophera*. Rheede's account (Hort. Malab. 2: 101–102 t. 52. 1679—*Ponnam-tagera*) reveals that *C. sophera* has been in use for long. But this is so closely similar to *C. occidentalis* that only trained taxonomists can distinguish them. This must be the reason why this distinction is not in vogue in current practice and both *C. sophera* and *C. occidentalis* are being taken as the source plant of this drug.

The two plants can be distinguished as follows.

Cassia sophera *Linn.* **(Caesalpiniaceae)**
Senna sophera (Linn.) Roxb.

Glabrous under-shrub; leaves alternate, pinnate, with a single gland near the base above the petiole; leaflets 6–8 pairs, opposite, elliptic-acute or acuminate, upto 4.5 × 1.5 cms, base oblique, membraneous, glaucous below; flowers bright yellow, showy, in short, few-flowered axillary or terminal corymbose racemes; calyx of 5 unequal sepals; petals 5, free, subequal; stamens 10, unequal; fruit a long, linear, subterete, glabrous pod upto 10 × 0.8 cms; seeds many, dark brown, 2-seriate.

Distribution: The plant is cosmopolitan in the tropics, found throughout all the plains districts of India, growing by roadsides and on waste lands.

Cassia occidentalis *Linn.* **(Caesalpiniaceae)** (Fig. 113)

Woody herb; stem purplish or green, smooth; leaves alternate, pinnate, stipulate with a sessile dark brown gland near the base of the petiole; leaflets 3–5 pairs, opposite, short-petioled, ovate-acuminate, 9 × 3.5 cms, base somewhat oblique, glabrous above, glaucous beneath; flowers yellow in axillary or terminal racemes; calyx 5-partite, segments creamy yellow; petals 5, free, subequal; stamens 10, unequal; fruit a linear-falcate, flat, glabrous pod; seeds many, 1-seriate.

Distribution: The plant is now pantropical in distribution. It is found throughout India from the Himalayas to Cape Comerin.

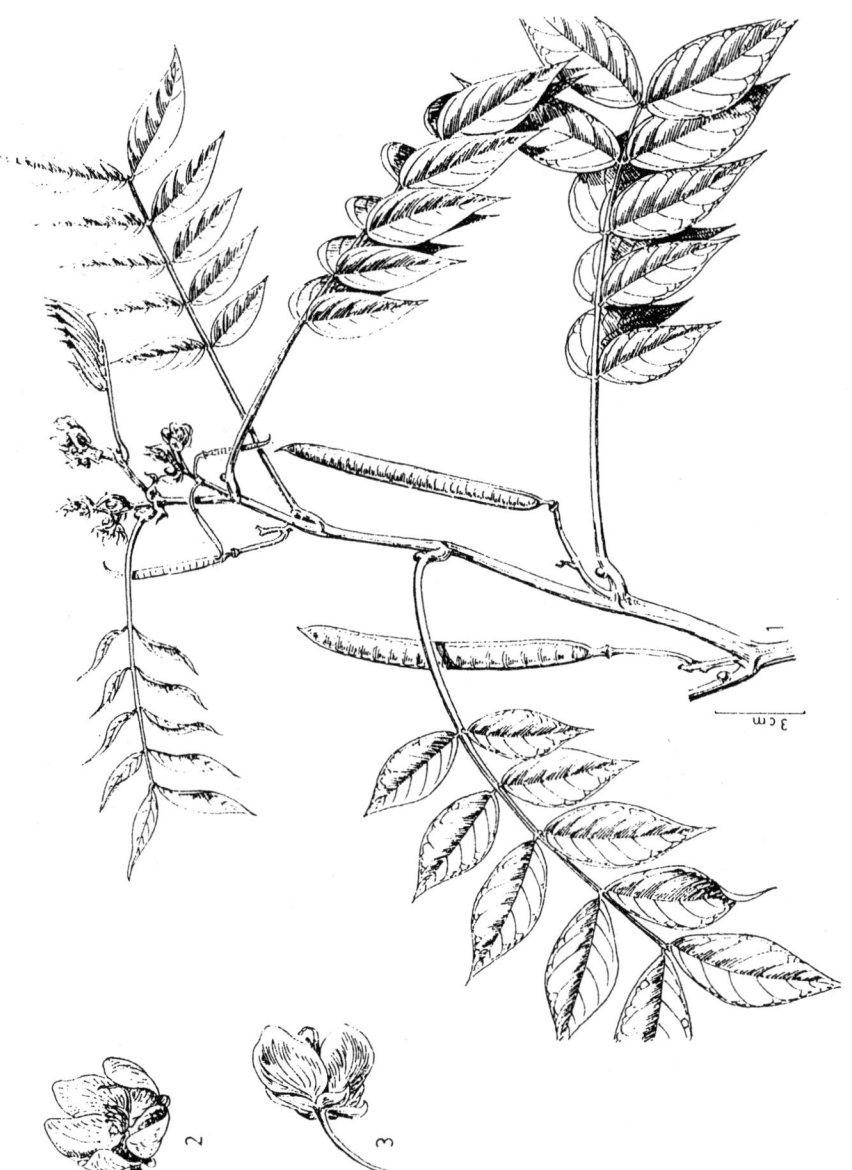

Figure 113: **Cassia occidentalis** L. 1, Twig; 2–3, Flowers.

KĀŚMARĪ (Mal. KUMIḶU, KUṀBIḶ)

Kāśmarī is an important ingredient of the group *daśamūla* (group of ten roots) which enters into the composition of many Āyurvēdic formulations. It is astringent, bitter, digestive, cardiotonic, diuretic, laxative and pulmonary and nervine tonic. It promotes digestive power, improves memory, overcomes giddiness and is useful in burning sensation, fever, thirst, emaciation, heart diseases, nervous disorders and piles. The fruits are bitter, cooling, tonic and overcome thirst, *vātarakta, pitta*, pleural and lung diseases. It produces corpulency, promotes sexual power and is good for growth of hair. It is useful in difficult urination, vitiation of blood and rheumatism and improving memory. Leaves are good for healing ulcers and headache (Kolammal, 1978: 2: 47).

The synonymy suggests that the plant is characterised by a thick bark (*sthūlatvacā*), dark petiole (*kṛṣṇavṛntā*), sweet leaves (*madhuparṇikā*) and yellowish flowers/fruits (*pītarōhiṇī*) (cf. Kolammal, 1978. 2: 47). These characters are not adequate to trace the accurate identity of the plant. But, fortunately, there is no dispute as to the plant source of the drug. *Gmelina arborea* Roxb. (Verbenaceae), locally called *kumiḷu* or *kuṁbiḷ* is the accepted source of the drug throughout India. That in Kerala also, this has been in use since long is testified by Rheede (Hort. Malab. 1: 75–76. t. 41. 1678, *Cumbulu*).

Gmelina arborea *Roxb.* **(Verbenaceae)** (Fig. 114)
Gmelina rheedii Hook.

Moderate-sized, unarmed deciduous tree; leaves simple, opposite, long-petioled, broadly ovate-acuminate, to 22 × 19 cms, glabrous, green above, soft, fulvous-tomentose beneath; flowers showy, yellow tinged with brown outside, in dense terminal pedunculate panicles; calyx campanulate, pubescent outside; corolla tube short, limb oblique; stamens 4, didynamous, included; ovary 4-chambered with one ovule in each, style slender, stigma bifid; fruit an ovoid or oblong succulent drupe, orange yellow when ripe.

Distribution: The plant is found wild throughout India from the foot of Himalayas to Kerala, in moist. semideciduous and open forests. Also distributed in Sri Lanka and Philippines.

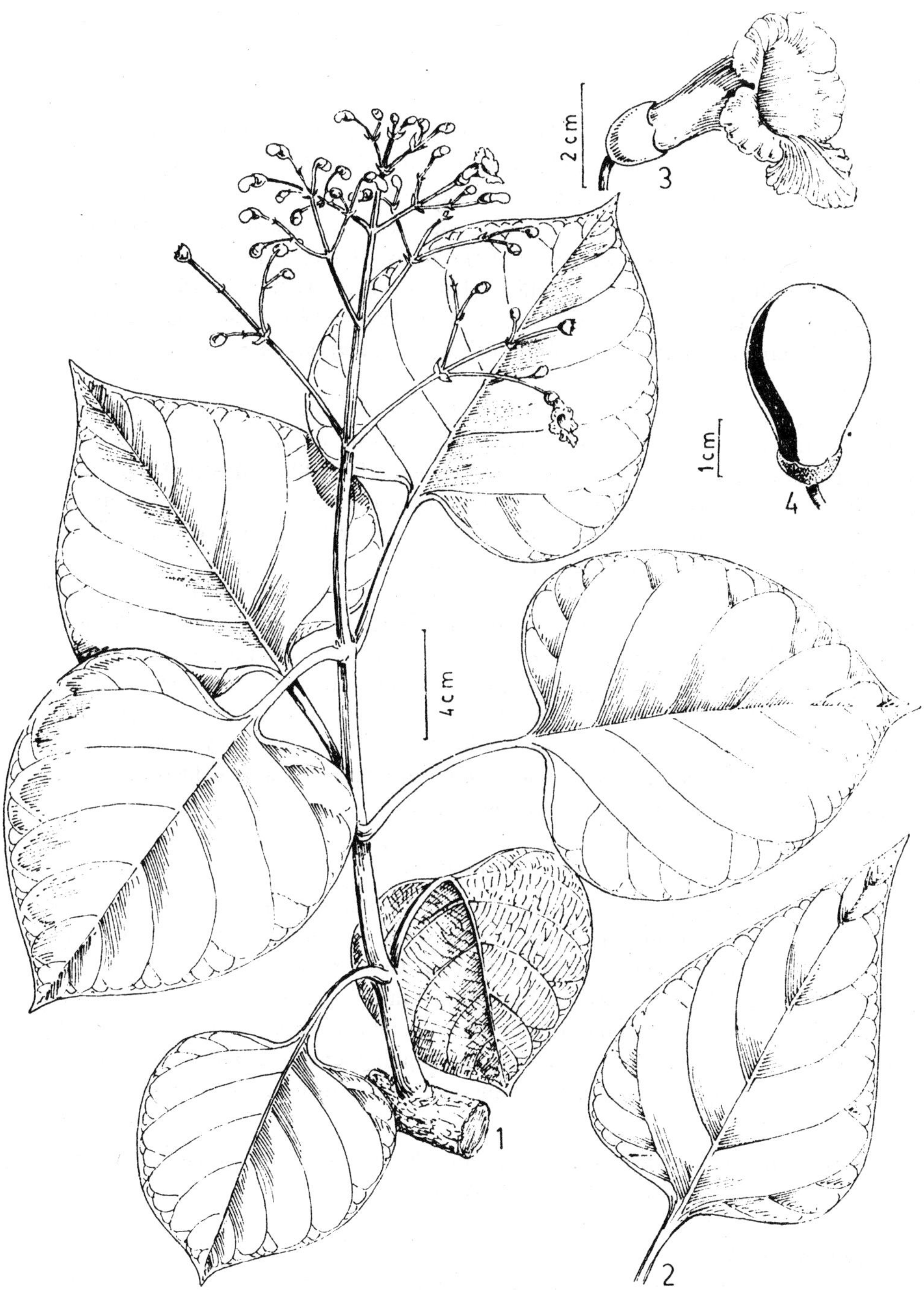

Figure 114: Gmelina arborea Roxb. 1, Flowering twig; 2, Leaf; 3, Flower; 4, Fruit.

KĒTAKĪ (Mal. PŪKKAITA)

Kētakī (i.e. the abode of beetles) is reported to be bitter, cooling, aromatic, antiseptic, aphrodisiac, carminative, stomachic and abortifacient. It overcomes the *tridōṣās* especially ***kapha*** and ***pitta***, cures earache, headache, eye diseases, ulcers, scabies and other skin diseases. It is also indicated in constipation, hysteria, debility, sterility and burning sensation of the body. It strengthens heart and liver, improves complexion, hair and intellect (Kurup *et al.*, 1979: 117; Dey, 1980: 82; Sharma, 1983: 143). The roots are used in formulations like *Teṅginpuṣpādi tailaṃ, Çeṛiya Candanādi tailaṃ, Kaccōradi tailaṃ, Mahārājapṛasāriṇī tailaṃ, Abhṛaṃ (101),* etc.

Bhāvaprakāśa describes two varieties of *kētakī* i.e. white and yellow. The yellow variety, called *suvarṇakētakī*, has golden yellow flowers which are smaller but more aromatic than that of the other variety (Chunekar, 1982: 498). Most authors equate the drug with *Pandanus odoratissiums* (now *P. fascicularis* Lam.) of Pandanaceae (Kirtikar & Basu, 1918: 1328, Nadkarni, 1954: 894; Kapoor and Mitra, 1979; 64; Kurup *et al.* 1979: 117; Dey, 1980: 82; Sharma, 1983; 141).

However, *Pandanus* is so difficult a genus for species identification that even seasoned taxonomists like Linneaus filius included every thing from the Malabar Coast in a single species. In practice, the herb collectors and pharmacists also are not equipped to make a distinction between the different species, as they are almost indistinguishable by the officinal part, the root. All the available species are taken. Hence, only a generic description is provided here followed by a key to the Malabar species of the genus, as they are understood currently, for the benefit of those who would like to have more accurate identifications.

Pandanus *Linn. ex Stickman* **(Pandanaceae)** (Fig. 115)

Shrubby or arborescent, often branched palm-like plants with stout stilt roots from the base of the prominently annulate fibrous stem; leaves trifariously spiral, in terminal crowns, long-lanceolate acuminate with three rows of prickles each on the margins and on midrib beneath, highly fibrous; inflorescence in spadices, unisexual, with prominent, yellowish foliaceous bracts; male flowers represented by naked stamens producing large amount of anemophilous pollen grains; female flowers solitary or clustered; carpels free or adnate, 1-ovuled; fruits ripening as individual drupes or syncarps.

Distribution: A large genus of about 600–700, terrestrial or semiaquatic species, wild and at times cultivated in the Old World.

Taxonomic Note

In Kerala there are 4 species of this genus. Rheede (Hort. Malab. 2. tt. 1–8. 1679) has portrayed all the four species. Linneaus filius, as mentioned earlier, considered all of them to be conspecific and assigned them to *Pandanus odoratissimus* L.f.

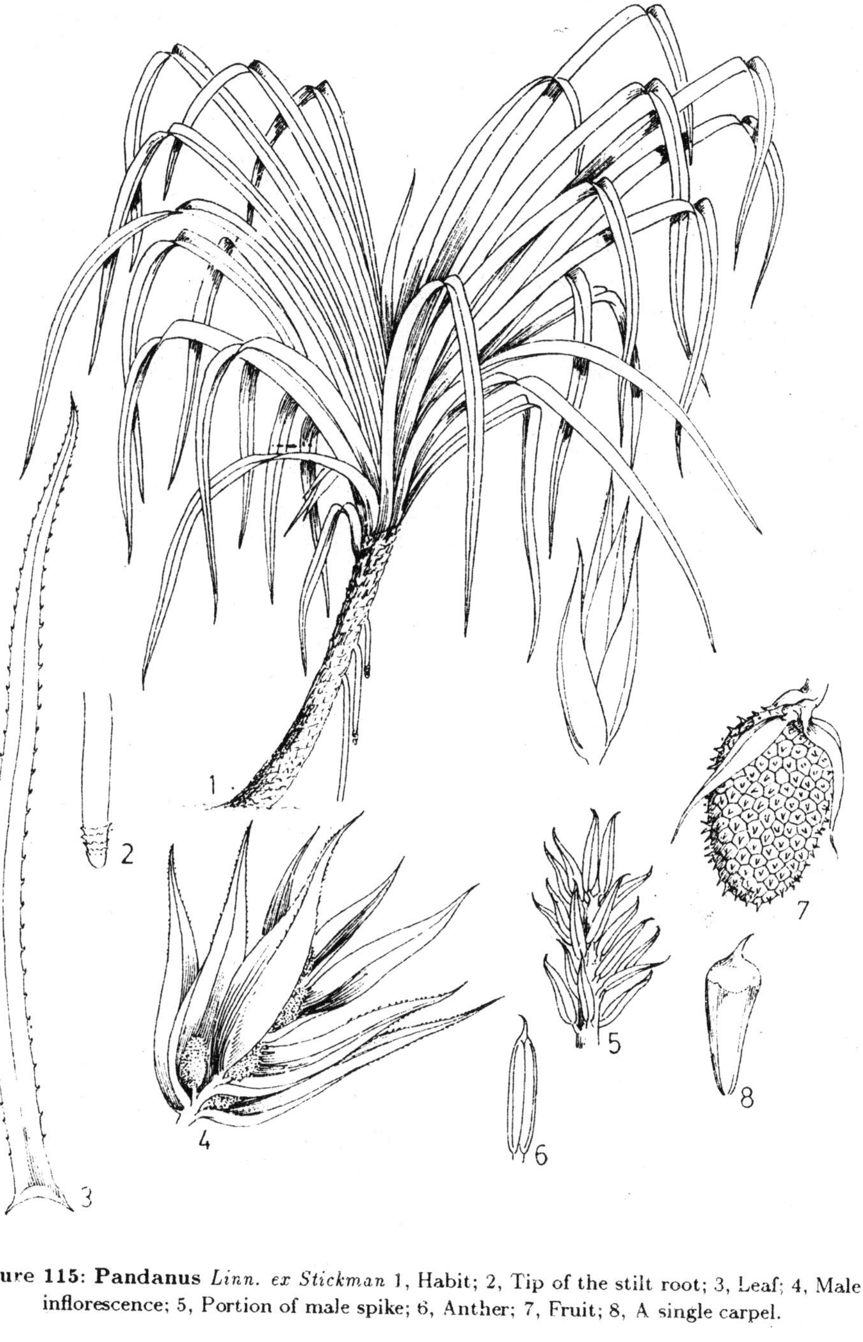

Figure 115: Pandanus *Linn. ex Stickman* 1, Habit; 2, Tip of the stilt root; 3, Leaf; 4, Male inflorescence; 5, Portion of male spike; 6, Anther; 7, Fruit; 8, A single carpel.

which is an illegitimate name (See Nicolson *et al.*, 1988. 304–305). The four species growing wild in Kerala and adopted as the source of this drug can be discriminated by the following key.

1. Ovary 5-many celled, carpels confluent in groups of 4–10, apex rounded with a depressed centre. . . . **P. fascicularis** Lam. (= *P. tectorius Soland, P. odoratissimus* auct. non. L.f.)
1. Ovary 1-celled;
   2. Drupes club shaped. . . . .
      P. unipapillatus Dennst. (= *P. canaranus* Warb.)
   2. Drupes cylindric:
      3. Bracts and spikes yellow, carpels simple, ripening as 1-seeded drupes. . . . . **P. furcatus** Roxb.
      3. Bracts and spikes white or cream, carpels in 2(-4) celled phallanges. . . . . .
         P. kaida Kurz.

(For illustrations of these species, readers may please see the following in Rheede's Hortus Malabaricus).

1. Pandanus kaida *Kurz.*	Hort. Malab. 2. t. 1–5. 1679 *'Kaida'*
2. P. fascicularis *Lam.*	Hort. Malab. 2. t. 6. 1679 *'Kaida-taddi'*
3. P. unipapillatus *Dennst.*	Hort. Malab. 2. t. 7. 1679 *'Perin Kaida taddi'*
4. P. furcatus *Roxb.*	Hort. Malab. 2. t. 8. 1679. *'Kaida-tsjeria'*

KIRĀTATIKTAḤ (Mal. KIRIYĀTTA)

The drug is reported to be a specific remedy for all types of fevers especially intermittent fevers. It is laxative, dry, cooling, bitter, light and overcomes ***sannipāta*** type of fever, difficulty in breathing, hemopathy due to the morbidity of ***kapha*** and ***pitta***, burning sensation, cough, oedema, thirst, skin diseases, fever, ulcer and worms. It is also useful in acidity and liver complaints (Aiyer & Kolammal, 1962. 5: 65). The entire plant is medicinal. The important preparations using the drug are *Tiktakaghṛtaṃ, Gōrōcanādi guḷika, Candanāsavaṃ, Pañcatiktaṃ kaṣāyaṃ*, etc.

The synonyms do not give any clue that would help the accurate identification of the plant except that the plant grows in the forest (*kirātaḥ, kirātikaḥ, kirātatiktaḥ*) and that it is a small plant growing close to the ground with qualities similar to that of Neem (*bhūniṁbaḥ*). Other terms only indicate the bitter taste of the drug (*tiktaḥ, mahātiktaḥ, kaṭutiktaḥ, anāryatiktaḥ*, etc.) and its property to cure fever (*jvarāntakaḥ, sannipātakaḥ*) (Aiyer & Kolammal, 1962. 5: 64).

Classical literature mention a second type of *kirāta* belonging to Nepal (*naipāḷaḥ*) which has the same properties, but less bitter (*ardhatiktaḥ*) (cf. Chunekar, 1982: 73), but this is not in use in Kerala.

Most of the books on Indian materia medica equate the drug *kirātatikta* with *Swertia chirata* Buch.-Ham. of Gentianaceae (Vaidya, 1936: 136, Kurup *et al.*, 1979: 119: 1980: 86; Sharma, 1983: 631) while others consider both *Swertia chirata* and *Andrographis paniculata* Nees (Acanthaceae) as the source of the drug. The Malayalam equivalents of the drug namely *kiriyāttu* and *nilavēppu* are given to both the plants by these authors (Kirtikar & Basu, 1918: 851, 965; Nadkarni, 1954: 1184, 101, Chopra *et al.*, 1956: 234, 18). In Kerala, however, *Andrographis paniculata*, locally called *kiriyāttu* is being used under the name *kirātatikta*. The plant has a strong bitter taste and it is found to be efficaceous in curing fever, thus agreeing well with the synonyms. It has been reported that *Andrographis paniculata* is popularly known as *bhūnimbaḥ* in central India and as *chirāyata* in Bihar. *Kālmegh* is another common name given to this plant. This indicates its use in place of *kirātatikta* since long (Singh & Chunekar, 1972: 287).

Andrographis paniculata (*Burm. f.*) *Wallich ex Nees* (**Acanthaceae**) (Fig. 116)
Justicia paniculata Burm. f..
Andrographis subspathulata C.B. Clarke

Much branched herb; stem and branches sharply 4-angled; leaves simple, opposite, short-petioled, glabrous, elliptic to lanceolate, narrowed at both ends, 10.5×2.5 cms; flowers small, white with purplish blotches in terminal and axillary panicles; calyx 5-partite, glandular-pubescent; corolla bilabiate, hairy outside, the lower lip deeply 3-lobed, deflexed, upper oblong, slightly 2-fid; stamens 2, filaments hairy, anthers 2-celled, connate, deep purple; fruit a linear compressed capsule; seeds 8–10 on retinacula.

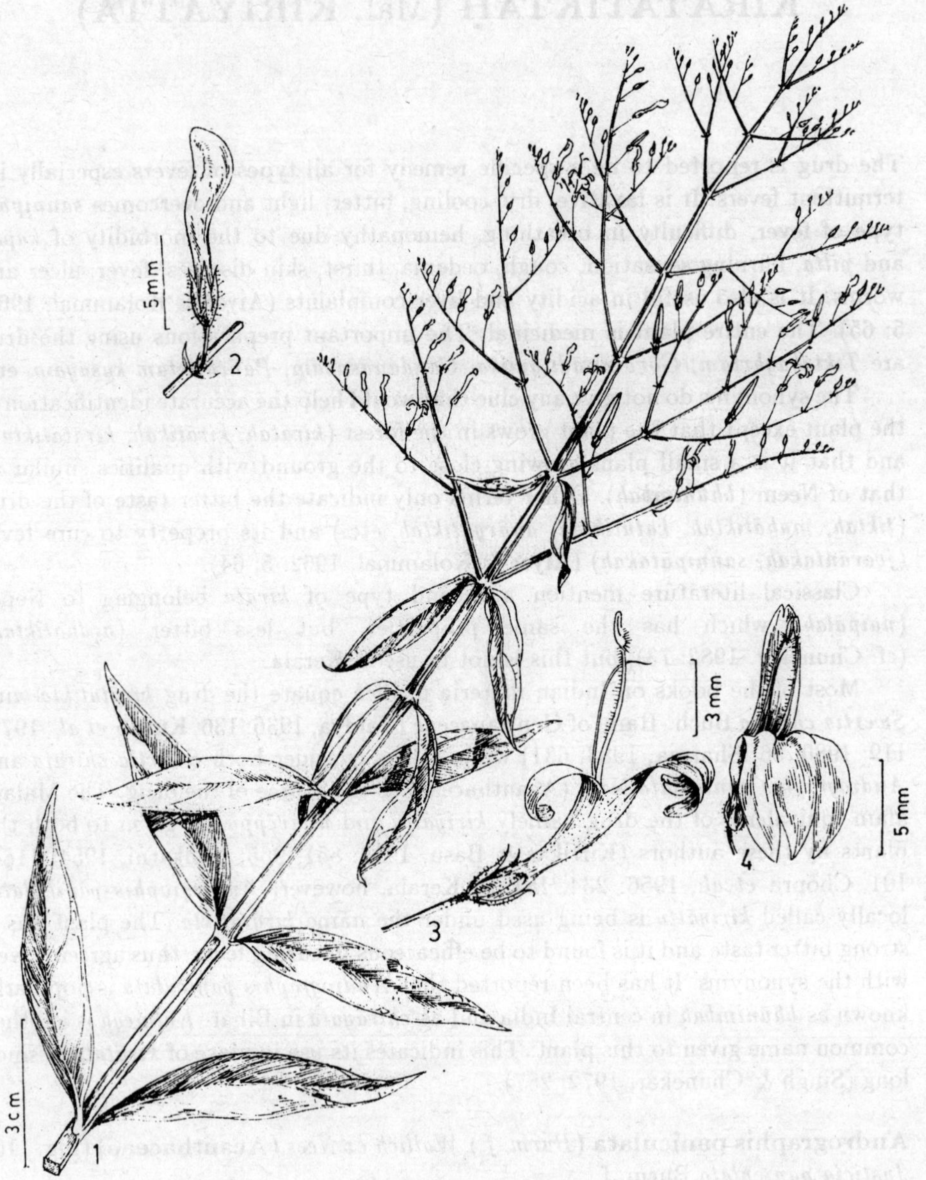

Figure 116: Andrographis paniculata (Burm. f.) Wallich ex Nees. 1, Twig; 2, Flower bud; 3–4, Flowers.

Distribution: The plant is found wild throughout tropical India and Sri Lanka. It is common in uncultivated ground and also as an undergrowth in forests.

Swertia chirayita (Roxb. ex Flem.) Karsten (Gentianaceae) (Fig. 117)
Swertia chirata (Wall.) C.B. Clarke

Erect robust herb; stem terete except near the top; leaves broadly lanceolate-acute, 10 × 3.75 cms; flowers in corymbosely paniculate cymes; calyx and corolla 4-lobed; corolla greenish-yellow tinged with purple with two glands on each lobe, fringed with long hairs; stamens 4–5, inserted at the base of the corolla; capsule sessile, oblong.

Distribution: The plant is found in eastern temperate Himalayas, Himachal Pradesh and Uttar Pradesh.

Note: The anti-inflammatory activity of the aqueous extract of *Andrographis paniculata* Ness (*chirayata*) has been clinically proved by Tajuddin *et al.* (1983). A decoction of the plant has been found to be effective in the treatment of infective hepatitis (Chaturvedi, *et al.*, 1983).

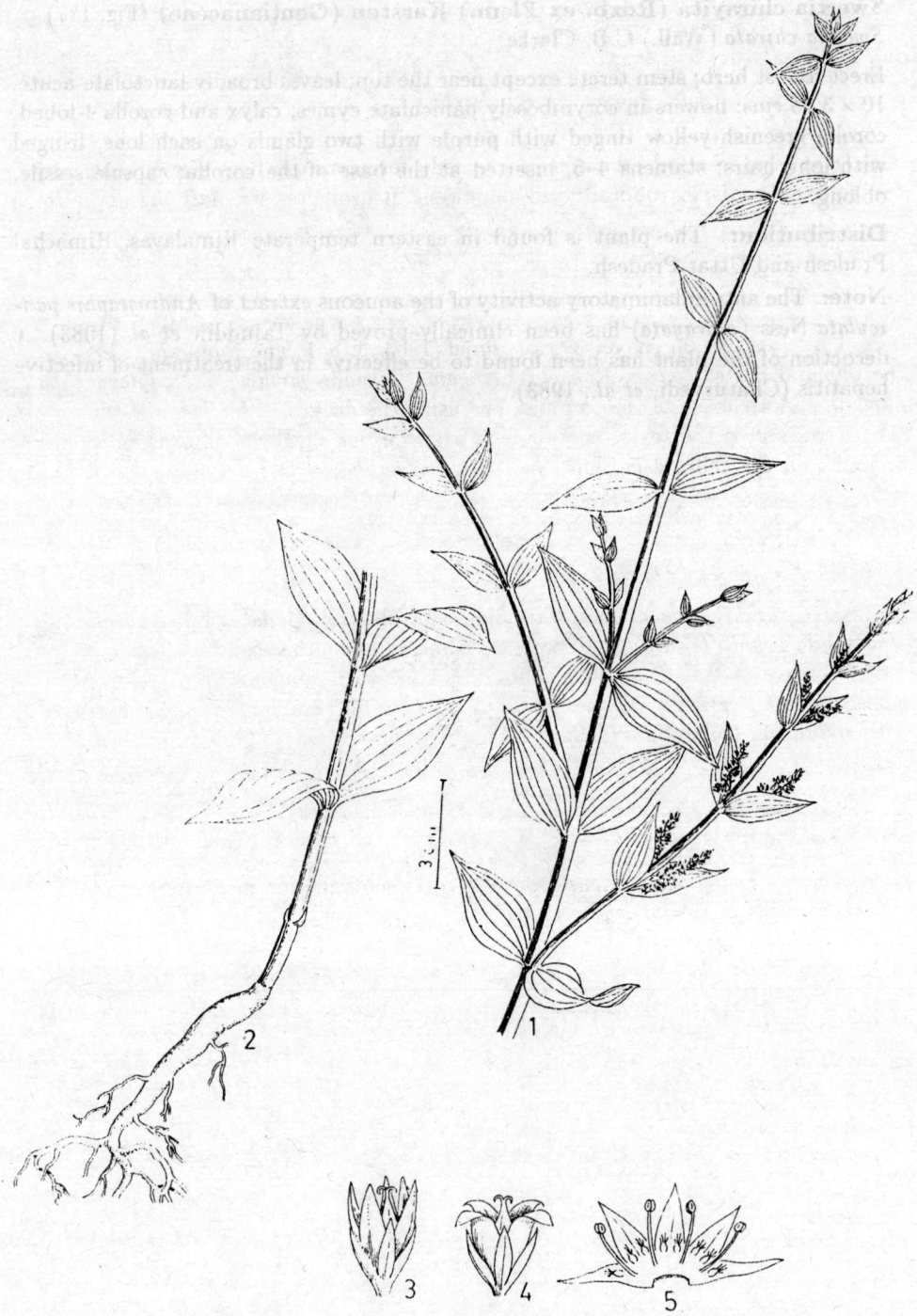

Figure 117: **Swertia chirayita** (Roxb. ex Flem.) Karsten. 1–2, Habit; 3–4, Flowers; 5, Corolla tube opened.

KŌKILĀKṢAḤ (Mal. VAYALCUḶḶI)

Kōkilākṣa is considered as a reputed remedy for arthritis. It is sweet, sour, bitter, cold, aphrodisiac, roborant and demulcent. It promotes strength and appetite, overcomes *āmavāta* and morbid *pitta*, cures oedema, ascites, thirst, bladder stones, eye-diseases and dysentery on account of *pitta*. Its leaves are good for toxicosis, flatulence and anaemia. Seeds are sweet and astringent. They promote sexual vigour and strength, arrest abortion, augment *kapha* and *vāta* and cure impurity of blood and burning sensation (Aiyer & Kolammal, 1963. 6: 88). The roots and seeds are the officinal parts. *Ceṟiya Rāsnādi kaṣāyaṃ, Rāsnādi ghṛtaṃ, Vastyāmayāntaka ghṛtaṃ*, etc. are some of the formulations using the drug.

According to the texts, the plant is a gregarious shrub having several nodes or joints on the shoot (*śṛṅkhalā, śṛṅkhalī, śṛṅkhalikā*) with a resemblence to *ikṣu* viz. sugarcane (*ikṣuraḥ, ikṣugandhā, kāṇḍēkṣuḥ*) and sharp thorns (*vajrakaṇṭakaḥ, kaṇṭakī*). The plant grows in marshy areas (*nādēyī*) and its flowers are deep blue like the eyes of the *kōkila* (*kōkilākṣaḥ*) (Aiyer & Kolammal, 1963. 6: 88).

There is little controversy about the identity of the plant source of this drug, among Kerala physicians. The Malayalam equivalent of *kōkilākṣa* is *vayalcuḷḷi* and *Hygrophila schulli* (Ham.) M.R. & S.M. Almeida (Acanthaceae) has been the accepted source of this drug in Kerala since long, as is obvious from the work of Rheede (Hort. Malab. 2: 87–88, t. 45. 1679). Some authors have equated this drug with *Artanema longifolium* (Linn.) Vatke (Scrophulariaceae) (Nadkarni, 1954: 141; Chopra *et al.*, 1956: 25; Aiyer & Kolammal, 1963. 6: 95). However, this plant (widely known as *nīrmuḷḷi* in Tamil) is not known to be in use as the source of *kōkilākṣa*, in any part of Kerala.

Śāligrāmanighaṇṭu mentions two varieties, viz., white-flowered and blue-flowered (cf. Aiyer & Kolammal, 1963. 6: 88). This distinction has been obliterated in present day practice and only the blue flowered variety is in use.

Hygrophila schulli (*Ham.*) *M.R. & S.M. Almeida* (**Acanthaceae**) (Fig. 118)
Bahel schulli Ham.
Hygrophila auriculata (Schum.) Heine
Asteracantha longifolia (Linn.) Nees
Hygrophila spinosa T. Anderson

Gregarious subshrubs, strigose-hispid all over; stem purplish, thickened at nodes; leaves simple, subsessile, narrowly lanceolate, 11 × 2.5 cms, in whorls of 6, with sharp axillary spines, the two outer leaves of each whorl larger and others much smaller; flowers bluish purple, in sessile axillary whorls; calyx deeply 4-partite, lobes unequal, clothed with soft hairs; corolla blue, distinctly 2-lipped, the upper 2-lobed and the lower 3-lobed; stamens 4, didynamous, filaments connate in pairs at base, anthers 2-celled; ovary 2-celled with 4 ovules in each cell, style filiform, pubescent, stigma simple; fruit a linear capsule, with orbicular seeds on retinacula.

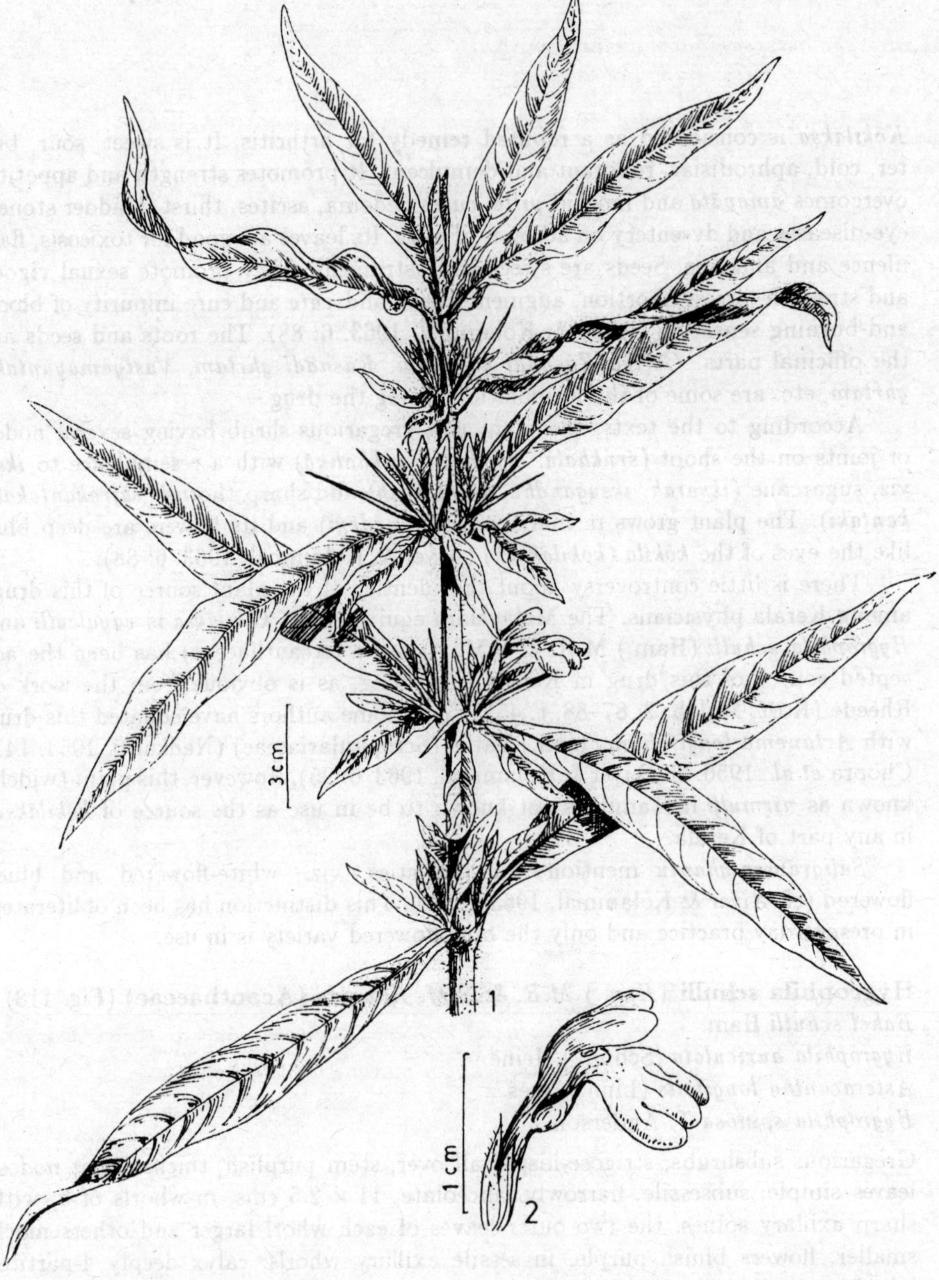

Figure 118: Hygrophila schulli (Ham.) M.R. & S.M. Almeida. 1, Habit; 2, Flower.

Distribution: The plant grows throughout the plains districts of India, in damp areas such as marshy margins of canals, rice fields etc. Also seen in tropical Himalaya, Burma, Indochina and Malaya.

Artanema longifolium (*Linn.*) *Vatke* **(Scrophulariaceae)** (Fig. 119)
Columnea longifolia Linn.
Artanema sesamoides (Vahl) Benth.

Glabrous herbs to 1.5 m tall; stem 4-angled; leaves opposite, short-petioled, lanceolate or ovate-lanceolate, to 26 × 7.5 cm, green above, pale below; flowers lilac in terminal bracteate racemes; calyx accrescent, 5-lobed; corolla blue or purple, gamopetalous, 2-lipped; stamens 4, didynamous, the posterior pair shorter with a small scale at the base of the filaments; ovary superior, 2-celled with many ovules on axile placenta, style slender ending in a bilamellate stigma; capsule globose; seeds many, small.

Distribution: The plant is found in W. Coast, in Malabar and Travancore, up to 3,000 ft in semi-evergreen forests, especially near streams or other water sources.

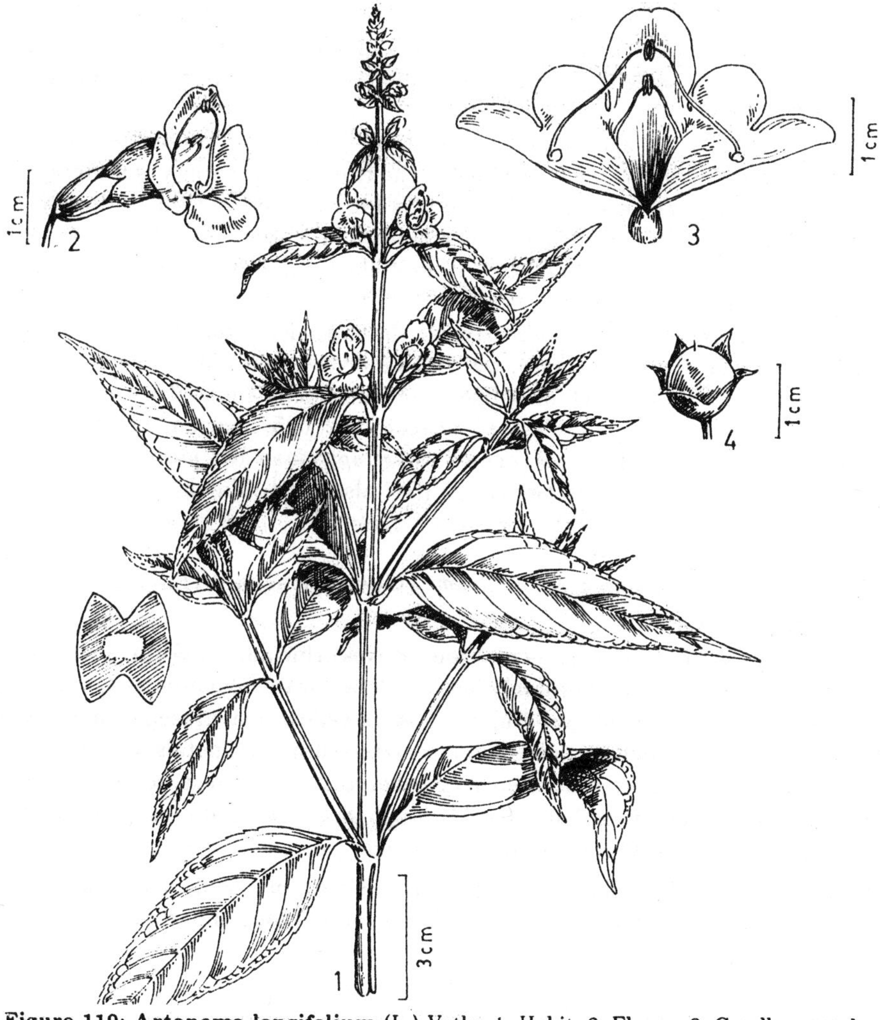

Figure 119: Artanema longifolium (L.) Vatke. 1, Habit; 2, Flower; 3, Corolla opened; 4, Fruit.

KŌŚĀTAKĪ
(Mal. PĪCCIṄṄA, PUṬṬALPĪRAṂ)

The term *kōśātakī* appears to be used in general for all the fruit drugs of the family Cucurbitaceae which have a fibro-vascular network enclosing the seeds (Singh & Chunekar, 1972: 121). Two types of the drug viz. *mahākōśātakī* and *rājakōśātakī* are described in the texts (cf. Chunekar, 1982: 685–686). Both the varieties, together known as *kōśavatau*, form ingredients of the *Madanādi gaṇa* of Vāgbhaṭa or the group of emetics (cf. Mooss, 1980: 2).

Mahākōśātakī is reported to be light, hot, bitter, acrid, emetic and laxative. It purifies blood and cures morbid *kapha* and *pitta*, oedema, intestinal disorders, flatulence, cough, asthma and poisonous affections. The fruit, flowers and leaves are used in medicine.

Rājakōśātakī is also reported to have the same properties as that of *mahākōśātakī* (Sharma, 1983: 382, 384). The fruit of this variety is a highly valued, well known culinary vegetable. The root is laxative and is used in dropsy. Leaves are applied locally in splenitis, haemorrhoids and leprosy. Juice of the fresh leaves is dropped into the eyes of children in granular conjuctivitis, (cf. Nadkarni, 1954: 752; Chunekar, 1982: 685).

The synonyms are not indicative of the botanical identity of the drug. Two species of *Luffa* (Cucurbitaceae), viz. *L. cylindrica* (Linn.) M.J. Roem. (=*L. aegyptiaca*) and *L. acutangula* (Linn.) Roxb. are commonly equated with *mahākōśātakī* and *rājakōśātakī* (Mooss, 1980: 6; Chunekar, 1982: 685; Sharma, 1983: 381, 383). In practice also, these two species, known as *kāṭṭupīcciṅṅa* and *pīcciṅṅa* in vernacular, are the plant sources of the two drugs (See also Hort. Malab. 8: 15, t. 8. 1688; 8: 13–14, t. 7. 1688).

Luffa cylindrica (*Linn.*) *M. J. Roem.* **(Cucurbitaceae)** (Fig. 120)
L. aegyptiaca Mill.

Monoecious climber, branchlets glabrous; leaves orbicular-reniform, acute or acuminate, 8–14 × 8–13.5 cm, palmately 5-lobed, lobes ovate, gland-dotted, scabrid, margin serrate; tendrils 3-fid, puberulous; flowers yellow, male racemes axillary; calyx tube broadly campanulate, lobes 5, lanceolate-acuminate; petals 5, yellow; stamens 5, filaments free, inserted at the calyx tube, anthers 1-celled, connectives dilated. Female flower solitary, axillary; fruit oblong, 18 × 6 cm, glabrous, green with white stripes when young, fibrous within; seeds many, ovoid.

Distribution: The plant is cultivated and also run wild in all plain districts, especially near the coast. Also reported from other tropical parts of the Old World.

Luffa acutangula (*Linn.*) *Roxb.* **(Cucurbitaceae)** (Fig. 121)
L. amara Roxb.
Very similar to *L. cylindrica*, but can be easily distinguished by its oblong clavate fruits with 10 sharp ridges; seeds not winged, slightly rugose on the sides.

Distribution: The plant is seen in most plains districts especially near the E. Coast, often cultivated as a vegetable.

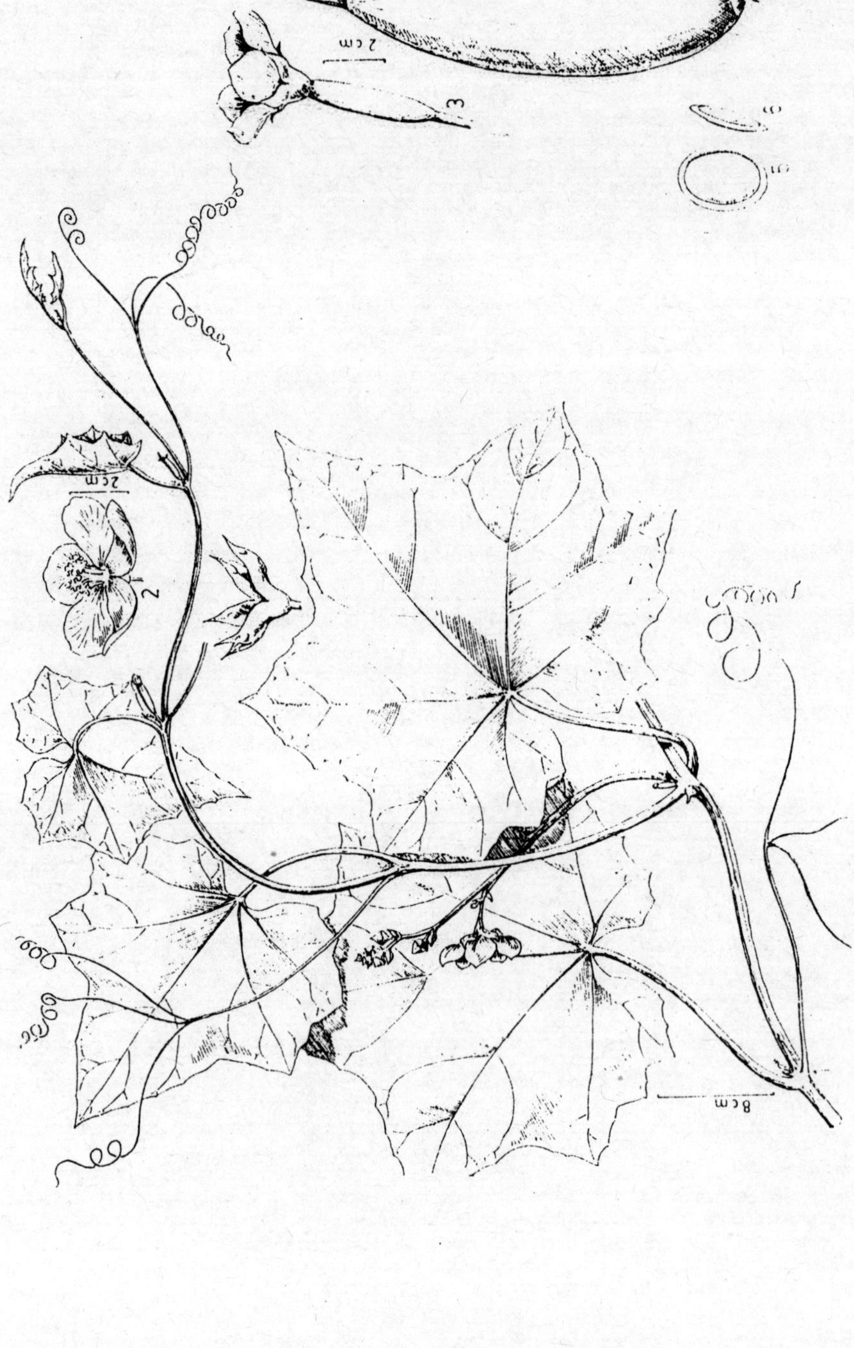

Figure 120: Luffa cylindrica (L.) M.J. Roem. 1, Flowering vine; 2, Male flower; 3, Female flower; 4, Fruit; 5–6, Seeds

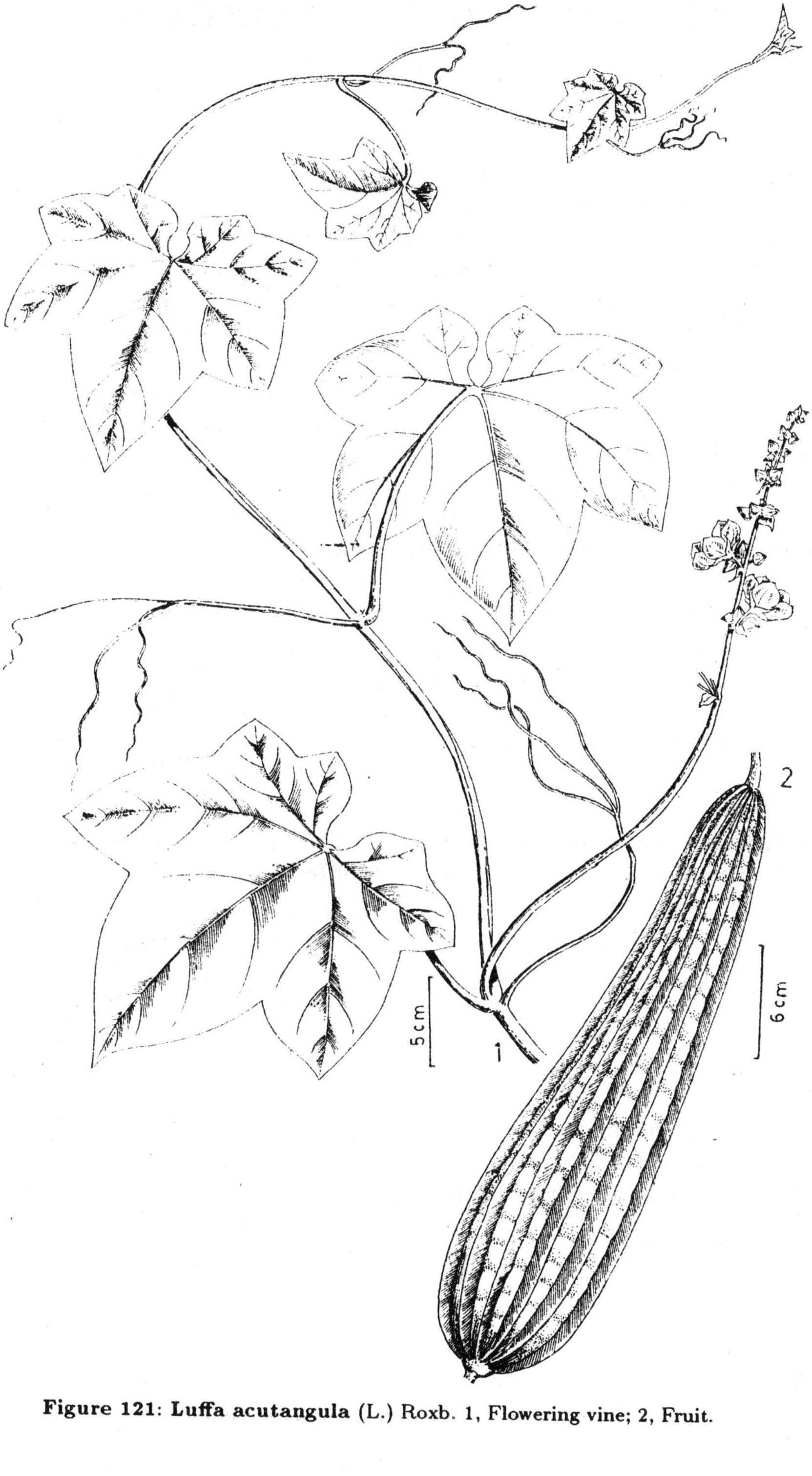

Figure 121: Luffa acutangula (L.) Roxb. 1, Flowering vine; 2, Fruit.

KṚṢṆABĪJAḤ (Mal. TĀḶIYARI)

The drug is reported to be a good purgative, anthelmintic, blood purifier, acrid, light and hot and useful in vitiated conditions of *kapha* and *vāta*. Seed is the officinal part. It is used as a purgative in cases of gastric disorders, flatulence, oedema, fever, headache and worms. It is also beneficial in rheumatism and paralytic affections. Seed paste is a good application to cure skin diseases (Dey, 1980: 87; Sharma, 1983: 423) *Pañcagavyaghṛtaṃ* is an important preparation using the drug.

Except for the black colour of the seeds (*kṛṣṇabīja* - *kṛṣṇa* = black, *bīja* = seed), the texts do not provide any descriptive hints that may help to identify the plant. *Ipomoea nil* (Linn.) Roth. (Convolvulaceae), locally known as *tāḷiyari* or *vaṭṭappūntāḷi* is the accepted source of this drug throughout the country (Kapoor & Mitra, 1979: 77; Dey, 1980: 87; Chunekar, 1982: 818; Sharma, 1983: 422).

Ipomoea nil (*Linn.*) *Roth.* (Convolvulaceae) (Fig. 122)
Convolvulus nil Linn.
Ipomoea hederacea auct. non (Linn.) Jacq.

Hispid vine; leaves simple, alternate, ovate-cordate, acuminate, entire or 3-lobed, to 11 x 9 cms, adpressed hairy above, puberulous below; flowers large, showy, solitary or in axillary few-flowered cymes; calyx lobes 5, subequal; corolla funnel-shaped, tube 5 cm long, white, limb purple; stamens 5, unequal, attached to the base of the corolla tube; ovary conical, style filiform, stigma capitate; capsule subglobose; seeds black, glabrous.

Distribution: A native of America, introduced in India by Portuguese by about 1500 A.D. This is now naturalised in all parts of India.

Note: There is some confusion in the taxonomy of this species. While some consider it to be polymorphic, Austin (1986) has segregated it to 4 different species (Key given below). All of them are available in India and are possibly used as the source of *kṛṣṇabīja*.

1. Sepals soft-pilose or glabrous .... *I. indica*
1. Sepals hispid-pilose:
    2. Sepals acute .... *I. purpurea*
    2. Sepals long acuminate:
        3. Sepals gradually narrowed, tips erect or suberect .... *I. nil*
        3. Sepals abruptly narrowed; tips strongly spreading .... *I. hederacea*

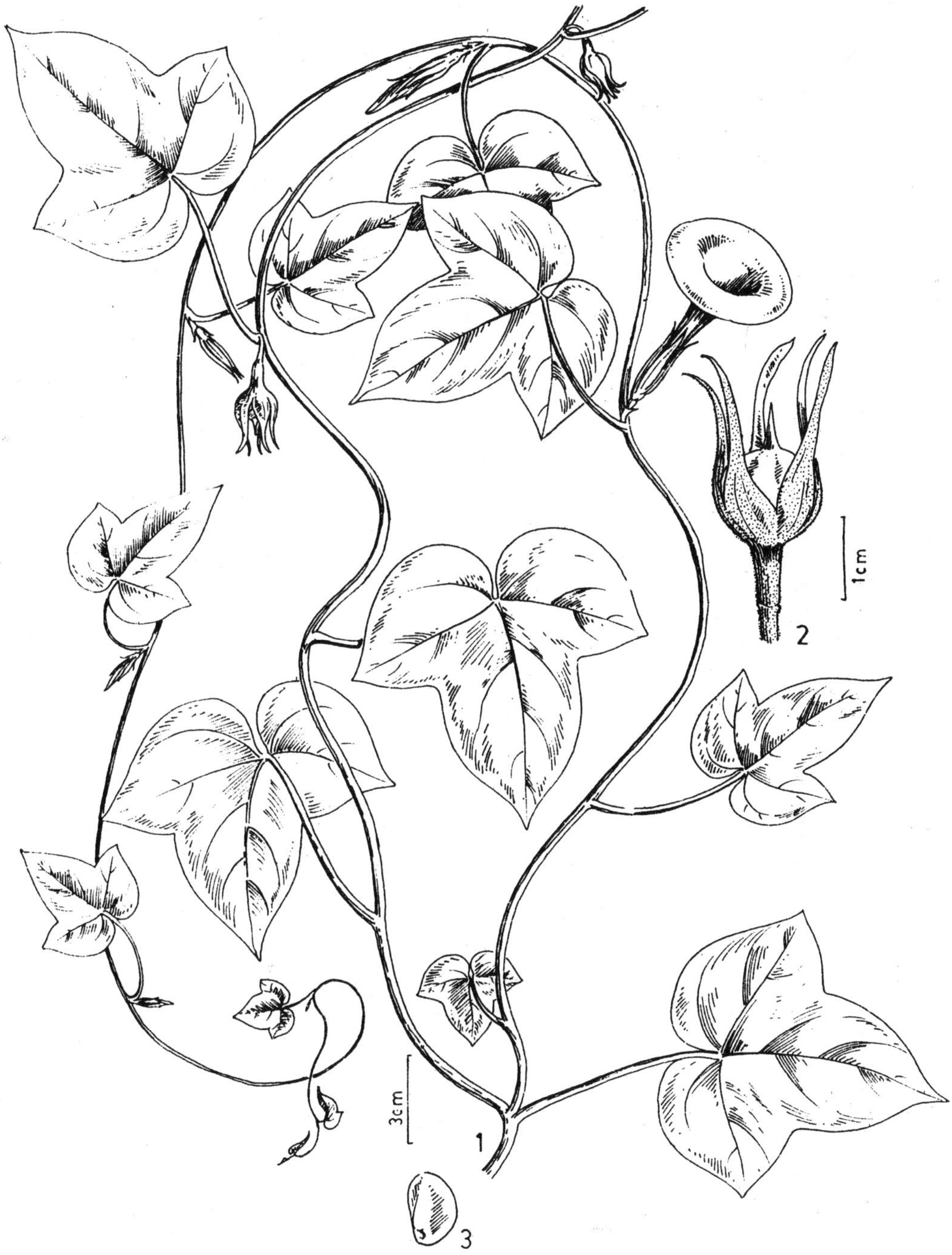

Figure 122: **Ipomoea nil** (L.) Roth. 1, Habit; 2, Fruit; 3–4, Seeds.

KUBĒRĀKṢĪ (Mal. KAḶAÑCI)

Kubērākṣī is reported to be bitter, germicidal, anti-pyretic, febrifuge and emmenagogue. The seed kernel is extensively used for intestinal worms, hydrocele and also against anasarca, liver and spleen diseases, malarial fever and mental disorders. The seeds promote digestive power, heal ulcers and cure vomiting, hiccough, diabetes, leprosy, piles and phantom tumour (*gulma*). It is a good remedy for diseases caused by the morbidity of *vāta* and *kapha*. Powder of the burnt seeds in hot water or buttermilk is taken internally to remove the obstructions of *apāna-vāyu* (Kolammal, 1979. 10: 54; Kurup *et al.*, 1979: 123). Seeds, leaves and rootbark are used in medicine. It forms an ingredient of preparations like *Cāṅgēryādi guḷika, Poṅkārādi guḷika, Ceṛiya Aantṛakuṭāram guḷika, Paphaṇādi tailam*, etc.

Ancient texts reveal that the fruits are thorny (*kaṇṭakinī, kaṇṭaphalā, viśalyakā*) and hence difficult to handle (*dusparśa, vārasu*). The seeds are ashy or grey-coloured like the eyeballs of a cow or deer or those of *kubēra* (*kubērākṣī*) and are very hard (*vajṛabījakaḥ*) (cf. Kolammal, 1979: 53–54). These synonyms go well with the plant that is being used as the source of the drug i.e. *Caesalpinia bonduc* (Linn.) Roxb. of Caesalpiniaceae, known as *kaḷañci* in vernacular. *Caesalpinia jayabo* Maza, on account of its striking resemblance to *C. bonduc* is also reported to be used along with the latter when available (cf. Kolammal, 1979. 10: 58).

Bhāvaprakāśa equates this drug with *pūtīkarañja* (cf. Chunekar, 1982: 352). This has been followed by some others also (Kapoor & Mitra, 1979: 67; Dey, 1980: 126; Sharma, 1983: 706). Singh & Chunekar (1972: 75) have discussed the matter in some detail and have concluded that *kubērākṣī* cannot be considered as the same as *pūtīkarañja*.

Caraka has mentioned the latter as a purgative bark and nowhere in the trio of classics (*Bṛhatrayi-Carakasaṁhita, Suśrutasaṁhita* and *Aṣṭāṅgahṛdaya*) one can find the fruits or seeds recommended as the officinal part. The drug *kubērākṣī* is the seeds of *Caesalpinia bonduc* and moreover, the plant does not have any particular odour, as the name *pūtika* or *pūtīkarañja* implies. These facts, probably vindicate the Kerala practice of considering them as different drugs.

Caesalpinia bonduc (*Linn.*) *Roxb.* **(Caesalpiniaceae)** (Fig. 123)
Guilandia bonduc Linn.
Caesalpinia bonducella (Linn.) Fleming

Large, thorny scrambling shrub; stems, branches and petioles armed with yellow falcate thorns; leaves large, alternate, bipinnate, the rachis and its branches armed with recurved prickles; leaflets ovate-oblong obtuse, mucronate, glabrous above, puberulous beneath; flowers dull yellow in dense terminal as well as supraaxillary, long-peduncled simple or panicled raceme; calyx gamosepalous, fulvous hairy; petals distinctly clawed; stamens 10, free, declinate, filaments flattened at base and clothed

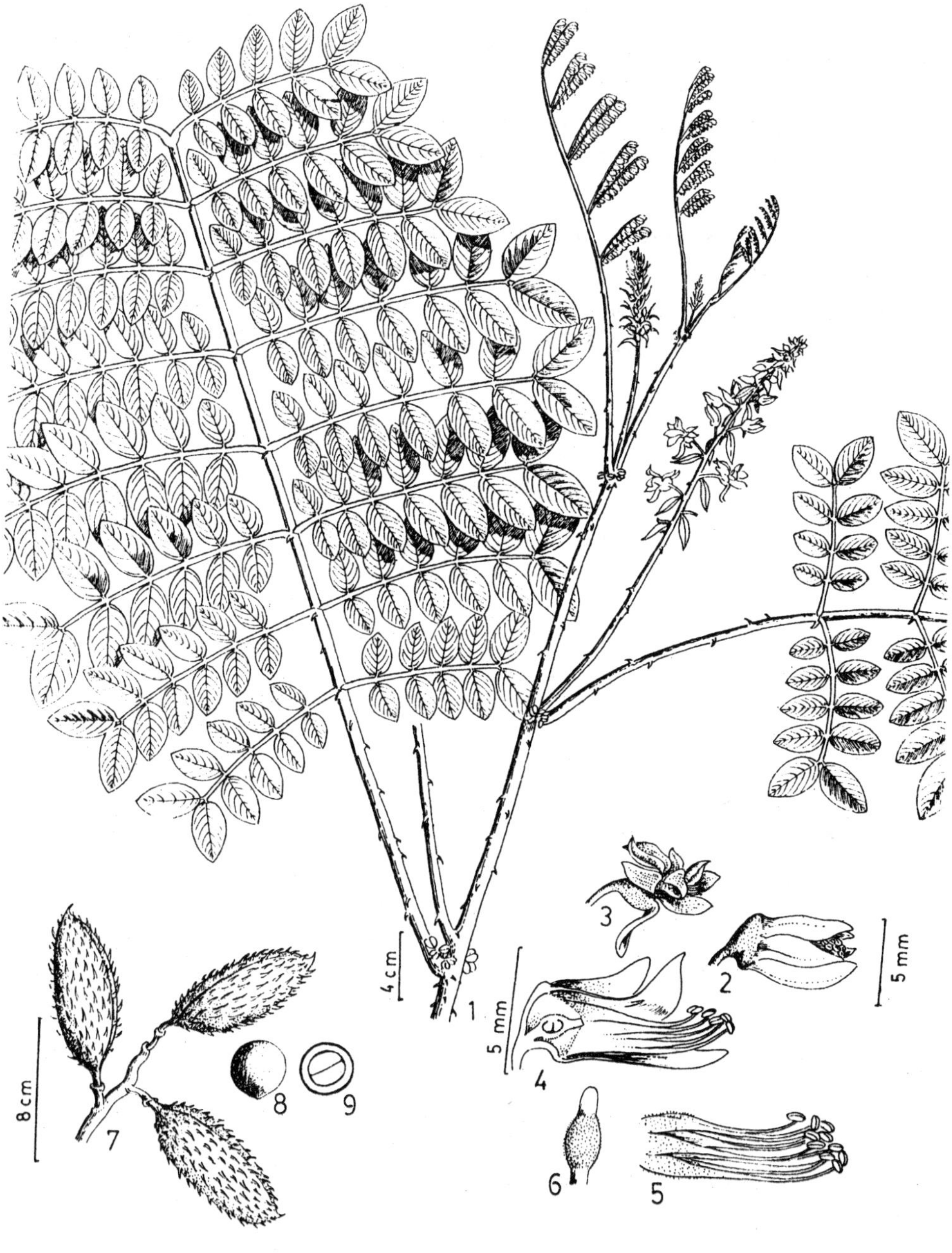

Figure 123: **Caesalpinia bonduc** (L.) Roxb. 1, Flowering twig; 2–3, Flowers; 4, Flower L.S.; 5, Stamens; 6, Pistil; 7, Fruits; 8, Seed; 9, Seed, T.S.

with white tomentum; pod 2-valved, oblong or ovate, inflated, densely prickly; seeds large, globose, hard, grey-coloured.

Distribution: A pantropical species, the plant is found naturalised in most plains districts of India.

Note: Clinical studies show that the seeds of *C. bonduc* are effective in the treatment of amoebiasis (Anonymous; 1978b).

Taxonomic notes: Many taxonomists have erroneously treated *C. bonduc* and *C. crista* as conspecific. They represent two different species and can be recognised as follows:

Stipules foliaceous, pinnate, pod prickly .... *C. bonduc*
Stipules simple, pod smooth .... *C. crista*

Rheede has clearly described them as two distinct taxas. *C. bonduc* as *Caretti* (Hort. Malab. 2: 35–36. t. 22. 1679) and *C. crista* as *Kaka-Moullou* (Hort. Malab. 6: 33. t. 19. 1686).

KUMĀRĪ (Mal. KAṬṬĀṚVĀḶA)

This is a reputed remedy for intestinal worms in children. It forms an important ingredient of Āyurvēdic formulations like *Kumāryāsavaṃ, Valiya candanādi tailaṃ, Annabhēdisindūraṃ, Mañjiṣṭhādi tailaṃ*, etc. Expressed and dried juice of the leaves forms the officinal part. It is reported to be bitter, cooling, anthelmintic, aphrodisiac, hepatic stimulant, purgative and emmenagogue. The drug is used in haemophilia, skin and uterine disorders, liver and spleen enlargement, eye affections, painful inflammations of the body, chronic ulcers and disorders due to ***kapha*** and ***pitta***. ***kumārī*** stimulates the growth of hair and it cures dyspepsia, flatulence, intestinal colic, dysuria, general debility, cough and asthma (Nadkarni, 1954: 74; Kurup *et al.*, 1979: 125; Sharma, 1983: 449).

Aloe barbadensis Mill. (= *Aloe vera* (Linn.) Burm. f.) of Liliaceae, locally called *kaṭṭāṛvāḷa* is the accepted source of the drug throughout India. (See also Rheede, Hort. Malab 11: 7, t. 3. 1692. *Catevala*).

Aloe barbadensis *Mill.* **(Liliaceae)** (Fig. 124)
Aloe vera (Linn.) Burm. f.

Dwarf, succulent plants; leaves in radical rosettes, ensiform, 40–60 × 2–8 cms succulent, base truncate, margin spiny, apex gradually tapering, spine-tipped; flowers orange in terminal racemes on axillary scapes; perianth tube somewhat curved, lobes 6, oblong, 3-nerved; stamens 3 + 3; ovary 3-celled, ovules many on axile placentae; capsule ellipsoid-oblong, to 1.5 × 1 cm.

Distribution: Introduced and now runs wild throughout India in drier localities. Naturalised in Florida, W. Indies, C. America and Asia.

Note: Moosa, J. S. (1985) found that *Aloe barbadensis* exhibits significant hypoglycaemic activity in experimental mice. The antiatherosclerotic activity of *A. barbadensis* extract has been studied by Dixit and Jain (1985).

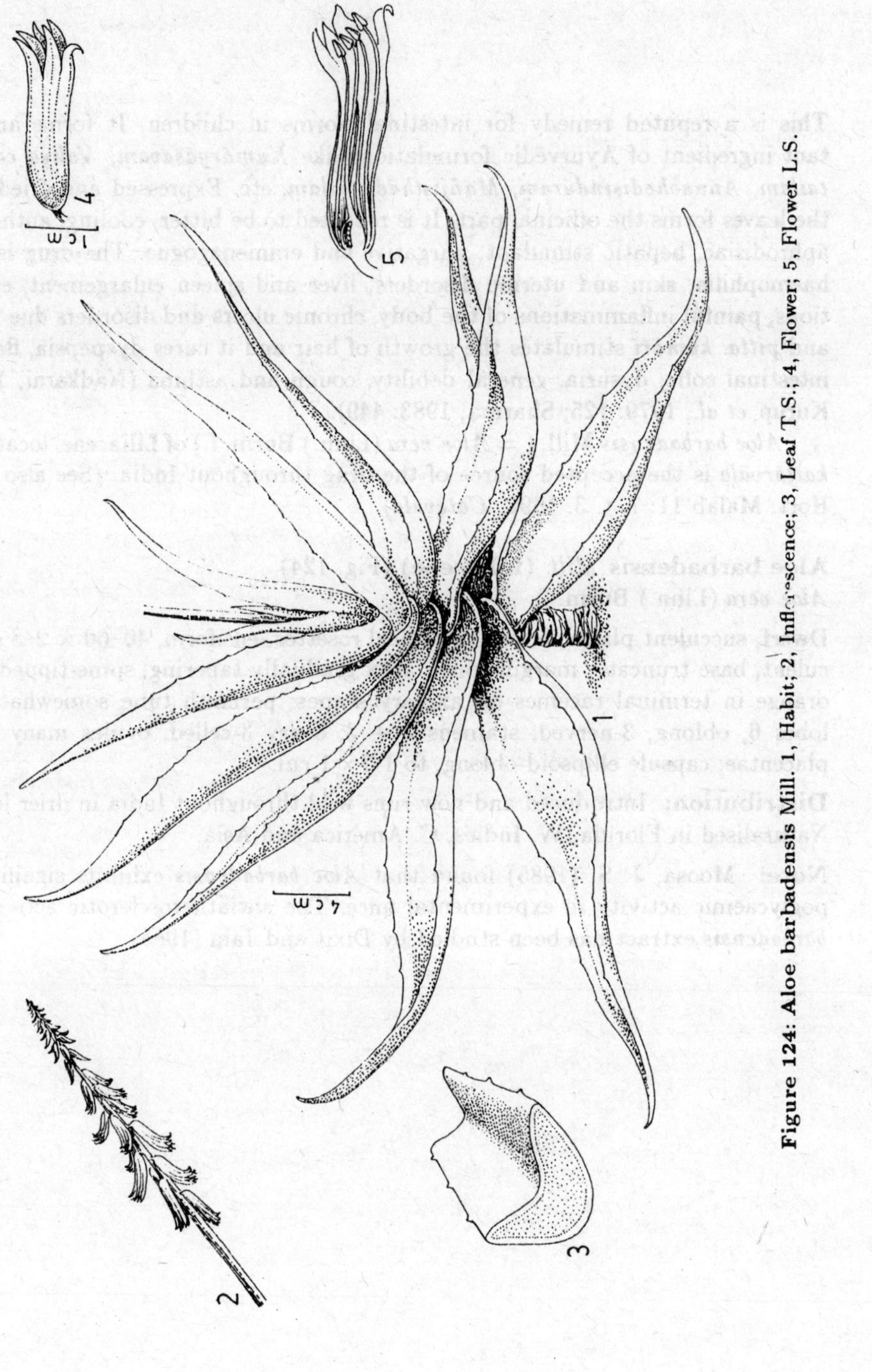

Figure 124: Aloe barbadensis Mill. 1, Habit; 2, Inflorescence; 3, Leaf T.S. 4, Flower; 5 Flower L.S.

KURŪṬAKAḤ (Mal. VĒLIPPARUTTI)

One of the twenty one drugs that constitute the *Vīrataradi* (*Vēllantarādi*) *gaṇa* of Vāgbhaṭa, which cures *vātadōṣa*, as well as vesical calculus, gravels, dysuria and anuria (Mooss, 1980: 63). The leaf juice of *kurūṭaka* is an expectorant in catarrhal affections and is an emetic. It is used in infantile diarrhoea, asthma, rheumatism, amenorrhoea and dysmenorhoea. Leaves are applied externally to rheumatic swellings and to carbuncle with good effect. Root bark is used as a purgative in rheumatic patients (Nadkarni, 1954: 431; Chunekar, 1982: 813). The important preparations using the drug are *Vīratarādi kaṣāyaṃ*, *Vīratarādighṛtaṃ*, etc.

Āyurvēdic texts reveal that the plant has *yugmaphala* and *phalakaṇṭaka* (having paired spiny fruits) *Pergularia daemia* (Forsk.) Choiv. belonging to Asclepiadaceae, locally called *vēlipparutti* is used as the source of the drug, and these synonyms suit it pretty well (See Kirtikar & Basu, 1918: 820; Nadkarni, 1954: 430; Mooss: 1980, 66 Chunekar, 1982: 813). Some people consider *vṛścikāḷi* as a synonym of this drug (cf. Singh & Chunekar, 1972: 377). But, Kerala physician treat *vṛścikāḷi* as a different drug, locally known as *tēḷkaḍa*, with *Heliotropium indicum* as the botanical source.

Pergularia daemia (*Forsk.*) *Choiv.* **(Asclepiadaceae)** (Fig. 125)
Daemia extensa (Jacq.) R. Br.
Pergularia extensa (Jacq.) N.E.Br.

Slender hispid climber; leaves simple, opposite, broadly ovate-acuminate, deeply cordate at base, upto 14 × 11 cms, flowers greenish white in axillary pedunculate corymbose cymes; calyx 5-partite, glandular within; corolla tube short, lobes 5, lanceolate acute, hairy on margins; corona double, the outer 5 lobes entire and the inner fleshy and spurred; pollinium, one in each cell; ovary of 2 distinct carpels; follicles 2, lanceolate, echinate.

Distribution: Hotter parts of India, tropical Africa, Burma, Malaya and Sri Lanka.

Note: For pharmacognostic studies on this drug, See Raghunathan and Mitra (1982: 983–995).

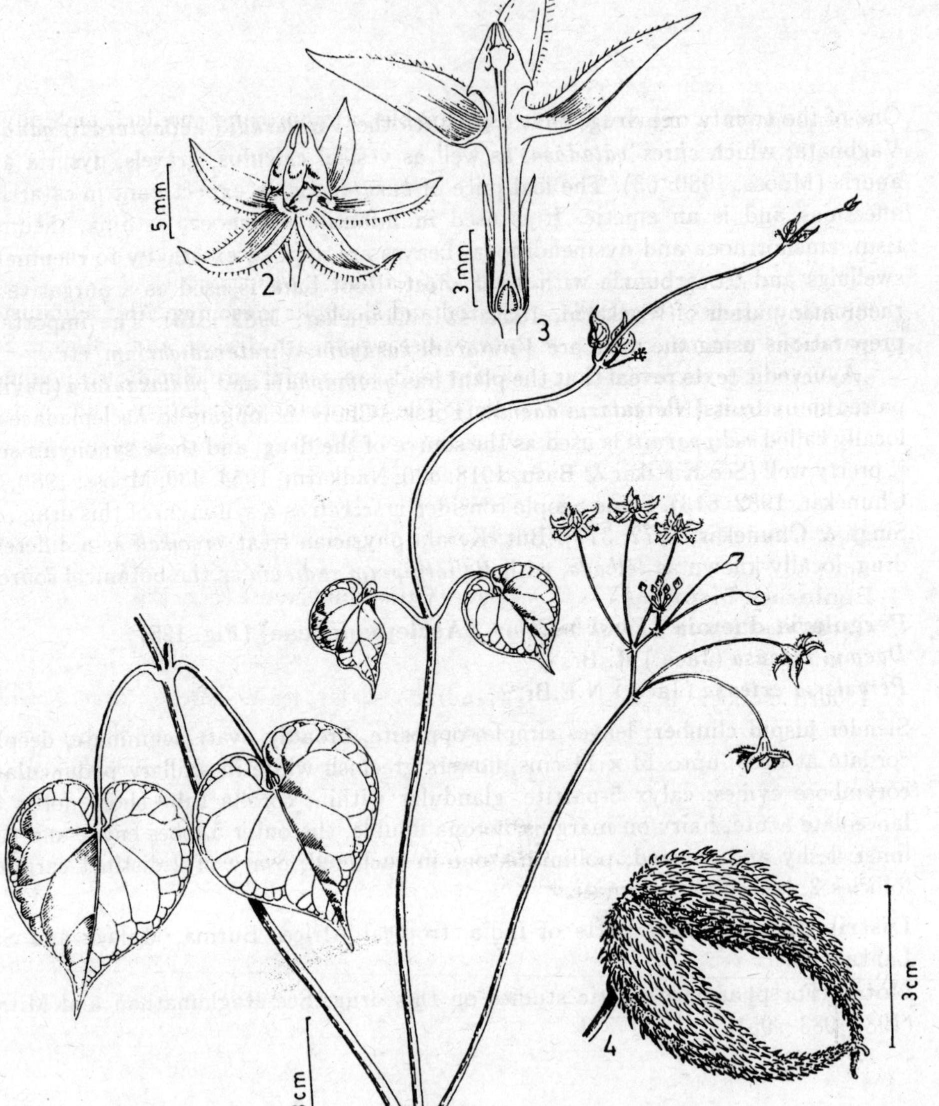

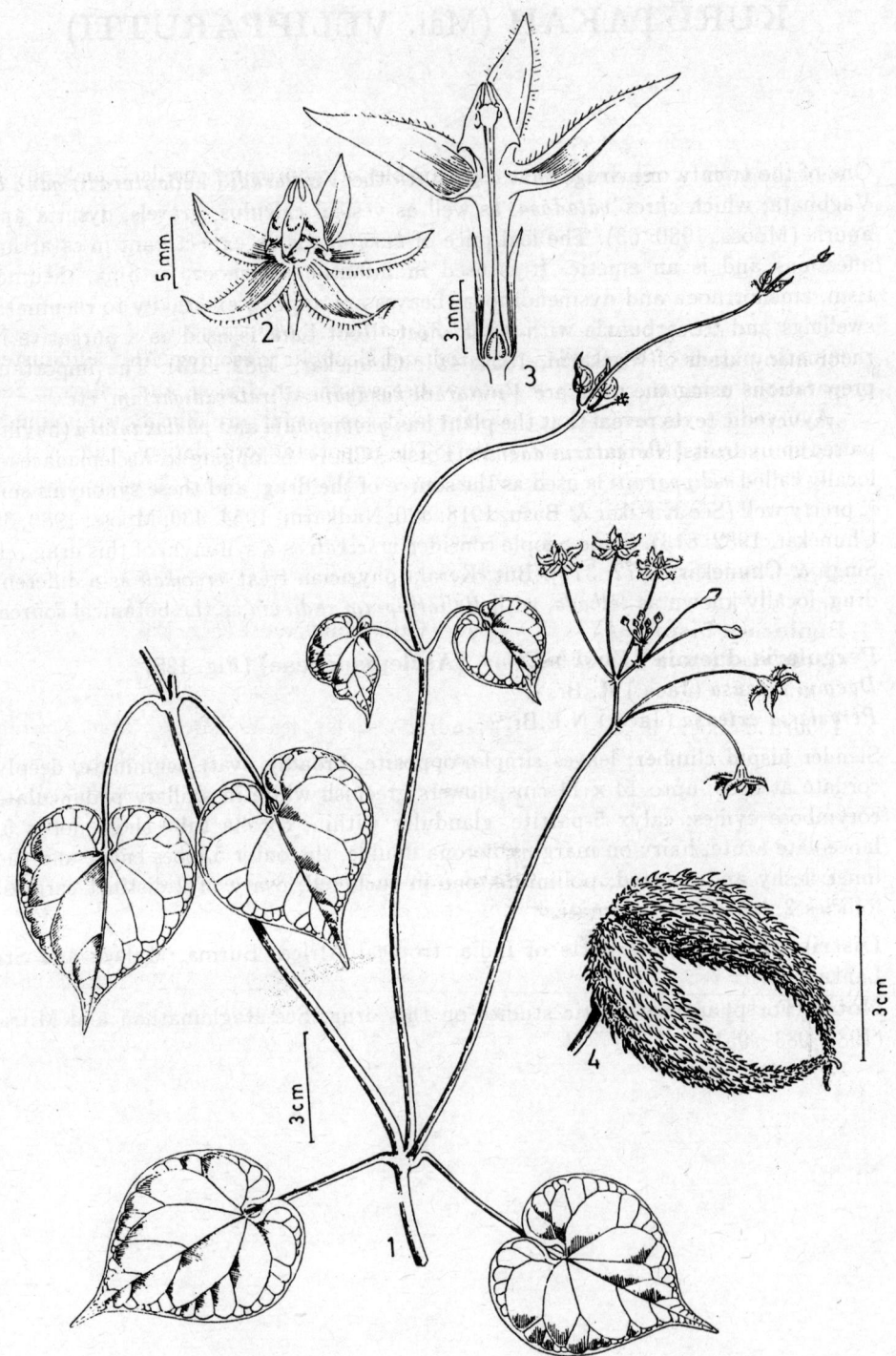

Figure 125: Pergularia daemia (Forsk.) Choiv. 1, Habit; 2, Flower; 3, Flower L.S.; 4, Fruits.

KŪŚMĀṆḌAḤ (Mal. KUṀBAḶAṀ)

Kūśmāṇḍa is a rejuvenative drug capable of improving intellect and physical strength. It is a highly nutritious food and is an important drug in naturopathy. In Āyurvēda, the fresh juice of the fruit is administered as a specific in haemoptysis and other haemorrhages from internal organs. The fruit is nutritive, tonic, diuretic, alterative and is useful in insanity, epilepsy and other nervous diseases, burning sensation, diabetes, piles and dyspepsia. It is a good antidote for many kinds of vegetable, mercurial and alcoholic poisoning. Also administered in cough, asthma, other respiratory diseases, heart disease and catarrh. Seeds are vermifuge expelling tape worms and are useful in difficult urination and bladder stones (Nadkarni, 1954: 186). The important formulations using the drug are *Kūśmāṇḍarasāyanaṃ, Himasāgaratailaṃ, Dhātryādi ghṛtaṃ, Vastyāmayāntaka ghṛtaṃ, Mahākūśmāṇḍakaghṛtaṃ*, etc.

Benincasa hispida (Thunb.) Cogn. (Cucurbitaceae) is the plant source of the drug. Rheede portrays this under the name *Cumbalam* (Hort. Malab. 8: t. 3, 1688).

Benincasa hispida (*Thunb.*) *Cogn.* **(Cucurbitaceae)** (Fig. 126)
Cucurbita hispida Thunb.
Benincasa cerifera Savi

Tendril climber; hispid all over, tendrils 2–3 fid, leaves simple, large, alternate, orbicular-cordate, palmately 5–7 lobed, to 50 cm across; flowers unisexual, large, yellow, axillary, solitary, long-pedicelled, pedicel upto 10–15 cm long; calyx tube broadly campanulate, lobes lanceolate; petals 5, obovate, softly pilose; stamens 3, inserted at the calyx tube, anthers sigmoid flexuose, connectives broadly 3-lobed, pistillode short; ovary densely pubescent in female, ovules many; style thick, stigmas large, undulate; staminodes 3; fruit large, succulent, densely white hairy when young and with a thick white waxy deposit when mature.

Distribution: The plant is widely cultivated in tropical Asia, including India for the fruits which are used as a vegetable and drug; seldom found wild.

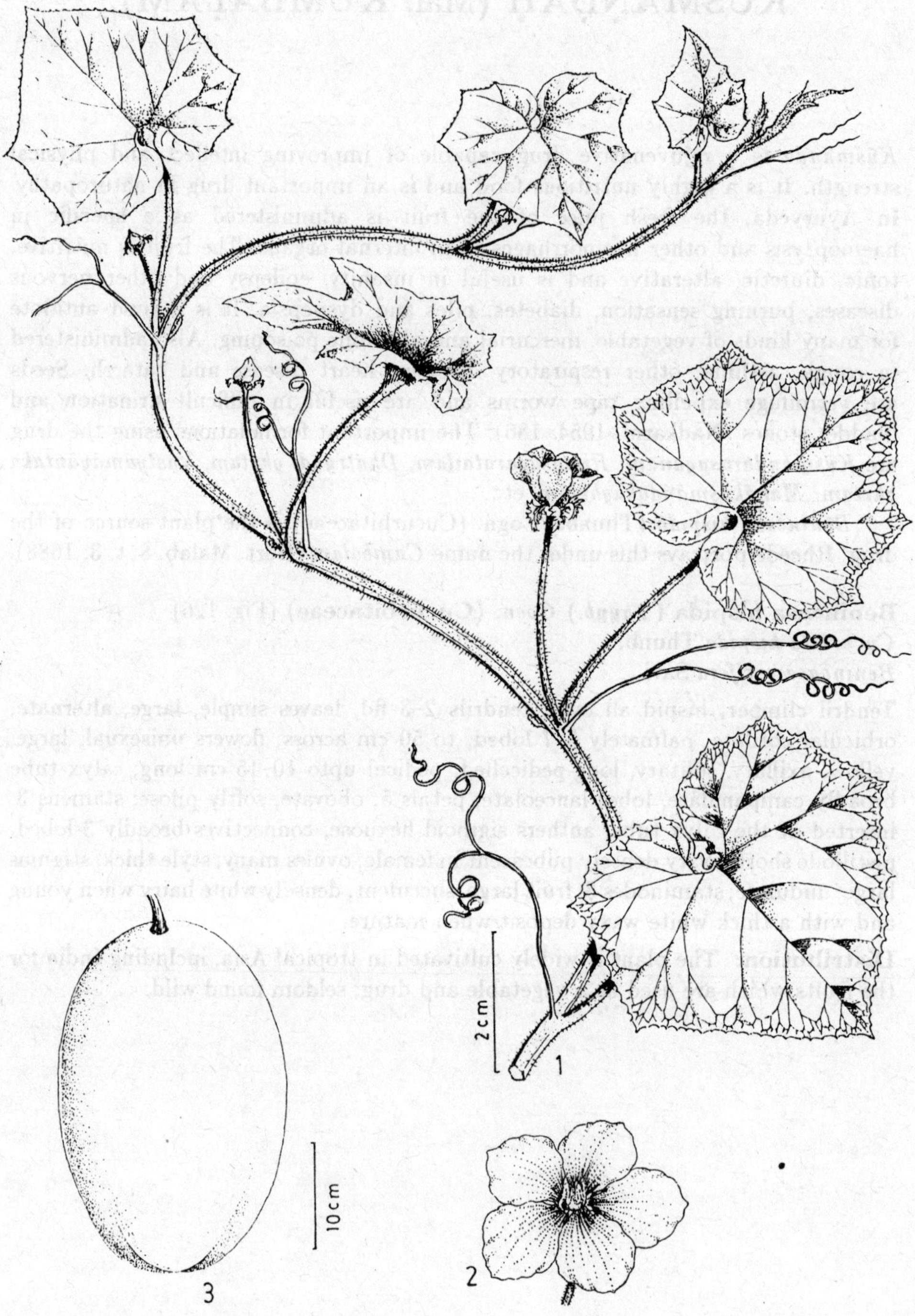

Figure 126: Benincasa hispida (Thunb.) Cogn. 1, Habit; 2, Male flower; 3, Fruit.

KUṬAJAḤ (Mal. KUṬAKAPPĀLA)

Kuṭaja is a reputed single drug remedy for chronic dysentery and diarrhoea. The officinal parts are the root bark and seeds. The root bark is bitter, astringent, cooling in action and carminative. It cures piles, diarrhoea, haemorrhage, indigestion and skin diseases. It is also reported to be useful in heart diseases, fever, *vātarakta, visarpa*, vomiting and disorders due to the morbidity of *tridōṣās*. The seeds known as *indrayava, bhadrayava*, etc. are considered to be astringent, febrifuge, anthelmintic and alleviative of all the three *dōṣās* and cure bleeding piles, diarrhoea and colic (cf. Aiyer & Kolammal, 1960. 4: 49; Mooss, 1976: 76). *Kuṭajāriṣṭam, Kuṭajatvagādi lēhaṃ, Ayaskṛti* etc. are some of the preparations using the drug.

According to the texts, the plant grows generally on mountain tops (*kuṭajaḥ, kūṭajaḥ, kauṭaḥ, girijaḥ*) and springs up in the rainy season (*prāvṛṣyaḥ, prāvṛṣēṇyaḥ*). Its flowers resemble that of *mallika*, i.e. *Jasminum* sp. (*girimallikā, mallikāpuṣpaḥ*) and are fragrant (*mahāgandhā*) The seeds are elongated like those of *yava* (*yavaphalaḥ*) (cf. Aiyer & Kolammal, 1960. 4: 47).

Caraka has mentioned two varieties of *kuṭaja*, viz. the male *kuṭaja* having glabrous leaves, white flowers and larger fruits and *strīkuṭaja* (*Strī* = female) which is darker in colour and have reddish flowers and smaller fruits (As any student of history of biology knows, ancient concepts of male and female among plants have been based on vegetative character difference rather than on the differential distribution of essential organs among them. We had to wait a long time for this erroneous idea to be corrected). Subsequent authors have, however, preferred to recognise them as *śvētakuṭaja* (the white flowered variety) and *kṛṣṇakuṭaja* (the dark coloured variety) (See Sharma, 1983: 464).

Holarrhena pubescens (Buch.-Ham.) Don (Apocynaceae) has been the most widely accepted source of the drugs *kuṭaja* and *indrayava* throughout the country (See Rheede, Hort. Malab. 1. 85–86, t. 47. 1678. *Kodagapala*). But some species of the closely related genus *Wrightia*, have also been accepted as the botanical source in some parts. However, doubts about this choice have been expressed by Aiyer and Kolammal (1960. 4: 45) and Chunekar (1982: 349). Singh and Chunekar (1972: 102) have unequivocally stated that *Holarrhena pubescens* is the right choice for *kuṭaja* and that *Wrightia tinctoria* and *W. arborea* might be considered as the sources of *strīkuṭaja* or *kṛṣṇakuṭaja.*

Sharma (1983: 464) has ruled out *W. tinctoria* as its source because it has got white flowers, and would prefer *W. tomentosa* to be the source plant of *kṛṣṇakuṭaja.*

Some consider *Wrightia tinctoria* as the source of *śvētakuṭaja* (See Nadkarni, 1954: 1296; Chopra *et al.*, 1956: 259; Kurup *et al.*, 1979: 203). The seeds of this species are sold in the market as *indrayava* along with those of *Holarrhena pubescens*. But the former can easily be recognised by its sweet taste as against the bitter seeds of the latter (Singh & Chunekar, 1972: 102).

The various plant sources of these drugs are briefly described as follows.

Holarrhena pubescens (*Buch.-Ham.*) *Wallich ex Don* **(Apocynaceae)**
Holarrhena antidysenterica (Linn.) Wall. ex DC. (Fig. 127)

Shrubs or small trees; leaves simple, opposite, short-petioled, broadly ovate-oblong acuminate, to 29 × 12 cms, glabrous above, pale and pubescent beneath; flowers white, fragrant, in axillary cymes; calyx 5-partite, lobes small, lanceolate-acuminate, hairy outside; corolla gamopetalous, salver-shaped, puberulous outside, tube 3 cm long, lobes 5, elliptic-obtuse with yellowish base; stamens 5, included, filaments very short; carpels 2, free, ovules many in each, style short, stigma oblong-fusiform; fruits paired, terete, 20–30 cm long; seeds oblong, to 2 cm long with an apical coma.

Distribution: The plant is found throughout the drier parts especially in deciduous forests upto 3,000 ft. Also distributed in tropical Himalaya, Burma, Indo-China and Malesia.

Note: Root bark of *H. pubescens* has been found to be efficaceous against Amoebiasis and Giardiasis (Singh, 1986). It helps dispel *Entamoeba hystolytica* cysts.

For pharmacognostic work on ***kutaja*** and ***indrayava*** see Satyavathy *et al.* (1987) and Anandakumar *et al.* (1984) respectively.

Wrightia tinctoria (*Roxb.*) *R. Br.* **(Apocynaceae)** (Fig. 128)
Nerium tinctorium Roxb.

Small deciduous tree; leaves simple, opposite, short-petioled, elliptic-oblong, to lanceolate-acuminate, to 14 × 15 cms, glabrous; flowers white, fragrant in terminal panicles; calyx 5 lobed, persistent, glandular inside; corolla gamopetalous, salver-shaped. 5-lobed, corona scales 2–3 series, filiform, fimbriate; stamens 5, filaments very short, anthers exserted, arrow-shaped, tip barbed; pistil bicarpellary, style equal to the length of corolla tube, stigma bilobed; fruit of two linear cylindric follicles tapering at both ends; seeds numerous, linear, slender with a deciduous coma of fine silky hairs.

Distribution: The plant is distributed in all forest districts, in deciduous forests, especially in Peninsular India and also in Burma and Timor.

Note: The plant is widely used in the Siddha system of medicine for the treatment of psoriasis and other skin diseases. Pharmacognosy, phytochemistry, and Pharmacology of *Wrightia tinctoria* have been discussed in detail (Anonymous, 1987). An oil (777 oil) prepared out of the fresh leaves of this plant is reported to have analgesic, anti-inflammatory and anti-pyretic activities (Ghosh *et al.*, 1985) and to be effective in the treatment of psoriasis. (Krishnamurthy *et al.*, 1981). Pharmacognostic features of *W. tinctoria* bark have been discussed by Atal and Sethu (1962).

Wrightia arborea (*Dennst.*) *Mabb.* **(Apocynaceae)**
Wrightia tomentosa Roemer & Schultes

Trees; branchlets tomentose; leaves simple, opposite, short-petioled, elliptic-oblong, 6–15 × 3–6 cm, thinly pubescent along nerves above, tomentose below; flowers creamy yellow in terminal corymbose cymes; calyx 5-lobed, tawny pubescent without, corolla-tube 6 mm, lobes 5, broadly oblong-acute, appressed pubescent; corona scales oblong, entire; stamens 5, anthers mucronate; fruit of two cylindrical, connate follicles, 15–20 cms long; seeds numerous, oblong, slender, tapering at apex with a white deciduous coma of fine silky hairs.

Distribution: The plant is found in all forest districts in deciduous forest, chiefly in the Circars, Deccan and Carnatic and also in Sri Lanka, Burma, Thailand.

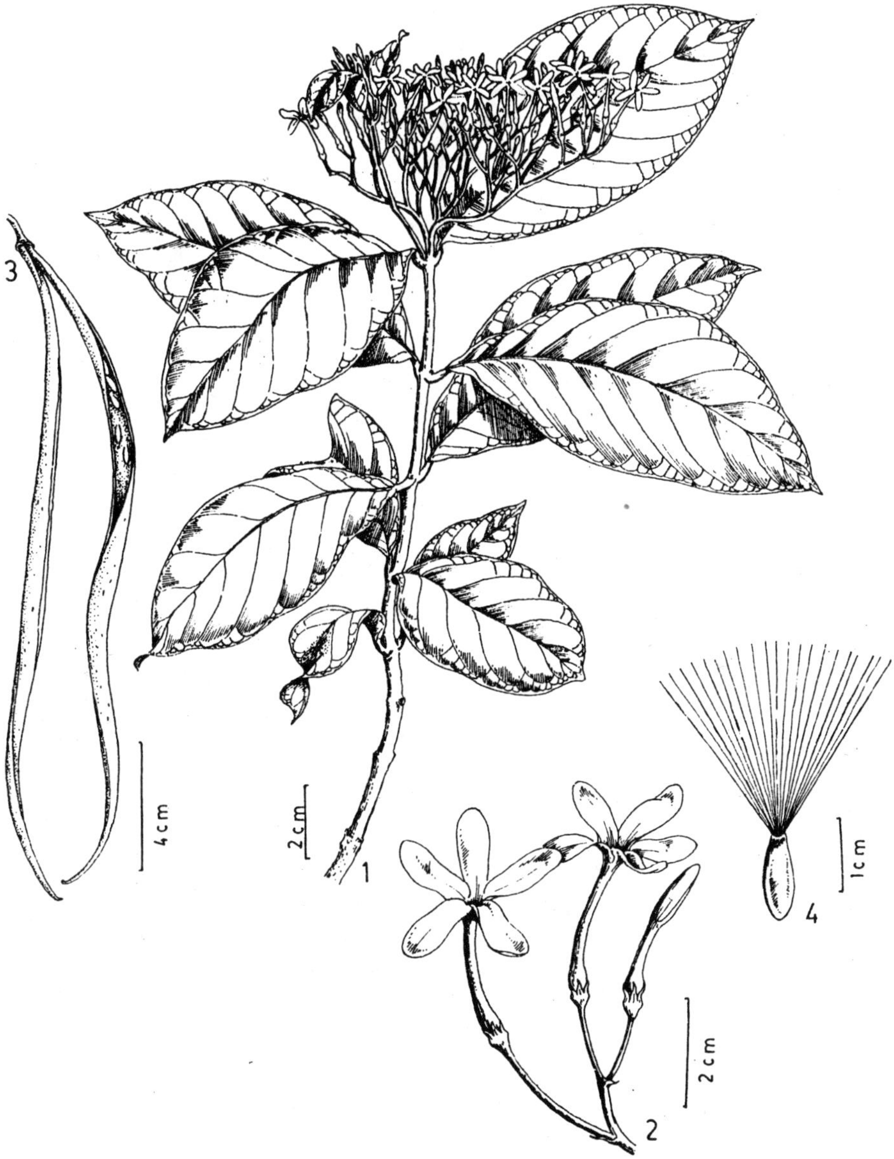

Figure 127: **Holarrhena pubescens** (Buch.-Ham.) Don. 1, Twig; 2, Flowers; 3, Fruits; 4, Seed.

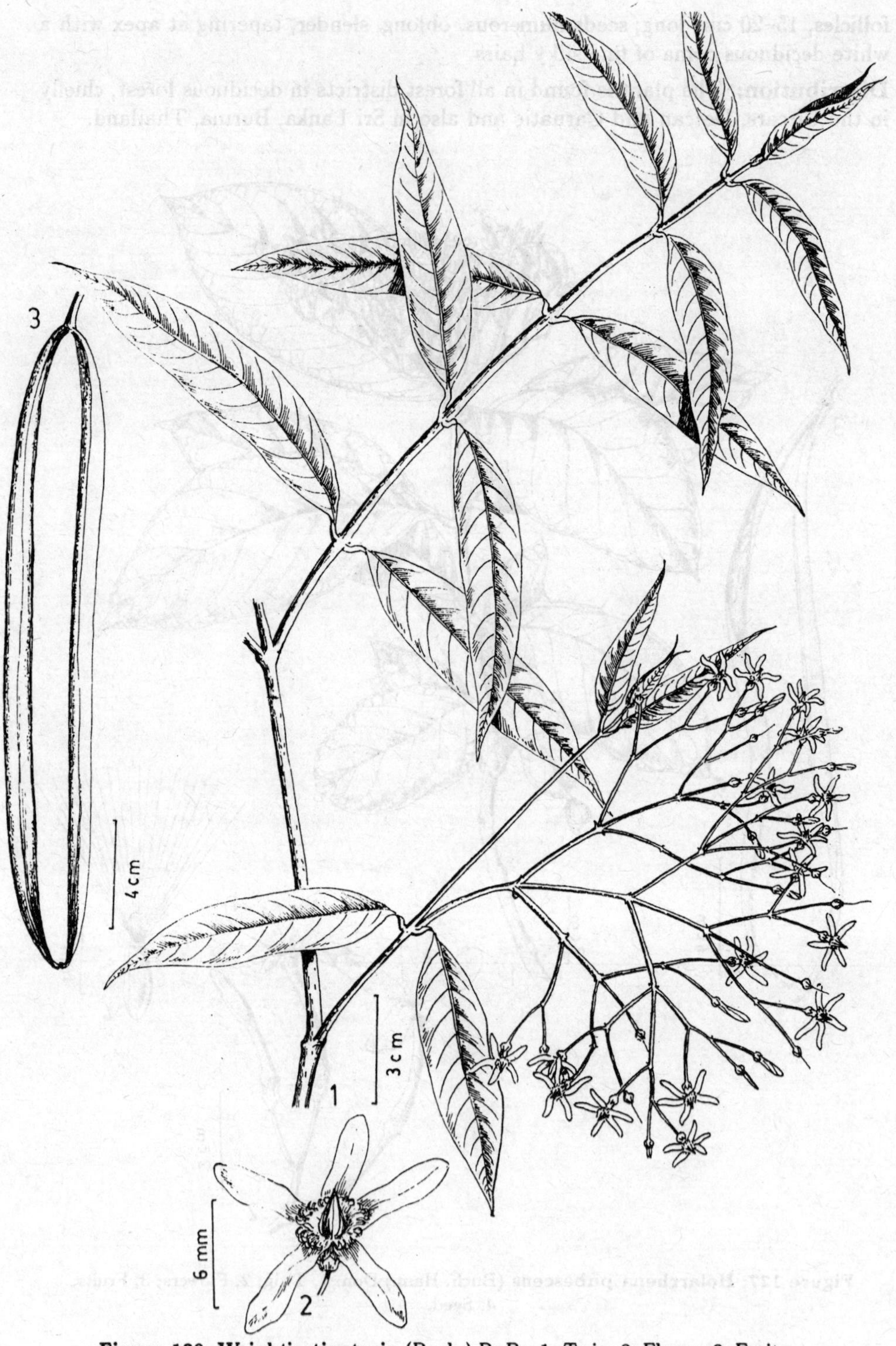

Figure 128: Wrightia tinctoria (Roxb.) R. Br. 1, Twig; 2, Flower; 3, Fruits.

LAJJĀLU (Mal. TOṬṬĀVĀṬI)

As the synonyms (*lajjālu, sparśasaṅkōcaparṇikā, añjalikārikā*) indicate, the plant has very sensitive leaves which fold on touching and has reddish roots (*raktapādī*) (cf. Aiyer & Kolammal, 1963. 6: 27). This description is well applicable to the plant that is being used as the drug source in Kerala, namely *Mimosa pudica* Linn. of Mimosaceae.

The whole plant is used medicinally. It is astringent, cooling, antiseptic, alterative and blood purifier. It is used in burning sensation in the body, diarrhoea, dysentery, haemophilic conditions, leucorrhoea, morbid conditions of vagina, wounds, skin diseases and snake poison (Kurup *et al.*, 1979: 131). *Yuvatyādi tailaṃ* and *Rajatabhasmaṃ* are some of the preparations using the drug.

Some of the synonyms like *lajjālu, añjalikārikā* are sometimes applied to another plant, *Biophytum sensitivum* (Oxalidaceae) which also, has sensitive leaves. However, in Kerala, this is the source of another drug, viz. *mukkuṟṟi*, which is discussed elsewhere. In practice, *Mimosa pudica* Linn. is the one which is commonly used as the source of *lajjālu* (Kirtikar & Basu, 1918: 495; Nadkarni, 1954: 799; Kurup *et al.*, 1979: 131; Chunekar, 1982: 457; Sharma, 1983: 749).

Mimosa pudica *Linn.* **(Mimosaceae)** (Fig. 129)

Diffuse, prickly, trailing herb; stem terete with recurved prickles; leaves alternate, stipulate, bipinnate; leaflets 10 to 12 pairs, folding obliquely upwards on touching, small, sessile, linear-oblong, clothed with appressed hairs below; flowers 4-merous, pink, in pedunculate, polygamous, globose heads; calyx minute; corolla pinkish, lobes 4, ovate oblong obtuse; stamens 4, filaments free, rose coloured, much exserted; ovary superior, oblong, unilocular, style filiform, ending in a small terminal stigma; fruit a lomentum, flat, bristly, slightly curved with 3–5, 1-seeded joints.

Distribution: A native of S. America, now naturalised throughout the hotter parts of India in the plains districts as a troublesome weed.

Note: For clinical and pharmacological details see Satyavati *et al.* (1987: 255).

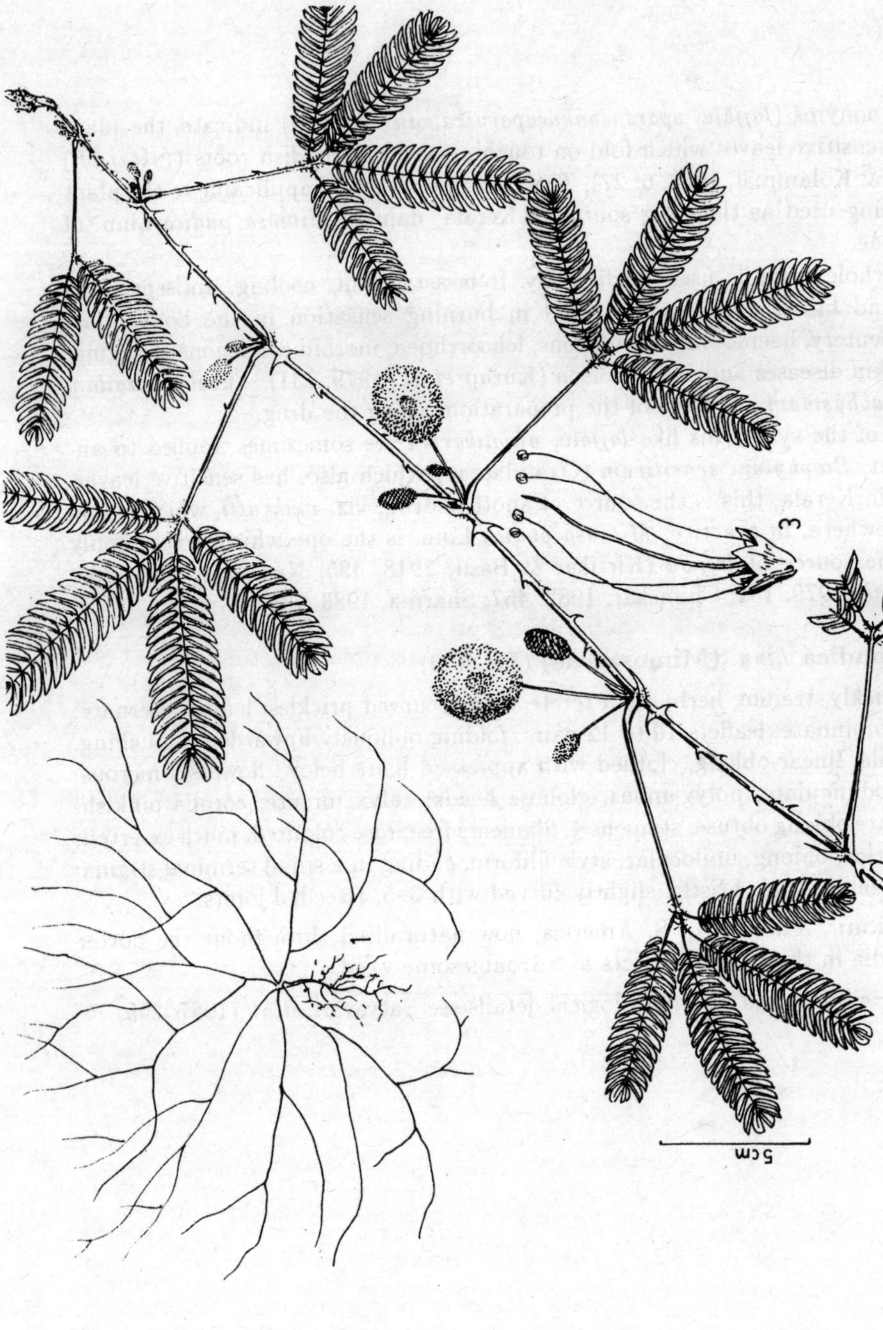

Figure 129: Mimosa pudica L. 1, Habit (diagrammatic); 2, Flowering twig; 3, Flower.

LAKṢMAṆĀ (Mal. TIRUTĀḶI)

The term *lakṣmaṇā* means the one having lucky signs or marks. This plant is described as having leaves with blood like (reddish) marks on them, (*raktālpabindubhirlāñchitachadā, asrabinduchadā, raktabindusamam patram, kaḷaṅkaparṇī*). The synonyms like *putradā, putrajananī*, etc. also indicate the property of the drug to bestow a male child. (It may be recollected that according to ancient Indian scriptures, the sex of the child can be altered by diet and medication). The plant is also described as a rhizomatous (*sukandā*) creeper with a hairy stem (*rōmavallīsamanvitam*) and flowers which are as white as cow's-milk. (*gōkṣīrasadṛśam puṣpam*) (Aiyer *et al.*, 1957. 3: 58; Chunekar, 1982; 372).

Lakṣmaṇā is cool. It promotes bodily strength, corrects vitiation due to *tridōṣa* and reduces *pitta*. In Āyurvēdic practice, *lakṣmaṇā* is a reputed single drug to cure sterility in women. (Aiyer *et al.*, 1957. 3: 59). Root, which is the officinal part, is an ingredient of *Mānasamitra vaṭakam*.

It is strange that some authors on Āyurvēdic materia medica have equated this drug with the famous Mandrake, *Mandragora officinalis* of Solanaceae (See Vaidya, 1936: 486 Nadkarni, 1954: 764). This plant, a native of the mediterranean, which resembles a distorted human body, has been associated with a lot of superstition and magical powers and was prescribed as a purgative and an emetic. It is still reported to be in use in the Middle East, where the fruit (called abore ruhr—'the giver of life') is thought to be useful in pregnancy. It is probably due to this similarity in use that this has come to be mistaken as *lakṣmaṇā*. It was also a notorious painkiller, the only anaesthetic available in Europe in the middle ages, but seldom used now because of its addictive property and side effects. This plant is not available in India and had never been in use in the Āyurvēdic medicine.

Lakṣmaṇā is equated with the vernacular name *tirutāḷi* by most of the commentators. In Kerala, a convolvulaceae creeper, *Ipomoea marginata*, locally called *tirutāḷi*, is used as the source of the drug. The reddish brown patches on the leaves of this plant and the hairy nature of the stem agree well with the description in the texts. As the plant is not rhizomatous, as mentioned in the texts, Menon (1976: 504) is of opinion that it cannot be equated with *lakṣmaṇā*. Anyway, Rheede's illustration of this plant under the name *Tirutali* (Hort. Malab. 11: 109–110, t. 53. 1692) is ample testimony to the fact that it has been in use in Kerala since the last few centuries. Our field studies have revealed that another species of *Ipomoea* namely, *I. obscura* with similarly blotched leaves and whitish flowers is also used as the drug source in Kerala.

Ipomoea marginata (*Desr.*) *Verdc.* **(Convolvulaceae)** (Fig. 130)
Convolvulus marginatus Desr.
Ipomoea sepiaria Koenig ex Roxb.

Slender twiner with slightly thickened or tuberous perennial root; leaves simple, alternate, ovate-acuminate, base cordate-hastate with acute lobes, entire, blotched

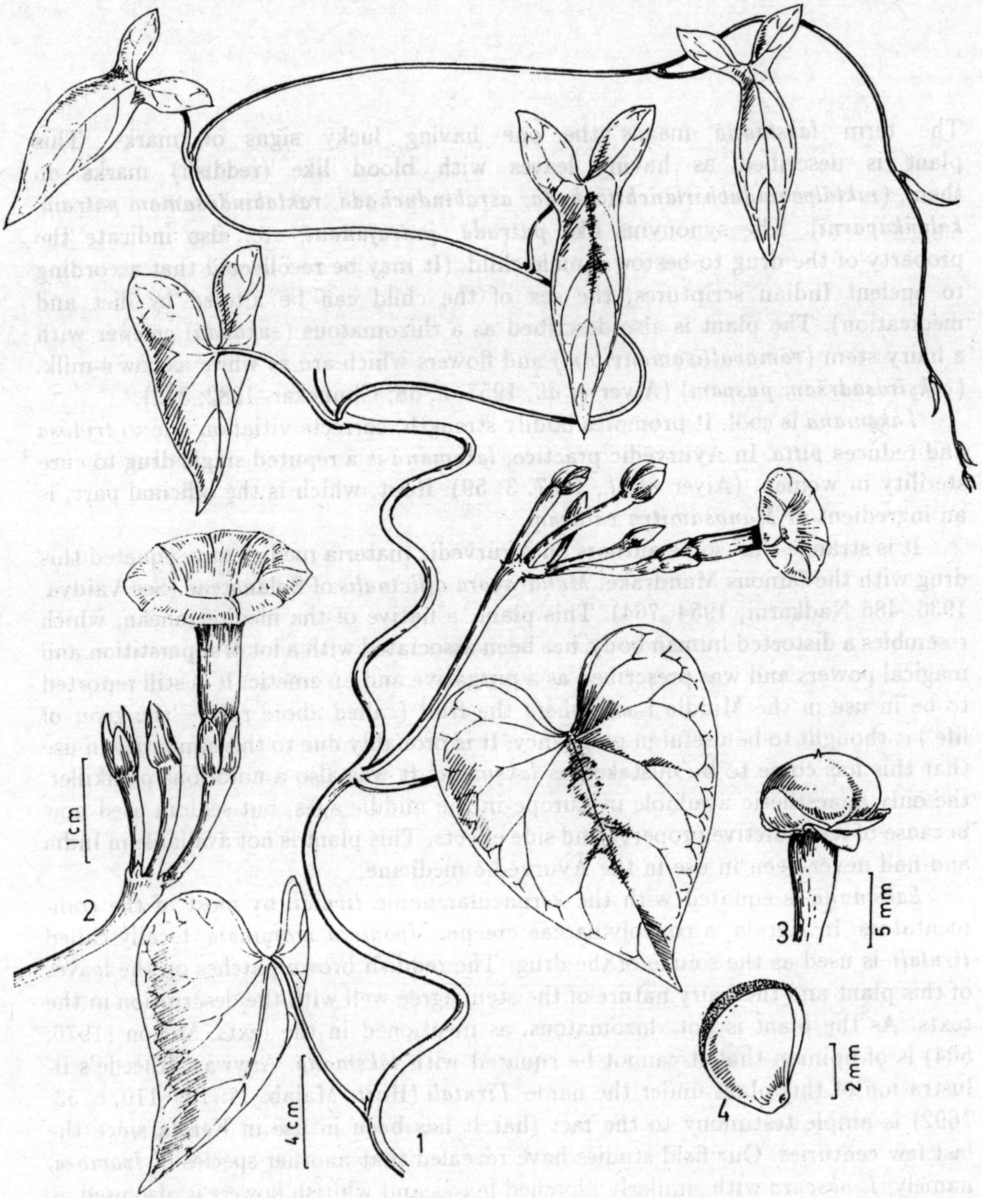

Figure 130: Ipomoea marginata (Desr.) Verdc. 1, Habit; 2, Inflorescence; 3, Fruit; 4, Seed.

with brownish patches towards the middle; flowers few at the tops of long axillary peduncles, pedicels short, thickened in fruit; sepals 5, subequal; corolla light pink with a dark eye, funnel-shaped; stamens 5, unequal; fruit an ovoid capsule.

Distribution: **The plant occurs throughout India in the plains, especially on the**

banks of streams and rivers, growing over hedges and thickets. Also distributed in tropical Africa, tropical Asia, Malesia, Formosa, Queensland and Australia.

Ipomoea obscura (*Linn.*) *Ker-Gawler* **(Convolvulaceae)** (Fig. 131)
Convolvulus obscurus Linn.

More or less glabrous slender twiner; leaves simple, alternate, broadly ovate-cordate, acuminate, often speckled with red, 8 x 7 cm, membraneous; flowers creamy yellow on 1--2 flowered slender axillary peduncles; sepals 5, subequal, ovate-oblong acute; corolla funnel-shaped, light yellow or white; stamens 5, unequal; fruit an ovoid capsule; seeds softly velvetty.

Distribution: The plant occurs all over India in the plains and low hills from sea level to 3,000 ft growing on hedges and other supports. Also reported from tropical and S. Africa, Madagascar, Queens Land, Fiji, China, Formosa.

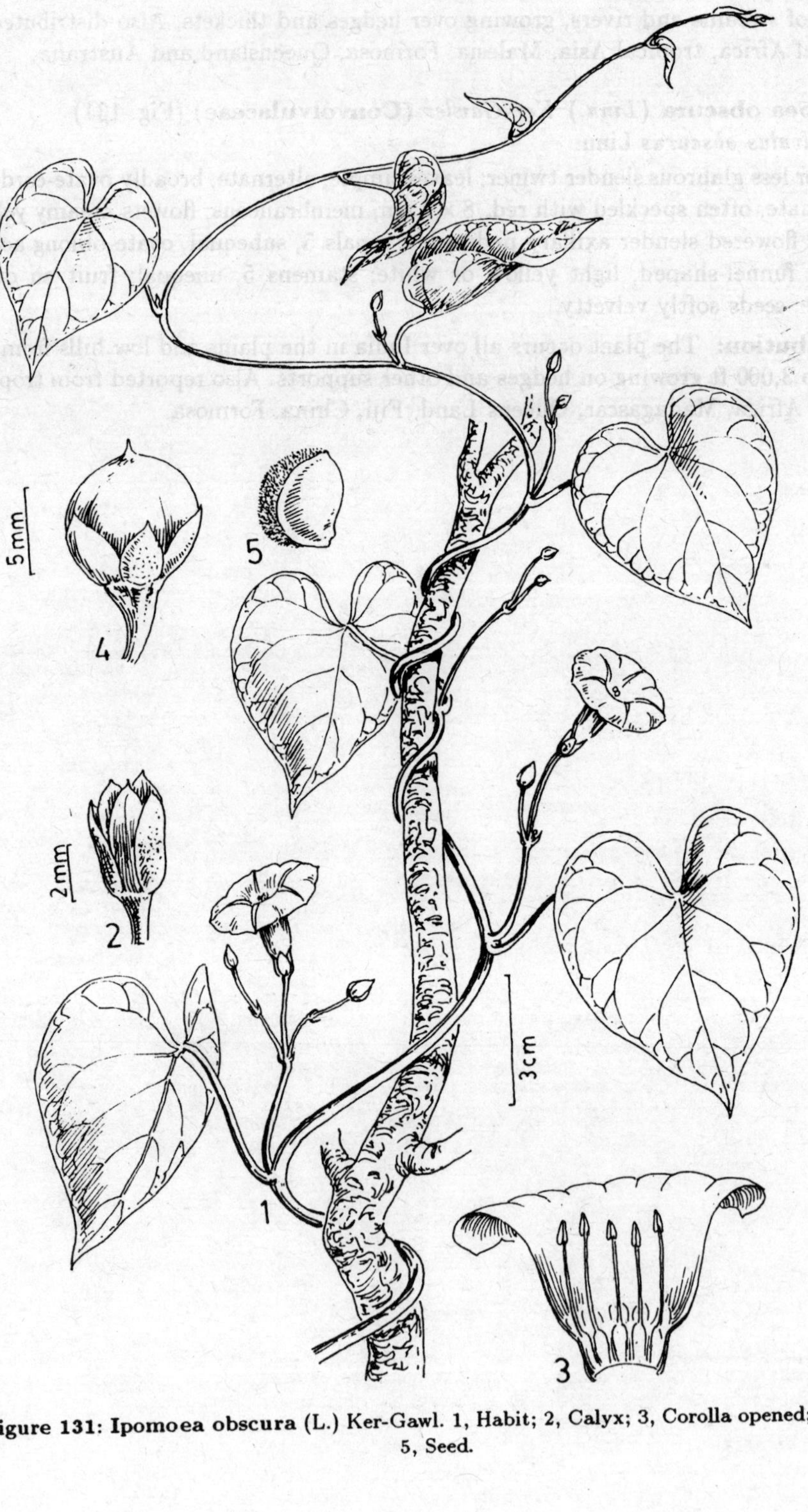

Figure 131: Ipomoea obscura (L.) Ker-Gawl. 1, Habit; 2, Calyx; 3, Corolla opened; 4, Fruit; 5, Seed.

LĀṄGALĪ (Mal. MĒNTŌNNI)

This herb with a plough-like root-stock (*lāṅgalī*) and reddish flame-coloured flowers at the tips of shoots (*agnijihvā, agniśikhā, vahniśikhā*) is a good abortifacient (*gaṛbhaghātinī*) causing expulsion of foetus from the womb (*kalikārī*). Because of this property, traditional healers apply the paste of the root-stock to the suprapubic navel region of vagina for easy and quick expulsion of the placenta after delivery. *Lāṅgalī* is bitter, acrid, astringent, anthelmintic and germicidal. It cures laprosy or dermatosis of any kind, swelling, piles, chronic ulcers, colic pain in the bladder, toxicosis, consumption and itching (Aiyer & Kolammal, 1963. 6: 35). The root, given internally is said to be an effective antidote against cobra poison. A paste of the root is also used as an anodyne application in bites of poisonous insects, snake-bites, scorpion sting, parasitic skin diseases and leprosy (Nadkarni, 1954: 579). *Jyōtiṣmatyādi tailaṃ, Mahābhūtarāvaghṛtaṃ*, etc. are prepared using the drug.

The accepted source of the drug throughout the country is *Gloriosa superba* Linn. belonging to Liliaceae.

In North Indian markets, however, the rhizomes of *Costus speciosus* (Koen.) Sm. (Zingiberaceae) are also sold in the name of *lāṅgalī*. Tewari *et al.* (1967: 196–202) have studied the comparative action of the two plants on uterus and have found them to be almost similar in action (Singh & Chunekar, 1972: 349).

In Kerala, the root-stock of *Gloriosa superba* Linn. locally called *mēntōnni*, has been used as the drug source. (See also Rheede Hort. Malab. 7: 107–108. t. 57. 1688).

Gloriosa superba *Linn.* **(Liliaceae)** (Fig. 132)

Glabrous climbing herb with tuberous root-stock, leaves simple, alternate or whorled, sessile, ovate-lanceolate, 17 × 4.5 cms, tip elongating into a spirally coiled tendril, base cordate, margin entire; flowers large in terminal racemes; perianth segments 6, linear, flexuosus and deflexed, basal half bright yellow, upper half red; stamens 6; ovary glabrous, 3-celled; capsule linear-oblong, greenish-yellow, septicidal, seeds subglobose.

Distribution: The plant is distributed throughout tropical India from sea level to about 2000 M. elevation, growing under a variety of soil conditions. Also distributed in tropical and S. Africa, Madagascar, Indonesia and Malesia.

Note: The antispermatogenic activity of the drug has been demonstrated by Dixit *et al.* (1983) in male gerbil. The drug administration caused degenerative lesions in the testes of gerbil.

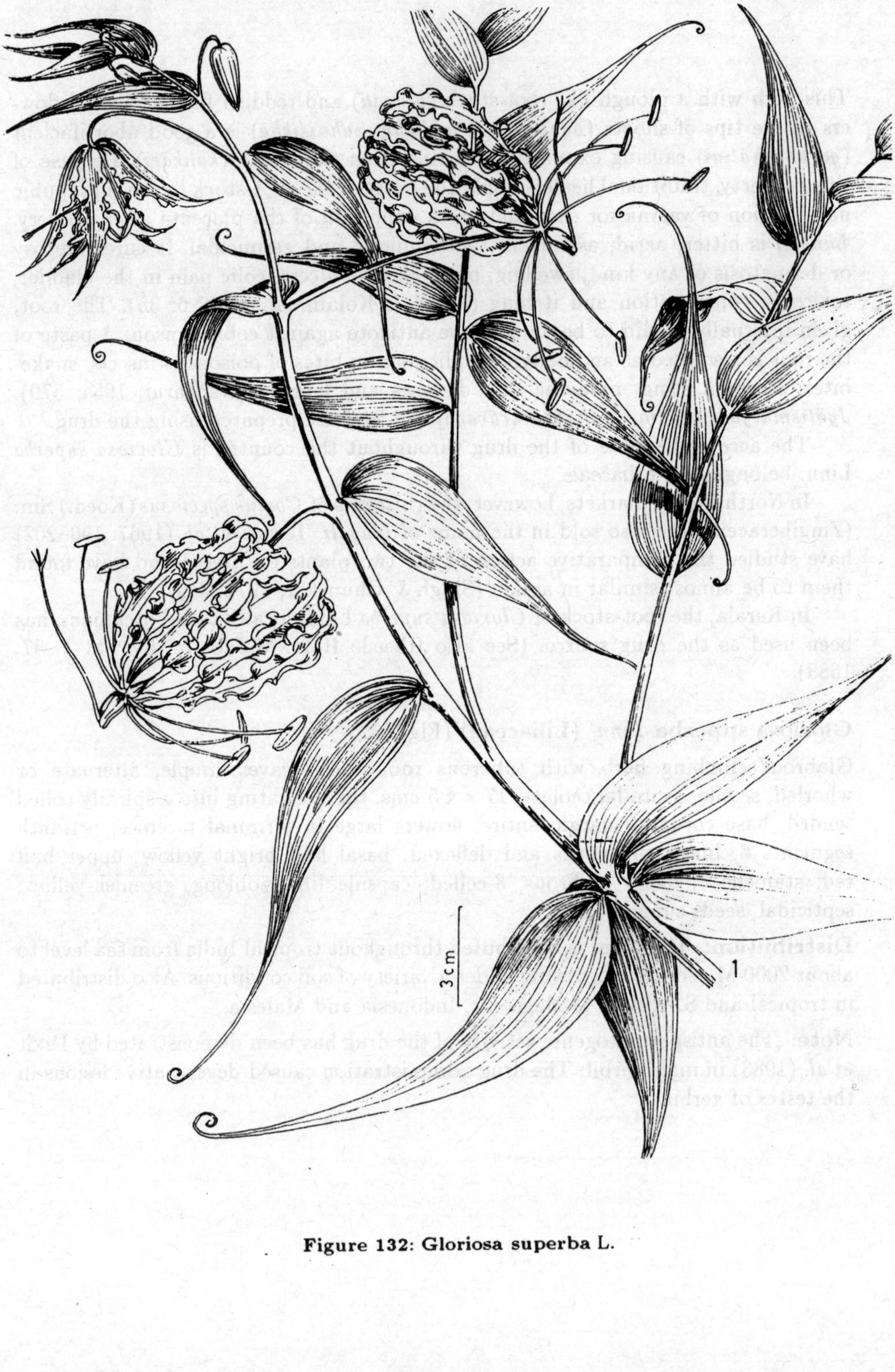

Figure 132: Gloriosa superba L.

LŌDHRAḤ (Mal. PĀCCŌṬṬI)

This is considered to be a specific remedy for uterine complaints, vaginal diseases and menstrual disorders. Bark is the officinal part. It is light, cool, astringent, carminative and a uterine tonic. It overcomes vitiated *kapha* and *pitta* and is useful in bowel complaints such as diarrhoea and dysentery, dropsy, eye diseases, fevers, cough, ulcers and swellings. The drug is recommended in cases of menorrhagia and leucorrhoea. A decoction of the bark is used as a gargle for giving firmness to spongy and bleeding gums (Nadkarni, 1954: 1187; Kurup *et al.*, 1979: 135, Sharma, 1983: 616). The important preparations using the drug are *Lōdhrāsavaṃ*, *Gandhatailaṃ*, *Daśamūlāriṣṭaṃ*, *Drākṣādi kaṣāyaṃ*, *Puṣyānugacūrṇaṃ*, etc.

Except for the thick nature of the bark (*sthūlavalkalaḥ*) the synonyms do not give any indication that may help to identify the botanical source.

Two varieties of *lōdhra* are described in the texts viz. *śābara lōdhra* and *paṭṭikā lōdhra*. The former is equated with *Symplocos racemosa* Roxb. and the latter with *Symplocos crataegoides* Buch.-Ham. (Symplocaceae) by the modern writers (Singh & Chunekar, 1972: 352; Chunekar, 1982: 128–130). But these two are exclusively North Indian species and are not available in Kerala. The varietal distinction is not observed in Āyurvēdic practice and in Kerala *Symplocos cochinchinensis* (Lour.) S. Moore (= *Symplocos spicata* Roxb.), localled called *Pāccōṭṭi*, is being used as the drug source (Aiyer *et al.*, 1957: 68; Mooss, 1980: 104). This is considered as the white variety by some, the red variety being *S. racemosa* (Nesamony, 1985: 343). Rheede's account of *S. cochinchinensis* in his Hortus Malabaricus (5: 9–10, t. 5. 1685, *Patsjotti*) proves that it has been the source of the drug since his period. The plant is described below.

Symplocos cochinchinensis (*Lour.*) *S. Moore* **(Symplocaceae)** (Fig. 133)
Drupatris cochinchinensis Lour.
S. spicata Roxb.

Medium-sized tree; leaves simple, alternate, short-petioled, elliptic-obovate or broadly lanceolate, acute or acuminate, crenate-serrate, 6–15 x 3–5 cm; flowers small, white, fragrant, in rusty-pubescent axillary spikes; calyx tube closely adnate to the ovary with 5 ovate, obtuse lobes; corolla 5-partite; stamens 2, unequal; ovary inferior, (sub) globose, with an annular fleshy disc; fruit drupaceous, globose or ampulliform, 5 mm across, with an apical ring; seeds oblong.

Distribution: South and Southeast Asia and Malesia. In India it is common on hills, more abundantly in tropical Shola forests.

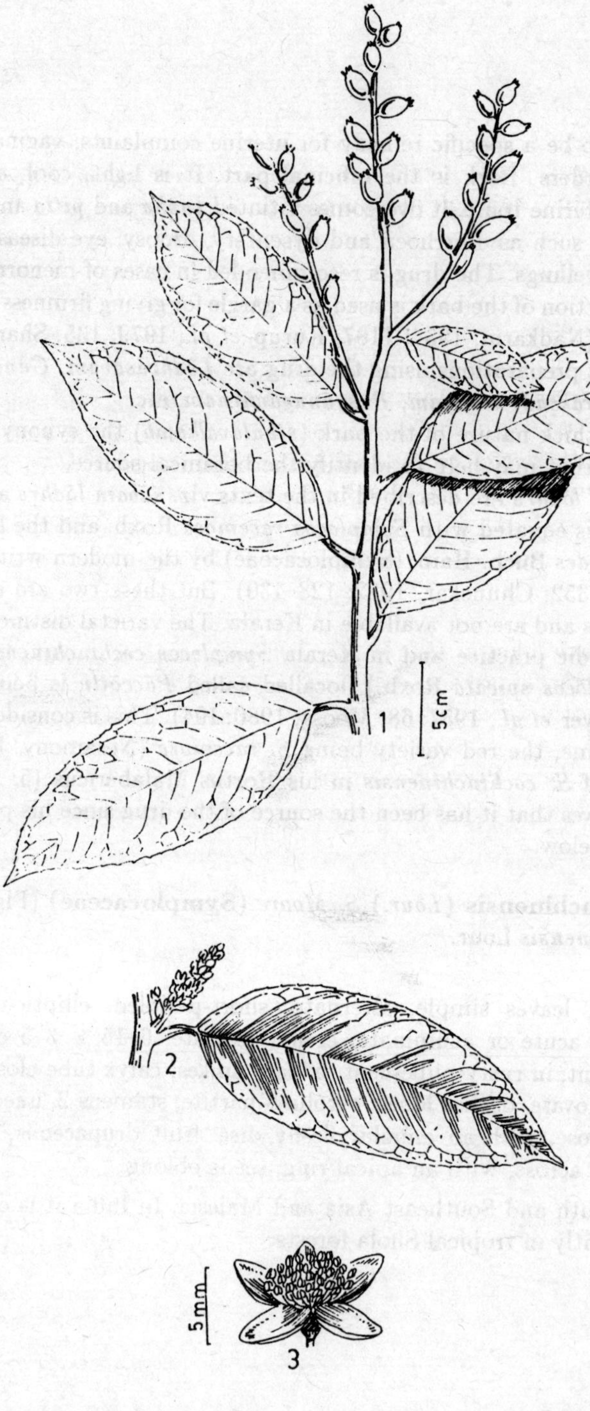

Figure 133: Symplocos cochinchinensis (Lour.) Moore. 1, Twig; 2, Inflorescence; 3, Flower.

LŌṆIKĀ (Mal. KOḶUPPA)

The drug forms an ingredient of preparations like *Āṛukālādi tailaṃ*, *Kaccōrādi oil*, *Valiya maṛmaguḷika*, etc. The whole plant is medicinal and is reported to be cooling, sour, blood purifier and alleviative of *kapha* and *pitta*. The seeds are diuretic and anthelmintic. The drug cures wounds, flatulence, cough, bronchitis, dysphonia and diabetes. It is also useful in eye diseases, inflammation of the bladder and kidney, fever, *raktapitta*, piles, burning sensation of the body, and thirst (Chunekar, 1982: 670).

Two varieties, viz. a smaller variety called *laghu lōṇikā* or *lōṇi* and a bigger type *bṛhallōṇi* or *ghōṭikā* are mentioned in the texts. Most of the authors have equated the former with *Portulaca quadrifida* Linn. and the latter with *Portulaca oleracea* Linn. of Portulacaceae (cf. Kirtikar & Basu, 1918: 137, 135; Nadkarni, 1954: 1007, 1005; Chunekar, 1982: 670, 671). However, as is obvious from Rheede's account (Hort. Malab. 10: 21–22. t. 11. 1690 *Coluppa*), it seems that *Alternanthera sessilis* of Amaranthaceae has been the source of this drug in Kerala, since long. Our field studies have revealed that at least three different plants are currently being used as the source plant of this drug in different parts of Kerala. They are *Alternanthera sessilis* (Amaranthaceae), *Glinus oppositifolius* (Molluginaceae) and *Portulaca oleracea* (Portulacaceae).

Portulaca oleracea *Linn.* **(Portulacaceae)** (Fig. 134)

Prostrate or erect, succulent herb; branchlets glabrous, green or purplish; leaves alternate or subopposite, obovate-spathulate, obtuse or retuse, 0.7–2 × 0.4–1.5 cm, fleshy, glabrous; flowers bright yellow, clustered at the tips of branches; sepals 2, lanceolate, subequal; petals 5, obovate-retuse, mucronate; stamens 12, filaments unequal, pubescent at base; ovary obovoid, 1-celled, style 4–5 fid; capsule ovoid, glabrous; seeds many, tubercled.

Distribution: A pantropical weed, seen wild throughout India in moist, shady localities. This is often used as a leafy vegetable.

Alternanthera sessilis (*Linn.*) *R. Br. ex DC.* **(Amaranthaceae)** (Fig. 135)
Alternanthera triandra Lam.

Diffuse or prostrate herb; leaves opposite, elliptic to lanceolate, 1.5–3 × 0.5–1 cm, glabrous; flowers minute, white in axillary capitate clusters; bracts ovate or obovate, 1 mm; bracteoles shorter, persistent; tepals 5, subequal, ovate, 1-nerved, acute; stamens 3, staminodes subulate; ovary depressed globose; utricle cordiform, strongly compressed; seeds orbicular.

Distribution: In wet places, in all districts, both in the plains and in the hills in India. Widespread in the tropics and subtropics of both Old and New Worlds.

Glinus oppositifolius (*Linn.*) *A. DC.* **(Molluginaceae)** (Fig. 136)
Mollugo oppositifolia Linn.

Prostrate or diffuse herb; leaves in whorls of 3–5, oblong-oblanceolate, acute, unequal, 0.5–3 × 0.2–0.6 cm, glabrescent; flowers small, white, fascicled in the axils; sepals 5, free, elliptic-obtuse; petals 0; stamens 5, alternating with sepals; staminodes 2-fid; ovary 2 lobed, many ovuled, styles 3; capsules 3 valved; seeds dark brown, reniform.

Distribution: Pantropical weed, common in moist shady places throughout India.

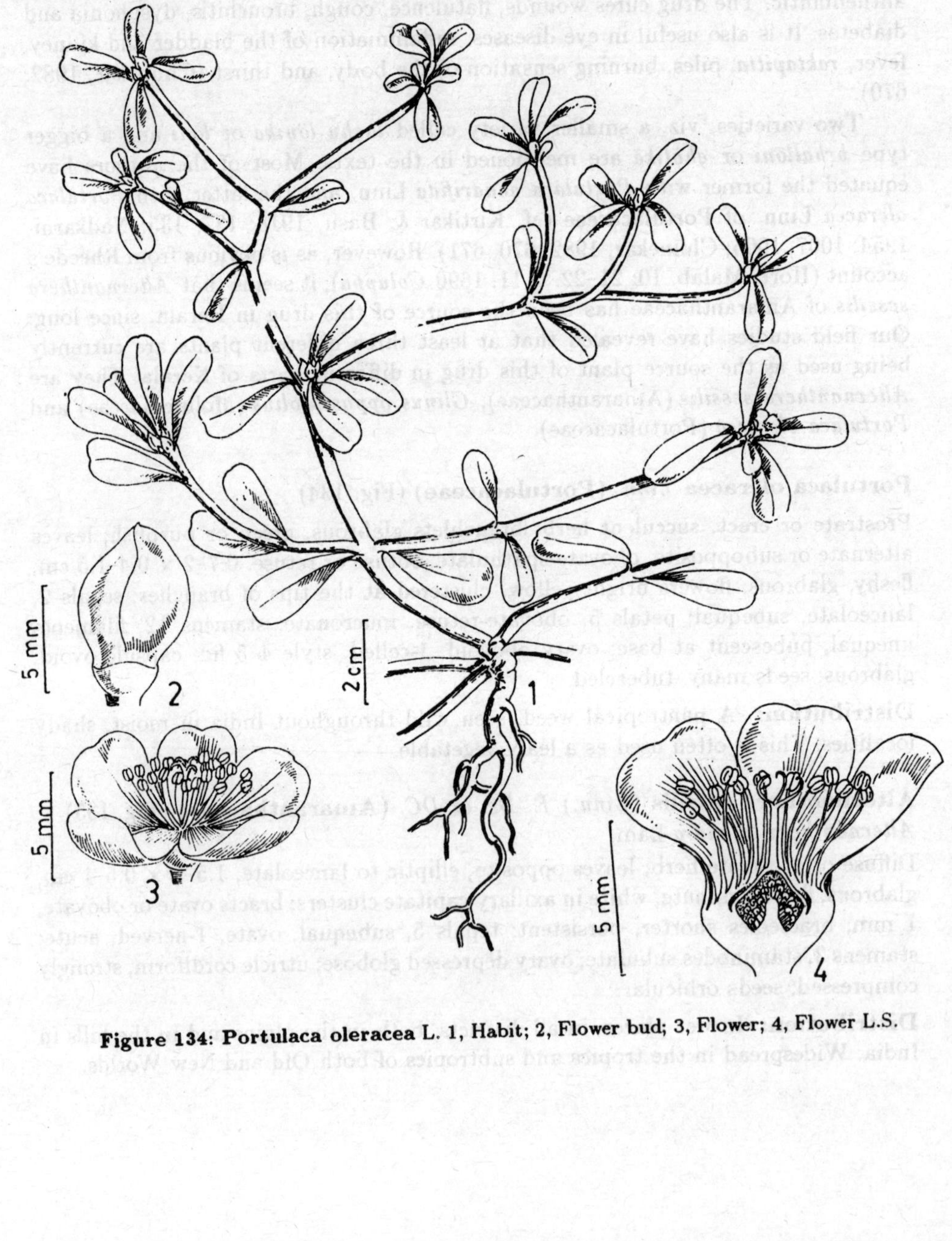

Figure 134: Portulaca oleracea L. 1, Habit; 2, Flower bud; 3, Flower; 4, Flower L.S.

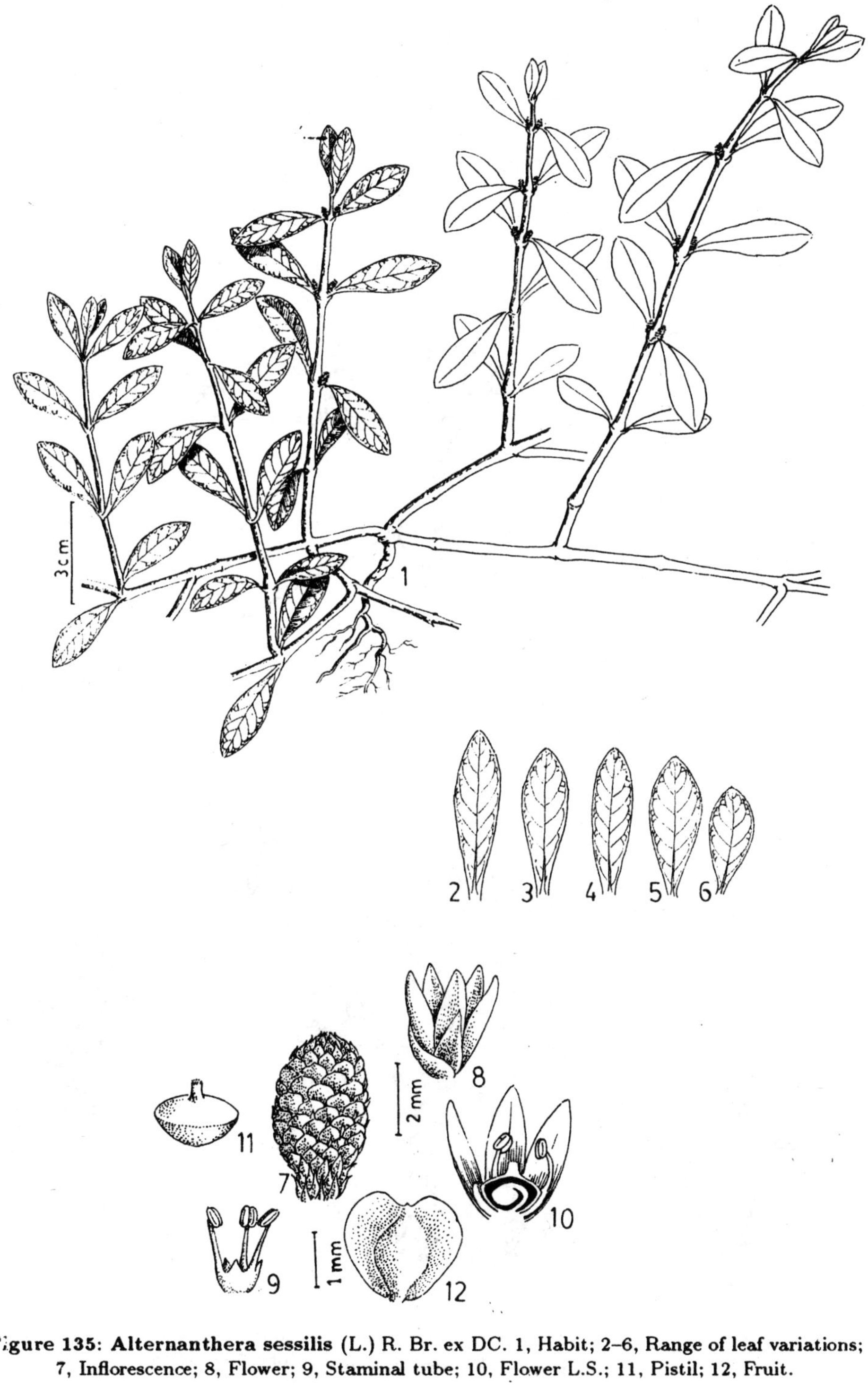

Figure 135: Alternanthera sessilis (L.) R. Br. ex DC. 1, Habit; 2–6, Range of leaf variations; 7, Inflorescence; 8, Flower; 9, Staminal tube; 10, Flower L.S.; 11, Pistil; 12, Fruit.

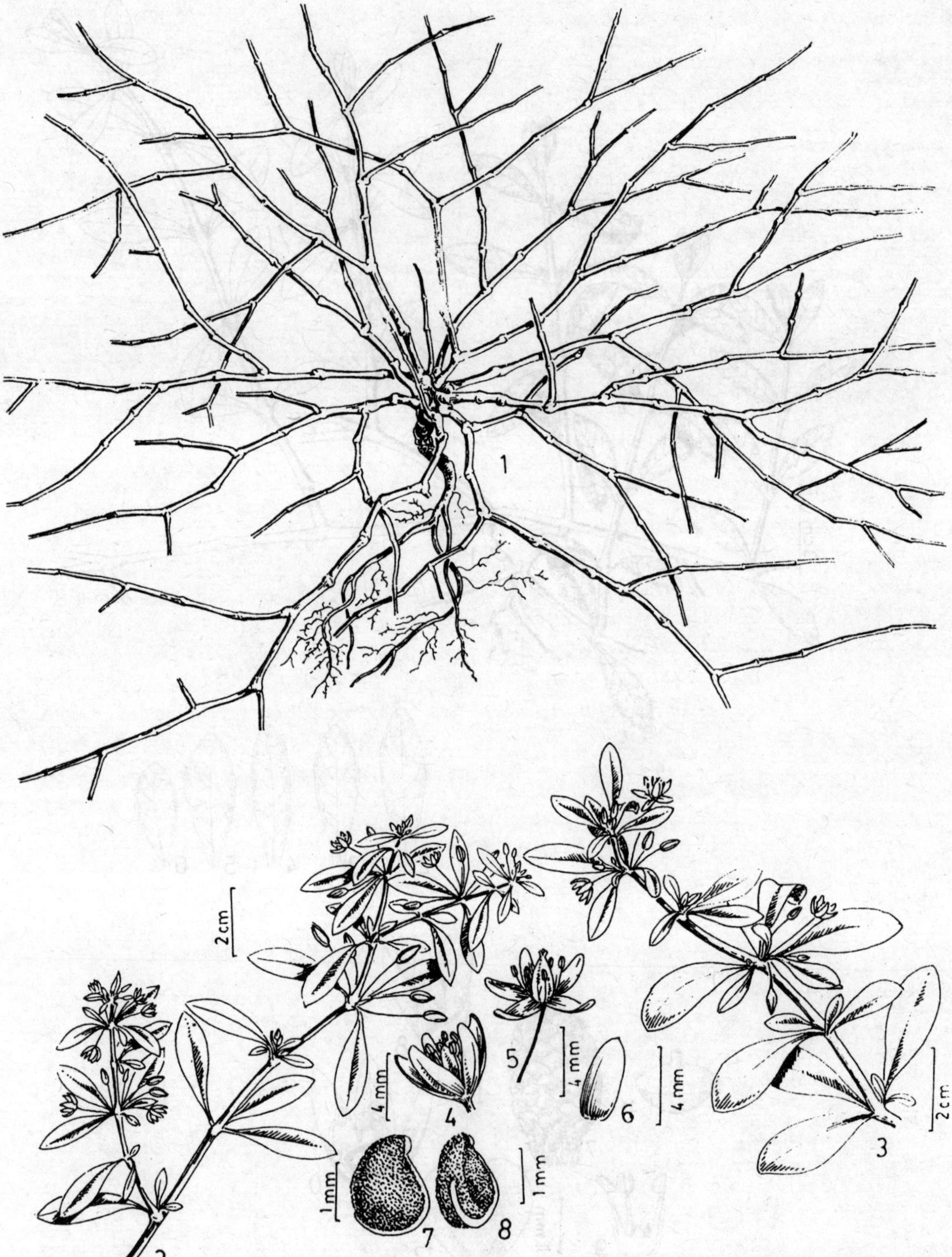

Figure 136: Glinus oppositifolius (L.) A. DC. 1, Habit (diagrammatic); 2–3, Flowering branch; 4–5, Flowers; 6, Perinath lobe; 7–8, Seeds.

MĀLATĪ (Mal. PICCAKAṂ)

The drug is reported to be good for healing chronic ulcers, skin diseases and poisonous affections. Leaves, flowers and sometimes the whole plant are used in medicine. The drug is bitter, astringent, anthelmintic, diuretic and emmenagogue. Leaves are chewed in aphtae and ulcers in the mouth, throat and gums. It also forms a good external application to ulcers. The oil prepared from the flowers is cooling and applied in skin disorders, headache and eye troubles. Flowers and leaves are aphrodisiac and overcome menstrual irregularities (Nadkarni, 1954; 702; Chunekar, 1982: 491; Nesamony, 1985: 360). The drug enters into the composition of preparations like *Mālatyādi tailaṃ, Jātyādi ghṛtaṃ, Jātyādi tailaṃ, Kalyāṇaka ghṛtaṃ, Āraṇyātuḷasyādi* coconut oil, etc.

Except for one or two synonyms like *hṛdyagandhā, mālatī* etc. which refer to the sweet smell of the flowers, the texts do not give any character detail of the plant. Most of the authors equate the drug with *Jasminum grandiflorum* Linn. of Oleaceae (Kirtikar & Basu, 1918: 765; Nadkarni, 1954: 701; Chopra *et al.*, 1956: 144; Chunekar, 1982: 491; Sharma, 1983: 178). In practice also, this plant, locally called *piccakaṃ* is the most popularly accepted source of the drug. Some authors mention a yellow-flowered variety called *svarṇajātī* or *hēmapuṣpikā* and identify it with *Jasminum humile* Linn. (Kirtikar & Basu, 1918: 764; Nadkarni, 1954: 702; Chopra *et al.*, 1956: 144; Chunekar, 1982: 492; Sharma, 1983: 178). But this is not used in practice. *Jasminum angustifolium* Vahl. called *kānanamallikā, āsphōtā* etc. in Sanskrit and *kāṭṭumallika* in Malayalam (Kirtikar & Basu, 1918: 763; Nadkarni, 1954: 700; Chopra *et al.*, 1956: 143) is also used in plenty as the source of the drug in Āyurvēdic formulations.

Classical texts mention another type of the drug viz. *gandhamālatī* or *madhumālatī*. Some of the practitioners consider this to be the same as *mālatī*, but most others treat it as a different plant, equating it with *Aganosma dichotoma* (Apocynaceae) (Singh & Chunekar, 1972: 307; Kapoor & Mitra, 1979: 71).

Rheede identifies *Jasminum grandiflorum* as *Pitsjegam-mulla* (Hort. Malab. 6: 91, t. 52, 1686) and *J. angustifolium* as *Katu-pitsjegam mulla* (Hort. Malab. 6: 93, t. 53. 1886). The two plants can be distinguished as follows:

Jasminum grandiflorum *Linn.* **(Oleaceae)** (Fig. 137)

Climbing shrub; leaves imparipinnate, 7–9 foliolate, the odd one ovate-acuminate, 3.5 x 2 cm, others ovate-obtuse, mucronate, 2.5 x 2.2 cm, glabrous; flowers white, sweet-scented in terminal corymbose panicles; calyx lobes linear; corolla tube upto 2 cm long, lobes spreading, lanceolate-acute, reddish beneath; stamens 2, included in the corolla tube, anthers oblong; ovary 2-celled, ovules 2 in each cell, style filiform, stigma bifid; fruit a didymous berry; seed 1 in each carpel.

Distribution: Subtropical N.W. Himalaya. The plant grows in N. Circars, Mahendragiri in Ganjam, hills of Vizagapatam, W. Ghats, Nilgiris, Pulneys and Hills of Tinnevelly above 5,000 ft. Probably introduced and run wild, often cultivated.

Jasminim angustifolium *Vahl.* **(Oleaceae)** (Fig. 138)

Climbing shrub; leaves simple, opposite, elliptic-ovate, acuminate, glabrous, upto 1–3 × 0.7–2 cm; flowers white, sweet-scented in terminal 1–3 flowered cymes; calyx lobes unequal, linear, sparsely ciliate, acute; corolla tube 1 cm long, lobes 5–9, oblanceolate; stamens 2, included, filaments short, anthers oblong; ovary 2 celled, style filiform, stigma 2-fid; berry globose, 0.8 cm across.

Distribution: The plant is found in Circars, Deccan & Carnatic on eastern side down to S. Travancore. Distributed also in Sri Lanka.

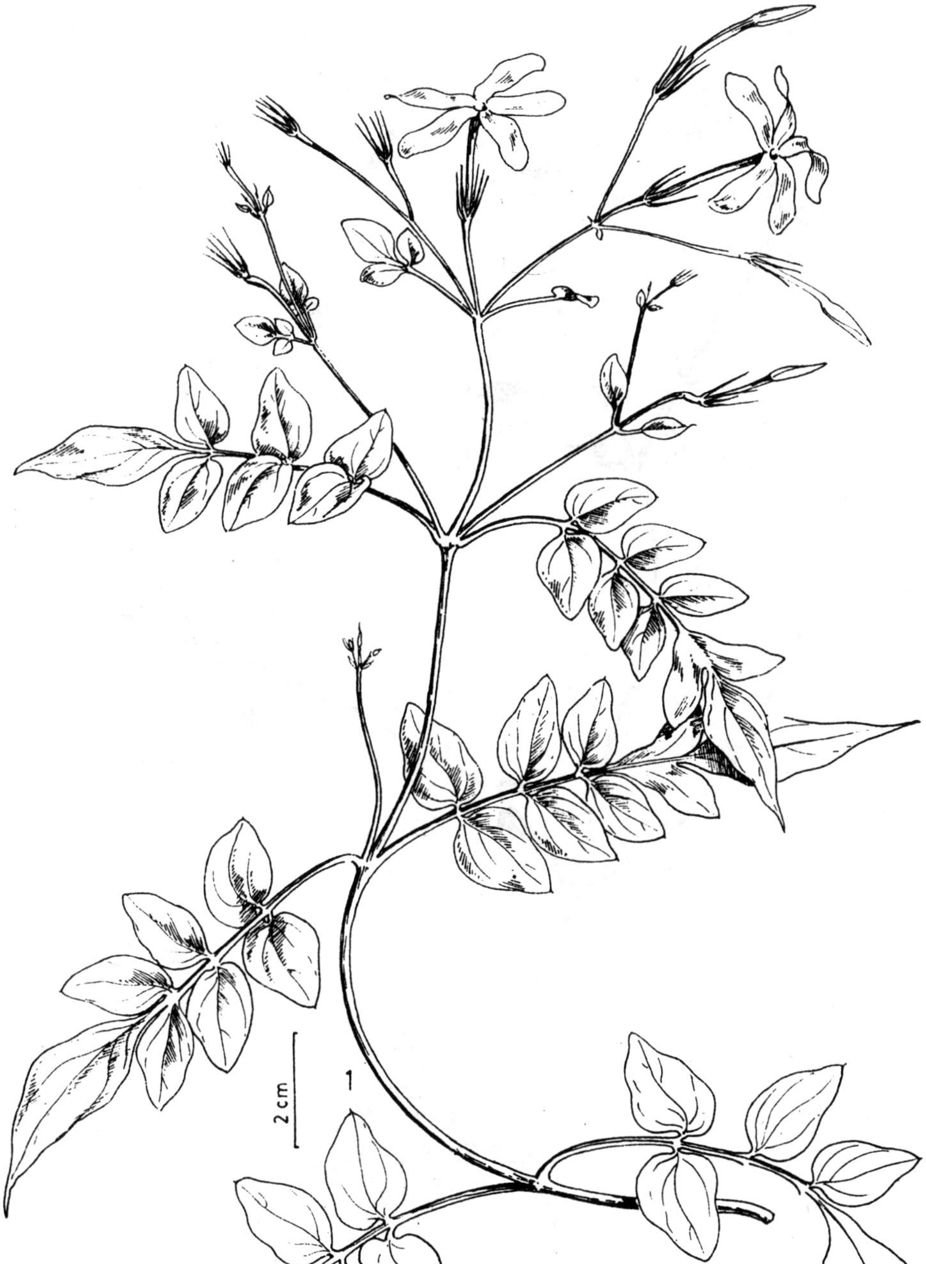

Figure 137: Jasminum grandiflorum L.

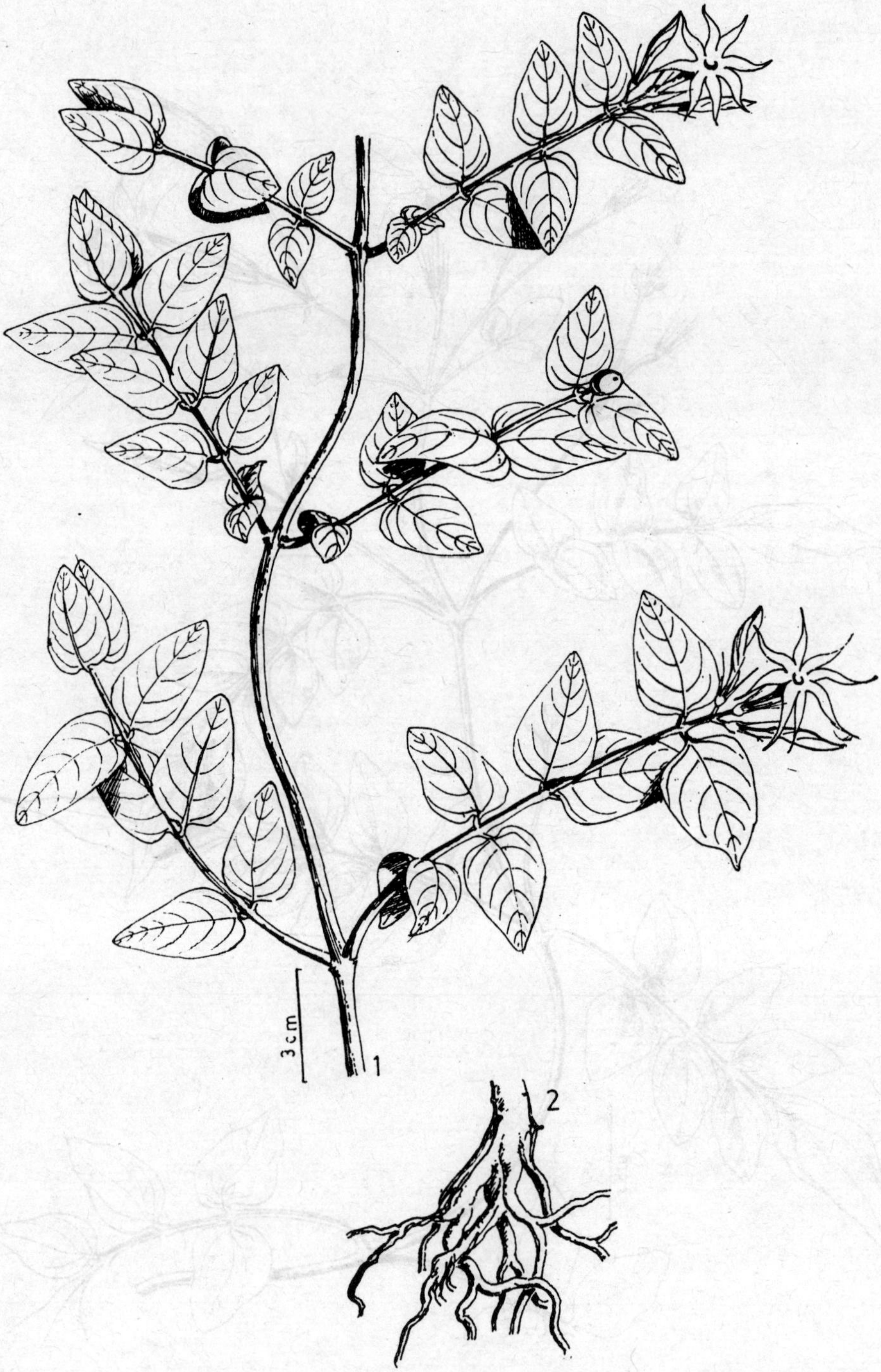

Figure 138: Jasminum angustifolium Vahl. 1, Habit; 2, Roots.

MAṆḌŪKAPARṆĪ (Mal. MUTTIḺ, KUṬAṄṄAL)

The etymology of the name *maṇḍūkaparṇī*, like that of many other names, is a matter of speculation. The literal meaning of the term i.e. plant having leaves resembling the shape of frogs (Aiyer & Kolammal, 1964. 8: 26) does not seem to make any sense. The name either owes to its occurance in wet or moist, shaded areas, preferred also by frogs (*maṇḍūka*) or because the drug has been brought into use by the sage *Maṇḍūka* (Sharma, 1983: 3).

Caraka includes this drug in his *Vayasthāpana varga*, the group of drugs that are capable of maintaining the youthful vigour and strength. *Maṇḍūkaparṇī* is also a *mēdhya* drug which improves the receptive and retentive capacity of mind. The whole plant is reported to be a nervine and cardiotonic, astringent and diuretic, capable of improving memory power, physical strength, voice, complexion and digestive power. The drug is also useful in dermatosis, anaemia, diabetes, cough, dyspnoea, emaciation and insanity. It dispels poisonous affections, splenic disorders and impurity of blood (Aiyer & Kolammal, 1964. 8: 26; Mooss, 1978: 68). The important formulations using the drug are *Valiya Ciñcādi tailaṃ, Brāhma rasāyanaṃ, Paphaṇādi tailaṃ, Paphaṇādi ghṛtaṃ*, etc.

The plant is described in the texts as one which bears solitary lamina on each stalk (*ēkaparṇī*) resembling the shape of an open umbrella (*chatrānuvartinī*) (Aiyer & Kolammal, 1964. 8: 26).

There is, however, some confusion with regard to the drugs *maṇḍūkaparṇī* and *brāhmī*. This may be due to the lack of description of the two drugs in the texts, attribution of similar properties to them (Chunekar, 1982: 462) and also application of the same synonyms. An analytical study of Āyurvēdic literature reveals that in the three great Āyurvēdic classics of *Caraka, Suśruta* and *Vāgbhata, brāhmī* and *maṇḍūkaparṇī* are always spoken of as two different drugs and are not held synonymous anywhere. The inclusion of both the drugs in one and the same formulation, *Aṣṭāṅga Ghṛta yōga* of *Aṣṭāṅgahridaya*, also shows that they are two independent drugs (Usman Ali, *et al.*, 1981).

Caraka holds that both the drugs are promoters of general mental ability *(mēdhya)* but, *brāhmī* is regarded superior to *maṇḍūkaparṇī* in that the former is specified in mental diseases like *unmāda, apasmāra*, etc., whereas the latter promotes general mental ability through its *rasāyana* effect.

Bhāvaprakāśa records that they are of different *rasa, brāhmī* of *tiktarasa* (bitter in taste) and *maṇḍūkaparṇī* of *kaṣāyarasa* (astringent). The phytochemical and pharmacological studies conducted on the two drugs also prove that they are two different plants i.e. *brāhmī* as *Bacopa monnieri* (Linn.) Pennel (Scrophulariaceae) and *maṇḍūkaparṇī* is *Centella asiatica* (Linn.) Urb. of Apiaceae (Usman Ali *et al.*, 1981).

Centella asiatica, known as *muttiḷ* or *kuṭaṅṅal* in the vernacular, is the accepted source of *maṇḍūkaparṇī* in Kerala. The same plant is reported to be used as *brāhmī* in North India. Kerala physicians use *Bacopa monnieri* as the source of *Brahmi* or *nīrbrahmi*, as it is called in Malayalam.

Rheede has described *Centella asiatica* under the name *codagen* (Hort. Malab. 10. 91. t. 46. 1690).

Centella asiatica (*Linn.*) *Urban* (Apiaceae) (Fig. 139)
Hydrocotyle asiatica Linn.

Stoloniferous, creeping herb, rooting at nodes; leaves simple, orbicular-reniform, base cordate with angular sinus, margin crenate-dentate, apex rotund, 2–4.5 × 3–6.5 cms, basally 5–7 nerved, petioles long, 2.5–25 cms, fascicled at the nodes; flowers small, brownish in axillary few-flowered umbels. Calyx truncate, fused with the ovary, 5-teethed; petals 5, minute, ovate-acute, red; stamens 5, epigynous, filaments incurved; ovary inferior, bicarpellary with a single ovule in each, styles 2, stigmas capitate; fruit of two, compressed prominently ridged mericarps.

Distribution: The plant is found in all plains districts in wet places, banks of streams and ponds, in the neighbourhood of rice fields, etc. It is distributed throughout the tropical and subtropical regions of India and throughout the world.

Note: *Centella asiatica* has been found to have considerable sedative action (Ramaswamy *et al.*, 1970; Agarwal, 1981). The drug showed significant improvement in cases of anxiety neurosis (Singh *et al.*, 1981) and peptic ulcer (Chao *et al.*, 1981). It has also been found to cure general debility (Rao *et al.*, 1973) and improve the faculty of memory in mentally retarded children (Sharma *et al.*, 1985).

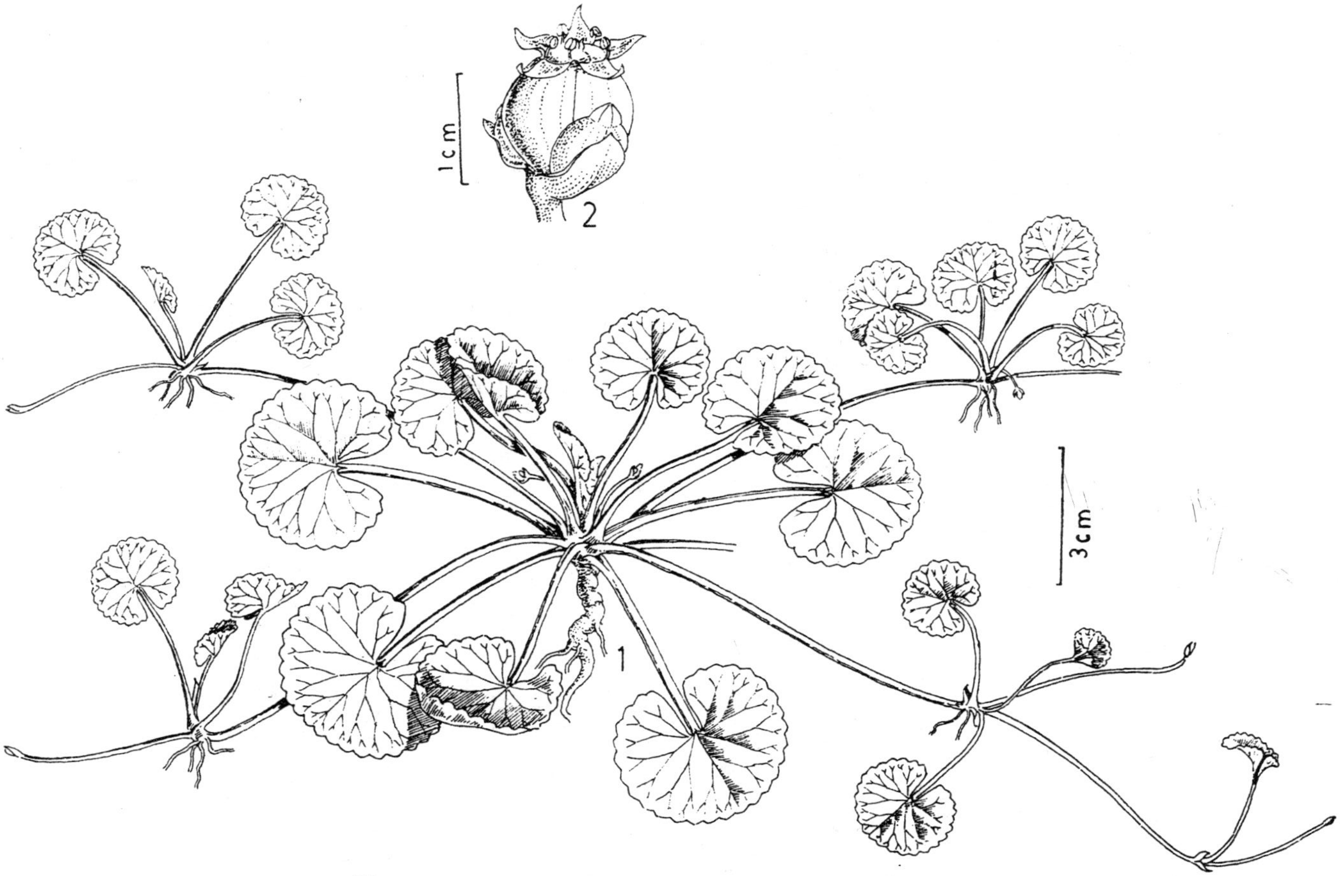

Figure 139: **Centella asiatica** (L.) Urb. 1, Habit; 2, Flower.

MAÑJIṢṬHĀ (Mal. MAÑJAṬṬI)

Mañjiṣṭhā is reputed as an efficient blood purifier and hence is extensively used against blood, skin and urinary diseases. It is alterative, antiseptic, astringent, bitter, pigment-stimulator and tonic. The drug is used in diseases of blood, dysentery, ear and eye diseases, ulcers, inflammation and swellings, poison, leprosy and other skin diseases and urinogenital disorders. It clears voice, improves complexion and cures hepatic obstruction, indigestion, jaundice and paralytic affections. Root is the officinal part. Root paste is a valuable application to freckles, external inflammations, ulcers and discolouration of the skin (Nadkarni, 1954: 1076; Kurup *et al.*, 1979: 140; Dey, 1980: 101). The important preparations using the drug are *Dhānvantarāriṣṭaṃ, Dhānvantaraṃ kuḻaṁbu, Mañjiṣṭhādi tailaṃ, Kalyāṇakaghṛtaṃ*, etc.

The source plant is described as an extensive climber (*samaṅgā*) having long jointed stem (*yōjanavallī*) and leaves which look like frogs (*maṇḍūkaparṇī*). The terms like *mañjiṣṭhā, bhāṇḍīri, bhāṇḍi*, etc. indicate the property of its root for imparting colour (Moosad, 1983: 334). This description agrees well with the plant *Rubia cordifolia* Linn. (Rubiaceae), known as *mañjaṭṭi* in vernacular, which is the accepted source of the drug throughout the country.

Rubia cordifolia *Linn.* **(Rubiaceae)** (Fig. 140)

Scabrous climber; stem 4-gonous; leaves whorld, ovate-acuminate, 10 × 4 cms, 5-nerved from base, scabrid, base rounded-cordate, margin entire; flowers small, greenish, in axillary and terminal cymes; calyx truncate, glabrous; corolla rotate to shortly campanulate, lobes 5, united in the middle into an inflated, short tube; stamens 5, exserted; ovary depressed globose with one ovule per cell, styles 2, stigmas capitate; drupe globose, fleshy, purplish.

Distribution: The plant is seen in the evergreen forests of peninsular India. Also reported from Greece, Africa and other Asiatic countries like China, Japan, Afghanisthan, Vietnam and Malesia.

Note: The anticancer activity of *Rubia cordifolia* has been studied by Adwankar *et al.* (1979) and Adwankar and Chitnis (1982). Antarkar *et al.* (1983) have proved the anti-inflammatory activity of the plant.

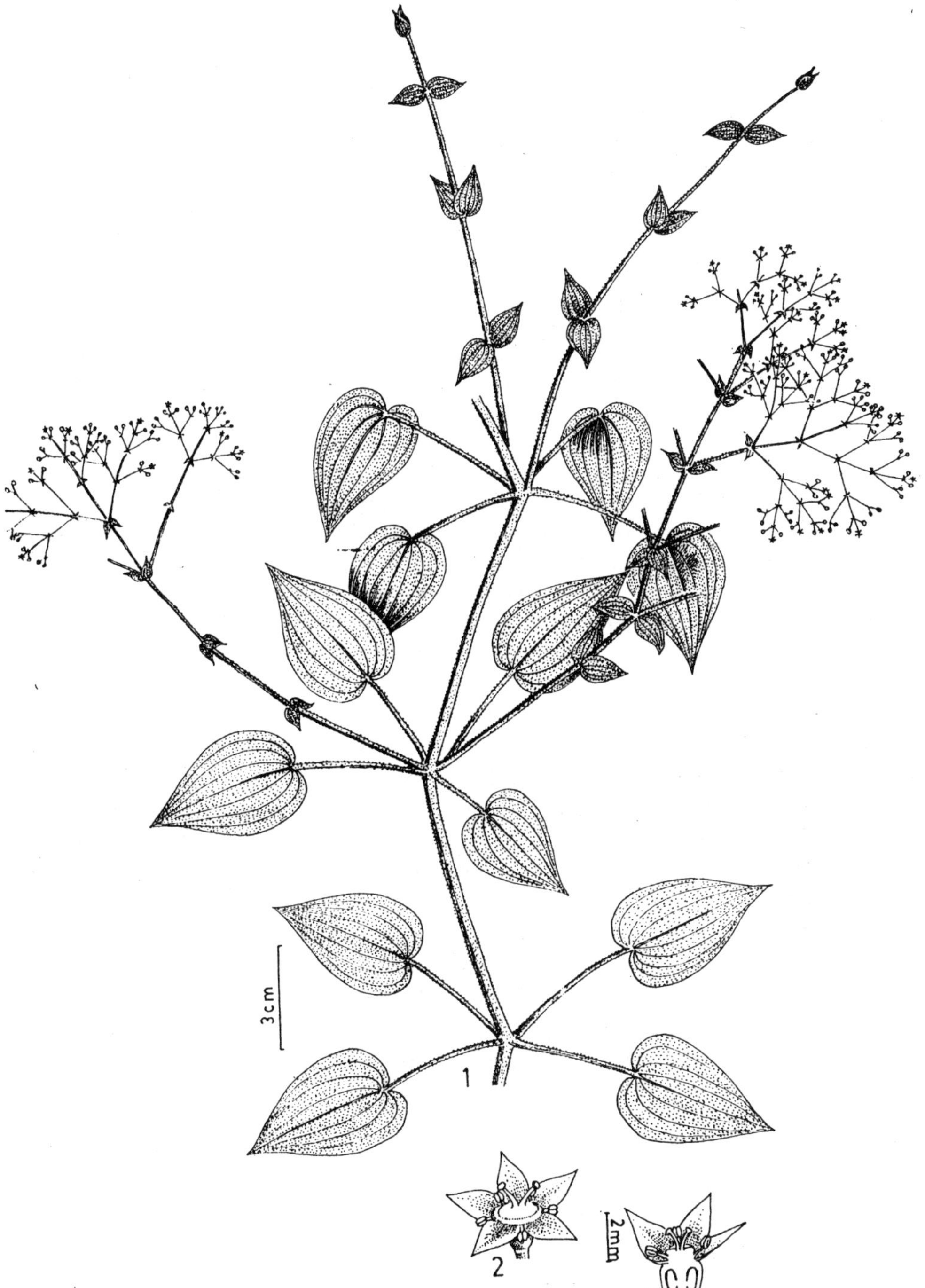

Figure 140: Rubia cordifolia L. 1, Habit; 2, Flower; 3, Flower L.S.

MARICAṂ (Mal. KURUMUḶAKU)

Maricam forms an ingredient of *trikaṭu*—the three spices, the other drugs being *pippali* and *śuṇṭhi.* The drug is acrid, bitter, hot, light, alterative, carminative, anthelmintic and appetizer. It increases the digestive power, improves appetite and cures cold, cough, dyspnoea, cardiac diseases, colic, worms, diabetes, piles and the diseases caused on account of the morbidity of *vāta, pitta* and *kapha.* It is also used in blood diseases, eczema, intermittent fevers, neurites, night blindness and dysentery. Fruits and roots are used in medicine (Aiyer & Kolammal, 1966. 9: 63; Kurup *et al.*, 1979: 143). The important formulations using the drug are *Daśamūlakaṭutrayādi kaṣāyam, Aṣṭacūrṇam, Amṛtāriṣṭam, Maricādi tailam, Daśamūlarasāyanam, Gulgulutiktaka ghṛtam*, etc.

The texts describe the plant as a creeper (*vallijam*), growing abundantly in Travancore (*dharmapaṭṭaṇam*)—The erstwhile Travancore had the name (*dharmarājya*) and which has spherical (*vṛttaphalam*), black (*kṛṣṇam, syāmam*) fruits in clusters *(kōlakam, kōlam).* The term *maricam* indicates the property of the drug to dispel poison (Aiyer & Kolammal, 1966. 9: 62).

Piper nigrum Linn. (Piperaceae), known as *kurumuḷaku* in vernacular, is the source of the drug throughout India (See also Rheede, Hort. Malab. 7: 23–24, t. 12. 1688).

Piper nigrum *Linn.* **(Piperaceae)** (Fig. 141)

Stout, woody, perennial climber, clinging to the support by several adventitious roots arising from the nodes; leaves simple, alternate, broadly ovate-acuminate, 10–20 × 6–9 cms, 7-nerved, entire, glabrous above, glaucous beneath; flowers minute, bisexual, in leaf-opposed, simple, pendulous slender spikes; bracteoles in a hood-like ridge, partly covering the pistil; stamens 2, filaments flat, anther-lobes widely separated, partly embedded in fleshy filament; ovary globose-ovoid; berry ovoid-globose, 4 × 3.5 mm.

Distribution: Widely cultivated in various parts of India from Konkan southwards, especially N. Canara and Kerala. Also reported from Sri Lanka.

Note: Piperine from *Piper nigrum* has been found to have diverse pharmacological activities like CNS depressent activity and antipyretic, analgesic and anti-inflammatory activities Lee *et al.* (1984).

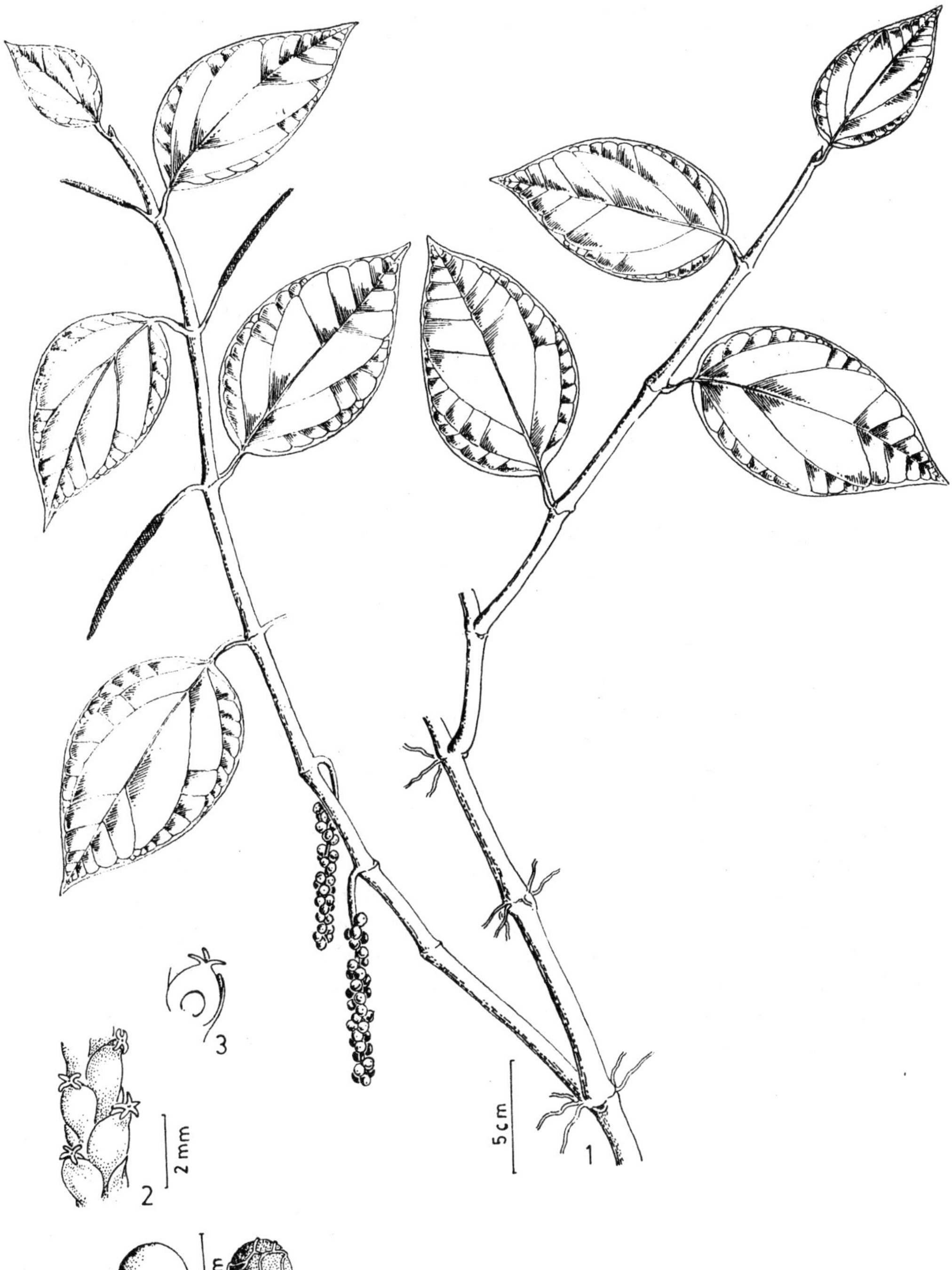

Figure 141: **Piper nigrum** L. 1, Habit; 2, portion of spike enlarged; 3, Flower L.S.; 4–5, Fruits.

MĀṢAPAṚṆĪ (Mal. KĀṬṬUḶUNNU)

Māṣaparṇī and *mudgaparṇī* together form what is called *sūpyaparṇī-dvayaṃ*. These two drugs are important ingredients of the *Jīvanīyagaṇa*, the group of rejuvenating drugs. *Māṣaparṇī* is bitter, cold, sweet on digestion, constipating, roborant, aphrodisiac and cures diseases caused by the vitiation of *vāta* and *pitta*, cough, emaciation, pyrexia and haemetemesis. It relieves pain in wounds on account of impure blood, promotes lymphatic circulation, increases bodily strength, colour of the skin, breast milk and hair growth. (Aiyer & Kolammal, 1963. 7: 69). The root is used in the preparations like *Dhānvantaraṃ kaṣāyaṃ, Dhānvantarāriṣṭaṃ, Balātailaṃ, Cyavanaprāśa lēhaṃ, Vidāryādyāsavaṃ*, etc.

According to the synonymy, the plant is a common (*sulabhā*) perennial (*ātmōtbhavā, svayambhūḥ*) creeper (*sāriṇī*) covered with whitish hairs (*pāṇḍu, pāṇḍulōmaśā*). The plant has tough roots (*vajṛamūlī*), dark coloured stem (*kṛṣṇavṛntā*) and hairy leaves (*lōmaśaparṇī*) which resemble the leaves of *māṣa* or blackgram i.e. *Phaseolus mungo* Linn. (*māṣaparṇī, māṣapatṛikā*). The term *mahāsahā* refers to its capacity to withstand severe adverse conditions or it may indicate the property of the drug to give necessary strength or vigour to withstand the evil effects of vitiated *dōṣās*, thus bestowing happiness to the consumer (*maṅgalyā, kalyāṇī*) (cf. Aiyer & Kolammal, 1963. 7: 69).

There is considerable controversy regarding the botanical source of *māṣaparṇī* which is called *kāṭṭuḷunnu* in vernacular. Most of the authors equate the drug with *Teramnus labialis* Spr. of Papilionaceae (See Kirtikar & Basu, 1918: 435; Vaidya, 1936: 444; Nadkarni, 1954: 1198; Chopra *et al.*, 1956: 241; Chunekar, 1982: 297; Sharma, 1983: 747). *Atylosia goensis* Dalz. (Papilionaceae) is equated with the drug by some other experts on Indian materia medica (See Nadkarni, 1954: 161; Chopra *et al.*, 1956: 31). But in Kerala, though these plants are available, they are seldom used as *māṣaparṇī*. Different species of the genus *Vigna*, viz. *Vigna radiata* var. *sublobata, Vigna dalzelliana, Vigna mungo, V. umbellata* and *Rhyncosia nummularia*, all belonging to Papilionaceae, are the ones used here. According to Rheede, *Vigna mungo* (Linn.) Hepper is the source of *Katu-ulunnu* (Hort. Malab. 8: 95, t. 50. 1688).

The various plant sources can be identified as follows:

Vigna radiata (*Linn.*) *Willczek. var.* **sublobata** (*Roxb.*) *Verdc.* **(Papilionaceae)**
Phaseolus sublobatus Roxb. (Fig. 142)

Diffuse or twining herb; branchlets hispid; leaves alternate, stipulate, stipules ovate-oblong, acute, hairy, 8 × 5 mm; petiolate, petiole clothed with reddish brown hairs, trifoliolate, leaflets broadly ovate-acute, 5.5 × 5 cm, tomentose on either side, terminal leaflet sometimes 3-lobed, laterals inequilateral; flowers yellow on very short pedicels borne on long peduncled, axillary, few-flowered short racemes; calyx campanulate; corolla papilionaceous; stamens diadelphous; ovary subsessile, many

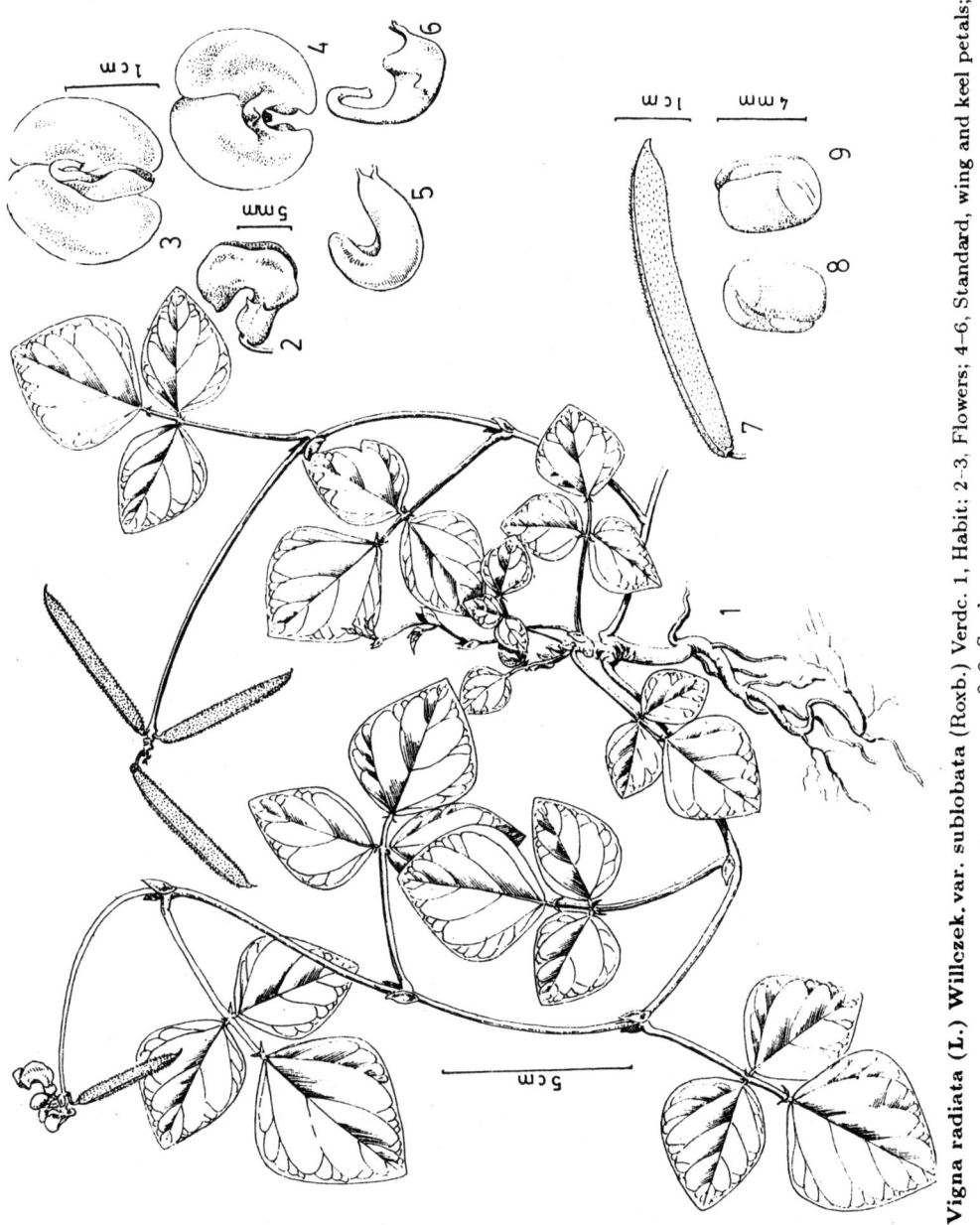

Figure 142: Vigna radiata (L.) Willczek. var. sublobata (Roxb.) Verdc. 1, Habit; 2–3, Flowers; 4–6, Standard, wing and keel petals; 7, Pod; 8–9, Seeds.

ovuled, style long, bearded down the side below the very oblique stigma; fruit a cylindric pod, hairy.

Distribution: Most parts of India, a weed on roadsides and waste lands.

Vigna dalzelliana (*O. Kze.*) *Verdc.* **(Papilionaceae)**
Phaseolus dalzelli T. Cooke
P. pauciflorus Dalz.

Herbaceous twiner; leaves alternate, long-petioled, petiole 4 cm long, 3-foliate, leaflets ovate or rhomboid-ovate, acute or shortly acuminate, margin entire, sparsely hairy on both surfaces, 2.5–6 × 2–5 cm, laterals inequilateral; flowers short-pedicelled, yellow, in axillary, long-peduncled, 2–3 flowered capitate racemes; calyx gamosepalous, campanulate; corolla papilionaceous; stamens diadelphous; ovary subsessile, many ovuled, style located within the beak of the keels and bearded down the side below the stigma which is very oblique; fruit a linear, subcylindric, slightly recurved, two valved pod, 3–6 cm long and 2 mm thick.

Distribution: Western Ghats, in the Nilgiris and Pulney hills at about, 3,000 ft.

Vigna umbellata (*Thunb.*) *Ohwi* & *Ohashi* **(Papilionaceae)**
Phaseolus calcaratus Roxb.
Slender, hairy climber, very similar to earlier species; stem clothed with stiff deflexed hairs, stipules lanceolate, hispid, leaflets broadly ovate, 5–10 cms long, scarsely lobed, acuminate; flowers yellow; pods more or less compressed.

Distribution: W. Ghats, in the Nilgris, Pulney and Travancore Hills, upto 7,000 ft.

Vigna mungo (*Linn.*) *Hepper* **(Papilionaceae)** (Fig. 143)
Phaseolus mungo Linn.

Erect herb, branchlets strigose; leaves 3-foliolate, leaflets not lobed, oblong-lanceolate or ovate, subacute, terminal one 7 × 4 cm, laterals smaller, scattered strigose; inflorescence axillary or leaf opposed; pod to 5 × 0.6 cms, with stiff-elongate hairs; seeds black.

Distribution: Native of India, cultivated in tropics in Africa, Asia.

Rhyncosia nummularia (*Linn.*) *DC.* **(Papilionaceae)**
Nomismia nummularia W. & A.
Trailing herbs; leaves 3-foliolate, leaflets broadly ovate-cuneate, obtuse, the terminal one truncate or emarginate; flowers small in elongate racemes; calyx lobes linear, the lowest the longest; pod 1-seeded, orbicular, with few branching transverse veins.

Distribution: Carnatic, Tinnevelly, also Shevaroy Hills of Salem.

Teramnus labialis (*L.f.*) *Spreng.* **(Papilionaceae)** (Fig. 144)
Glycine labialis L.f.

Extensively spreading, perennial, shrubby twiner; stem short, woody, young branches slightly hairy; leaves alternate, pinnately trifoliolate, long-petioled, petioles 1–2 to 3.8 cm long, hairy and channelled above; leaflets ovate or ovate-oblong, entire, acute or subobtuse, 5 × 2.3 cm, nearly glabrous above, sparingly hairy below; flowers small, pinkish on slender axillary peduncled racemes; calyx gamosepalous, campanulate with short white silky hairs outside; corolla papilionaceous; stamens 10, monadelphous; ovary sessile, many ovuled with a short, thick, curved, beardless style ending in a capitate stigma; fruit narrow, linear, cylindric or slightly flattened, 2-valved pod, hairy when young but glabrous when ripe.

Distribution: Pantropical Peninsular India. Also reported from Sri Lanka, Bangladesh, Burma, Penang, Thailand, Indo-china, Vietnam, Indonesia, Philippines, New Guinea, Miconesia and Madagascar.

Atylosia goensis *Dalz.* **(Papilionaceae)**
Atylosia barbata (Benth.) Baker.

Twiners with stem and branches densely clothed with greyish hairs when young; leaves alternate, pinnately 3-foliate, stipulate; leaflets deltoid to roundish ovate, shortly acuminate, 7.5 to 10 cms long, thinly pubescent, greyish green above, paler beneath with scattered reddish-brown resinous glands; flowers yellow, streaked with purple on long-peduncled, densely pilose, axillary racemes; calyx gamosepalous, tube campanulate, slightly 2-lipped, 5 toothed; corolla papilionaceous, slightly exserted; stamens 10, diadelphous, filaments unequal; ovary sessile, style filiform, incurved, hairy below, stigma capitate; fruit a straight, oblong, few seeded pod, densely clothed with grey hairs.

Distribution: W. Ghats, from S. Canara to Travancore, at low elevation and upto 3,500 ft.

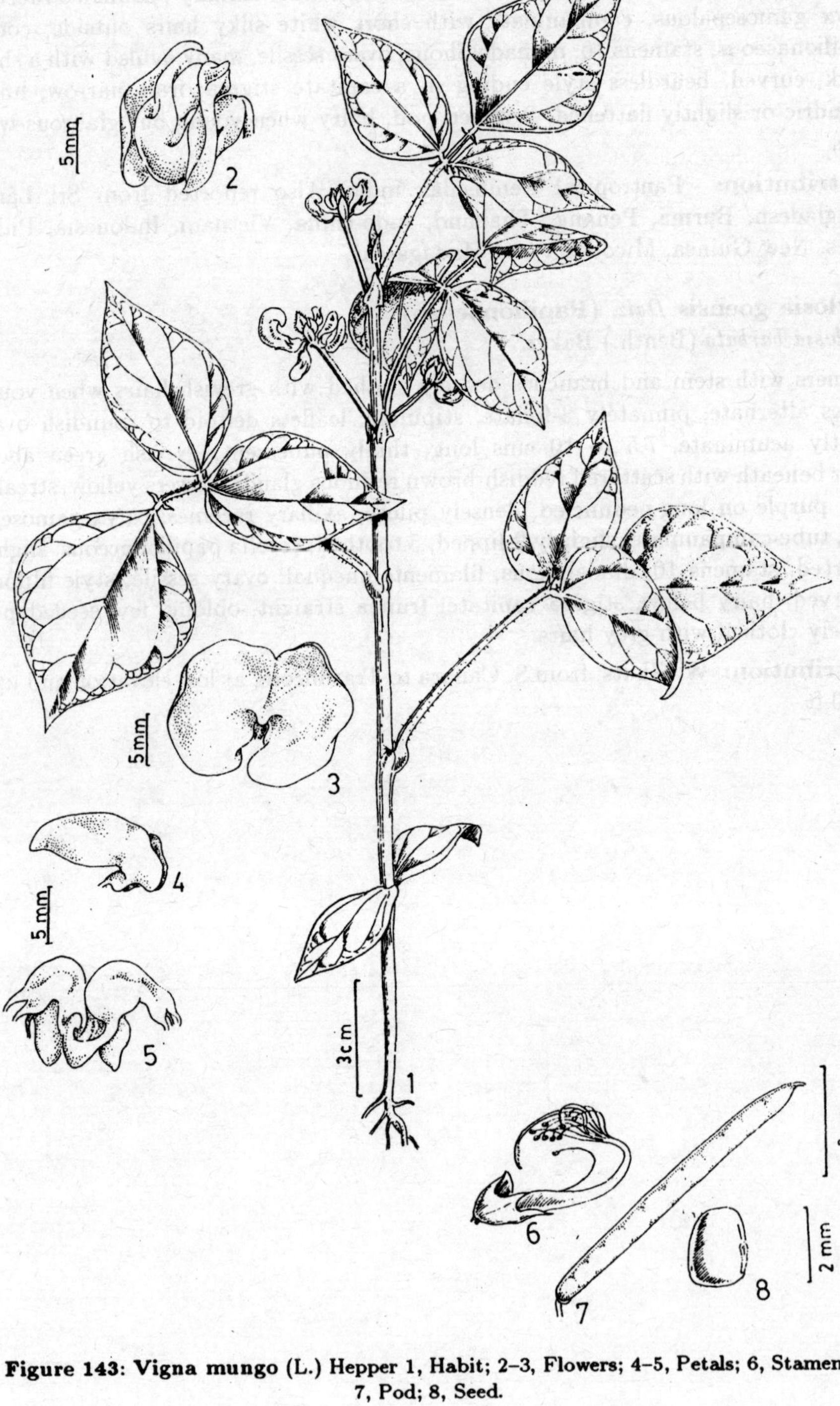

Figure 143: Vigna mungo (L.) Hepper 1, Habit; 2–3, Flowers; 4–5, Petals; 6, Stamens; 7, Pod; 8, Seed.

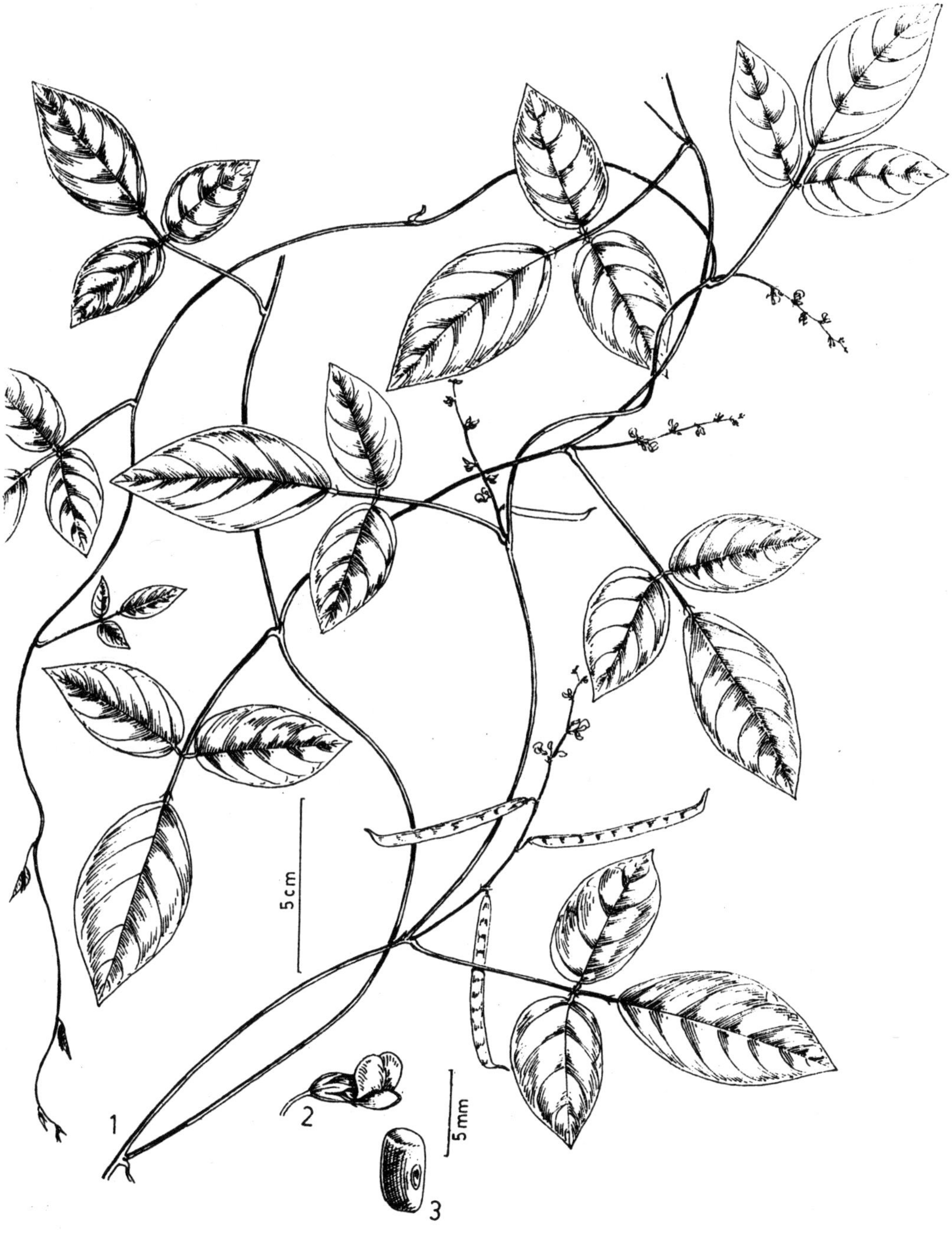

Figure 144: **Teramnus labialis** (L.f.) Spreng. 1, Habit; 2, Flower; 3, Seed.

MĀTULUṄGAḤ (Mal. GAṆAPATINĀRAKAṂ)

The drug is reported to be light, cooling, digestive, carminative, anthelmintic, stomachic, tonic and is useful in asthma, bilious vomiting, blood purification, cold, cough, fever, dyspepsia, thirst, hiccough, lumbago and sciatica. It overcomes diseases due to the morbidity of the three *dōṣās*, flatulence, piles, dysentery, diarrhoea, cardiac disorders, blood disease (*raktapitta*) and menstrual disorders. Application of the leaves reduces pains. Seed paste is used in swellings, skin disease and scorpion bites. (Dey, 1980: 104; Sharma, 1983: 344). The drug enters into the composition of preparations like *Pūtīkarañjāsavaṃ, Tēḷviṣaparihāriguḷika, Kṣārataīlaṃ, Ārdrakaghṛtaṃ, Sūraṇādi lēhaṃ*, etc.

According to the synonymy, the plant sets profuse fruits (*phalapūraḥ*) which have many seeds (*bījapūraḥ*). (Moosad, 1983: 327).

Most of the authors equate the drug with *Citrus medica* Linn. of Rutaceae. (Kirtikar & Basu, 1918: 265; Nadkarni, 1954: 348; Kapoor & Mitra, 1979: 74; Dey, 1980: 103; Chunekar, 1982: 593; Sharma, 1983; 343). This plant, locally called *gaṇapatinārakaṃ*, is being used as the drug source in Kerala.

Citrus medica *Linn.* **(Rutaceae)** (Fig. 145)

Small trees; leaves unifoliolate, elliptic-oblong, obtuse, crenate, petiole narrowly winged; flowers white in axillary cymes; calyx white, cupular, 5-lobed; corolla 5, linear oblong, thick, gland-dotted; stamens numerous, inserted round an annular disc, filaments irregularly polyadelphous, anthers oblong; ovary many-celled, style stout, stigma capitate; fruit a large ovoid berry, conspicuously warted.

Distribution: The plant is often cultivated.

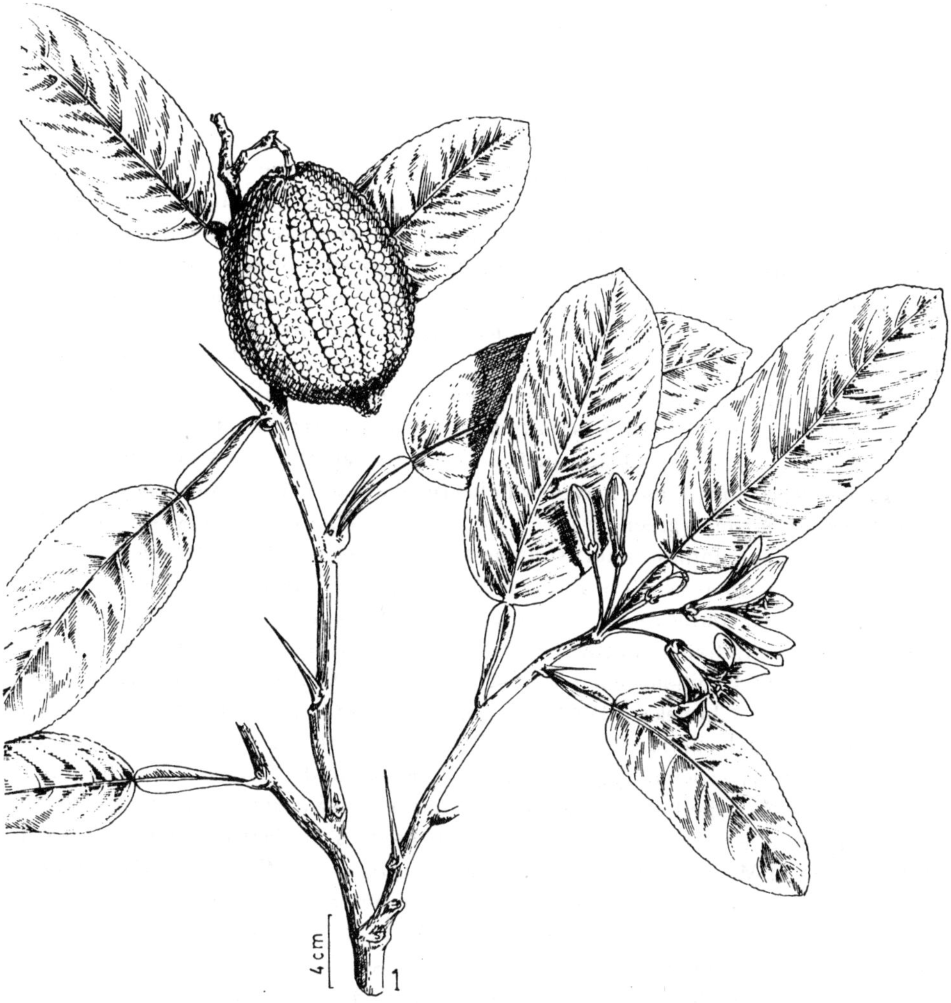

Figure 145: Citrus medica L.

MUDGAPARṆĪ (Mal. KĀṬṬUPAYAṚ)

Mudgaparṇī is often used along with *māṣaparṇī*, the two together known as *sūpyaparṇīdvayaṃ* and forms an important ingredient of the *Jīvanīyagaṇa* or the group of rejuvenating drugs that are indicated in general debility. *Mudgaparṇī* is bitter, cold, light, germicidal and aphrodisiac. It arrests bleeding from wounds, cures eye diseases, consumption, swelling, indigestion, piles, diarrhoea, cough, rheumatism, fever, burning sensation and is effective in all diseases caused by the discordance of *vāta, pitta* and *kapha* (Aiyer and Kolammal, 1963. 7: 81). Roots and sometimes the whole plant are used in medicine. The drug enters into the composition of preparations like *Dhānvantaraṃ kuḻambu, Vidāryādi lēhaṃ, Mahākalyāṇakaghṛtaṃ, Mahāmāṣatailaṃ, Amṛtaprāśa ghṛtaṃ*, etc.

According to the description in the texts, the plant thrives on semi-dry areas (*kākamudgā*) and it has leaves which are black in colour (*kākaparṇī*) resembling those of *mudga* (green gram, *Vigna radiata* (Linn.) Wilczek var. *radiata*) (*mudgaparṇī*). The names *śiṁbī, śiṁbiparṇikā* etc. refer to the resemblence of the leaves to that of *śiṃbī* which is *Dolichos lablab* (Aiyer & Kolammal, 1963. 7: 81).

There is much confusion with regard to the botanical identity of the drug. Most of the books on Indian materia medica equate the drug with *Phaseolus trilobus* Ait. belonging to Papilionaceae (Vaidya, 1936: 447; Nadkarni, 1954: 942; Chopra *et al.*, 1956: 190; Chunekar, 1982: 297; Sharma, 1983: 745) Monier Williams in his Sanskrit-English dictionary equates *P. trilobus* with *kākaparṇī* and *sūrpaparṇī* which are synonyms of *mudgaparṇī* (Aiyer & Kolammal, 1963: 7: 90). The plant, though available in the Cape Comerin area and in other parts of the Madras State, is not very common in Kerala and is seldom used as *mudgaparṇī* here. Nadkarni (1954: 938) and Mooss (1980: 27, 29) equate *Vigna adenantha (Phaseolus adenanthus* G.F. Meyer) with *mudgaparṇī.* Rheede also describes and portrays this plant as the source of *Katu-paeru* (Hort. Malab.8: 79–81, t. 42. 1688). In practice, *Centrosema pubescens* and different species of *Vigna* like *Vigna pilosa, Vigna angularis, V. umbellata, V. vexillata* and *V. adenantha* are used as the source of the drug. The important distinguishing features of the various plant sources are described below.

Centrosema pubescens *Benth.* **(Papilionaceae)** (Fig. 146)

Climber, branchlets pubescent; leaves 3-foliolate, leaflets ovate-lanceolate, 4.9 × 1.5–5 cm, thin-coriaceous, pubescent, base obtuse, margin entire, apex acuminate, mucronate; stipules persistent; flowers pink in axillary racemes; calyx-tube campanulate, glabrous, lobes unequal; corolla exserted, papilionaceous; pod oblong, compressed, 4-ribbed, glabrescent.

Distribution: A native of tropical America, now widely cultivated and often naturalised.

Distribution: The plant is found in W. Ghats, in the S. Canara, Nilgiri and Pulney Hills, upto 7,000 ft.

Vigna angularis (*Willd.*) *Ohwi & Ohashi*
Phaseolus angularis Willd.

Some authors have identified this as *V. angularis* but it is known from cultivation only in China and Japan. So this must be a wrong identification.

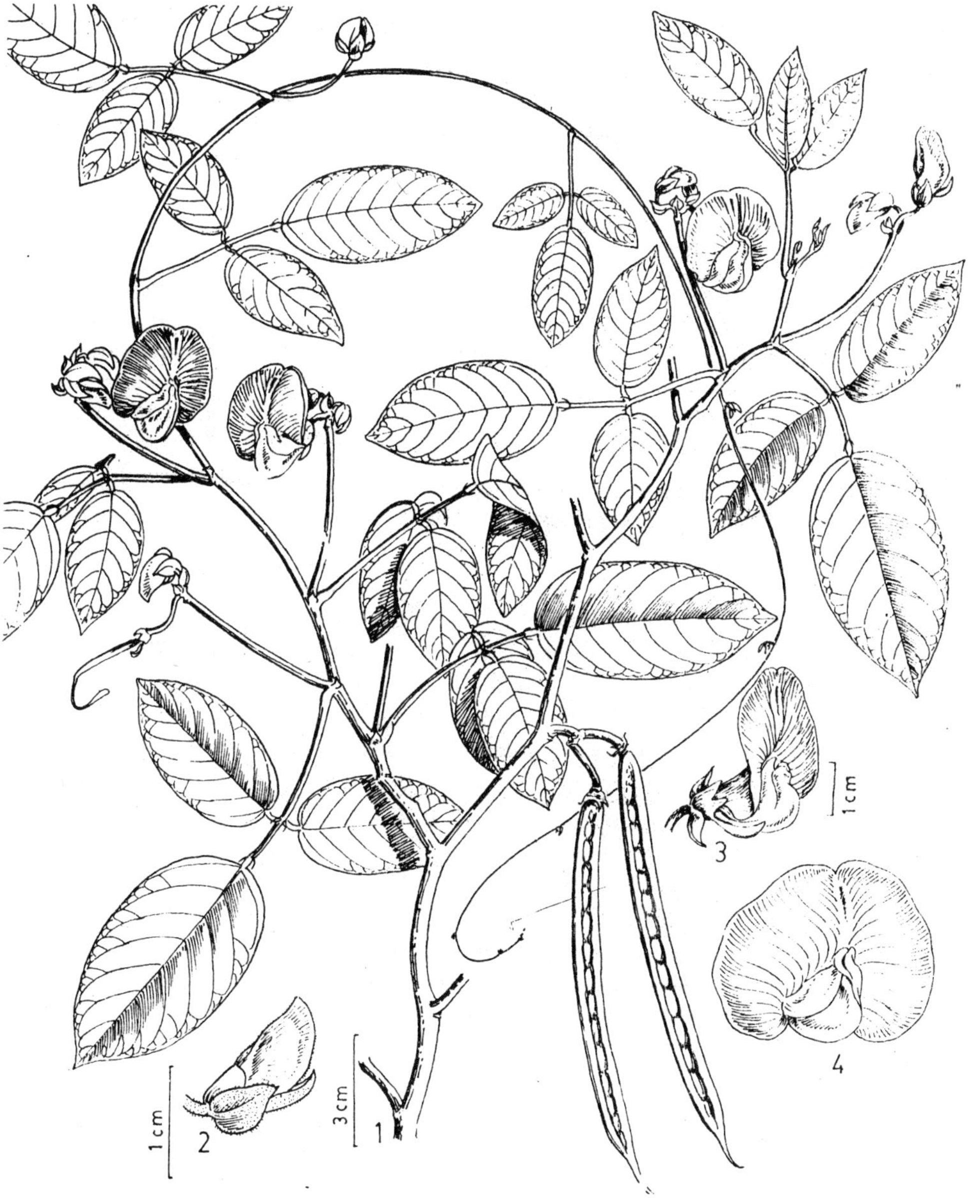

Figure 146: Centrosema pubescens Benth. 1, Habit; 2–3, Flowers; 4, Flower front view.

Vigna trilobata (*Linn.*) *Verdcourt* **(Papilionaceae)** (Fig. 147)
Phaseolus trilobus Ait.

Twining, hispid herb; leaves alternate, trifoliolate, long-petioled, petioles longer than the leaflets and channeled; leaflets small, ovate or rhomboid 2.5 to 5 cm, long, membraneous, glabrous, shallowly or deeply lobed; flowers yellow, short pedicelled, borne in pairs in 4 to 8 flowered, closely compressed racemes at the ends of long slender axillary peduncles; calyx gamosepalous, campanulate, pale yellow; corolla papilionaceous, exserted; stamens 10, diadelphous; ovary sessile, many-ovuled, style filiform, stigma oblique; fruit a linear subcylindrical, glabrous, recurved pod, more or less distinctly septate.

Distribution: The plant is found wild throughout India from the Himalayas to Cape Comerin but chiefly in Bengal, Deccan and Coromandal. It grows in all plains districts on fallow lands, waste places, river banks and the seacoast.

Vigna adenantha (*Meyer*) *Marechal* **(Papilionaceae)**
Phaseolus adenanthus G.F. Meyer

Subglabrous, twining shrub with a long tuberous tap root and semiwoody stem; leaves alternate, trifoliate; leaflets entire, ovate, subacute, 7.5 to 10 cm long with subulate stipels; flowers large and showy, rose-purple in a few-flowered axillary racemes; calyx gamosepalous, campanulate; corolla papilionaceous; stamens 10, diadelphous; ovary sessile, many ovuled, style bearded down the side below the oblique stigma; fruit a linear, flat, slightly curved, pendulous pod, 10 to 15 cm long.

Distribution: The plant is found throughout the plains districts of India, chiefly in Bengal, Konkan, Circars, Kerala, etc. It grows scrambling over hedges or twining on small trees.

Vigna pilosa *Baker* **(Papilionaceae)** (Fig. 148)

Slender, hairy twiner; stem short, densely covered with soft, whitish hairs; leaves alternate, pinnately trifoliolate; leaflets large, ovate-acute, 5 to 10 cm long × 2.5–4 cm broad, with a few, short, adpressed hairs; flowers many, blue, borne in fascicles at the distal end of axillary racemose peduncles; calyx campanulate, thinly silky; corolla papilionaceous, exserted; stamens 10, diadelphous; ovary sessile, many ovuled, style filiform, longitudinally bearded on the inner face and ending in a very oblique stigma; fruit a pendulous, linear, subterete pod, densely brown villous, septate between the seeds; seeds reniform, dark brown.

Distribution: The plant is found in most parts of tropical India. It has been recorded as occuring in Assam, Bengal, Orissa, S. Canara and in the Western Peninsula. It grows at low altitudes in evergreen, semievergreen and deciduous forests.

This is the most commonly accepted botanical source of *mudgaparṇī* in Kerala.

Vigna vexillata (*Linn.*) *A. Rich* **(Papilionaceae)** (Fig. 149)

Pretty climber, leaves 3-foliolate, leaflets small, ovate or lanceolate, acute; flowers reddish purple, in racemes at the end of axillary peduncle; calyx strigosely hirsute, teeth subequal, as long as the tube; petals long-clawed; pod linear, septate between the seeds, hairy when young, glabrous later.

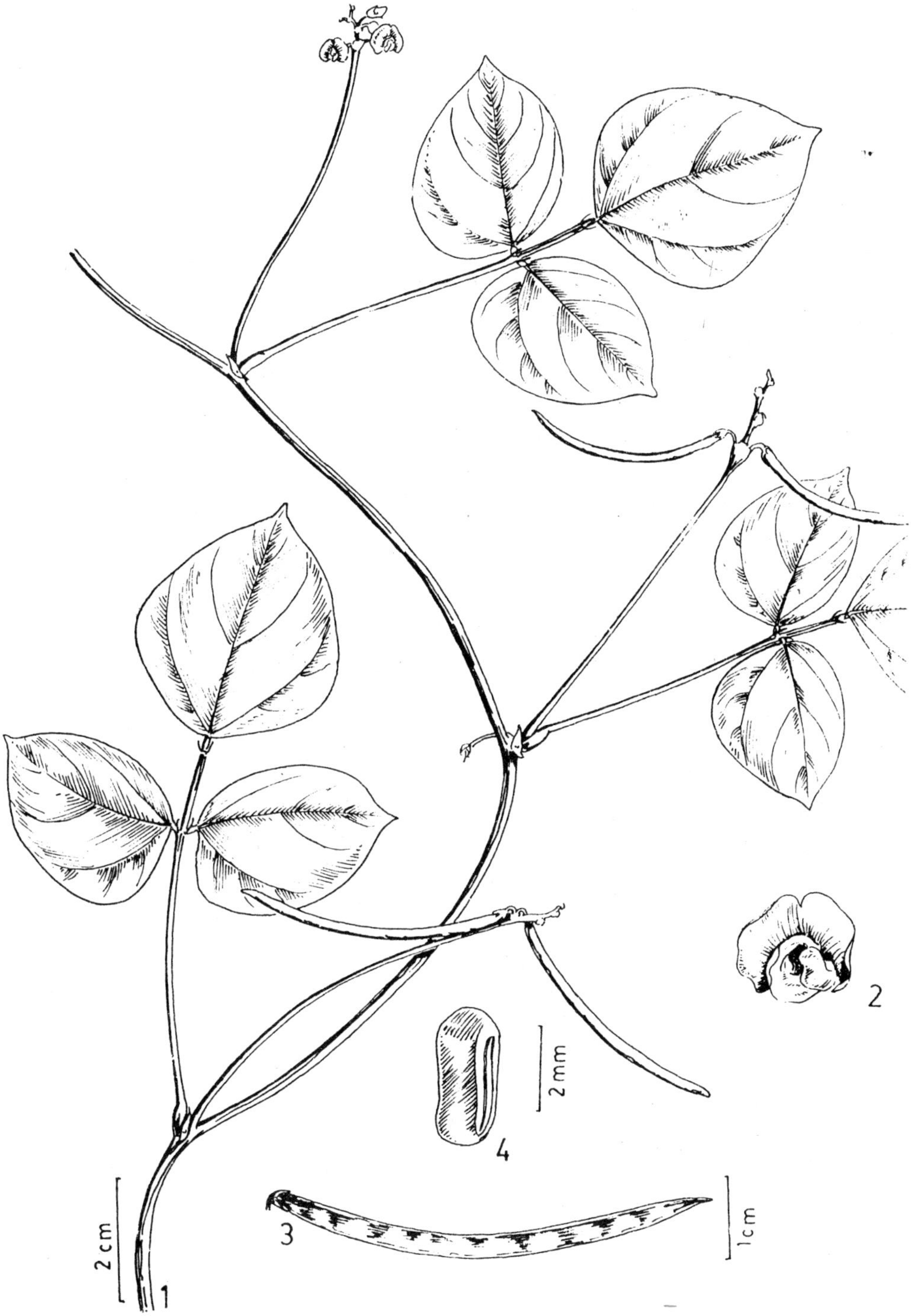

Figure 147: **Vigna trilobata** (L.) Verdc. 1, Habit; 2, Flower; 3, Pod; 4, Seed.

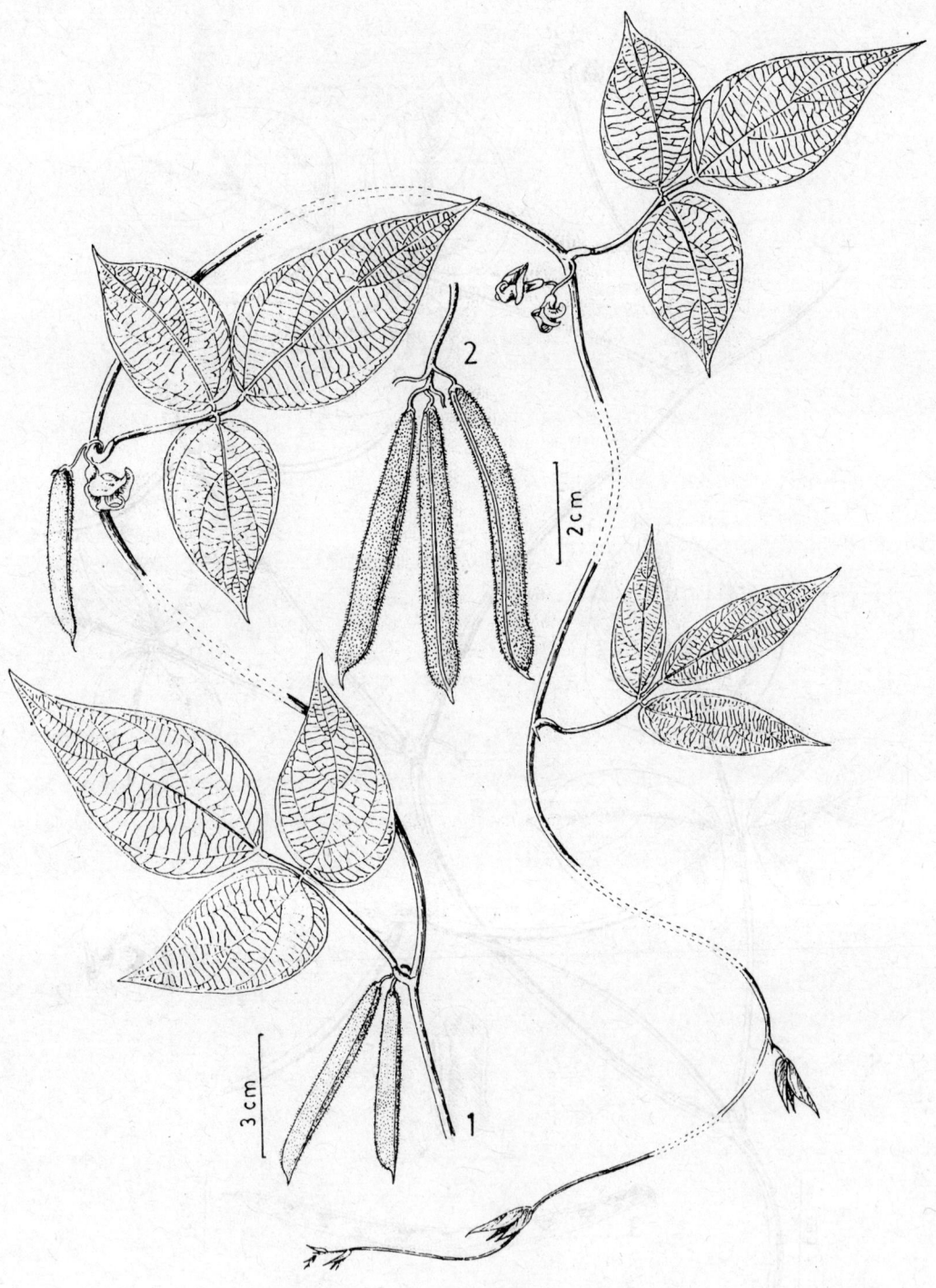

Figure 148: Vigna pilosa Baker. 1, Habit; 2, Pods.

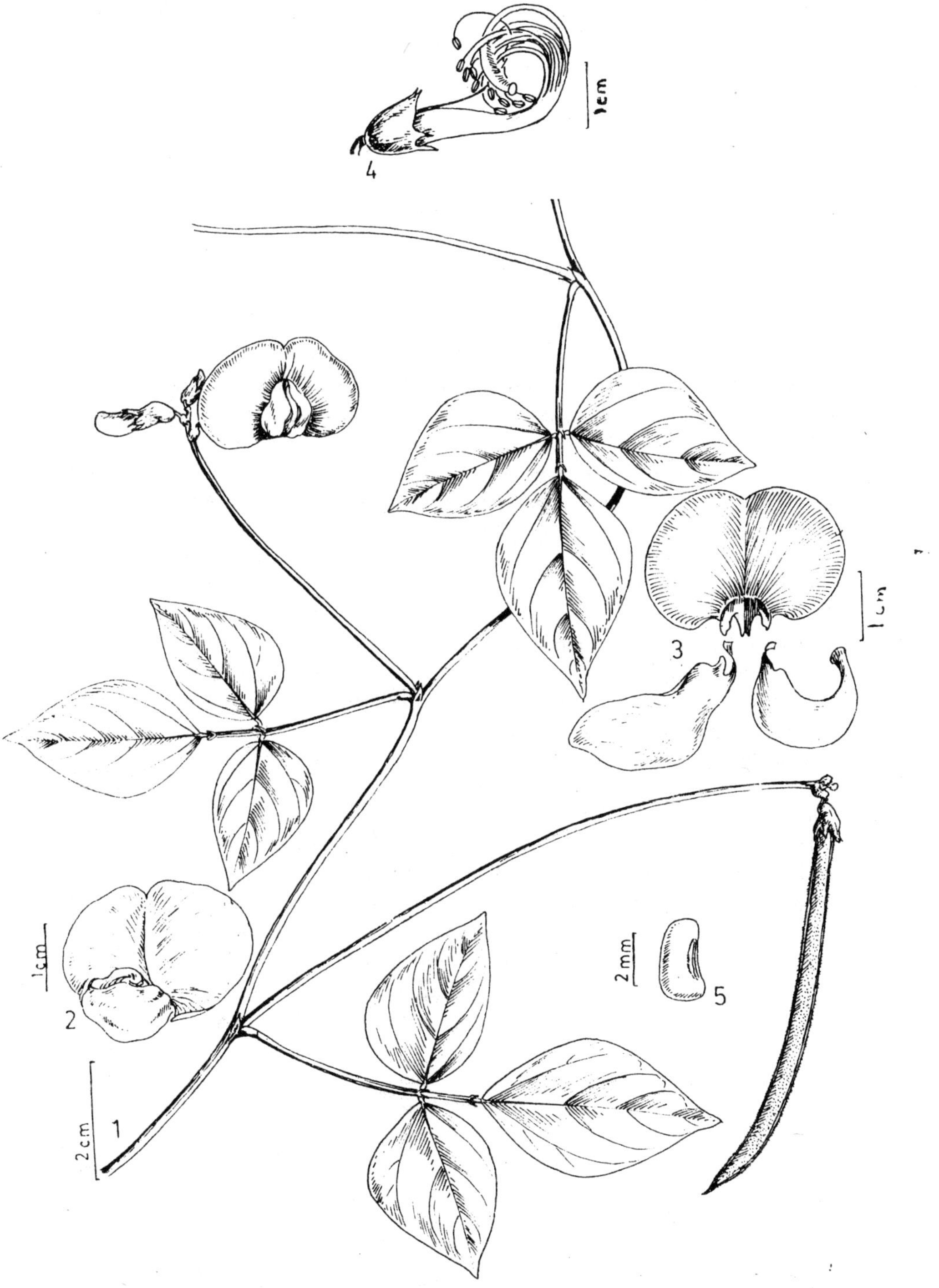

Figure 149: Vigna vexillata (L.) A. Rich. 1, Habit; 2, Flower; 3, Petals; 4, Stamens; 5, Seed.

MŪṚVĀ (Mal. PERUṀKURUṀBA)

Mūṛvā is one of the twenty two drugs that constitute the emetic group, *Madanādi gaṇa*. It is reported to be bitter, heavy of digestion, laxative and useful in urinary, heart and skin diseases and intermittent fevers. It controls morbid *kapha* and *vāta*, cures vomiting and purifies blood (Kolammal, 1978. 2: 1). Root, which is the officinal part, is an ingredient of preparations like *Ayaskṛti, Varaṇādi kaṣāyaṃ, Yōgarājaguggulu, Ceriya Lākṣādi tailaṃ*, etc.

Important synonyms attributed to the drug indicate that it is a climber (*mūṛvā, mōraṭā*) having a characteristic exudate (*sṛavā, sṛuvā*), an easily separable bark (*pṛthaktvacā*) and leaves resembling cow's ears (*gōkaṛṇī*). The plant is highly fibrous and is useful in making bow strings (*dhanuṛmālā, dhanuṛguṇā*) (cf. Kolammal, 1978. 2: 1; Moosad, 1983: 329–330). Despite this information, the identity of the actual plant source of this drug has been highly controversial. It has been equated with *Clematis triloba* (Ranunculaceae), *Maerua oblongifolia* (Capparaceae), *Bauhinia vahli* (Caesalpiniaceae), *Marsdenia tenacissima* (Asclepiadaceae), *Chonemorpha fragrans* (Apocynaceae), *Argyreia nervosa* (Convolvulaceae) and species of *Sansevieria* (Agavaceae), even though none of these fully tallys with the character indications implicit in the synonyms. In any case, practitioners in Kerala have not accepted the first four plants as the source of this drug, nor is there any mention of these four in Rheede's *magnum opus*. Rheede, however, has described the other three plants mentioned above but under different vernacular names, among which the name *peruṁkuruṁba*, currently widely used in the Āyurvēdic parlance, does not figure anywhere.

Literature has it that Bengali Kavirajas accept *Sansevieria roxburghiana* as the source of *mūṛvā* which they locally call *sūcīmukhī mūṛvā*. Rheede's work (Hort. Malab. 11: 83, t. 42. 1692) bears testimony for the fact that it was used by Kerala physicians as the drug source called *'Katukapel'* or *'Cadenaco'*. However, this plant is neither a climber nor has any exudate as has been implied in the synonymy.

Āyurvēdic formulary of India (Anonymous, 1978a: 254) accepted *Marsdenia tenacissima* as the source of *mūṛvā* and this has been followed by many authors (Mooss, 1980: 4; Chunekar, 1982: 435; Sharma, 1983: 699). The long, wiry, fibrous stem, milky exudate and the laxative property of the roots seem to vindicate this choice.

In Kerala, however, the accepted source of the drug is *Chonemorpha fragrans* which has been discussed by Rheede (Hort. Malab. 9: 7–8, t. 5–6. 1689, *Belutta Kaka-Kodi*). Like *Marsdenia tenacissima* this also has got a strong, wiry, fibrous stem and milky exudate, but is a suggested substitute for the former (Anonymous 1978a: 254) Mooss (1980:5), opines that this is probably one of the two varieties of *mūṛvā* called *mōraṭa*, recognised by Bhiṣagārya.

Argyreia nervosa (Burm. f.) Boj. is also found to be used as *mūṛvā* in some parts of Kerala. But the plant is equated with a different drug *vṛddhadaruka* in most of the works. (Aiyer & Kolammal, 1964. 8: 61; Kurup *et al.*, 1979: 232; Chunekar,

1982: 409; Sharma 1983: 766) and is described by Rheede (Hort. Malab: 11: 125. t. 61. 1692) with its local name as *Samudra-tsjogam*. Studies on market samples of Āyurvēdic drugs by Nair *et al.* (1982) have revealed that the stem of *Chonemorpha fragrans* and roots of *Marsdenia tenacissima* are being marketted as *mūrvā*.

The different plants used by Kerala physicians can be identified as follows:

1. Chonemorpha fragrans (*Moon*) *Alston* **(Apocynaceae)** (Fig. 150)
Echites fragrans Moon
C. macrophylla (Roxb.) G. Don

Large, laticiferous, climbing shrub covered with dense rusty tomentum; leaves large, simple, opposite, short-petioled, ovate or elliptic-acute, subcordate at base, tomentose, more densely beneath; flowers white turning yellow, fragrant, in terminal cymes; calyx campanulate, 5 lobed; corolla tube short, cylindrical, slightly expanded above the base, lobes 5, overlapping to the right; stamens 5, epipetalous, filaments short, villous, anthers included, sagitate; pistil bicarpellary, style filiform, ending in a hemispheric stigmatic head; follicles about 25 cm long.

Distribution: The plant occurs throughout India. It is common in the moist, semideciduous forests of Kerala from the plains upto 2,500 ft.

Marsdenia tenacissima (*Roxb.*) *Moon* **(Asclepiadaceae)**
Asclepias tenacissima Roxb.

Laticiferous climbing shrub, tender parts tomentose; leaves 8–11 × 7–11 cm, broadly ovate-cordate, acuminate; flowers small, yellowish green in axillary corymbose cymes; calyx lobes lanceolate, corolla campanulate, villous without; corona linear, hard, acuminate; stamens and pistil united to form a gynostegium; follicles oblong, terete, 12 × 2 cm.

Distribution: Sri Lanka, India, Burma, Indo-China, W. China.

Argyreia nervosa (*Burm. f.*) *Boj.* **(Convolvulaceae)** (Fig. 151)
Convolulus nervosus Burm. f.
Argyreia speciosa (L.f.) Sweet
Lettsomia nervosa (Burm. f.) Roxb.

Very large, extensively spreading, silky pubescent climber; leaves 22 × 23 cm, simple, alternate, long-petioled, broadly ovate-cordate, apiculate at tip, glabrous green above, densely white silky velvety beneath; flowers rose-purple in axillary, many-flowered, bracteate cymes borne on stout peduncles, bracts ovate-lanceolate, acuminate, 3–4 cm long; sepals persistent, densely white tomentose outside; corolla woolly outside; stamens 5, included, filaments enlarged and villous at base; ovary globose, 4-ovuled, style filiform, stigma biglobose; fruit globose, indehiscent berry.

Distribution: The plant grows on river banks, edges of lakes and as an undergrowth in semideciduous forests climbing over bushes, throughout most parts of India.

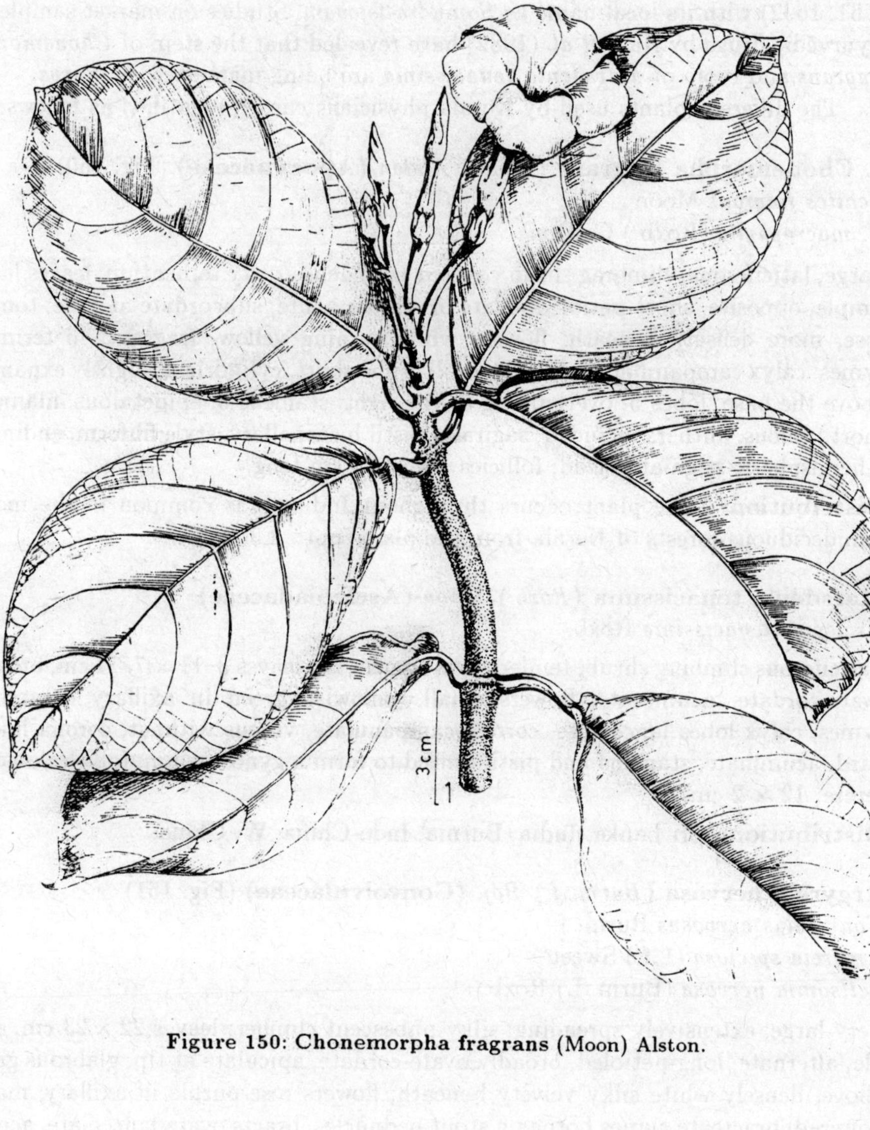

Figure 150: Chonemorpha fragrans (Moon) Alston.

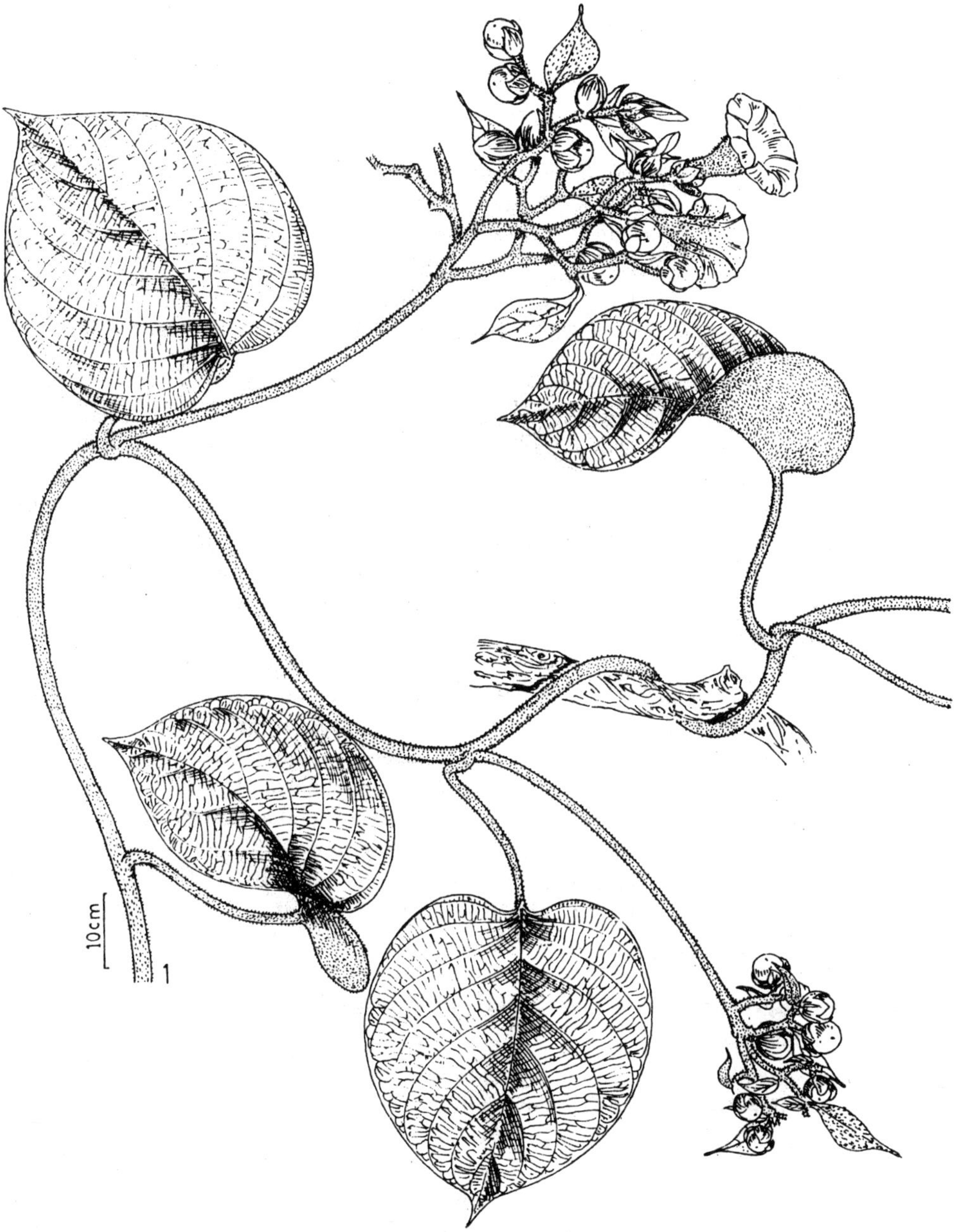

Figure 151: Argyreia nervosa (Burm. f.) Boj.

MUSALĪ (Mal. NILAPPANA)

Musalī is a reputed *rasāyana* (rejuvenative) drug and a good aphrodisiac. It is sweet, bitter, viriligenic, roborant, easily digestible, diuretic and tonic. It cures morbid *vāta* and *pitta*, improves complexion and is useful in general debility, cough, asthma, piles, skin diseases, impotence, jaundice, urinary diseases, leucorrhoea and menorrhagia (Mooss, 1978: 83; Sharma, 1983: 561). The tuberous root-stock is the officinal part. *Vidāryādi ghṛtaṃ, Vidāryādi lēhaṃ, Maṛmaguḷika*, etc. are some of the preparations using the drug.

According to the texts, the plant is a miniature *tāli* palm, growing close to the ground (*bhūtālī*) with its rootstock and leaves bearing resemblence to those of *tāli*, the Palmyra palm. (*tālamūlī, tālamūlikā, tālapatṛikā*). The root-stock is long and tuberous (*dīṛghakandikā*) resembling a *musala* —a wooden pestle used for husking and cleaning paddy—in shape (hence the name *musalī*) and it has golden yellow flowers (*hēmapuṣpī*). The term *paṛṇapuṣpikā* refers to that particular feature of the plant, the leaf tips of which function for vegetative propagation, giving rise to new plants on touching the ground (Aiyer & Kolammal, 1963. 6: 4; Mooss, 1978: 82). The description given in the texts agree well with the plant that is being used as the source of the drug viz. *Curculigo orchioides* Gaertn. of Hypoxidaceae.

Two types of *musali* are recognised in the texts i.e. a black and a white variety. The black variety is equated with *Curculigo orchioides.* The white variety has been equated with *Asparagus adscendens* of Liliaceae, by some (Nadkarni, 1954: 411, 151; Chopra *et al.*, 1956: 84, 28; Mooss, 1978: 79; Chunekar, 1982: 391; Sharma, 1983: 559) and with *Chlorophytum arundinaceum* Baker (Liliaceae) by others (Chunekar, 1982: 390; Sharma, 1983: 559). This distinction, however, is not in vogue in practice, at least in Kerala. *Curculigo orchioides*, locally known as *nilappana* or *nilappana kiḻan̈n̈u* is used for both (See also Rheede, Hort. Malab. 12: 111, t. 59. 1693. *Nella-pana kelangu*).

Curculigo orchioides *Gaertn.* **(Hypoxidaceae)** (Fig. 152)
C. malabarica Wight

Small, geophilous, perennial herbs with long, cylindric, root-stock; leaves basal, sessile, linear or lanceolate, acute, plicate, glabrous, upto 34 × 3 cm, the tips often bearing bulbils; flowers small, yellow on very short scape, hidden in the leaf sheath; perianth gamophyllous, yellow, rotate, 6-lobed; stamens 6, filaments short, adnate to the base of the perianth lobes; ovary inferior, tricarpellary, syncarpous with a fairly long slender beak—the stipe, style short, columnar, stigma 3-cleft; fruit a 1–4 seeded capsule.

Distribution: The plant is found in all districts of India from near sea level to 2,300 m, especially in rock crevices and lateritic soil. Also distributed in Sri Lanka, Japan, Malesia and Australia.

Note: The pharmacognosy of *C. orchioides* has been discussed by Raghunathan & Mitra (1982: 670–673).

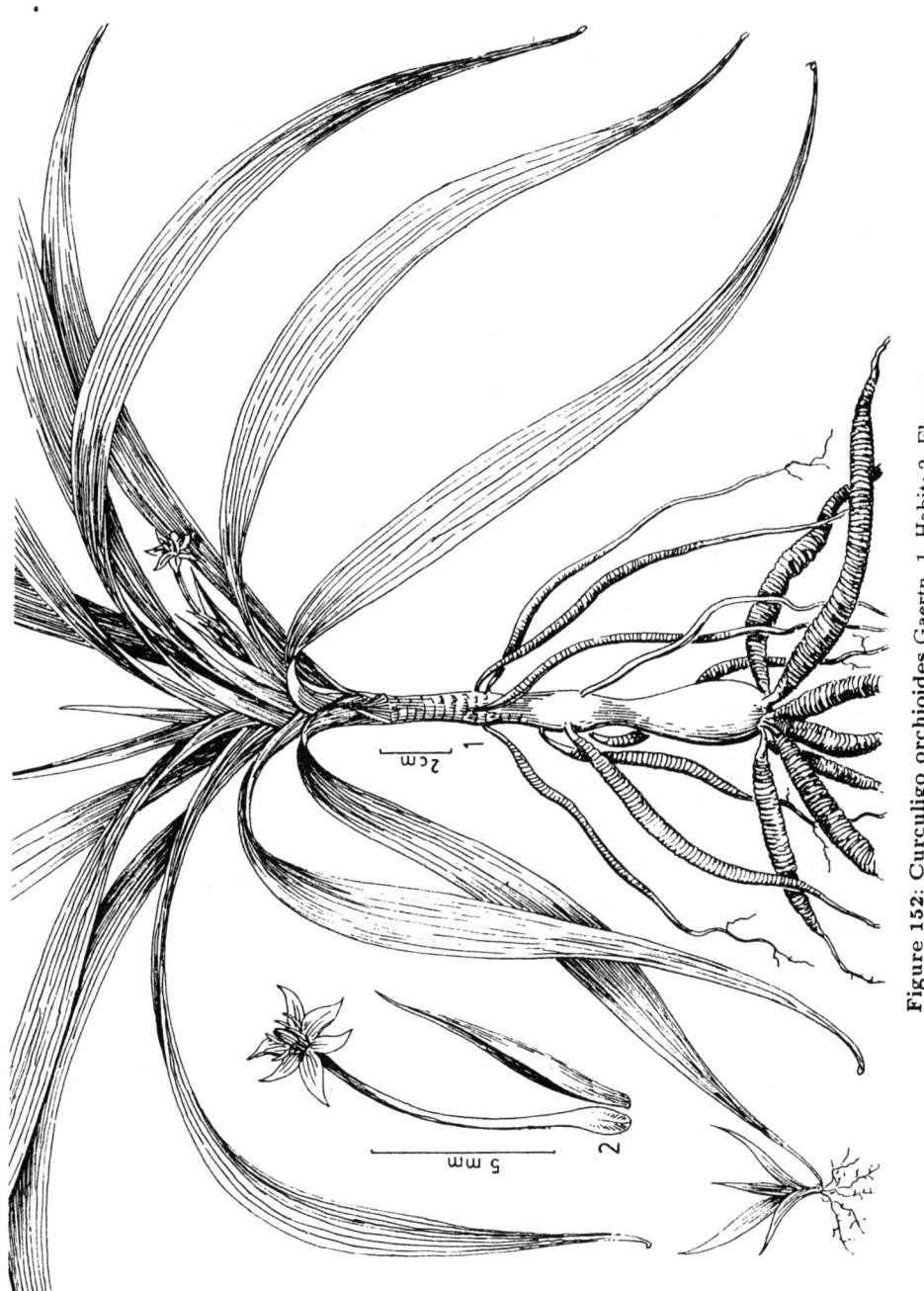

Figure 152: **Curculigo orchioides** Gaertn. 1, Habit; 2, Flower.

MUSTĀ (Mal. MUTTAṄṄA)

Mustā is an important home remedy for indigestion, sprue, diarrhoea and other intestinal problems of children. Root tuber is the part used in medicine. It is light, bitter, aromatic, astringent, carminative, diuretic, anthelmintic, galactagogue, emmenagogue and nervine tonic. It cures *kapha* and *pitta* disorders, dyspepsia, vomiting, indigestion, thirst, worm troubles, cough, bronchitis, dysuria, fever and poisonous affections. The drug is also used in epilepsy, loss of memory, blood diseases and general debility. The paste is applied in skin diseases and eye disease (Kurup, *et al.*, 1979: 147; Sharma, 1983: 372). *Mustāriṣṭaṃ, Ceṛiya Rāsnādi kaṣāyaṃ, Cāṛṅgēryādi ghṛtaṃ, Vyāghṛyādi lēhaṃ*, etc. are some of the preparations using the drug.

The Āyurvēdic texts mention two different types of *mustā* having almost similar properties, namely *mustā* and *bhadramustā*. The former, known as *muttaṅṅa* in vernacular, is invariably equated with *Cyperus rotundus* Linn. of Cyperaceae by all the authors. (See also Rheede, Hort. Malab. 12: 97, t. 52. 1693). This is the plant used as *mustā* throughout India. But in some places *Kyllinga nemoralis*, belonging to the same family, is also found used as the drug source, probably as an unauthorised substitute.

Cyperus esculentus (Cyperaceae), locally called *kaḷimuttaṅṅa*, is the plant used as *bhadramustā*. The various plant sources can be identified as follows.

Cyperus rotundus *Linn.* **(Cyperaceae)** (Fig. 153)

Perennial herb; rhizomes stoloniferous; stem sparsely tufted, erect, triquetrous; leaves several, flat, 9–15 × 0.1–0.2 cm, nerves prominent, scabrous, inflorescence simple or compound; involucral bracts 3, unequal; spikes 2–8 spikeletted, at right angles to the rachis, spikelets spicate, narrow, oblong, pale or purplish, stramineous, 10–20 flowered, glumes closely imbricating, ovate-membraneous, 5-nerved, margin hyaline, apex subobtuse, keel green, 3-nerved; stamens 3, anthers red-crested; stigmas 3; nut oblong, trigonous, stramineous, stipitate.

Distribution: A cosmopolitan weed found throughout India in all districts.

Note: The chemistry and pharmacology of *Cyperus rotundus* have been discussed by Satyavati *et al.* (1976: 324).

The root of *C. rotundus* has been found to be effective in the treatment of conjunctivitis (Saxena, 1980). Bambhole and Jiddewar (1984) found that oral administration of the root powder of *Cyperus rotundus* produces significant reduction in the body weight and that it lowers blood pressure in hypertensive obese patients.

Kyllinga nemoralis *Hutch.* & *Dalz.* **(Cyperaceae)** (Fig. 154)
Kyllinga monocephala Rottb.
Cyperus kyllingia Endl.

Glabrous herb; rhizome creeping, elongate; stem close or distant, 5–40 cms, erect,

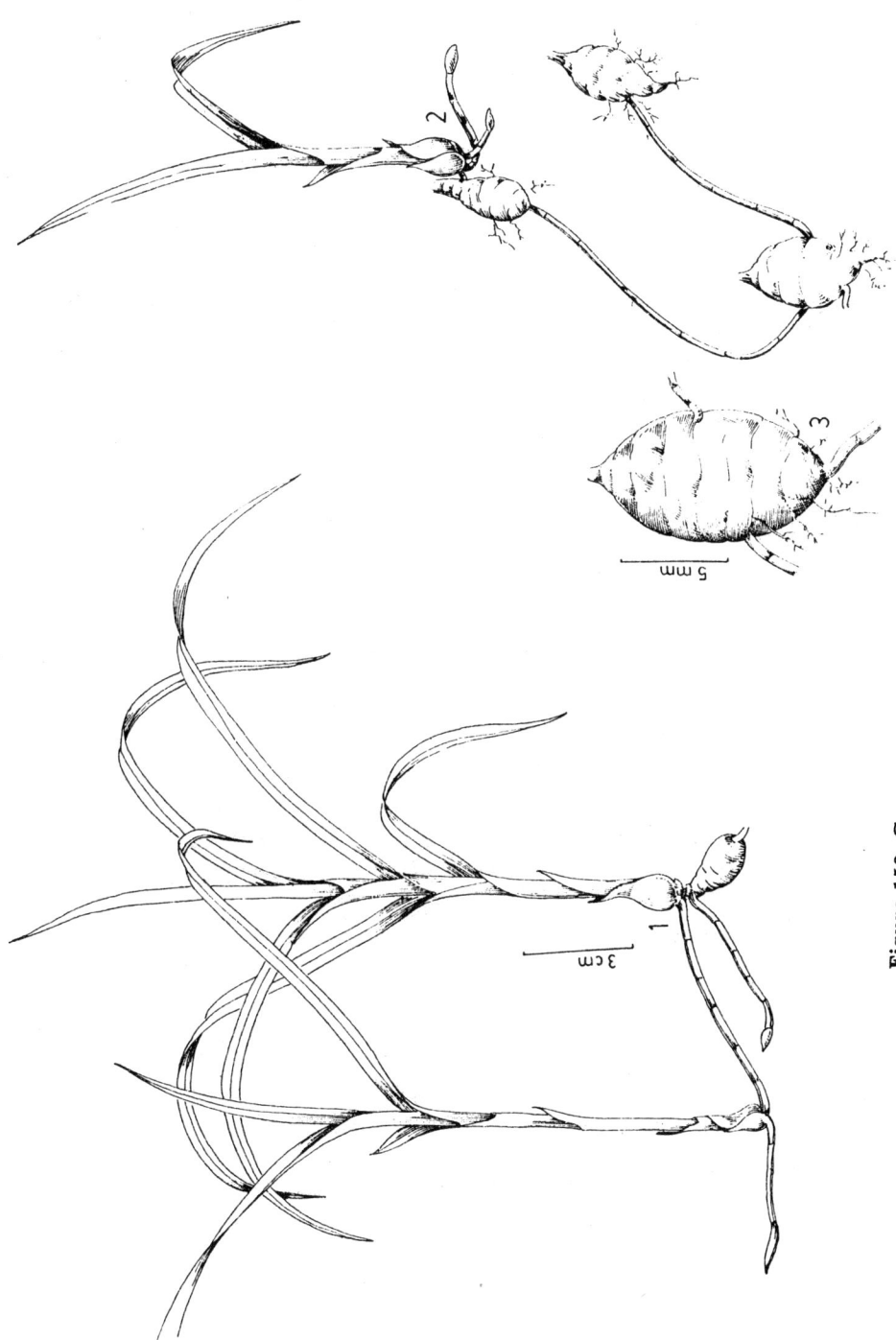

Figure 153: **Cyperus rotundus** L. 1–2, Habit; 3, Tuber.

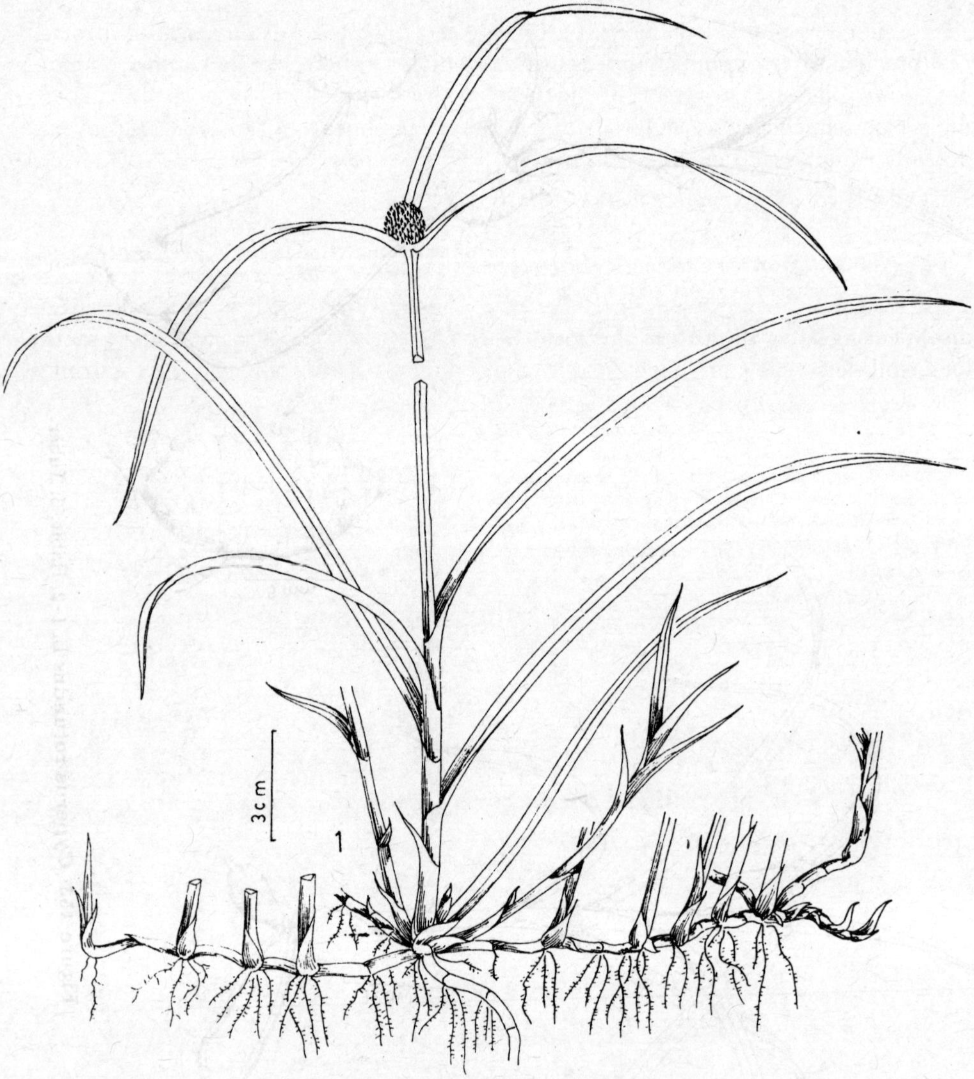

Figure 154: Kyllinga nemoralis Hutch. & Dalz.

slender, triquetrous; leaves several, flat or canaliculate, 15 × 0.4 cm flaccid, nerves strong above, scaberulous; sheaths grey; spikes globose, 4 × 8 mm, white; involucral bracts 3, overtopping; spikelets ovate or elliptic, suberect or spreading; glumes 4(5), lower ones narrow-linear, hyaline, keeled; 3rd bisexual, upper most bisexual or male, boat-shaped, mucronulate; stamens 3, anthers linear, nut obovoid, biconvex, dorsally compressed, apiculate, stipitate.

Distribution: A pantropical weed found in all districts throughout India.

Cyperus esculentus *Linn.* **(Cyperaceae)** (Fig. 155)

Perennial herb; stem at base erect; stolons slender, with small pale scales, often disappearing after the tubers are formed; tubers woody, zoned; leaves and bracts long; spikelets yellow or yellow-brown; glumes plicate-striate, slightly rigid in fruit.

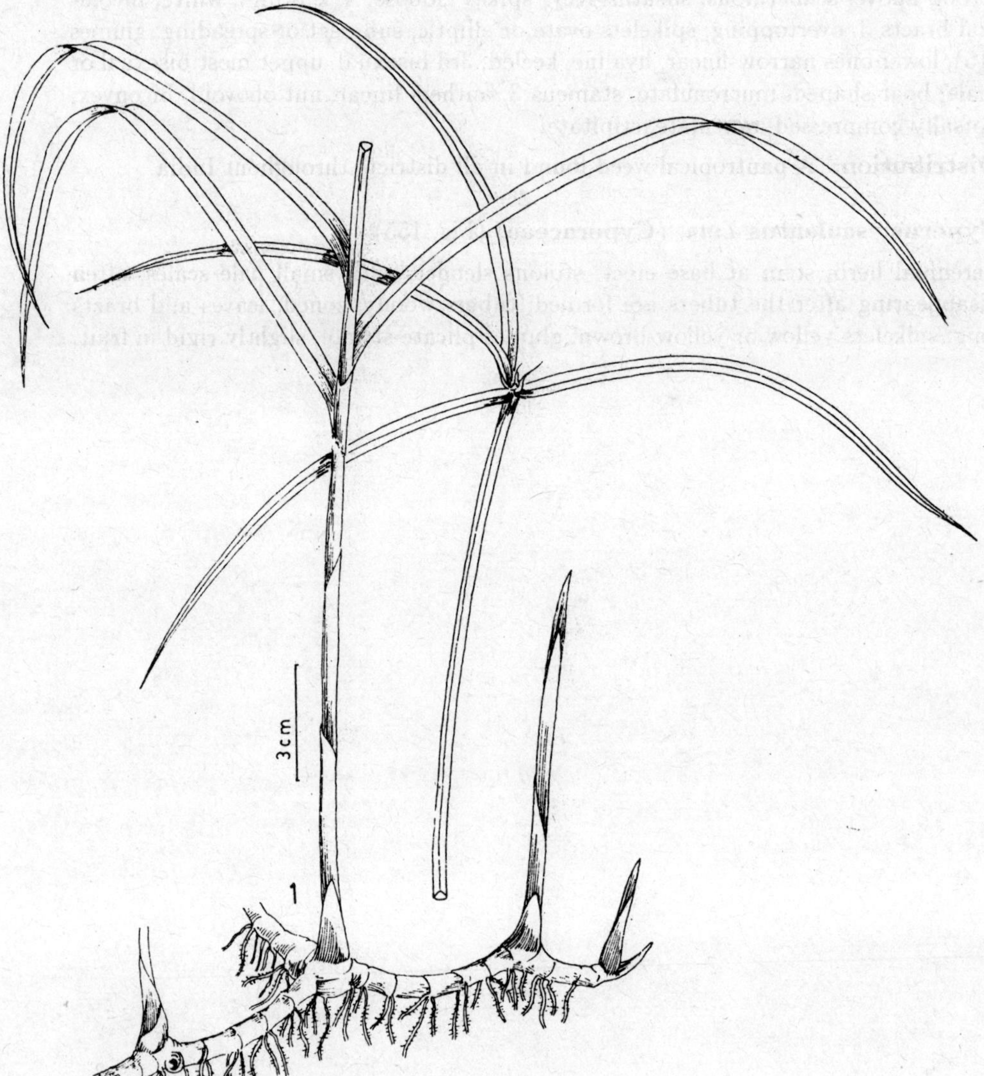

Figure 155: Cyperus esculentus L.

NANDYĀVAṚTAḤ (Mal. NANTYĀṚVAṬṬAṂ)

In traditional practice, the flower buds of this plant are used extensively in eye diseases. Juice of the flowers is used to relieve burning sensation in sore eyes and also in skin diseases. The root is acrid, bitter, anodyne, vermicide and tonic and is useful in toothache, opacity of the cornea and pain in the joints and limbs. The milky juice of the leaves is used as a cooling application for wounds to prevent inflammation (Nadkarni, 1954: 1189).

Most of the authors consider this to be synonymous with *nandīvṛkṣa* which is equated variously by various people. Some consider it to be one of the *kṣīrivṛkṣās* (trees with milky latex) and equated it with some species of *Ficus* of Moraceae, viz. *Ficus retusa* (Chunekar, 1982: 515) and *F. arnottiana* (Vaidya, K.M. 1936: 310; Anonymous, 1978a: 250). But most others consider *Tabernaemontana divaricata* (= *T. coronaria*) of Apocynaceae to be the plant source of this drug (See Kirtikar & Basu, 1918: 796; Nadkarni, 1954: 1189; Chopra *et al.*, 1956: 110) Kerala physicians also use this plant, known as *nantyāṛvaṭṭaṃ* in vernacular, as the drug source (see also Rheede, Hort. Malab. 2: 107. t. 55. 1679, 'Nandi-ervatam').

Tabernaemontana divaricata (*Linn.*) *Roem. & Schult.* **(Apocynaceae)**
T. coronaria (Jacq.) Willd. (Fig. 156)
Ervatamia coronaria (Jacq.) Stapf.
E. divaricata (Linn.) Burkill.

Glabrous laticiferous shrub; leaves elliptic-oblong to oblanceolate-acuminate, entire, 9–15 × 3–5 cm, shining green; flowers white, fragrant, in lax terminal, few-flowered cymes; calyx 5-lobed, lobes glandular-scaly within; corolla white, salver-shaped, tube 2 cm, inflated over stamens, lobes 5; stamens 5, included, anthers lanceolate; mericarps seldom seen here.

Distribution: Throughout tropical parts of the world and in the Himalayas. In Kerala, this is found only under cultivation in ornamental gardens.

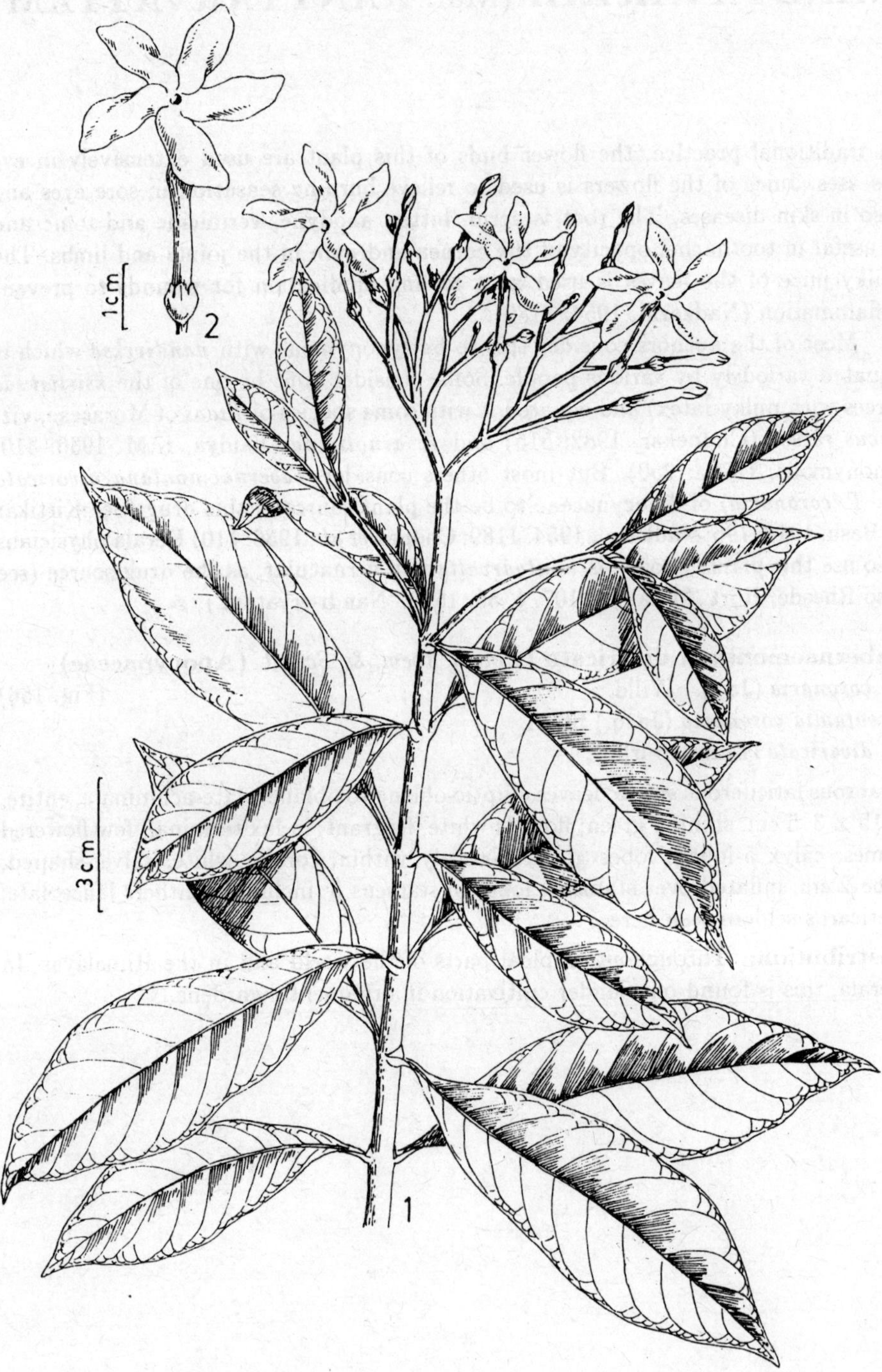

Figure 156: Tabernaemontana divaricata (L.) R. & S. 1, Twig; 2, Flower.

NIṀBAḤ (Mal. VĒPPU, ĀRYAVĒPPU)

All parts of the plant, especially bark, leaves and seeds have been extensively used against skin diseases and rheumatism since time immemorial. The stem bark is reported to be bitter, cooling, anthelmintic, antiperiodic and astringent. It rehabilitates vitiated *pitta* and *kapha* and is useful in intestinal worms, impurity of blood, eye diseases, intermittent fevers, thirst, vomiting, general debility, diabetes, leprosy, skin diseases, ulcers and insect poison. Leaves and flowers also possess the same properties. An infusion of the leaves forms a good wash for wounds and ulcers. Garcia da Orta (1563: 328–30) has recorded that the bruised leaves applied with lemon juice, cured ulcers in horses and men, and that the people of the then Malabar used it likewise against rheumatic complaints as well. A paste of fresh leaves is used for external application in the treatment of small pox, chicken pox and other cutaneous affections. Oil from the seeds form a useful application in ulcers, chronic skin diseases like ringworm, scabies and itch and rheumatism. Decoction of root bark gives complete relief in filarial fever. Nimbidin obtained from the bark and oil has been found useful in tropical eosinophilia (Nadkarni, 1954: 780; Aiyer & Kolammal, 1957: 3: 23; Kurup *et al.*, 1979: 151). Bark and leaves form important ingredients of preparations like *Dūrvādi tailaṃ, Jātyādi ghṛtaṃ, Niṁbādi tailaṃ, Tiktakaṃ kaṣāyaṃ*, etc.

The texts suggest that the drug is highly bitter (*tiktakaḥ*) and that it comes from a tree with pinnate leaves (*viśīrṇaparṇaḥ*), yellow or reddish heart wood (*pītasārakaḥ*) and an exudate with asafoetida-like odour (*hiṅguniryāsaḥ*).

Three varieties of *niṁbaḥ* have been mentioned in *Abhidhānamañjari* viz. *niṁbaḥ, mahāniṁba* and *kṛṣṇaniṁba*. Mooss (1978: 39) and Nesamony (1985: 39) equate these with *Azadirachta indica* A. Juss., *Melia azedarach* L. (Meliaceae) and *Murraya koenigii* Spreng (Rutaceae) respectively. It is doubtful whether the equation of *mahāniṁba* and *kṛṣṇaniṁba* is correct, but throughout the country *Azadirachta indica*, commonly called 'Neem-tree', is used as *niṁbaḥ*, the vernacular name being *āryavēppu*. (See also Rheede, Hort. Malab: 4: 107–108 t. 52. 1683) *Murraya koenigii* is described else where.

The other two plants can be identified as follows:

Azadirachta indica *A. Juss.* **(Meliaceae)** (Fig. 157)
Melia azadirachta Linn.

Trees; leaves alternate, imparipinnate, 7–13 foliolate; leaflets sub-opposite, falcate-lanceolate, oblique at base, coarsely serrate, acuminate, upto 7.5 × 2.5 cms, glabrous green above, pale beneath; flowers greenish white in axillary panicles; calyx 5 fid; petals 5, free, shortly ciliate, staminal tube cylindric, 8–10 lobed, lobes slightly toothed at the tip; ovary three-chambered, superior, style slender, elongate, ending in a three lobed cylindric stigma; drupes ellipsoid, fleshy, yellow when mature.

Distribution: A native of India and China, this species is now naturalised in Pakistan and Malesia. In India, this occurs throughout most parts of the country,

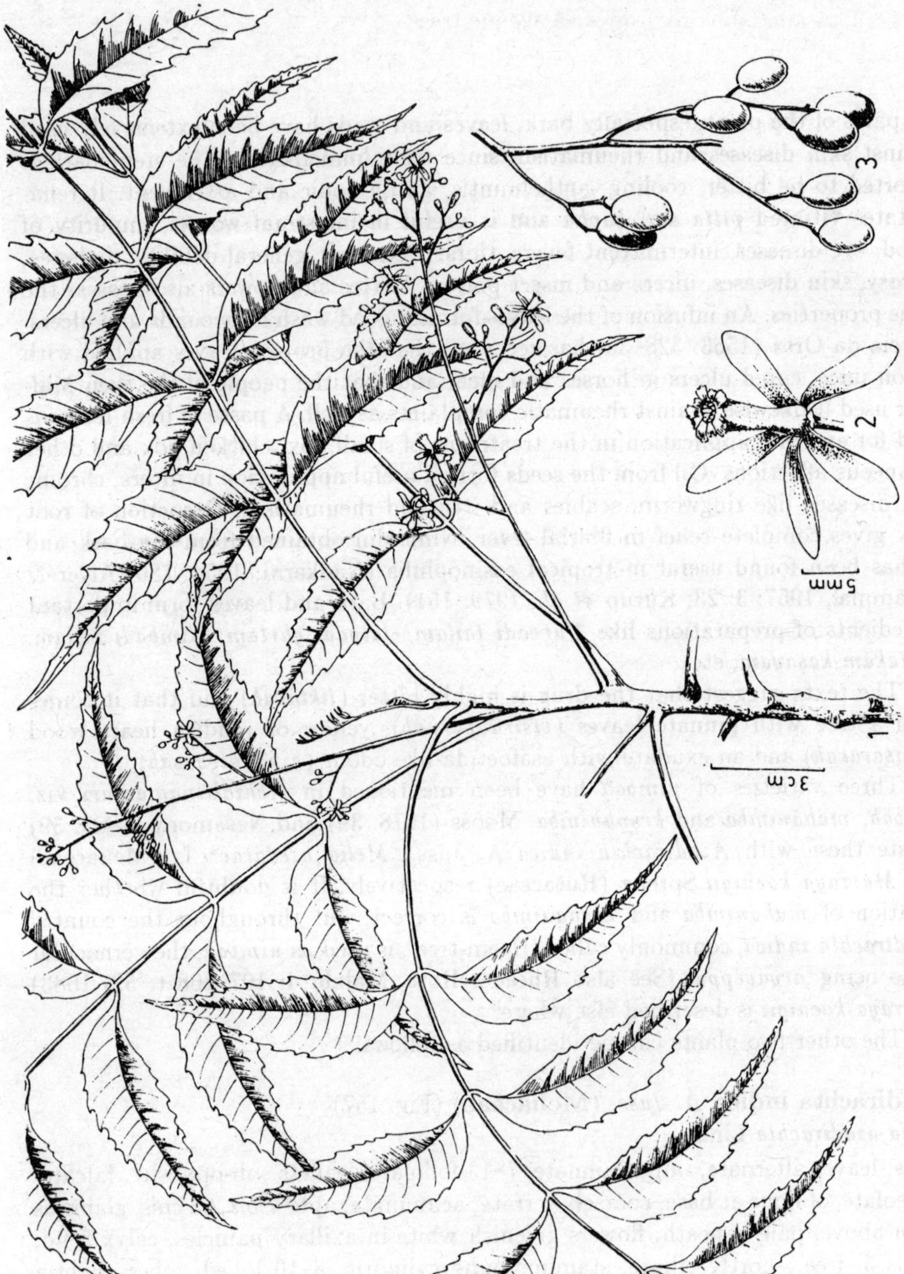

Figure 157. Azadirachta indica A. Juss. 1, Flowering twig; 2, Flower 3, Fruits.

to an altitude of 3,000 ft. Believed to be an auspicious tree, this is often cultivated in gardens and along roadsides as avenue trees.

Note: This is one of the few drugs that has been extensively studied as to their pharmacological and clinical properties. Water extracts of leaves and neem oil have been found to reduce blood sugar significantly and to prevent adrenalin-induced hyper-glycaemia in experimental animals (Moorthy *et al.*, 1978: Sharma *et al.*, 1983; Moosa, 1985).

Also they have been demonstrated to exhibit significant antifertility property in male rats without interfering with spermatogenesis (Deshpande *et al.*, 1980, Khare *et al.*, 1984, Sharma *et al.*, 1987). Alcoholic extracts of leaves were found to cure skin affections like eczema, ringworm, scabies, etc. (Singh *et al.*, 1979). The anthelmintic property of the drug has been studied by Singh *et al.* (1980).

Nimbidin, a bitter component from Neem oil has been found to possess significant analgesic and antipyretic activity (Pillai *et al.*, 1980) and to be effective in the treatment of psoriasis (Rajasekharan *et al.*, 1980) and chronic gastroduodinal ulcer (Pillai & Shantakumari 1984). Nimbatikta—total bitter principle of *Azadirachta indica*—was also found to cure completely chronic ulcers (Pillai *et al.*, 1983). Neem oil has been reported to prevent pregnancy when used intravaginally (Sinha *et al.*, 1984, Sinha & Riar 1985).

Melia azedarach *Linn.* **(Meliaceae)** (Fig. 158)

Medium sized tree; leaves alternate, exstipulate, bi-or tripinnate, 30 × 20 cm, pinnae three to four pairs; leaflets 1–5 pairs, opposite, ovate-obovate or lanceolate-acuminate, 4.5–6.5 × 1.5—3.5 cm, tomentose, base oblique, cuneate, margin entire; flowers lilac in long-peduncled axillary cymose panicles; calyx pubescent outside, deeply 5 lobed, petals 5, lilac, lanceolate-obovate, glabrescent; stamens 10, filaments united into a purple, puberulous, striate, staminal tube; ovary ovoid, 5-celled with 2 ovules in each; drupe oblong, 1-seeded.

Distribution: The plant is a native in W. Himalaya, and is naturalised in China, Burma, India, Pakistan, Iran and Turkey.

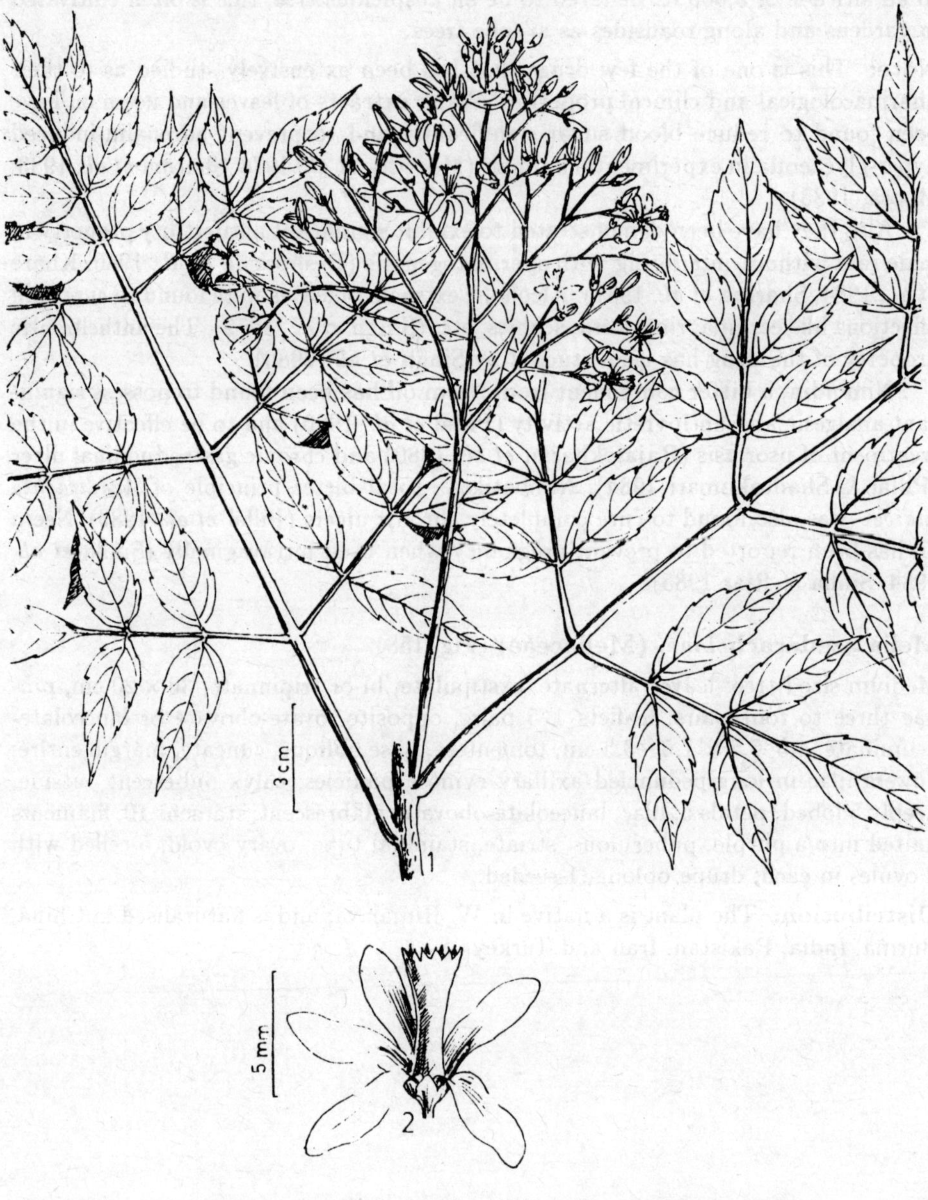

Figure 158: Melia azedarach L. 1, Flowering Twig; 2, Flower.

NĪLĪ (Mal. AMARI)

In Āyurvēdic practice, *nīlī* is considered as a reputed drug for the promotion of hair growth and forms a major ingredient of preparations like *Nīlībhṛṅgādi* oil etc. Due to the antitoxic property, it is also a good remedy against all poisonous affections. According to *Bhāvapṛakāśa, nīlī* is purgative in action, bitter, hot, cures *mēha* (urinary diseases with excessive urine), giddiness, abdominal enlargement (ascites), enlargement of spleen, *vātarakta*, gout and intestinal obstruction (*udāvarta*). The leaves are externally applied as a poultice in various skin affections like scabies and to cleanse and heal wounds and ulcers. Juice of leaves is given in asthma, whooping cough, palpitation of the heart, lung disease and kidney complaints. Root is useful in bladder stones and epilepsy (Nadkarni, 1954: 681; Aiyer & Kolammal, 1960. 4: 63). Root, leaves or the entire plant are used in medicine.

According to the texts, the plant is blue-black in colour (*nīlī, nīlā, kālā*) having bluish or dark coloured stem, leaves and flowers (*nīlayaṣṭī, nīlapatrī, nīlapuṣpī*) and containing a dye (*rañjanī*). The synonyms *viṣaghnī* and *śōdhanī* indicate the antitoxic and laxative properties of the drug respectively (Aiyer & Kolammal, 1960. 4: 62).

There is no confusion as far as the plant source of this drug is concerned. Most of the authors have equated this with *Indigofera tinctoria* Linn. (Papilionaceae), the original source of natural Indigo. In Kerala also, this has been the accepted source of the drug since long (See Rheede, Hort. Malab. 1: 101–102. t. 54. 1678). The synonyms attributed to this drug also seem to go well with the plant.

However, Aiyer and Kolammal (1960. 4: 61) refer to two distinct varieties of the drug, namely white and dark. But this distinction is not in vogue among practitioners of Kerala, who invariably take *Indigofera tinctoria* for this drug.

Indigofera tinctoria *Linn.* **(Papilionaceae)** (Fig. 159)

Erect shrub; stem and branches green, branchlets silvery pubescent; leaves alternate, stipulate, imparipinnate, leaflets 7–11, elliptic-oblong, membraneous, 1.7 × 0.9 cms, shortly mucronate, pale green or bluish; flowers small, rose-coloured, in axillary racemes; calyx 5-cleft, gamosepalous; corolla papilionaceous; stamens diadelphous; ovary sessile with a short incurved style ending in a capitate stigma; pods linear, cylindrical to 2.5 cms long, deflexed, 8–12 seeded.

Distribution: This plant is distributed in South and South East Asia, tropical Africa and is introduced in tropical America. In India, it is found almost throughout.

Note: The pharmacological studies conducted on *I. tinctoria* have been discussed in detail by Satyavati *et al.* (1987).

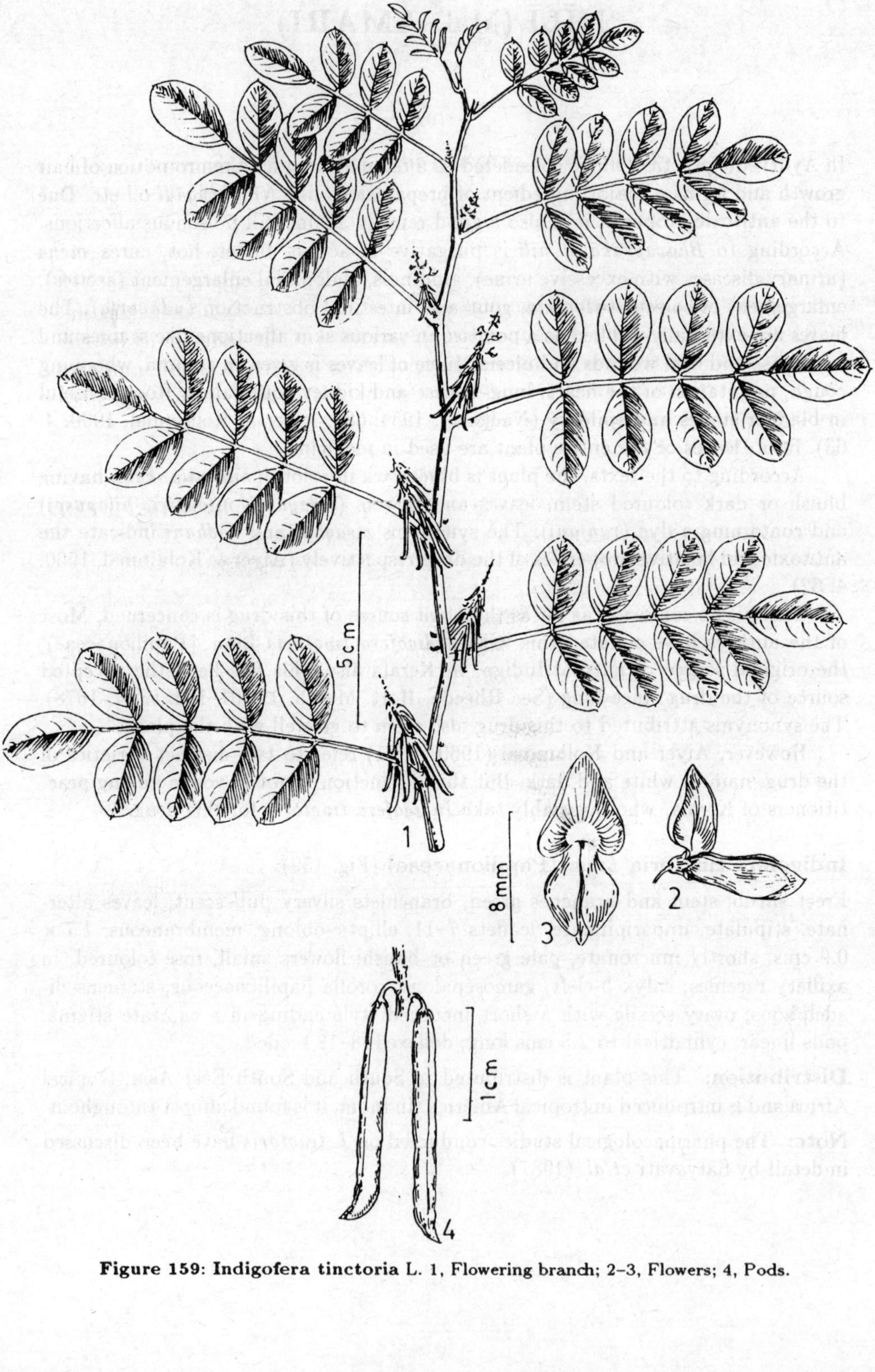

Figure 159: Indigofera tinctoria L. 1, Flowering branch; 2–3, Flowers; 4, Pods.

NIṚGUṆḌĪ (Mal. NOCCI, KARINOCCI)

Nirguṇḍī has been a reputed drug in Āyurvēdic medicine and is reportedly astringent, bitter and cold. Roots and leaves are the officinal parts. It has got germicidal properties. It is easily digestible and can cure morbid *vāta* and *kapha*. The drug cures cough, asthma, eye diseases, inflammatory, glandular and rheumatic swellings, intestinal worms, fever, ulcers, skin diseases, nervous disorders and leprosy. The leaves are aromatic, discutient, vermifuge and are very efficaceous in dispelling inflammatory swellings of the joints in acute rheumatism, of the testes in hydrocele and gonorrhoea, also sprained limbs and in splenic enlargement. *Nirguṇḍī* improves receptive and retentive power of mind, complexion and growth of hair. Oil prepared with the juice of leaves is effective in rheumatism, sinus, scrofulous sores and ulcers. Root is used in dyspepsia, colic, rheumatism, worms, boils and piles (Nadkarni, 1954: 1279; Mooss, 1978: 177; Sharma, 1983: 67). The leaves are used to prepare *Vacādi tailaṃ, Rāsnādi tailaṃ, Jātyādi tailaṃ*, etc. *Aṣṭavargaṃ kaṣāyaṃ* is an important preparation using the root of *nirguṇḍī*.

There are two varieties of this drug mentioned in some of the texts. viz. *śvētanirguṇḍī* (Mal. *veṇnocci*) and *nīlanirguṇḍī* (Mal. *karinocci*). Some authors have distinguished them in terms of the flower colour and have attributed different synonyms for them. viz. *sinduvārah, sindukaḥ* and *sinduvārakaḥ* for the white-flowered variety and *nirguṇḍī, śēphalī* and *suvahā* for the blue-flowered variety (Chunekar, 1982: 344). However, in Kerala, they are differentiated by the colouration of the whole plant and not by the flower colour. In fact, both the species that are adopted here have blue flowers.

Most of the authors and commentators do not make a distinction between these two varieties and equate *nirguṇḍī* with *Vitex negundo* Linn. (Verbenaceae). However, some authors have mentioned that *Vitex trifolia* is the source plant of *śvētanirguṇḍī* and *V. negundo* of *nīlanirguṇḍī* (Kirtikar & Basu, 1918: 998; Nadkarni, 1954: 1281; Chopra *et al.*, 1956: 257). They are also reported to have the same properties. Rheede has portrayed the two species but in the reverse order i.e. *Vitex negundo* for "Ben-nosi" and *Vitex trifolia* for "Cara-nosi" (Hort. Malab. 2: 13–14. t. 11 & 2: 15. t. 12. 1679). This can either be a mistake or it is equally possible that these two closely similar species had been in use in Kerala during that period.

Currently, however, only *'kari-nocci'* is widely used by practitioners in Kerala, and the accepted source of this drug is *Vitex negundo*. There are two varieties in this species, i.e. var. *negundo* in which the whole plant is covered with dense grey hairs, giving a white colour for the whole plant and var. *purpurascens* where the whole plants looks blackish due to the purplish tomentum on the plant body. It is the latter variety which is preferred in medicine, but occasionally var. *negundo* is used to substitute/adulterate the former. The various plant sources equated with the drug can be distinguished as follows.

Vitex negundo *Linn. var.* **negundo (Verbenaceae)** (Fig. 160)

Large shrub, tender parts grey-pubescent; leaves opposite, digitately 3–5 foliolate; leaflets lanceolate-acuminate, entire, green above, grey-pubescent beneath, terminal leaflet upto 17 × 3 cms; flowers blue in terminal thyrsoid, grey-pubescent panicle; calyx gamosepalous, campanulate, shortly 5-lobed; corolla gamopetalous, irregular, 2-lipped, upper lip 2-lobed, lower lip divided into 3; stamens 4, didynamous, epipetalous, exserted, filaments hairy at base; ovary 2–4 celled, 4-ovuled, style filiform ending in a bifid stigma; drupes ovoid, 1 cm long, black when ripe.

Distribution: Sri Lanka, India, Afghanistan, Himalaya, Burma, China, Indo-China, Malesia. It is found throughout India.

Vitex negundo *Linn. var.* **purpurascens** *Sivar. & Mold.* **(Verbenaceae)**

This is very similar to the former species, but differs in its purple pubescence, deep purple corolla and purple staminal filaments and style.

The plant is distributed throughout India in all districts, common on waste lands around villages, on roadsides and the banks of streams.

Vitex trifolia *Linn.* **(Verbenaceae)** (Fig. 161)

Shrub; tender parts softly pubescent; leaves 3-foliolate, leaflets elliptic or obovate-oblanceolate, obtuse, glabrous above, dense tomentose beneath, 5–9 × 2–4 cms, the middle leaflet much larger than the laterals; flowers pale purple in terminal panicle; calyx teeth 5, triangular; corolla bluish, tube 3 mm, lobes 5; stamens 4; drupes subglobose, purplish when ripe.

Distribution: Sri Lanka, India, Himalaya, China, Japan, Malesia and Australia. In India it is found in coast districts, especially the west in S. Canara and Malabar.

Note: The macroscopic and microscopic characters of the leaf and root of *Vitex negundo* have been described by Madan & Nayar (1959). The drug has been found to be effective in the treatment of *sandhigata vāta* (non-inflammatory type) (Bhattacharya, 1981). Pharmacological properties of *V. negundo* leaf extracts have been evaluated by Ravisankar *et al.* (1985). Bhargava (1986) has found that the flavanoids of *Vitex negundo* seeds possess antifertility activity in dogs.

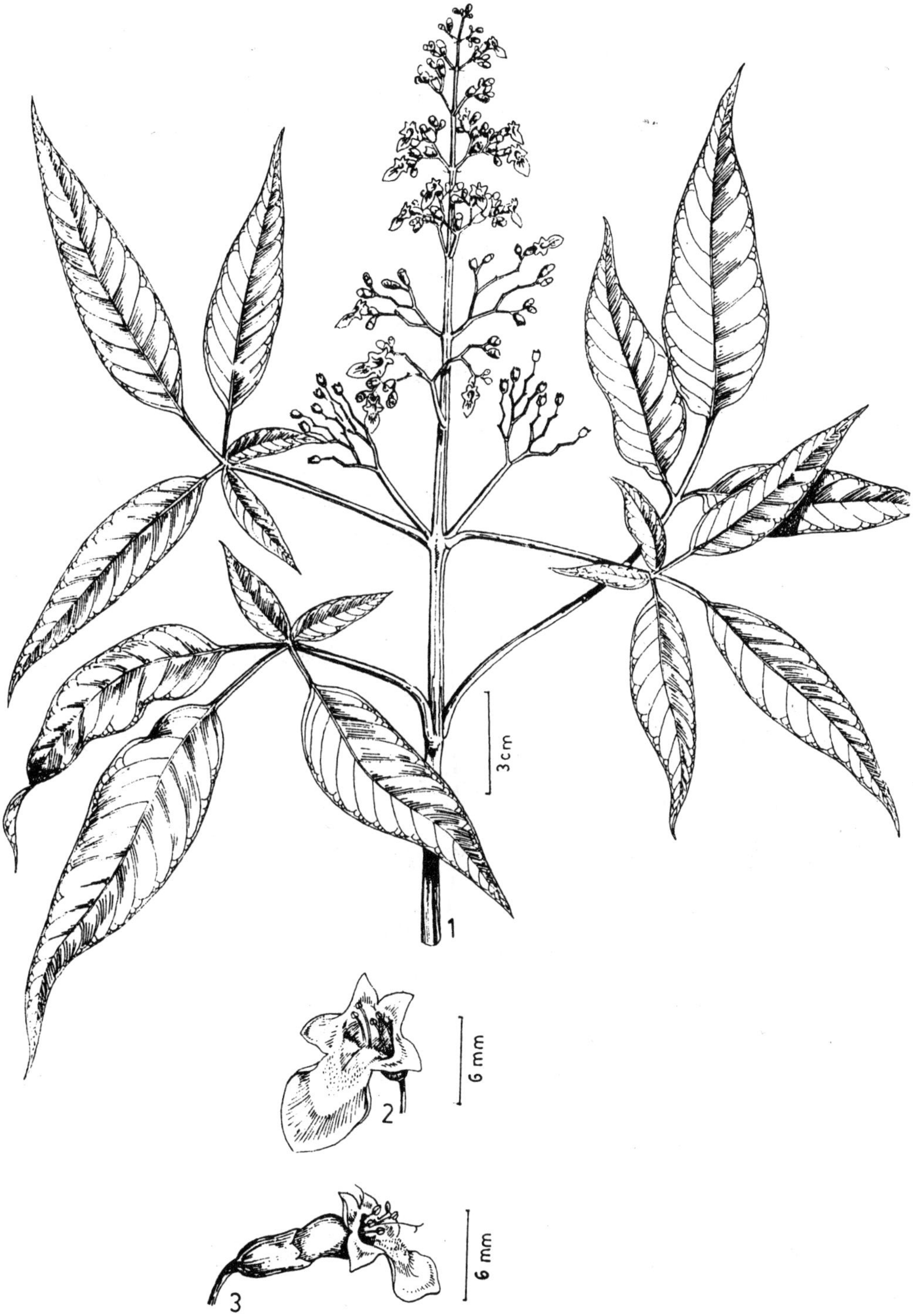

Figure 160: Vitex negundo L. var. **negundo.** 1, Flowering Branch; 2–3, Flowers.

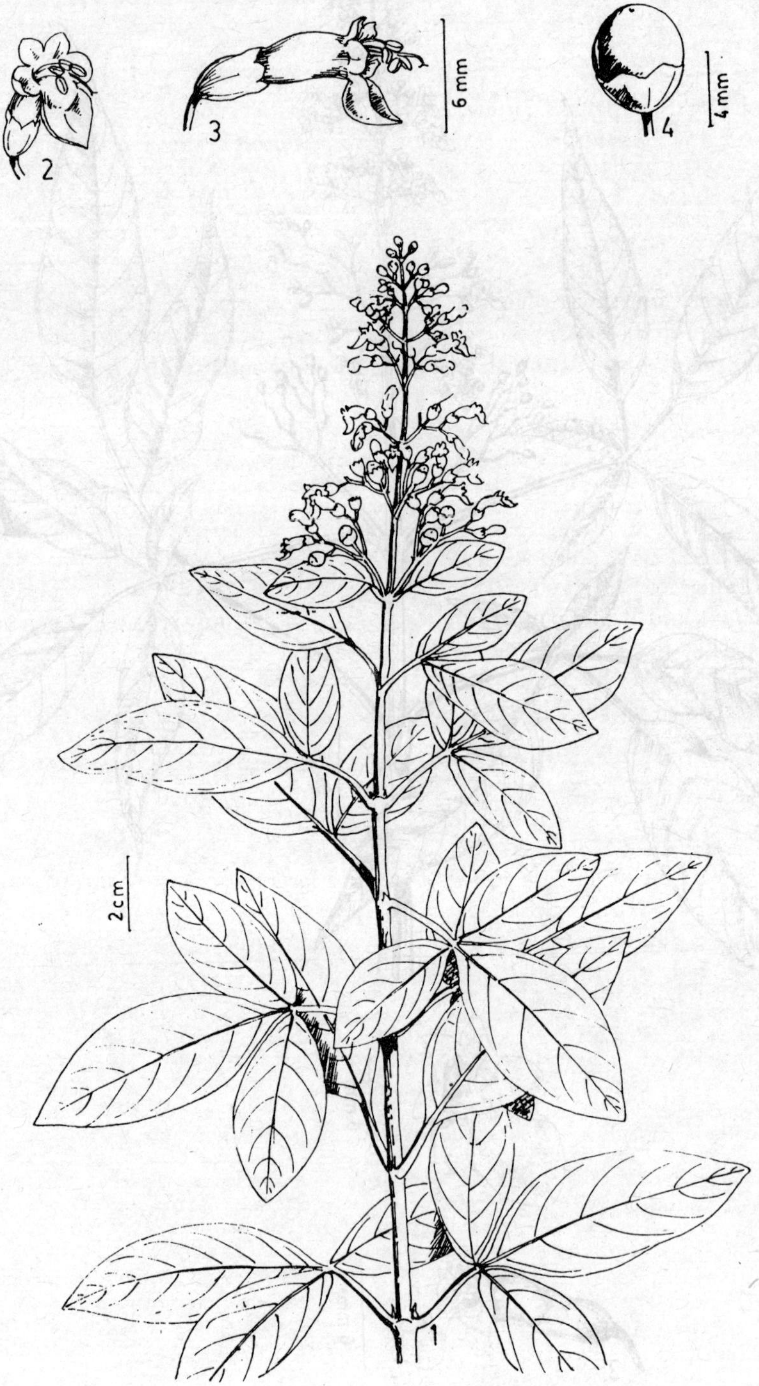

Figure 161: Vitex trifolia L. 1, Flowering Branch; 2–3, Flowers; 4, Fruit.

NYAGRŌDHAḤ (Mal. PĒRĀL)

This is one of the four laticiferous trees that constitute the *Ksīrivṛkṣās* (the others being *aśvatha, plakṣa* and *udumbaraḥ*). It is widely used in the treatment of skin diseases with *pitta* and *rakta* predominance. Stem bark, root bark, aerial roots, leaves, vegetative buds and milky exudate are used in medicine. The bark is astringent, cooling and alleviative of vitiated *kapha* and *pitta*. It improves complexion, cures erysepelas, burning sensation and vaginal disorders, while an infusion of the bark cures dysentery, diarrhoea, leucorrhoea, menorrhagia, nervous disorders and reduces blood sugar in diabetes. A decoction of the vegetative buds in milk is beneficial in haemorrhages. A paste of the leaves is applied externally to abscesses and wounds to promote suppuration, while that of young aerial roots cure pimples. Young twigs, when used as a tooth-brush, strengthen gum and teeth (Nadkarni, 1954: 544; Iyer & Kolammal, 1957: 85; Mooss, 1976: 67). The drug forms an important constituent of formulations like *Nālpāmarādi* coconut oil, *Śāribādyāsavaṃ, Kuṁkumādi tailaṃ, Khadiraguḷika, Valiya candanādi tailaṃ, Candanāsavaṃ, Dinēśavalyādi kuḷaṁbu*, etc.

According to the texts, this laticiferous tree (*kṣīri*) has reddish fruits (*raktaphalaḥ*) and it is wound round (*vaṭaḥ*) by aerial adventitious roots (*śriṅgī*) which look like many legs (*bahupādaḥ*) (Aiyer *et al.*, 1957. 3: 84). This description is well applicable to the plant source of the drug viz. *Ficus benghalensis* Linn. of Moraceae, known as *pērāl* in vernacular. (See also Rheede, Hort. Malab. 1: 49–50, t. 28. 1678, *Peralu*).

Ficus benghalensis *Linn.* **(Moraceae)** (Fig. 162)
Urostigma benghalense (Linn.) Gasp.

Large tree with many large aerial roots; leaves large, alternate, broadly elliptic to ovate, to 10–17 × 7–12 cm, rounded, subcordate or slightly narrowed at base, blunt or obtusely cuspidate at apex, entire, coriacious, glabrous above, puberulous below; figs monoecious, 1 or 2, axillary, depressed-globose, 2 cm across, sessile, greenish when young, brick red when ripe; bracts 4–5, cupular, 6 mm, shortly connate, obtuse, persistent, tepals 3–5, shortly connate, glabrous. Male flowers dispersed with female, stamen 1, anther oblong, parallel, unequal, shortly mucronate. Female sessile. Ovary obovoid-globose, 1.5 × 1 mm, style erect or curved, tapering, gall flowers similar to female, pedicellate, achenes globose-ellipsoid, 2 × 1.5 mm, dark brown.

Distribution: The tree is commonly found all over India from sea level to an elevation of about 3,000 ft. It is also reported from Sri Lanka, Pakistan, now widely cultivated.

Note: The prop roots of *Ficus benghalensis* had been found to be useful in checking the external as well as internal bleeding in cases of haemoptysis, menorrhagia and ulcers. (Atiane *et al.*, 1985).

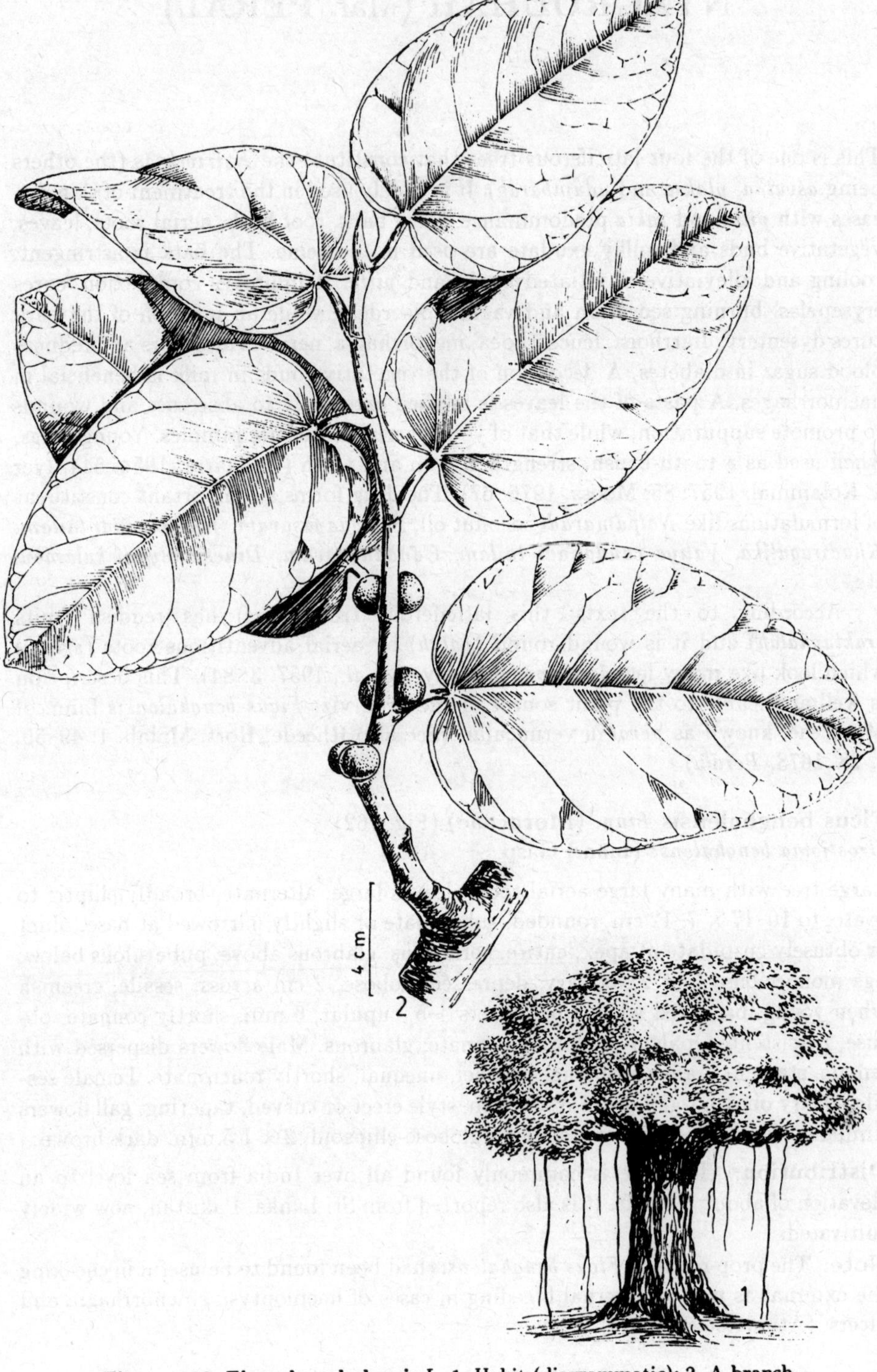

Figure 162: Ficus benghalensis L. 1, Habit (diagrammatic); 2, A branch.

PADMACĀRIṆĪ (Mal. ŌRILATTĀMARA)

The drug *padmacāriṇī* is reportedly hot, bitter and astringent. It overcomes morbid *kapha* and *vāta* and cures dysuria, colic, urinary calculi, cough, asthma and poison (Chunekar, 1982: 482). According to Rājanighaṇṭu, the drug is aromatic and it cures vomiting, epilepsy, *raktapitta*, diarrhoea, diabetes and diseases caused by evil spirits (cf. Moosad, 1983: 377). *Vasıyāmayāntaka ghṛtaṃ, Śatāvari ghṛtaṃ* etc. are some of the preparations using the drug.

Ancient texts describe this plant as one which spreads very fast (*aticarā*) like lotus (*padmacāriṇī*). Ironically, though, none of the plants that are used as the source of this drug has any similarity with the lotus plant, nor do they agree with the synonyms provided above. This does not find mention in the samhitās of Caraka and Suśruta, but is a constituent drug of *Priyaṅgvādi gaṇa* of Vāgbhaṭa (cf. Mooss, 1980: 93).

The botanical source of this plant is highly controversial. Most of the authors have equated it with *Hybanthus enneaspermus* (L.f.) Muell. (= *Ionidium suffruticosum*) of Violaceae (See Kirtikar & Basu, 1918: 115; Nadkarni, 1954: 683; Chopra *et al.*, 1956: 136; Chunekar, 1982: 482; Nesamony, 1985: 100). While a few have adopted *Habenaria grandiflora* (Orchidaceae) as the drug source (Vaidya, K.M. 1936: 337, Mooss, 1980: 93).

Kerala physicians have considered *ōrilattāmara* (i.e. single leaved lotus-like plant) to be the same as *padmacāriṇī*, and have accepted some species of orchids as the source plants. They include some three species of *Nervilia* (viz. *N. plicata, N. aragoana* and *N. prainiana*) and *Habenaria diphylla*. Despite the fact that *Hybanthus enneaspermus* does not suit the suggestive synonyms attributed to this drug, this is also being used by some (Nesamony, 1985: 100). Rheede (Hort. Malab. 9: 117. 60. 1689) has illustrated this plant under a different name, *Nelamparanda*. This again seems to be an inadvertent mistake, because the source plant of *nelaṁparaṇḍa* throughout Kerala is a leguminous plant, *Desmodium triflorum*.

The various plant sources of the drug can be identified as follows:

Nervilia plicata *Schltr.* **(Orchidaceae)**
Pogonia plicata Lindl.

Tuberous, 1-leaved herb; leaf lying flat on the ground, broadly ovate or suborbicular, obtuse or acute, base cordate, many ribbed, purplish hairy, 5–10 cms diam; flowers yellowish green in 1–3 flowered racemes; sepals and petals yellowish green, linear lanceolate acuminate; lip entire; apex emarginate, base slightly saccate, lilac with a yellow median line.

Distribution: Western Ghats

Nervilia aragoana *Gaud.* **(Orchidaceae) (Fig. 163)**
Pogonia flabelliformis Lindl.

Terrestrial, tuberous, 1-leaved herb; leaf appearing after the flowers, long-petioled, petiole 10–20 cms long, orbicular or subreniform, cuspidate, base cordate, 13 or more

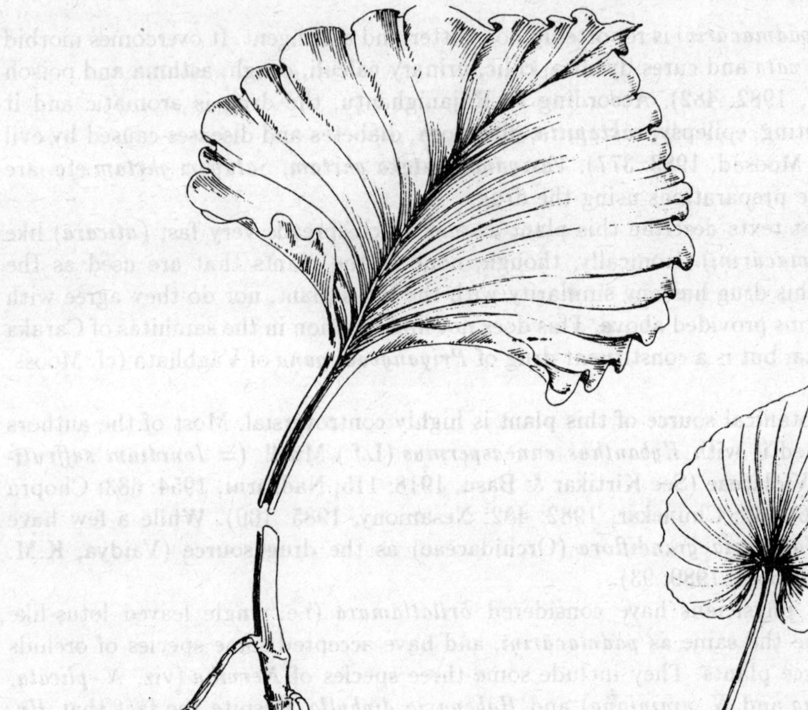

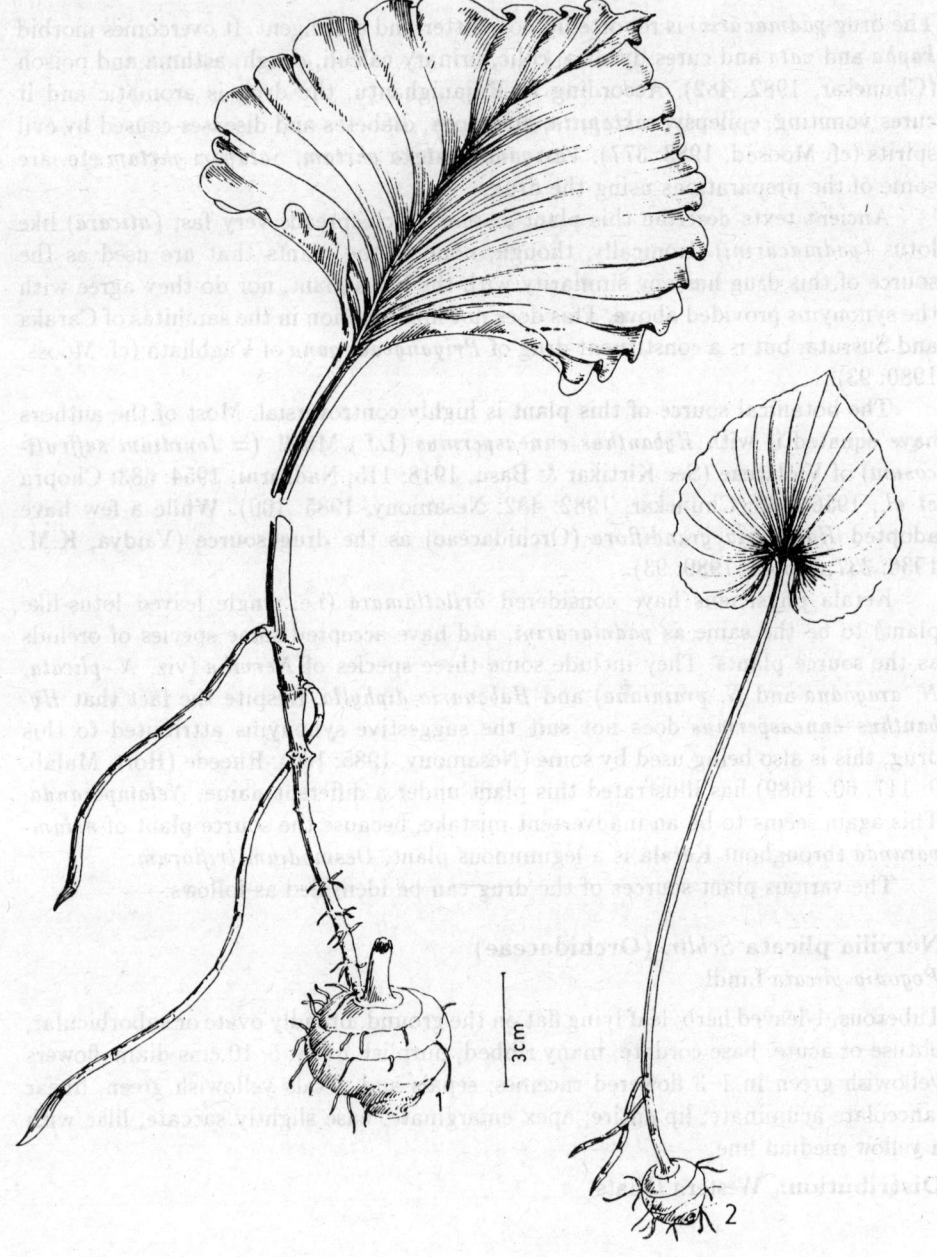

Figure 163: Nervilia aragoana Gaud. 1–2, Vegetative habit.

ribbed, margin wavy, coarsely dentate, and 10–29 cms diam; flowers in many-flowered racemes; sepals pale green, veined with purple, linear-lanceolate acute; petals narrower; lip white veined with purple, tinged with yellow near the base, 3-lobed.

Distribution: Western Ghats.

Nervilia prainiana (*King & Pantl.*) *Seiden f.* **(Orchidaceae)**
Pogonia prainiana King & Pantl.

Tuberous, 1-leaved herb; leaf orbicular obtuse, base cordate, coarsely hairy, green, usually spreading over the ground; inflorescence erect, 1-flowered, sepals and petals white with purple tinge.

Distribution: In Peninsular India, N.W. Himalaya, Sikkim, Manipur and Thailand.

Habenaria diphylla *Dalz.* **(Orchidaceae)** (Fig. 164)

Tuberous herb; leaves in unequal pairs, appressed to the ground, orbicular, or broadly ovate-obtuse, base cordate, 2–5 cms diam. glabrous; flowers greenish white in many-flowered racemes; bracts ovate, acuminate; sepals ovate-acute; petals linear, subfalcate acute, as long as the sepals; lip 3-partite, laterals much longer than the mid-lobe, spur as long as the ovary, inflated, acute.

Distribution: The plant occurs in W. Coast from Kanara to Travancore at low elevations.

Hybanthus enneaspermus (*L.f.*) *Muell.* **(Violaceae)** (Fig. 165)
Viola enneasperma Linn.
Ionidium suffruticosum (L.) Ging. ex DC.

Herb; leaves linearly lanceolate or elliptic, 2.5 × 0.7 cm, base attenuate, margin serrate, apex acute, subsessile; flowers rose, axillary, solitary; sepals 5, lanceolate, sub-equal, subconnate; petals 5, unequal, obovate, upper ones oblong, laterals falcate, lower ones orbicular, clawed, saccate at base; stamens 5, connate, anterior filaments appendaged, puberulous, anthers villous; ovary ovoid, ovules many on parietal placentae, style suberect, stigma oblique; capsule subglobose; seeds ribbed.

Distribution: Throughout widely distributed in Africa and Madagascar, Sri Lanka, China, New Guinea, and tropical Australia.

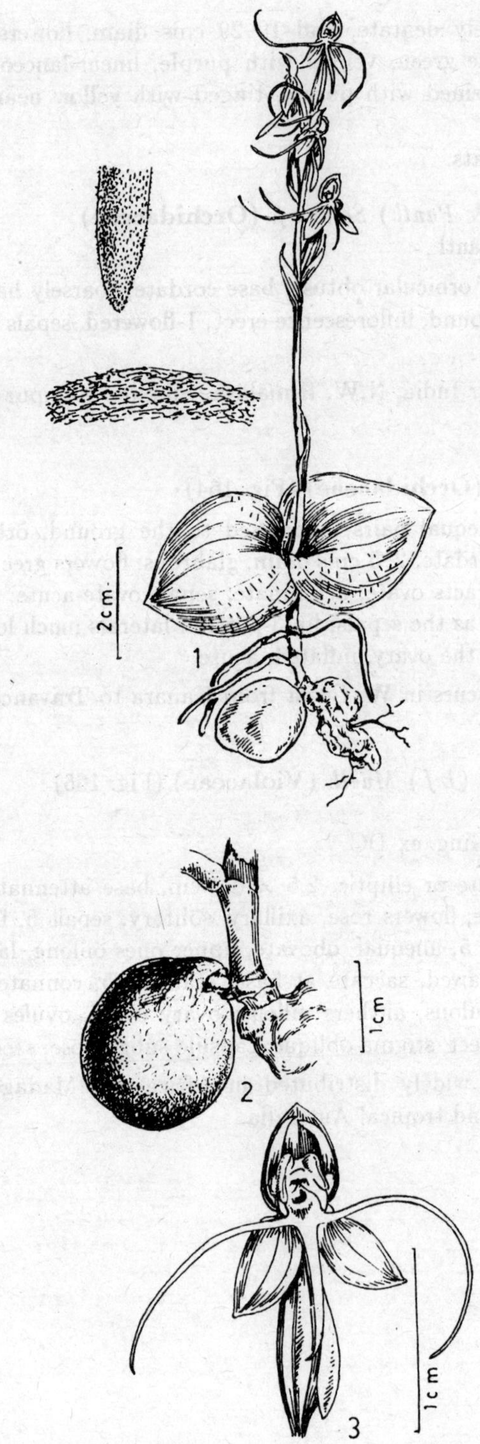

Figure 164: Habenaria diphylla Dalz. 1, Habit; 2, Tuber; 3, Flower (front view).

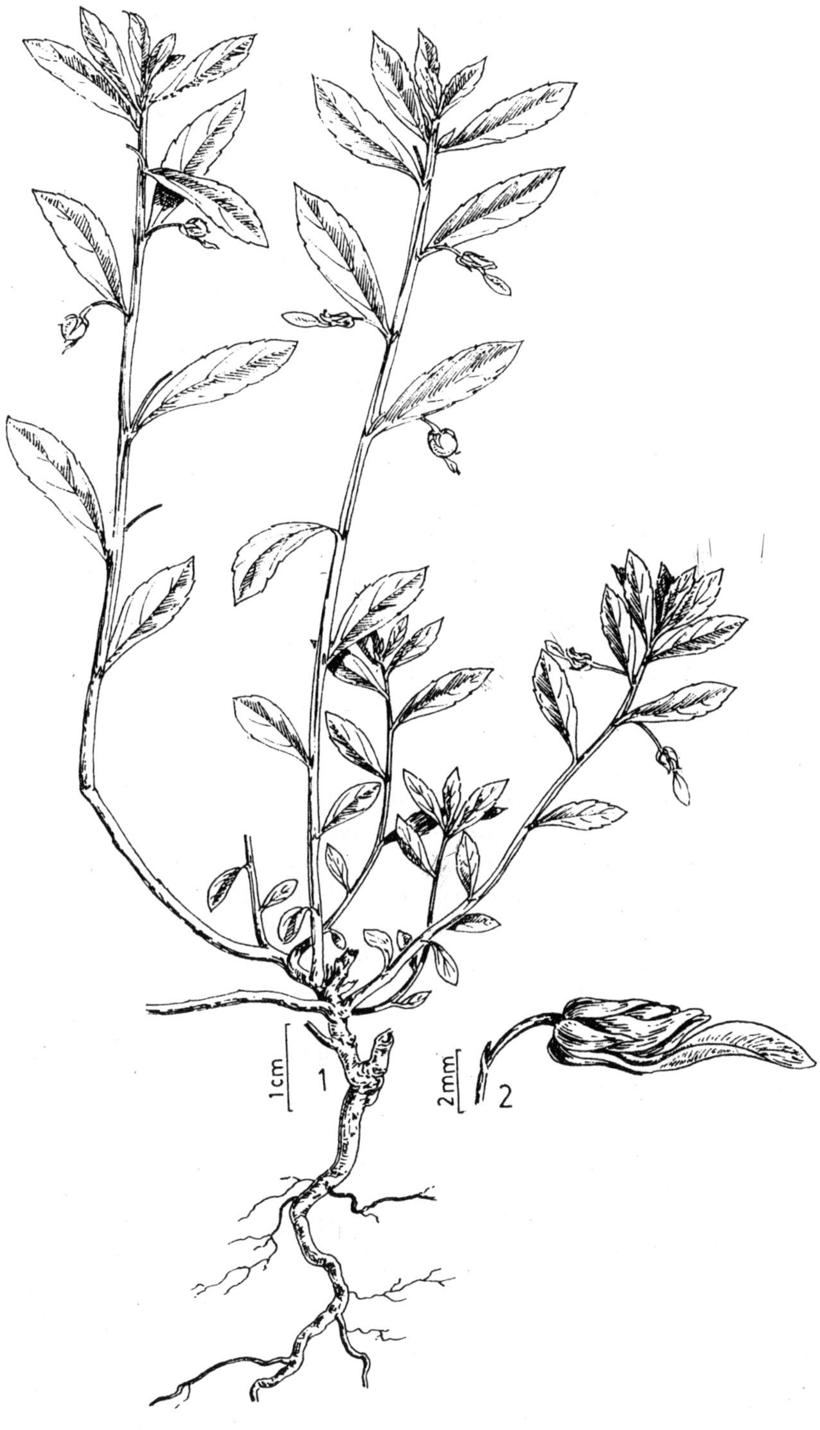

Figure 165: Hybanthus enneaspermus (L.f.) Muell. 1, Habit; 2, Flower.

PALĀŚAḤ (Mal. PLĀŚU)

The drug is considered to be efficaceous in the treatment of vaginal diseases, helminthic manifestations and haemorrhages. The bark of the tree is reported to be astringent, bitter, acrid, anthelmintic, aphrodisiac and alterative and is useful in abdominal tumours, colic, intestinal worms, bleeding piles, ulcers, haemorrhages, amenorrhoea and dysmenorrhoea. The gummy exudation from the bark which is called *Butea-gum* is an excellent astringent and is useful in diarrhoea, dysentery and also haemorrhage from the stomach and bladder. It is also applied to bruises, ulcers, ringworm and erysipelatous inflammations. The flowers are astringent, sweet, acrid and alleviate morbid *pitta* and *kapha* and cures burning sensation, thirst, skin diseases and painful micturition. The seeds alleviate deranged *vāta* and *kapha* and is useful in abdominal tumours, intestinal worms, urinary diseases, skin diseases and piles. (Nadkarni, 1954: 223). Bark, leaves, flowers, seeds and gum are used medicinally. It forms an important ingredient of preparations like *Ayaskṛti, Ceṛiya arimēdastailaṃ, Balātailaṃ, Palaśakṣāraṃ*, etc.

Believed to be a celestial tree, *pḷāśu* is associated with religious rites. This is reflected in its synonym *palāśaḥ* (possessing sacred leaves) and *parṇaḥ* (= ingratiating to those who strictly observe religious rites and ceremonies). The plant alleviates morbid *vāta* (*vātapōthaḥ*) and has flowers resembling the beak of parrots (*kiṁśukaḥ*) (cf. Moosad, 1983: 291, 292).

Madanapāla mentions four types of *palāśaḥ* with red, yellow, white and blue flowers (cf. Moosad, 1983: 292). Two varieties of *palāśaḥ* viz. *palāśaḥ* and *vallīpalāśaḥ* have been mentioned in Abhidhānamañjari and they are equated with *Butea monosperma* (Lam.) Taub. and *Butea superba* Roxb. (Papilionaceae) respectively (Mooss, 1978: 54). In practice, however, only the red-flowered *Butea monosperma*, known as *pḷāśu* in vernacular, is being used. Rheede has described and portrayed it under the name *Plaso* (Hort. Malab. 6: 29–30, t. 16–17, 1686).

Butea monosperma (*Lam.*) *Taub.* (Papilionaceae) (Fig. 166)
Erythrina monosperma Lam.
Butea frondosa Roxb.

Middle sized, deciduous tree; branchlets tomentose; leaves alternate, trifoliolate, leaflets large, 14–22 × 12–20 cms, coriaceous, obovate-obtuse, entire, glabrous above, sericeous below; flowers large, bright red, clustered on the trunk and older branches; calyx tube velvety; corolla red, papilionaceous; standard lanceolate, silk-pubescent without, wings falcate, adnate to keel, keel incurved, beaked; stamens diadelphous; staminal sheath thick, curved; ovary silky pubescent; fruit an indehiscent, flat, thin pod, to 16 × 5 cms.

Distribution: All dry districts of India, both in open country and deciduous forests. Distributed also in tropical Himalaya, Sri Lanka, S.E. Asia and Malesia.

Note: In ancient Āyurvēdic literature, there is extensive mention of the drug *palāśa*

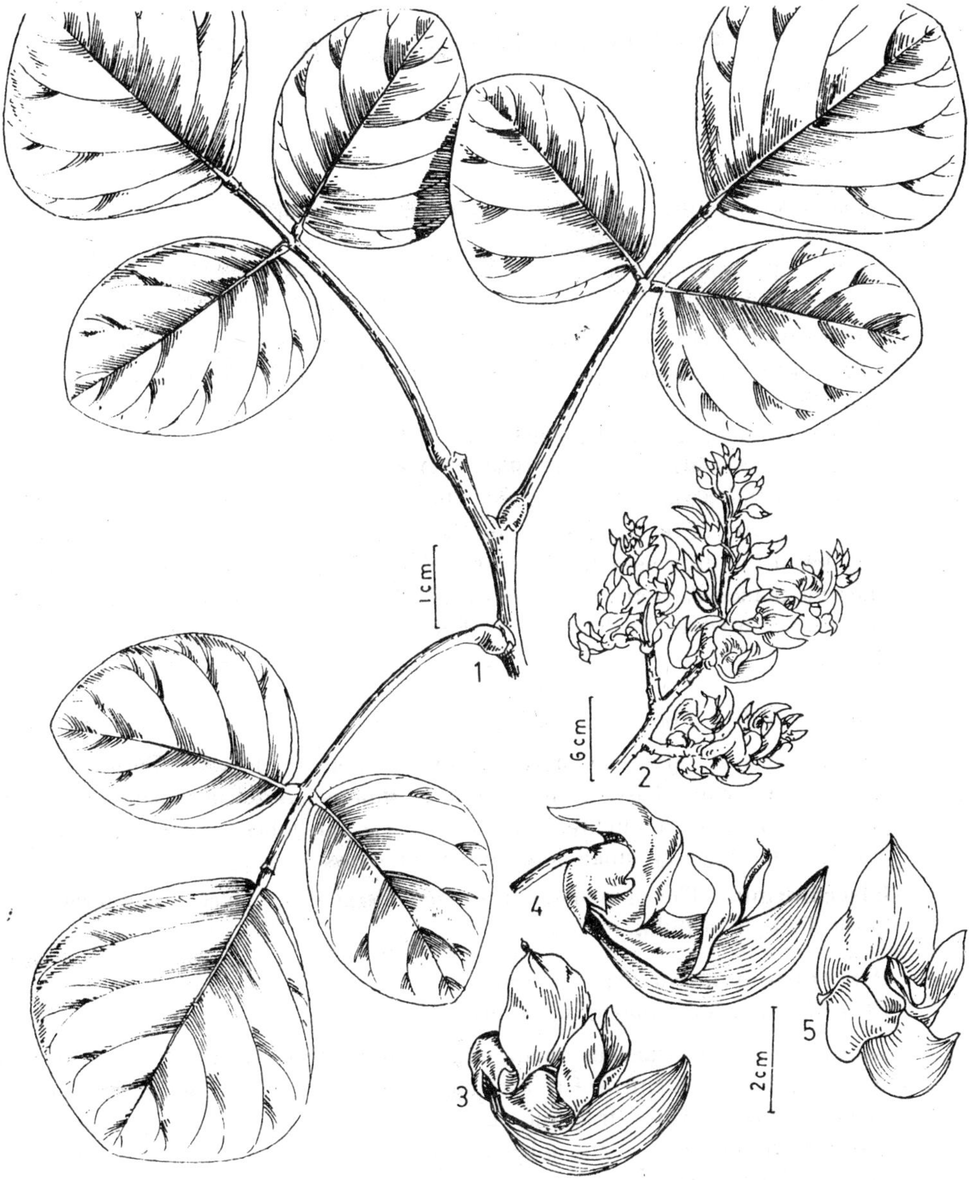

Figure 166: Butea monosperma (Lam.) Taub. 1, Vegetative branch; 2, Inflorescence; 3–5, Flower, different views.

in the treatment of worm infestations (*kṛmirōga*). This property has been clinically proved by many. The seeds have been found to be an effective cure for ascariasis (Shaw & Thripathi, 1982) and thread worm infestation (Jain & Naqvi, 1986). The antifertility activity of the seeds has been proved by Mehta *et al.* (1983), while the bark has been demonstrated to have significant antiasthmatic property (Phadke *et al.*, 1983).

PAPHAṆAḤ (Mal. PĀVEṬṬA)

Paphaṇaḥ is another drug which does not find mention in classical Āyurvēdic literature. Yet, this has been in use in Kerala since long (See Rheede, Hort. Malab. 5: 19–20. t. 10. 1685) and is a constituent drug of *Paphaṇādi tailaṃ* and *Phaphaṇādi ghṛtaṃ*. Leaves and root form the officinal part. Root is bitter, tonic, aperient and is prescribed in visceral obstructions, renal dropsy and ascites. Leaves form a good fomentation for haemorrhoidal pains and piles (Nadkarni, 1954: 925; Chopra *et al.*, 1956: 187).

The source plant is identified as *Pavetta indica* Linn. (Rubiaceae) by Kirtikar & Basu (1918: 659), Nadkarni (1954: 924) and Chopra *et al.* (1956: 187). Rheede's account of this plant (Hort. Malab. 5: 19–20, t. 10. 1685) also proves that this has been the source of the drug in Kerala since a long time. But a survey of the market samples of the drug used in different parts of Kerala reveals that some other Rubiaceous plants like *Pavetta tomentosa, Morinda pubcscens* and *Stylocoryne lucens* are also accepted as the drug source. The various plant sources can be identified as follows:

Pavetta indica *Linn.* **(Rubiaceae)** (Fig. 167)

Much branched, glabrous shrub; branches angular; leaves elliptic-obovate or oblanceolate-acute, base acute-attenuate; flowers white in terminal coymbose panicles; calyx teeth minute; corolla tube 1.5 cm, lobes 4, obovate; stamens 4; filaments short; berry subglobose, to 0.8 cm across.

Distribution: The plant is seen as an undergrowth of deciduous forests in all forest districts in India.

Pavetta tomentosa *Roxb. ex Smith*
P. indica Linn. var. *tomentosa* (Smith) Hook. f.

Tomentose shrub; branches quadrangular; leaves broadly elliptic to oblanceolate acute, 12–17 × 5–8 cms, softly tomentose above, densely so below, base acute or rounded; flowers white, fragrant, in terminal tomentose cymes; calyx tomentose outside; corolla tube 1.5 cm, lobes 4, oblong; stamens 4, filaments short, anthers linear-oblong; berries subglobose, 7 cm across.

Distribution: India and Indo-China in deciduous forests and in scrub jungles along hill slopes.

Morinda pubescens *Smith* **(Rubiaceae)** (Fig. 168)
Morinda coreia Buch.-Ham.
M. tinctoria Roxb.

Tree; leaves opposite, elliptic to oblanceolate-acuminate, upto 20 × 10 cms, glabrous above, pale beneath; flowers white in simple terminal, axillary or leaf opposed capitate, inflorescence; calyx truncate; corolla tube 1.5 cm lobes 5, oblong; stamens 5,

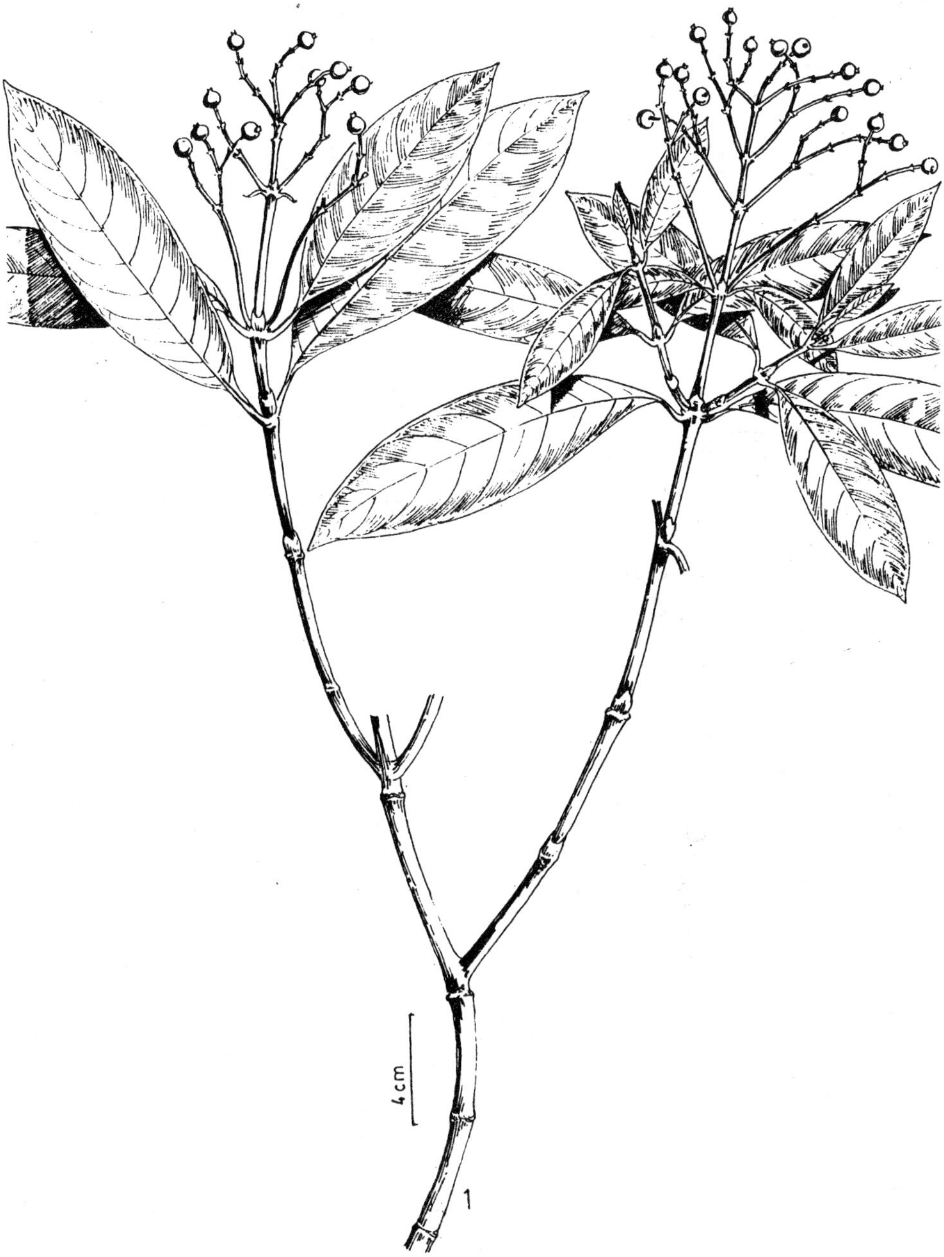

Figure 167: Pavetta indica L.

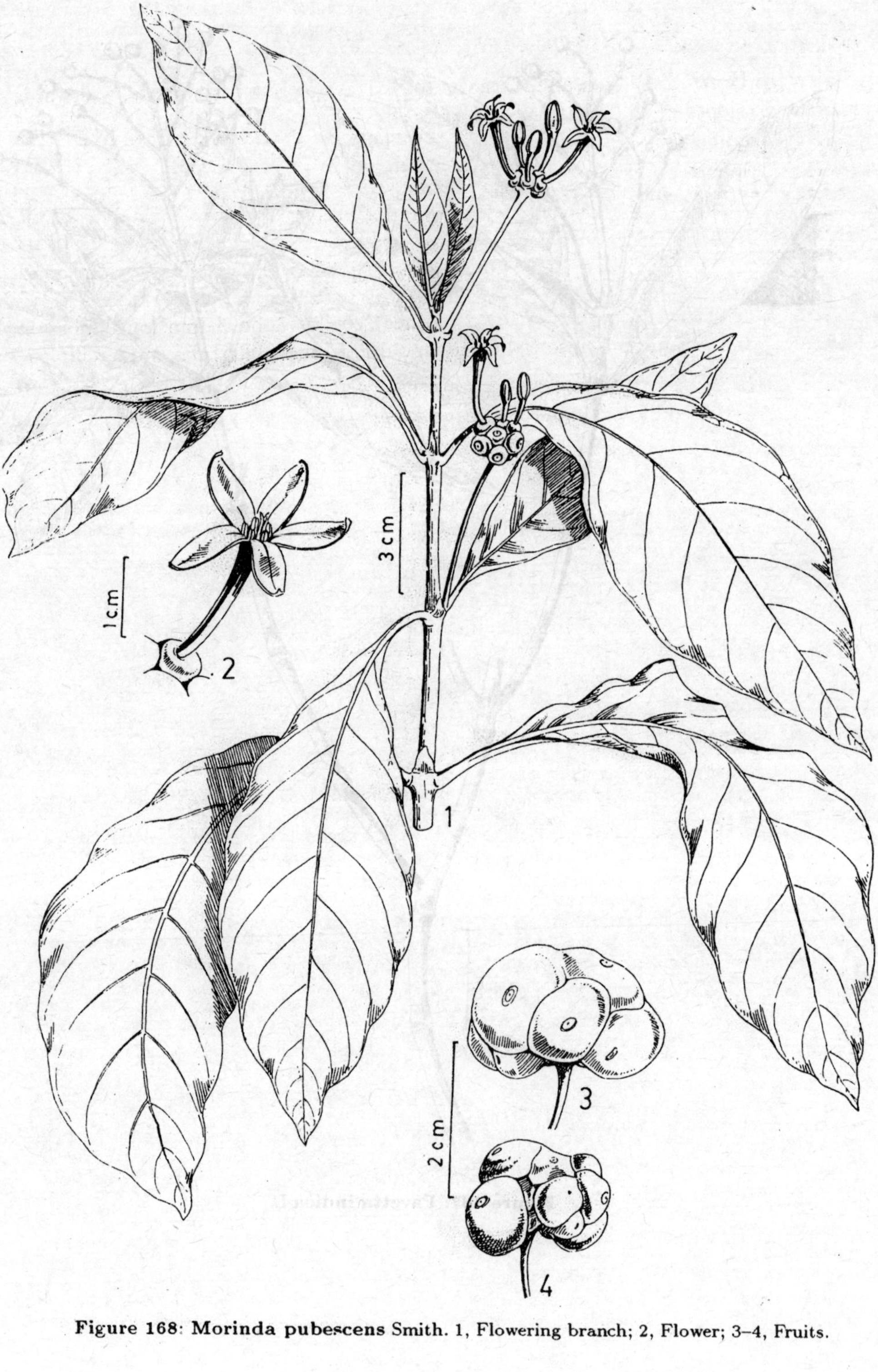

Figure 168: **Morinda pubescens** Smith. 1, Flowering branch; 2, Flower; 3–4, Fruits.

exserted; style forked from above the middle; fruit a syncarpium to 2 cm across; seeds oblong or obovoid.

Distribution: S. Deccan and Carnatic to S. Travancore in dry forests, westwards to the E. slopes of the Ghats at low levels. It is also reported from Sri Lanka and Malay Archipelago.

Stylocoryne lucens *Gamble* **(Rubiaceae)** (Fig. 169)
Webera lucens Hook. f.

Large glabrous shrub; leaves lanceolate or oblanceolate, obtusely acute, coriaceous, to 15 × 4.5 cms prominently veined, glabrous; flowers white, fragrant, in terminal corymbose cymes; calyx turbinate, 5-toothed; corolla tube 3 mm long, lobes 5, oblong, 5 mm; stamens 5, inserted on the mouth of the corolla tube, anthers linear; ovary 2 celled, style slender, stigma fusiform; berry ovoid.

Distribution: W. Ghats, especially in Shola forests.

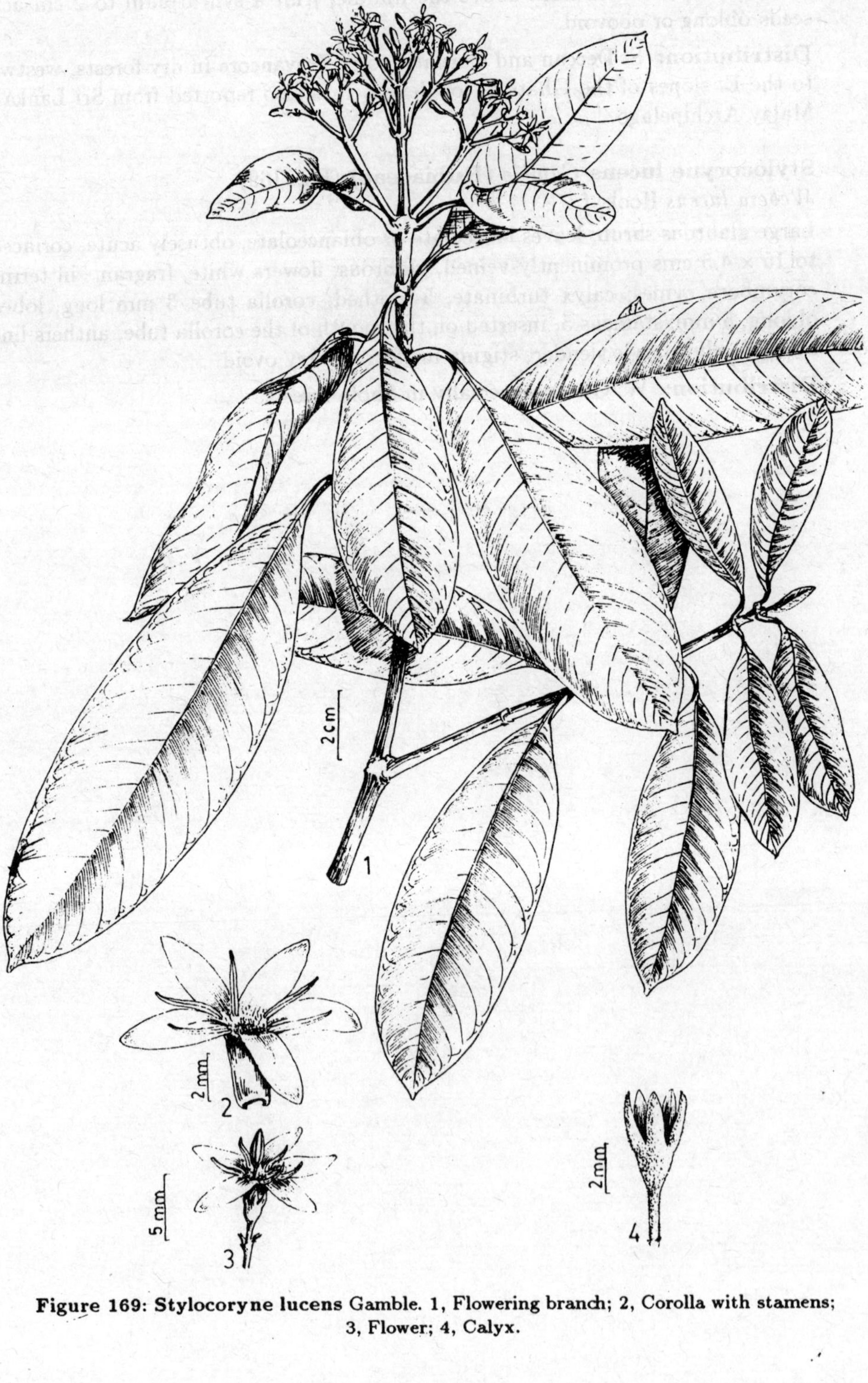

Figure 169: Stylocoryne lucens Gamble. 1, Flowering branch; 2, Corolla with stamens; 3, Flower; 4, Calyx.

PĀRANTĪ (Mal. TECCI, CETTI)

Pāranti is considered to be a good blood-purifier and hence beneficial in skin affections like itches, scabies, boils, etc. An infusion of leaves and stem is often used as an ablution for infantile skin ailments. It is astringent, antiseptic and sedative. Root is useful in diarrhoea, dysentery, gonorrhoea and fever. Flowers are administered externally to sores, chronic ulcers, scabies and some types of dermatitis and also given internally for cholera, dysentery, gonorrhoea and lencorrhoea (Nadkarni, 1954: 699; Mooss, 1978: 111, Nesamony, 1985: 286). The flowers form an ingredient of *Cemparutyādi* coconut oil. Roots are used to prepare *Pārantyādi tailaṃ*.

There is no mention of *pāranti* in classical Āyurvēdic literature and it seems to be an innovation of Kerala physicians, who have unanimously accepted *Ixora coccinia* Linn. (Rubiaceae) as the drug source. That this has been in use since very early times is obvious from Rheede's description (Hort. Malab. 2: 17–18, t. 13. 1679-*Schetti*).

Ixora coccinia *Linn.* **(Rubiaceae)** (Fig. 170)

Woody shrub; leaves glabrous, leathery, sessile, opposite, oblong or obovate, acute or obtuse, cordate at base, 8 × 4.5 cms, flowers red in terminal corymbose cymes; calyx teeth minute; corolla tube 3.5 cm long, lobes 4, spreading; stamens 4, inserted between the corolla lobes; berries subglobose, green when young and dark red when ripe.

Distribution: The plant is found throughout India, more common in the W. Peninsula in scrub jungles. Widely cultivated throughout the tropics.

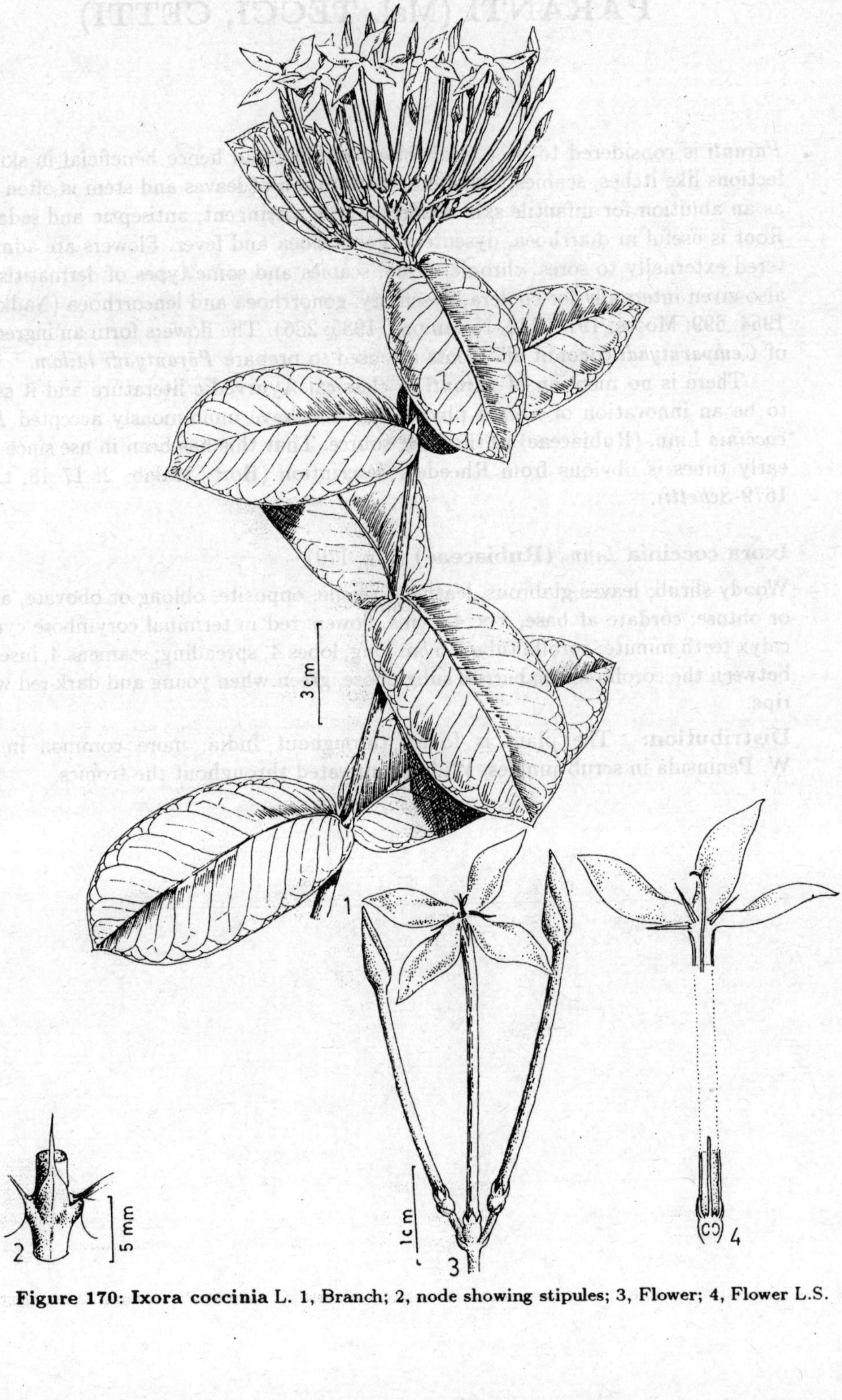

Figure 170: Ixora coccinia L. 1, Branch; 2, node showing stipules; 3, Flower; 4, Flower L.S.

PĀRIBHADRAḤ (Mal. MURIKKU)

Pāribhadra is acrid, hot, anthelmintic, carminative, diuretic, galactagogue, expectorant and febrifuge. Bark and leaves are used in medicine. It is used in anorexia, ear diseases, helminthic manifestations, inflammation, intestinal worms and obesity. The drug promotes appetite, destroys pathogenic parasites, arrests excessive micturition and cures oedema, flatulence, colic, arthritis, skin affections and diseases due to the morbidity of *vāta* and *kapha*. Decoction of the bark is used in dysentery, ophthalmia and other eye diseases. Fresh juice of the leaves is a good vermifuge. It cures dysmenorrhoea, reduces excess fat and increases secretion of milk. Crushed leaves are applied to rheumatic joints to relieve pain (Nadkarni, 1954: 508; Aiyer & Kolammal, 1963. 7: 4; Kurup *et al.*, 1979: 159) *Mahārājaprasāriṇi tailaṃ* and *Viḍaṅgamūlādi kaṣāyaṃ* are some of the preparations using the drug.

The texts describe the plant as one having small thorns or prickles all over (*kaṇṭakī, kaṇṭakiṁśukaḥ, mandāraḥ*) and possessing reddish flowers (*tāmrapuṣpaḥ, raktapuṣpī, rōhitaḥ*) (Aiyer & Ammal, 1963. 7: 4). Most of the authors equate the drug with *Erythrina variegata* L. var. *orientalis* Merr. belonging to Papilionaceae and locally known as *murikku* or *muḷḷumurikku* (Kirthikar & Basu, 1918; 439; Nadkarni, 1954; 507; Kurup *et al.*, 1979; 159; Kapoor & Mitra, 1979: 76; Dey, 1980: 114; Chunekar, 1982: 334; Sharma, 1983: 99) Rheede has described and portrayed *Erythrina variegata* Linn. as the source of *Mouricou, Muricu* (Hort. Malab. 6. 13–14, t. 7. 1686). This is the most commonly accepted source of the drug in Kerala. But occasionally, *E. stricta* is also found to be used as *pāribhadra*.

Abhidhānamañjari mentions two varieties of *pāribhadra*, namely a black or dark variety called *karimurukku* and a white variety *veṇmurukku*, having similar properties. (Aiyer & Kolammal, 1963. 7: 4). In practice, however, this varietal distinction is not observed.

Erythrina variegata *Linn. var.* **orientalis** *Merr.* **(Papilionaceae)**
Erythrina indica Lam.

Unarmed, large, deciduous tree, branchlets stellate-pubescent; leaves alternate, pinnately 3-foliolate, stipulate; leaflets rhomboid-ovate, acuminate, inequilateral, upto 17 x 17 cms, flowers bright red in clustered racemes at the tips of branches; calyx tubular, spathaceous, 5 toothed at apex in bud; corolla papilionaceous, much exserted; stamens 10, exserted; ovary superior, long stalked, unilocular with 10–15 or more ovules, style incured at the apex ending in a capitate, glutinous stigma; fruit a stipitate, falcate, linear, cylindrical, turgid pod, compressed between the seeds, with a sharp curved beak.

Distribution: The plant is found throughout India. It is common in Assam, Bengal, Konkan, N. Canara, Madras, Kerala. Also distributed in Africa, Madagascar, Sri Lanka, Burma, Thailand, Cambodia, Laos, Vietnam, China, through Malesia.

Erythrina stricta *Roxb.* (Papilionaceae) (Fig. 171)

Medium sized deciduous tree, armed with short dense sharp prickles; leaves alternate, pinnately 3-foliolate, stipulate; leaflets broadly deltoid-ovate, 8–12 × 9–20 cms, glabrescent on both surfaces, inequilateral; flowers scarlet-red, crowded in dense terminal unilateral racemes; calyx spathaceous, entire at the tip; corolla papilionaceous; stamens 10, monadelphous; ovary villous containing 4 to 6 ovules; fruit a stalked, linear, 1–3 seeded pod.

Distribution: The plant is found in Assam, Manipur, Chittagong and the West Coast of Kerala and also in Nepal, Burma, Thailand, Vietnam and China.

Note: The pharmacognosy, chemistry and pharmacology of ***Erythrina variegata*** var. ***orientalis*** have been described by Satyavati *et al.* (1976: 390–392).

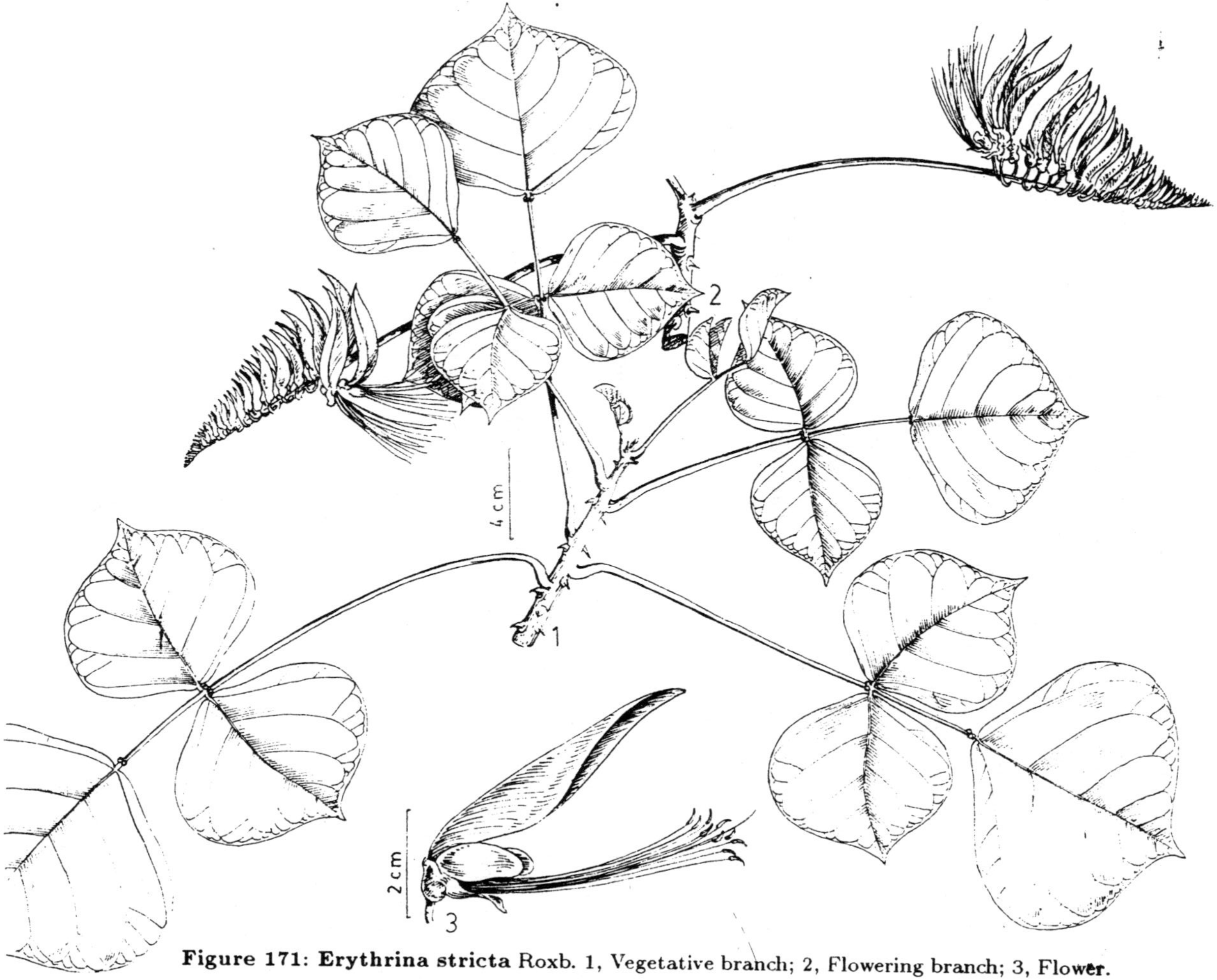

Figure 171: Erythrina stricta Roxb. 1, Vegetative branch; 2, Flowering branch; 3, Flower.

PĀRIṢAḤ (Mal. PŪVARAŚU)

Pāriṣa is a reputed remedy for skin diseases. According to the texts, it is light, acrid, cooling and astringent and is useful in disorders due to morbid *kapha* and *pitta*, dysentery, piles, diabetes, haemorrhoids, excessive thirst and poison. The drug cures ulcers, itching, scabies and other skin diseases and urinary disorders (Sharma, 1983: 680). Bark is the officinal part. It is an ingredient of *Āraṇyātuḷasyādi* coconut oil and *Yaṣṭimadhukādi tailaṃ*.

Most of the authors have equated the drug with *Thespesia populnea* (L.) Sol. ex. Corr. of Malvaceae. (Kirtikar & Basu, 1918: 186; Vaidya, 1936; 98; Nadkarni, 1954: 629; Chunekar, 1982: 515; Sharma, 1983: 680; Nesamony, 1985: 372). But some people consider it as a constituent of the group *pañcavalkala* i.e. group of five barks, others being *aśvattha, nyagrōdha, uduṁbara* and *pḷakṣa*, all equated with different *Ficus* species (Chunekar, 1982: 515). *Kapītanaḥ*, a synonym of *pāriṣa* is commented upon by Pāṭhyakara and Parameswara as *kallāl* which has been identified as *Ficus tjakela* of Moraceae (cf. Mooss, 1980: 104). Kerala physicians, however, consider them to be two different drugs and equate *pāriṣa* with *Thespesia populnea*, locally called *pūvaraśu* or *pūparutti* (see also Rheede, Hort. Malab. 1: 51–52, t. 29. 1678).

Thespesia populnea (*Linn.*) *Sol. ex. Corr.* **(Malvaceae)** (Fig. 172)
Hibiscus populneus Linn.

Tree; leaves alternate, long petioled, broadly ovate-cordate, acuminate, entire, 5–7 nerved from base, 5–13 × 4–10 cm; flowers solitary, axillary large, yellow, long peduncled; epicalyx segments 3–5; calyx cupular, lobes 5; petals 5, yellow, obovate, united at the base with the staminal column; capsule sub-globose, indehiscent, glabrescent; seeds obovoid.

Distribution: The plant is widely distributed in the tropics. In India it is seen wild in peninsular part, also grown as an avenue tree.

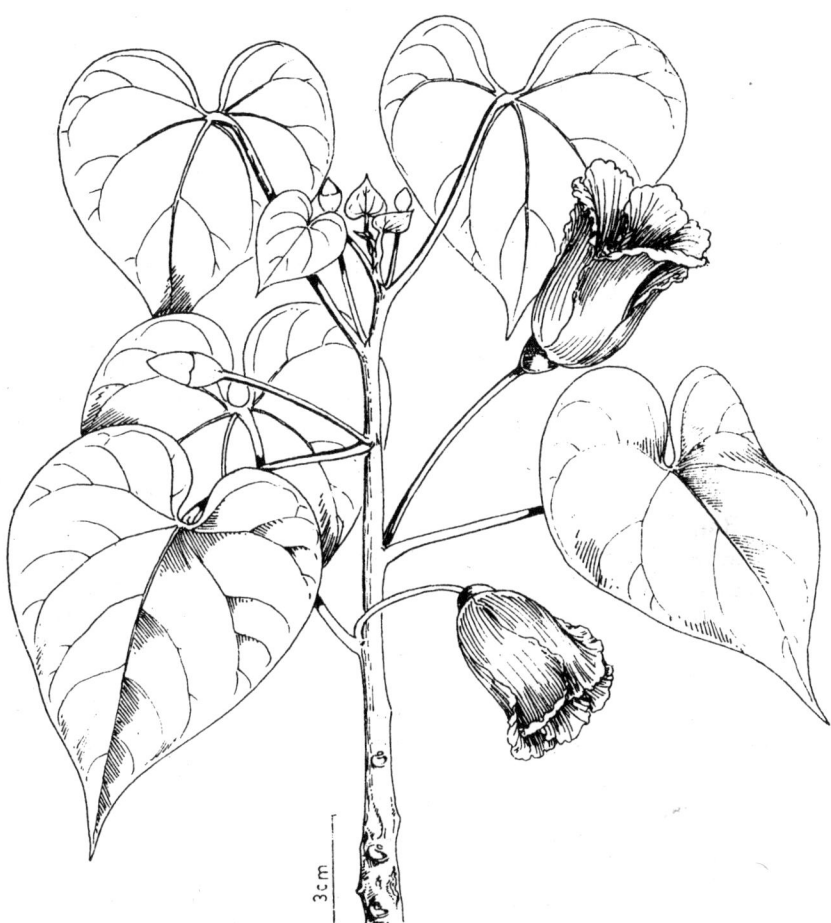

Figure 172: Thespesia populnea (L.) Sol. ex. corr.

PAṚPAṬAKAḤ (Mal. PAṚPAṬAKAṂ)

This is esteemed as a specific remedy for all types of fevers. It overcomes morbid *pitta* and *kapha*, purifies blood, improves digestion, stimulates the action of liver and cures burning sensation, thirst and skin diseases. The drug is diuretic, anthelmintic, digestive and constipating. The whole plant is medicinal (Sharma, 1983: 321, Nesamony, 1985; 339). The important preparations using the drug are *Amṛtāriṣṭaṃ, Candanāsavaṃ, Mahātiktakaghṛtaṃ, Jātyadi tailaṃ, Āraṇyātuḷasyādi* coconut oil, etc.

The synonyms do not help in the accurate identification of the plant source of this drug and consequently there is a lot of controversy regarding the botanical identity of the drug. Most of the authors equate it with *Fumaria indica* (Hausskn.) Pugsley of Fumariaceae (Kirtikar & Basu, 1918: 86; Chopra *et al.*, 1956: 122; Kurup *et al.*, 1979: 161; Dey, 1980: 115; Sharma, 1983: 320). The physicians of Punjab, Sindh, Rajputana, U.P. and Bihar use this plant as *paṛpaṭaka* (Chunekar, 1982: 324; Vaidya Bapalal, 1982: 209). According to the Ayurvedic formulary of India also, this is the accepted source of the drug (Anonymous, 1978a: 251). Some others equate it with *Rungia repens* Nees of the family Acanthaceae (Kapoor & Mitra, 1979: 66). This is the *paṛpaṭaka* of Gujarat and Saurashtra. It is believed to be efficaceous in slow fevers (Vaidya Bapalal, 1982: 209). Other plants equated with the drug are *Polycarpaea corymbosa* (Linn.) Lamk. (Caryophyllaceae), *Justicia procumbens* Linn. (Acanthaceae), *Glossocardia linearifolia* Cass. (Asteraceae) and *Mollugo stricta* Linn. (Molluginaceae) (Chunekar, 1982: 324).

In Kerala, however, none of these is the accepted source of the drug. Instead, three closely similar species of *Hedyotis* (=*Oldenlandia*), viz. *Hedyotis brachypoda* (=*O. brachypoda*), *H. corymbosa* (=*O. corymbosa*) and *H. diffusa* (=*O. diffusa*) are the ones which are generally accepted. That this has been the accepted practice here since long, is testified by Rheede's portrayal of *H. corymbosa* with its vernacular name *Parpadagam* (Hort. Malab. 10:69 t. 35. 1690). Kirtikar & Basu (1918: 645), Nadkarni (1954: 869), Chopra *et al.*, (1956: 180) and Chunekar (1982: 324) also have listed the name *paṛpada* under this species, among many others. In practice, however, Kerala physicians do not make a distinction and all the three species are generally found to be accepted as the source of this drug. The three species are very closely similar and there was confusion about their identity until recently when Sivarajan *et al.* (Taxon 39: 665–674. 1990) made an exhaustive revisionary study of this complex group.

Hedyotis brachypoda (*DC.*) *Sivar. et al.* **(Rubiaceae)** (Fig. 173:1–2)
Oldenlandia brachypoda DC.
Hedyotis diffusa auct., non Willd.

Diffuse or prostrate herbs; leaves linear-lanceolate; flowers axillary, solitary or in pairs, sessile or stout-pedicelled; calyx of 4 lobes, usually spreading in bud; corolla tube longer than calyx, 4-lobed, tube without a ring of hyaline hairs within; stamens

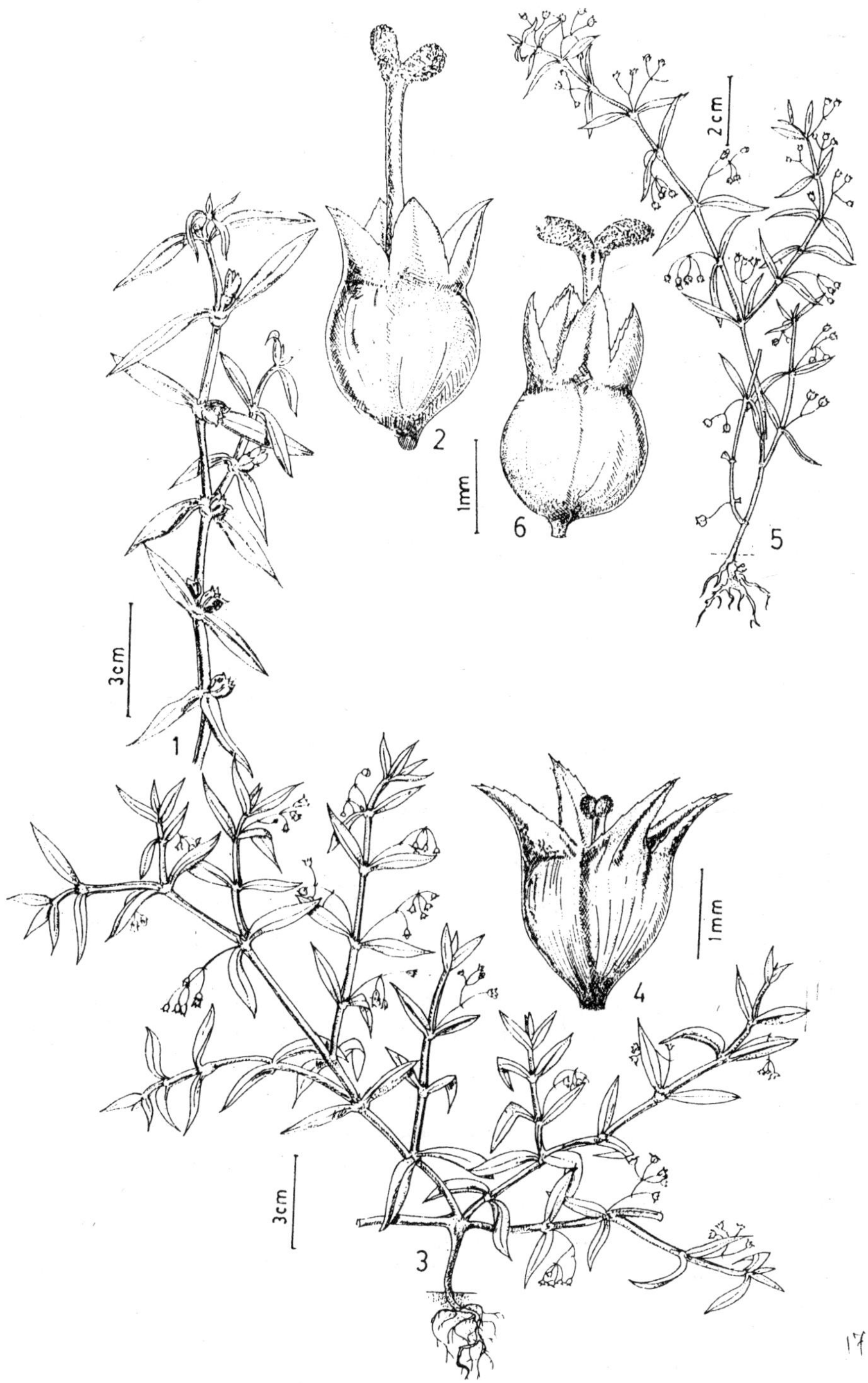

Figure 173: 1–2, **Hedyotis brachypoda** (DC.) Sivar. et al. 3–4, **Hedyotis corymbosa** (L.) Lam. 5–6, **Hedyotis diffusa** Willd.

4, inserted at the sinuses of the corolla lobes; style and stigma exceeding calyx; fruit subglobose; disc not raised.

Distribution: South and Southeast Asia and in America. In India it is a common weed in wet low lands and in cultivated fields.

Hedyotis corymbosa (*Linn.*) *Lam.* **(Rubiaceae)** (Fig. 173:3–4)
Oldenlandia corymbosa Linn.

Diffuse or prostrate herbs, often rooting at lower nodes; leaves linear to lanceolate; flowers in many flowered, axillary, corymbose cymes, distinctly pedicelled; calyx 4–5 lobed; corolla white or pinkish, 4–5 lobed, tube with a ring of hyaline hairs at the throat; stamens 4–5, inserted at the base of the corolla tube; style and stigma much shorter than calyx; capsule obovoid.

Distribution: Pantropical. Here it is a common weed in wet low lands and in cultivated fields.

Hedyotis diffusa *Willd.* **(Rubiaceae)** (Fig. 173:5–6)
Oidenlandia diffusa (Willd.) Roxb.

Erect or diffuse herbs; stem terete; leaves linear-lanceolate; flowers in axillary, pedunculate cymes or 1-2 nate; calyx 4–5 lobed; corolla tube without a ring of hyaline hairs inside, 4–5 lobed; stamens 4–5, inserted at the sinuses of the corolla lobes; style and stigma exceeding calyx; capsule subglobose with a prominently raised disc at the top.

Distribution: South and Southeast Asia and in America. Here it is usually found as a weed in fallow or cultivated low lands and in grasslands.

Fumaria indica (*Hausskn.*) *Pugsley* **(Fumariaceae)** (Fig. 174)
F. vaillantii Lois.
F. parviflora ssp. *vaillantii* (Lois.) Hook. f.

Diffuse annual herb; branchlets grooved, puberulous; leaves 2–3 pinnatisect, 5–7 cm, segments membraneous, entire; flowers small, white or pink with purple tips in terminal or leaf-opposed racemes; sepals 2, ovate; petals 2 + 2, oblong; stamens 3 + 3, staminal sheath subacute above; ovary ovoid, 1-celled, ovules 1 or 2 on parietal placentae, style filiform, stigma 2-lobed; fruit indehiscent, globose, nutlet, 1-seeded.

Distribution: A weed of cultivation, chiefly at somewhat high elevation, as on the Mysore Plateau and in the E. Nilgiris. Also found in Central Asia.

Note: Pharmacognostic studies on *Oldenlandia corymbosa* have been done by Datta & Sen (1969). The chemical and pharmacological studies on different species of the genus *Hedyotis* (= *Oldenlandia*) have been discussed by Satyavati *et al.* (1987). Mehra *et al.* (1968) have described the pharmacognosy of *Fumaria indica* and its adulterants.

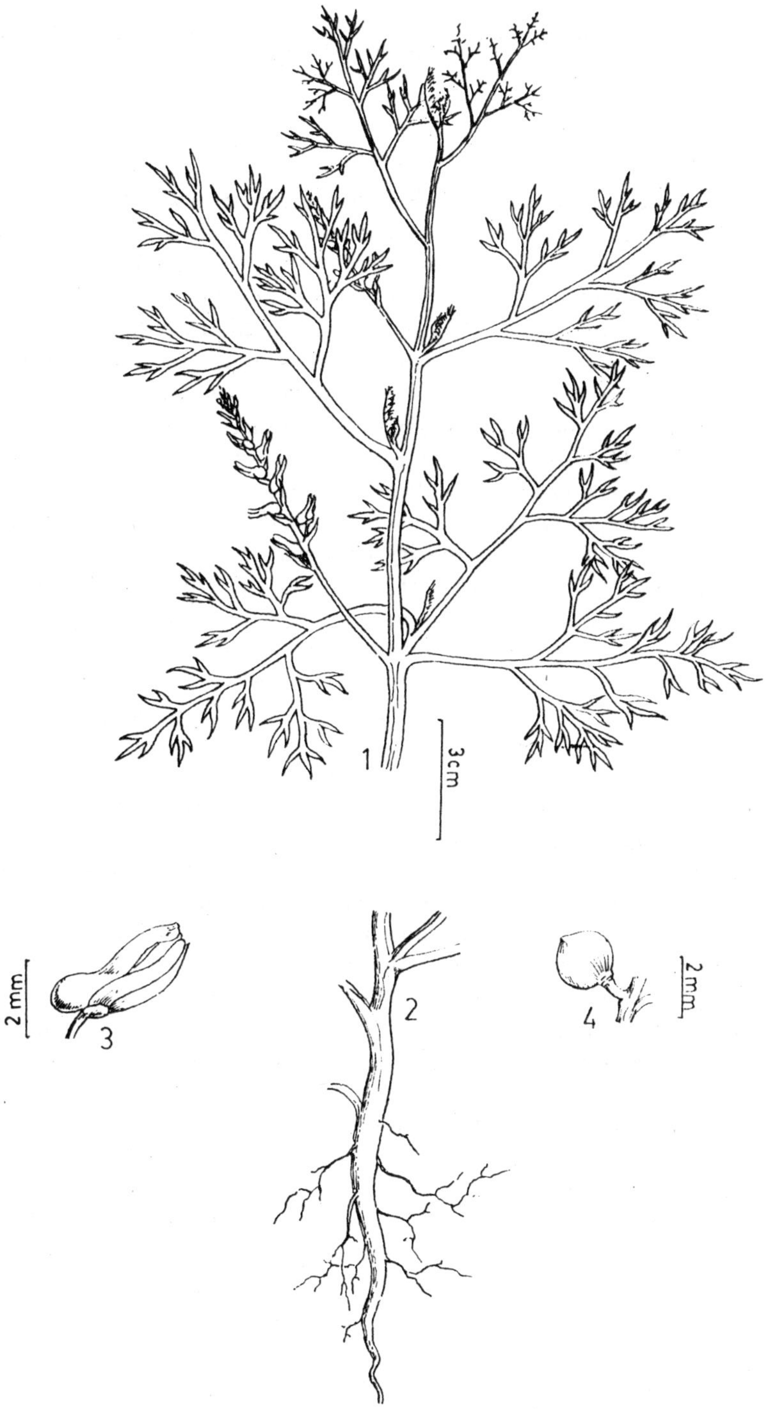

Figure 174: **Fumaria indica** (Hausskn.) Pugsley. 1, Habit; 2, Roots; 3, Flower; 4, Fruit.

PĀṢĀṆABHĒDAḤ (Mal. KALLŪṚVAÑCI)

Etymologically, the name *pāṣāṇabhēda* means that which breaks or destroys stones. As the name implies, it is considered a specific remedy against kidney and bladder stones. This is one of the twenty one drugs that constitute the *Vīratarādi* or *Vēllantarādi gaṇa* of Vāgbhaṭa which eradicates diseases due to *vāta*, vesical calculus, gravels, dysuria and anuria (Mooss, 1980: 63). Root is the officinal part and is reported to be light, cool, astringent, bitter, diuretic and useful in cough, cardiac disorders, dysuria, blood disorders (*raktapitta*), piles, fever, poison, ulcers, swellings, uterine disorders and diseases caused by the morbidity of the three *dōṣās* (Sharma, 1983: 652). The drug enters into the composition of preparations like *Pūtikarañjāsavaṃ, Traikaṇṭaka ghṛtaṃ, Valiya Marmaguḷika*, etc.

The various names (*pāṣāṇabhēdaḥ, aśmaghnaḥ, giribhid, bhinnayōginī*) attributed to this drug refer to its capacity to break or destroy stones. But one cannot be very sure whether they refer to the ability of the drug to cure stones and gravels in human body (like the bladder stones, kidney stones etc.) or they indicate the habitat characters of the plant itself, in which case it should be one which grows in crevices of rocks leading to its final disintegration (Vaidya Bapalal, 1982: 1).

However, there are no reliable indications regarding the identity of the herb in the texts and as a result, the plant source of this drug is highly disputed. To make matters worse, *Rājanighaṇṭu* has described four different types of the drug viz. *vaṭapatri, airāvati, śvētāśmabhēda* and *kṣudrapāṣāṇabhēda* which are supposed to have the same therapeutic properties (Chunekar, 1982: 105). In practice, anyway this varietal distinction is not in vogue, at least in Kerala. Yet, there is no unanimity of opinion among men of Āyurvēda regarding the plant source of this drug. Nadkarni (1954; 371, 652, 1054, 1113) and Chopra *et al.* (1956: 74, 135, 215, 37) attribute the name *pāṣāṇabhēda* to four different plants namely *Coleus ambonicus* Lour. (Lamiaceae), *Homonoia riparia* Lour. (Euphorbiaceae), *Rotula aquatica* Lour. (Boraginaceae) and *Saxifraga ligulata* Wall. (Saxifragaceae). According to Kirtikar & Basu (1918), *Coleus aromaticus* and *Saxifraga ligulata* are the sources of the drug. Kapoor & Mitra (1979: 66), Dey (1980: 116) and Sharma (1983: 651) equate the drug with the mountain species, *Saxifraga ligulata*. This plant is reportedly in use in Gujarat and North India as *pāṣāṇabhēda* (Vaidya Bapalal, 1982: 6). Singh and Chunekar (1972: 247) comment that its habitat (growing on rocks) and its clinical efficacy in dissolving stones formed in the urinary tract, fully justify its use as *pāṣāṇabhēda*.

There are a score of other plants equated with this drug. Kurup *et al.* (1979: 163) consider *Aerva lanata* (Linn.) Juss. of Amaranthaceae as the source of the drug and Vaidya Bapalal (1982: 1) has corroborated this by reporting that people of Madras and Andhra Pradesh have found it efficaceous. In some other places, *Kalanchoe pinnata* (= *Bryophyllum calycinum* Salisb.) of Crassulaceae, *Ocimum basilicum* Linn. (Lamiaceae), *Bridelia montana* (Euphorbiaceae) and *Ammania baccifera* (Lythraceae) are also reported to be used as the source plants of this drug.

(Bapalal Vaidya, 1982: 7). Nadkarni (1954: 91) equates *Ammania baccifera* Linn. with ***kallūrvañci***, the vernacular name for *pāṣāṇabhēda*. Vaidya Bapalal (1982: 6) has reported that this plant, known as *agnigarbha* (= pregnant with fire) probably due to its property of producing blisters, is used as the source of the drug in some parts of Kerala. But our field studies do not lend any support to this.

In Kerala, *Coleus ambonicus* and *Aerva lanata* are used as sources of some other different drugs, *kaññikkūrkka* and *cerūḷa* respectively. *Kalanchoe pinnata* is locally called *'elamuḷacci'* and is not in use. The two plants widely used as the sources of *pāṣāṇabhēda* in Kerala are *Rotula aquatica* Lour. (Boraginaceae) and *Homonoia reparia* Lour. (Euphorbiaceae)

They can be identified as follows:

Rotula aquatica *Lour.* **(Boraginaceae)** (Fig. 175)

Woody perennial herbs with trailing branches, often rooting at lower nodes and producing dwarf shoots in the axils of leaves; leaves simple, alternate, 1.5 × 0.8 cms, obovate-spathulate, glabrous; flowers pink, solitary, axillary, subsessile; calyx 5-partite; corolla tube short, campanulate, 5 lobed; stamens 5, alternating with the corolla lobes; fruits orange-red when ripe.

Distribution: Commonly growing along rocky riverbanks, this is a rhoeophyte widely distributed in India, Sri Lanka, tropical South East Asia and Latin America.

Homonoia riparia *Lour.* **(Euphorbiaceae)** (Fig. 176)
Adelia neriifolia Roth.

Woody herbs or shrubs with fibrous stems; leaves spiral, linear or lanceolate, acute, upto 25 × 2 cm, entire or serrulate, glabrous, glandular-scaly beneath; flowers unisexual, greenish in axillary, solitary or clustered spikes; capsule of 3–2 valued cocci, 4 mm across.

A rhoeophyte, abundant along rocky river banks and in riverbeds, usually growing in the crevices of rocks, often breaking them. Widely distributed in South and S.E. Asia including India.

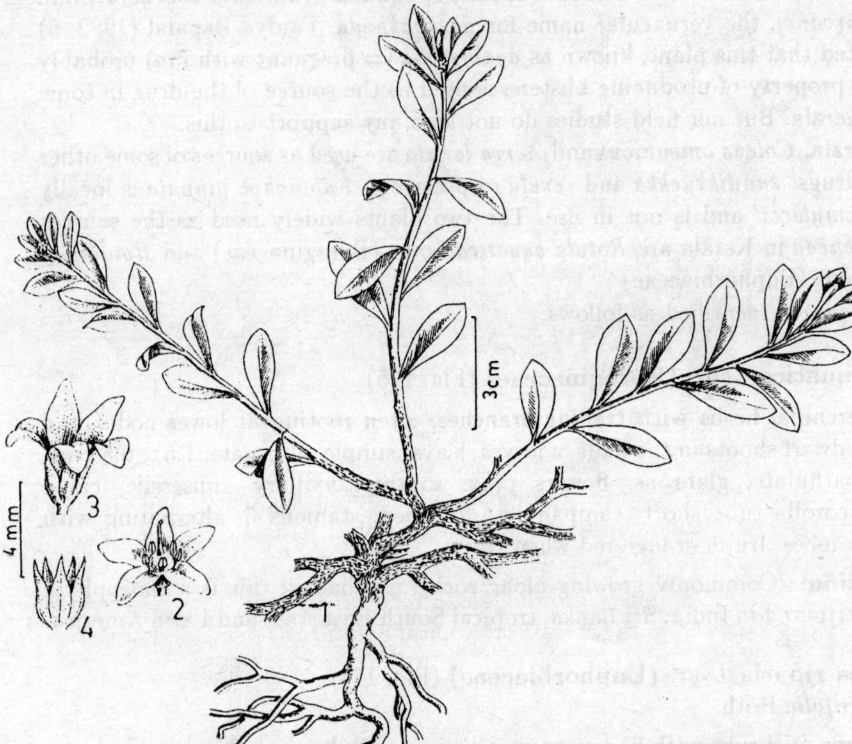

Figure 175: Rotula aquatica Lour. 1, Habit; 2–3, Flowers; 4, Calyx.

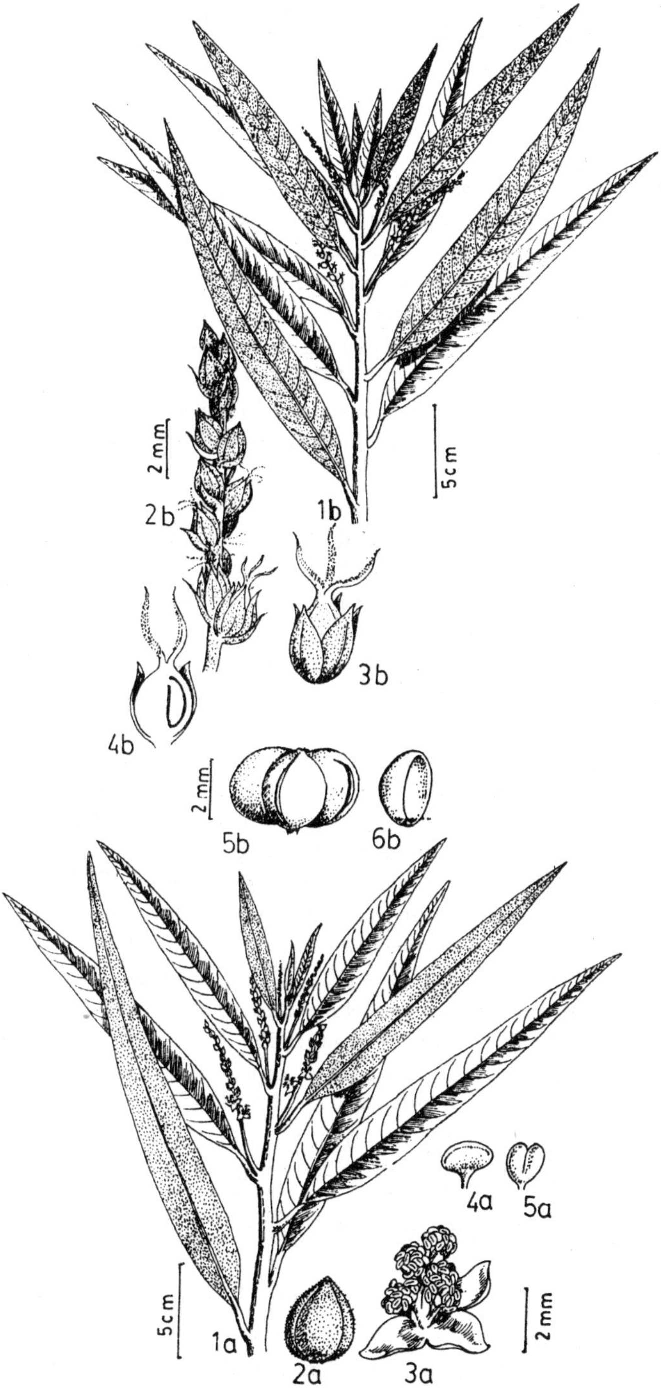

Figure 176: **Homonoia riparia** Lour. 1a, Male plant; 2a, Flower bud; 3a, Male flower; 4a-5a, anthers. 1b, Female plant; 2b, Female spike; 3b, Female flower; 4b, Female flower L.S.; 5b, Fruit; 6b, Seed.

PĀṬALĀ (Mal. PŪPPĀTIRI)

This is an ingredient of the reputed *daśamūla* (ten roots) and is used in many important Āyurvēdic formulations. *Pāṭalā* is reported to be bitter, astringent, cardiotonic, cooling, diuretic and tonic. It relieves the three *dōṣās*, overcomes anorexia, difficult breathing, anasarca, piles vomiting, hiccough and thirst. Flower is astringent, sweet, aggreeable to the heart, useful in vitiated *kapha*, bleeding diseases, diarrhoea of the *pitta* type and is good for the throat. The fruit is useful in hiccough and blood diseases (Kolammal, 1978. 2. 36, 37: Kurup *et al.*, 1979. 164). Root, root bark, flowers and tender fruits are used in medicine. The important preparations using the drug are *Daśamūlariṣṭaṃ, Dhānvantaraṃ tailaṃ, Cyavanapr̥āśaṃ, Agastyarasāyanaṃ*, etc.

Classical literature indicate that this is a woody plant (*kāṣṭhapāṭalā*) with a characteristic odour (*sthiragandhā*) and that it has dark trunk and branches (*kōkilā, kr̥ṣṇavr̥ntā, kālavr̥ntā*) and bell-shaped flowers (*ghaṇṭapāṭaliḥ*) which are either copper-red (*tāmrapuṣpī*) or greyish white (*kar̥burā*) or pale red or pinkish (*pāṭalā, pāṭaliḥ*) (cf. Kolammal, 1978. 2. 35–36). In flowers, it is a favourite of beetles (*aḷivallabhā*) and is a messenger of the spring (*madhudūtī*).

Śāligrāmanighaṇṭu recognises three types of *pāṭalā* viz. *bhūmipāṭalā, kṣudrapāṭalā* and *vallīpāṭalā*. Bhāvaprakāśa, however, has mentioned only two; the white flowered one (*pāṭalā*) and the copper-red flowered one (*tāmr̥apāṭalā*) (cf. Chunekar, 1982. 279–80). *Tāmr̥apāṭalā* is reportedly bitter, acrid, hot and relieves morbid *kapha*. It is also useful in *sannipāta*, difficult breathing, vomiting, oedema and flatus. The white variety purifies blood, increases appetite and cures oedema, thirst, vomiting, hiccough and morbid *kapha* and *vāta* (Kolammal, 1978: 36–37).

Chunekar (1982: 279–80) in his commentary on Bhāvaprakāśa has equated the white-flowered *pāṭalā* with *Stereospermum chelenoides* (Linn.f.) DC. (now *S. colais*) and the *tāmr̥apāṭalā* with *S. suaveolens* DC. of Bignoniaceae. *Radermachera xylocarpa* of the same family has also been referred to as the source of this drug in some texts (Kolammal, 1978: 2: 35). Most authors, however, do not make a distinction of these types and accept *S. suaveolens* as the drug source. (Nadkarni, 1954: 1168; Kapoor & Mitra, 1979: 66; Kurup *et al.*, 1979: 164; Dey, 1980: 117; Sharma, 1983: 223). Kerala physicians, however, rely on *S. colais* for this drug. Rheede, also portrays this plant i.e. *S. colais* as the source of 'Padri' (Hort. Malab. 6: t. 26).

The two species can easily be differentiated as follows:

Stereospermum suaveolens *DC.* **(Bignoniaceae)** (Fig. 177)

Large tree; branches and leaves glabrous; leaves opposite, imparipinnate; leaflets broadly elliptic, shortly abruptly acuminate, often serrulate, rough; flowers crimson in large terminal panicles; calyx campanulate; corolla tubular, campanulate, 2-lipped; stamens 4, filaments without a tuft of wooly hairs; capsule stout, straight, nearly terete, lenticellate upto 50 cm long.

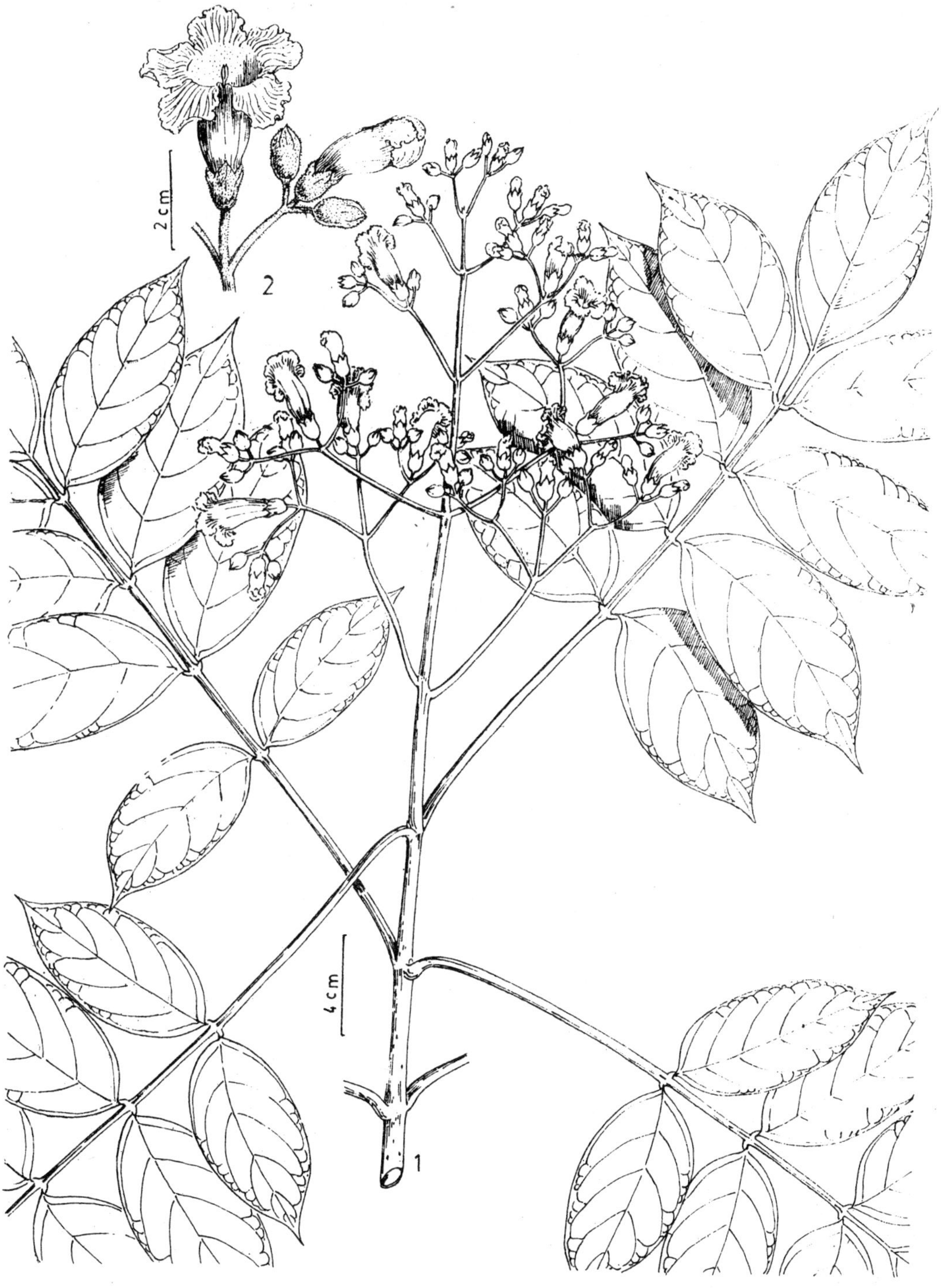

Figure 177: Stereospermum suaveolens DC. 1, Twig; 2, Flower.

Distribution: The plant grows in the deciduous forests of Western Ghats.

Stereospermum colais (*Dillwyn*) *Mabb.* **(Bignoniaceae)** (Fig. 178)
S. tetragonum DC.
S. personatum (Hassk.) Chatterjee
S. chelonoides auct. non (Linn. f.) DC.

Large, deciduous tree; branches and leaves pubescent, leaves opposite, imparipinnate; leaflets 7–9, 7–15 × 4–7 cms, thin coriaceous, obovate to lanceolate, acute or rounded, often unequal-sided at base, acute to caudate-acuminate at apex, entire or shortly serrate; flowers fragrant, yellow with reddish veins in lax terminal cymose panicle; calyx campanulate, glabrous; corolla bilabiate; stamens 4, filaments with a tuft of wooly hairs; capsule pendulous, 4-angled or ribbed, 30–40 × 1 cm.

Distribution: The plant is distributed throughout India and also reported from Sri Lanka, Thailand, Indo-China and Malesia.

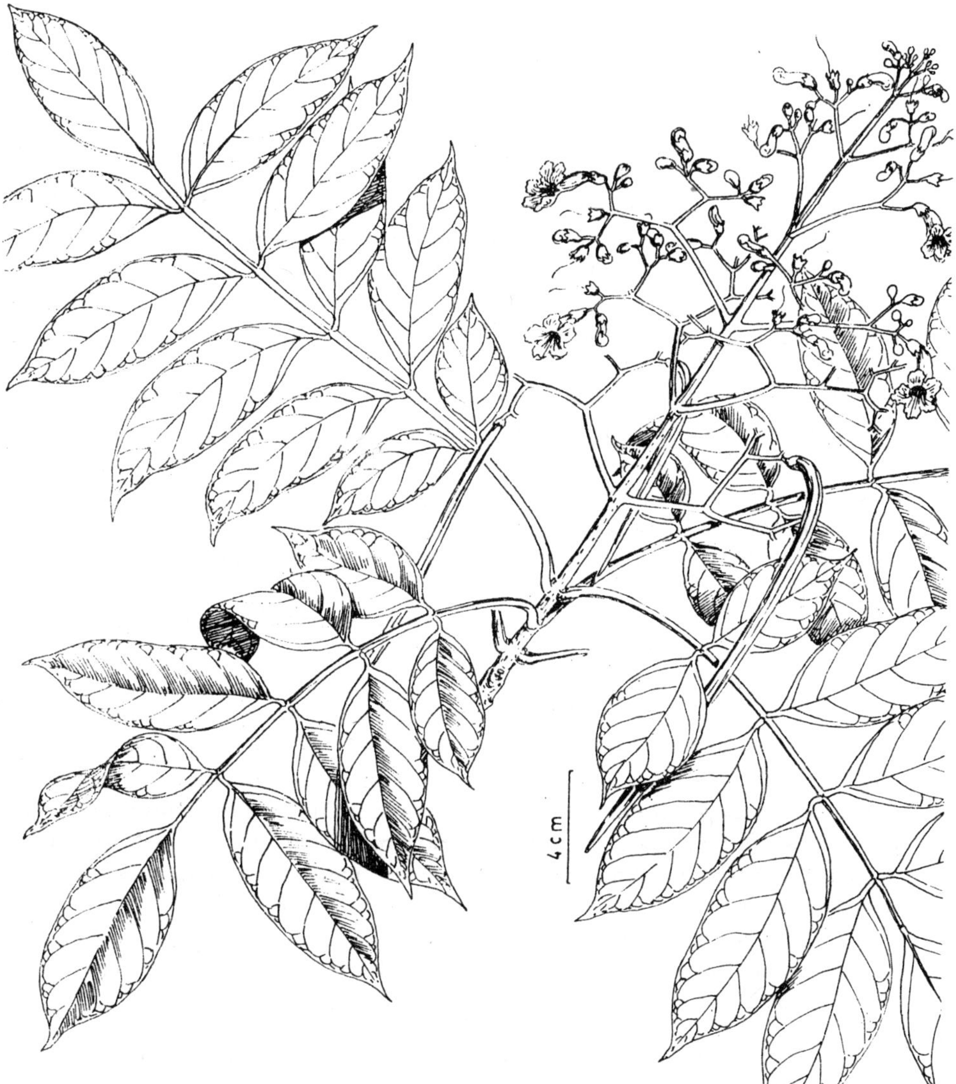

Figure 178: **Stereospermum colais** (Dillw.) Mabb.

PĀṬHĀ (Mal. PĀṬAKKIḶAṄṄU)

Due to the blood purifying property of the drug, it is considered to be beneficial in treating skin diseases and poisonous affections. Root is the officinal part. It is bitter, acrid, cardiotonic and is useful in colic pains, fevers, vomiting, diarrhoea, heart-diseases, burning sensation, pruritus, worms, respiratory disorders, *gulma* (internal tumour) and ulcers. In Kerala it is largely used as an internal remedy in inflamed piles (Aiyer 1951: 1; Nesamony, 1985; 348) *Ayaskṛti, Candanāsavaṃ, Pāṭhādi cūrṇaṃ, Paṭōlakaṭurōhiṇyādi kaṣāyaṃ*, etc. are some of the preparations using the drug.

The synonyms are indicative of only the properties of the drug. Suśruta and Vāgbhaṭa mention only one type of *pāṭhā* whereas two types are mentioned in *Caraka Samhita* and the later *Nighaṇṭus*. They are *laghupāṭhā* and *rājapāṭhā*. Almost all the authors equate *pāṭhā* or *laghupāṭha* with *Cissampelos pariera* Linn. of Menispermaceae. (Kirtikar & Basu, 1918: 61; Nadkarni, 1954: 334; Chopra *et al.*, 1956: 66; Kurup *et al.*, 1979: 165; Dey, 1980: 118; Chunekar, 1982: 395; Sharma, 1983: 627).

Ayurvedic formulary of India also recommends this as the source of *pāṭhā* (1978a: 251). *Rājapāṭhā* with bigger leaves and tubers is variously identified as *Cyclea peltata* (Lamk.) Hook. f. & Thoms. (Vaidya Bapalal, 1982: 136; Chunekar, 1982: 396), *Cyclea arnotii* Miers (Sharma, 1983: 627) and *Stephania japonica* (Thunb.) Miers (Kirtikar & Basu, 1918: 59: Chunekar, 1982: 396; Sharma, 1983: 627), all belonging to Menispermaceae. In practice, in Kerala there is no distinction of different varieties. *Cyclea peltata* known as *pāṭakkiḷaṅṅu* in Malayalam is invariably used as *pāṭhā* in all formulations. *Cissampelos pariera*, the plant used in North India, is available in Kerala but known under a different name *malatāṅṅi* and is not used in Āyurvēdic practice.

Rheede also describes and portrays *Cyclea peltata* as the source of *Pada-kelengu* or *Pada-valli* (Hort. Malab. 7: 93, t. 49. 1688). The various plant sources can be identified as follows.

Cyclea peltata (*Lam.*) *Hook. f.* & *Thomson* **(Menispermaceae)** (Fig. 179)
Menispermum peltatum Lam.

Slender, hispid climber with long tuberous roots; leaves simple, alternate, exstipulate, peltate, long-deltoid, coriaceous, entire, palmately veined, slightly cordate at base, acute or mucronate at apex, to 12.5 × 7.5 cms, dark green above covered with short stiff hairs, softly pubescent and pale beneath; flowers small, unisexual, greenish in axillary hispid panicles; Male flowers: calyx globose, broadly campanulate, sepals 4 to 6, connate, unequal; petals connate to form a semifleshy, saucer-shaped, lobed structure from the centre of which arises the staminal column; anthers 4 to 6 arranged on the top of the staminal column. Female flowers: perianth of 2 broadly ovate to orbicular, semifleshy structures; ovary single, style short ending in 3 stigmatic branches; drupe ovoid.

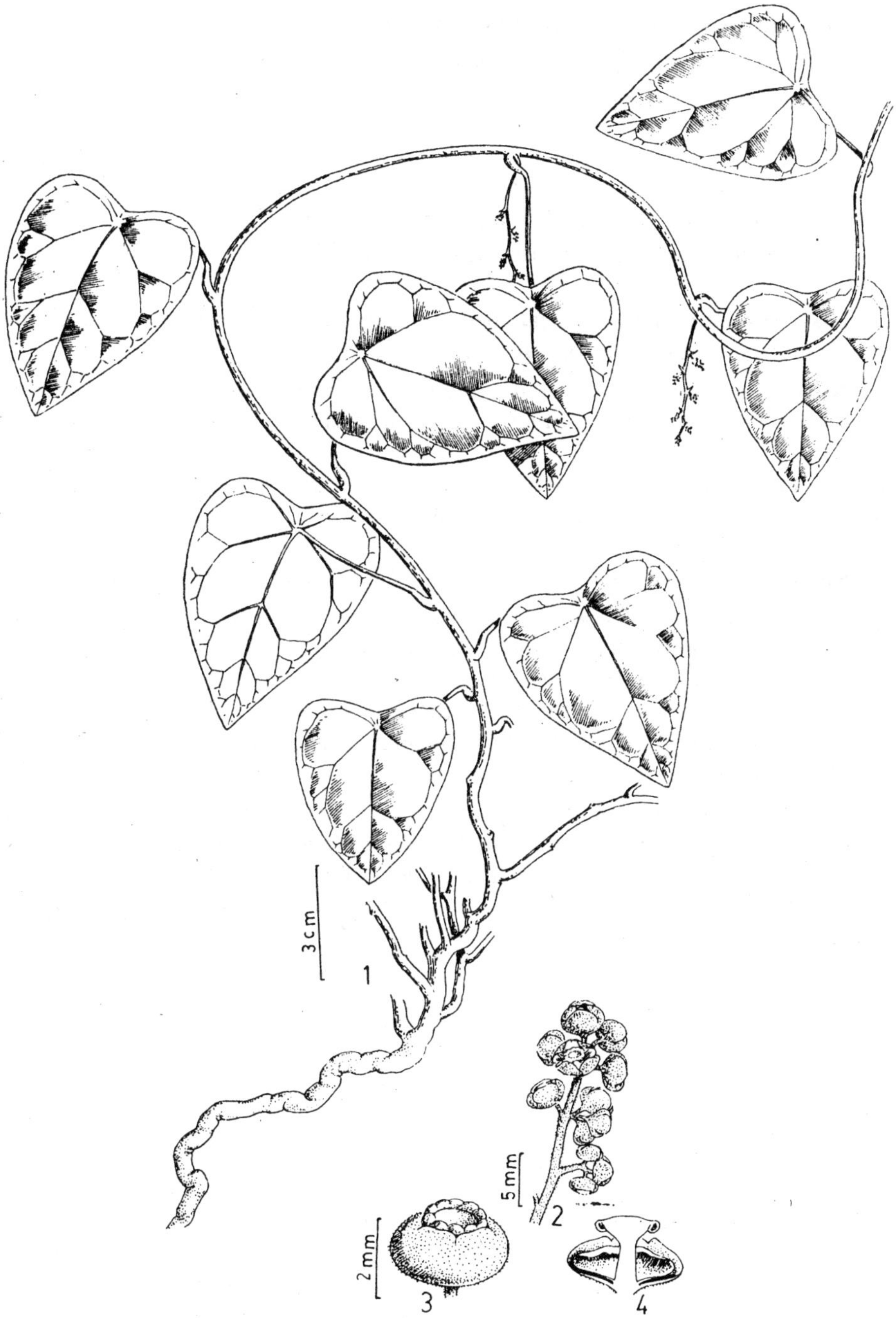

Figure 179: **Cyclea peltata** (Lam.) H. f. & Thoms. 1, Habit; 2, Male inflorescence; 3, Male flower; 4, Male flower L.S.

Distribution: The plant grows wild in the West Coast of India from sea level to about 3,000 ft. Also distributed in Sri Lanka and Malesia.

Cissampelos pariera *Linn.* **(Menispermaceae)** (Fig. 180)

Slender, perennial, glabrous twiner; leaves simple, alternate, exstipulate, long-petioled, orbicular-reniform to reniform-cordate, thin, 4 × 4.5 cms entire, mucronate at tip, pubescent when young; flowers small, greenish, unisexual, male flowers: cymose and female racemed, crowded in the axils of leafy bracts; Male: sepals 4, obovate-oblong, hairy outside; petals 4, connate forming a 4-lobed cup; stamens 4, connate round the flattened top of the staminal column; female: sepals broadly obovate; petal 1, greenish white; ovary 1, style short ending in a trifid stigma; drupe ovoid.

Distribution: A pantropical species, the plant is common in almost all districts of the tropical and subtropical India.

Note: The morphological and anatomical characters and chemical constituents of the roots of *Cyclea peltata* and *Cissampelos pariera* are described by Aiyer (1951: 4–13).

The chemistry and pharmacological and clinical studies of this plant have been discussed by Satyavati *et al.* (1976: 236–240).

Stephania japonica (*Thunb.*) *Miers.* **(Menispermaceae)**

Climbing shrub; leaves peltate, 5–7.5 × 5–6 cm, chartaceous, 9–11 nerved, glabrous; flowers small, unisexual, greenish in axillary stalked umbels; Male: sepals 4 + 4, free, oblanceolate, puberulous without; petals 4, free, suborbicular; stamens 6 connate to form a staminal column with the anthers arranged on the top; Female: sepals 3–5, oblong or elliptic; petals 3–5, suborbicular; carpels ovoid, stigma 3-lobed; drupe globose-obovoid.

Distribution: The plant is found in the forests of the W. Ghats, common from Coorg to Tinnevelly, upto 6,000 ft. Also distributed in Sri Lanka, Malesia, E. China, Korea, Japan, Tonga, Formosa and Society Isls.

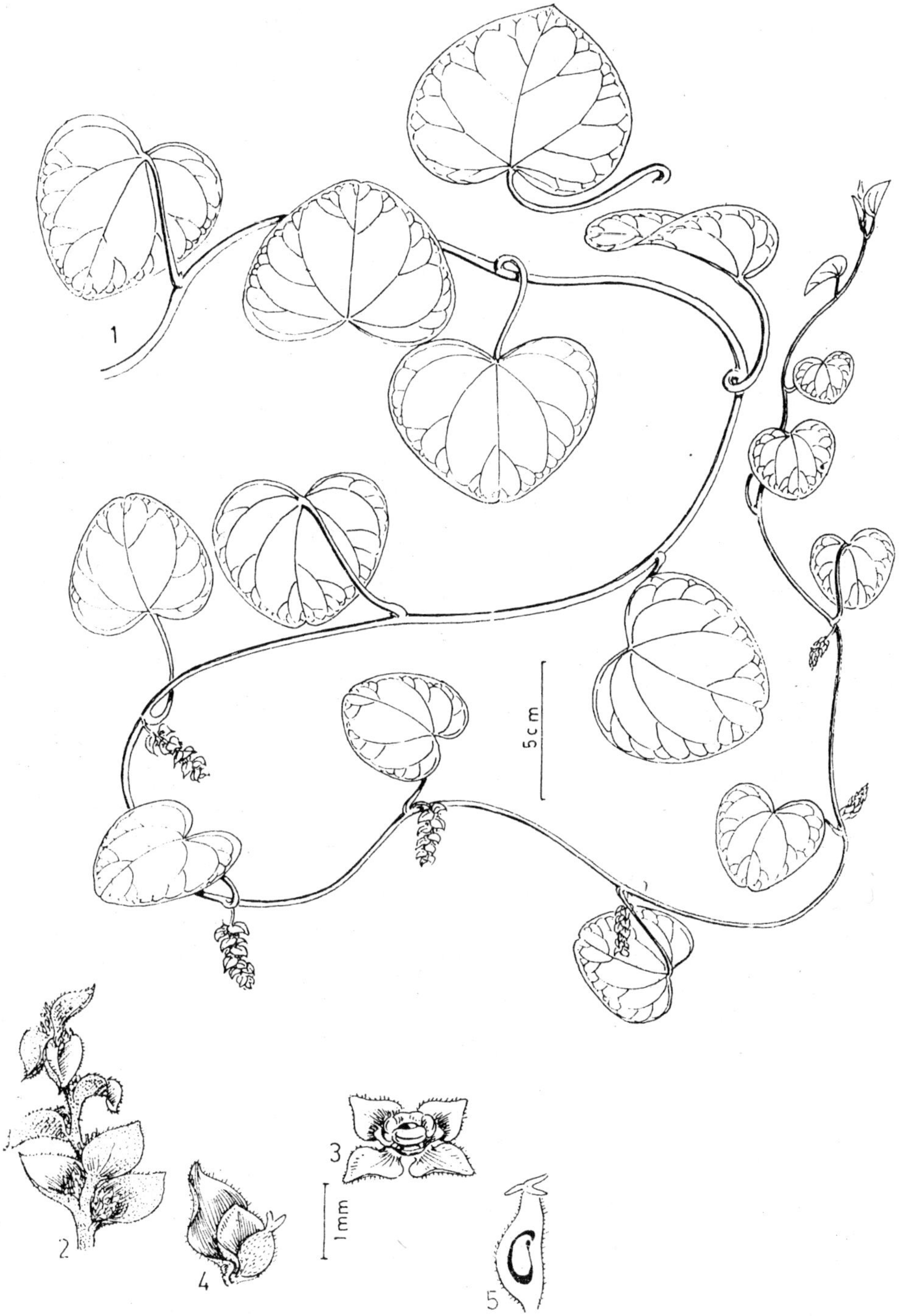

Figure 180: **Cissampelos pariera** L. 1, Habit; 2, Inflorescence; 3, Male flower; 4, Female flower; 5, Ovary L.S.

PAṬŌLAḤ (Mal. KAIPPANPAṬAVALAṂ or KĀṬṬUPAṬAVALAṂ)

Paṭōla is regarded as a good blood purifier and hence beneficial in the treatment of skin diseases. It is bitter, acrid in taste, hot in action, appetiser, digestive, germicidal, laxative and aphrodisiac. It aids digestion, cures haemetemesis, dermatosis, fever, cough and ulcers. It overcomes itching sensation, excessive thirst, intestinal disorders, concocted poisons, eye diseases and morbidity of the *tridōṣas*. Leaves are easily digested and cure diseases caused by *pitta*. The fruits are light and bitter, promote digestion and sexual vigour, keep the three humors in equilibrium and dispel the pathogenic organisms. The stem cures diseases caused by vitiation of *kapha*. Roots are good purgatives. The plant as a whole, along with roots, are used medicinally (cf. Aiyer & Kolammal, 1963. 7: 45). The important preparations are *Gulgulutiktakaṃ kaṣāyaṃ, Mahātiktaka ghṛtaṃ, Vajrakaṃ kaṣāyaṃ, Mahātiktakaṃ kaṣāyaṃ*, etc.

According to the synonyms in the text, the plant is very bitter (*tiktaḥ, tiktōttamaḥ*), rough to touch (*karkaśacchadaḥ, kachuraḥ*) and it usually grows spreading on the floor (*paṭōlaḥ, paṭōlakaḥ*). The fruits are variegated (*pāṇḍukaḥ, pāṇḍuphalaḥ*) with five longitudinal white streaks or bands (*rājīphalaḥ, rājīmān, pañcarājīphalaḥ*) (cf. Aiyer & Kolammal, 1963. 7: 45).

Āyurvēdic texts recognise two kinds of *paṭōla*, namely a small fruited bitter variety called *paṭōla* proper and a large fruited sweetish edible variety called *svādupaṭōla* (Mooss, 1976: 153). The former is highly bitter and is locally called *kaippan paṭavalaṃ* or *kāṭṭupaṭavalaṃ*. This is the one commonly used in medicine by the physicians of Kerala and is equated with *Trichosanthes cucumerina* of Cucurbitaceae (See also Rheede, Hort. Malab. 8: 29–30. t. 15 1688, *'Padvalam'*). The *svādupaṭōla*, the edible variety, reportedly has all the qualities of the bitter variety but is largely used as a vegetable. This variety, known as *paṭavalaṃ* in vernacular is *Trichosanthes cucumerina* var. *anguina*, the 'Snake-gourd' (see Fig. 182). Rheede (Hort. Malab. 8. t. 16. 1688) has described yet another variety of this drug, *Tsjerupadavalam* which is *Trichosanthes nervifolia* L. but this is not found to be in use at present.

The plant source of the drug in the northern provinces of India is said to be *Trichosanthes dioica* Roxb. (Dey. 1980: 119; Chunekar, 1982: 686; Sharma, 1983: 697). Many authors have conceded the use of both *T. dioica* and *T. cucumerina* as *paṭōla* (Kirtikar & Basu, 1918: 581–582; Nadkarni, 1954: 1235, 1236; Chopra *et al*, 1956: 248). Among Kerala physicians, however, *T. cucumerina* L. is the accepted source of the drug.

Trichosanthes cucumerina *Linn.* **(Cucurbitaceae)** (Fig. 181)

Slender, hispid, climbers; tendrils 2-fid, leaf-opposed, leaves broadly ovate or orbicular-reniform, 3–5 lobed, to 15 cms across, base cordate with a wide sinus, margin denticulate; flowers white, unisexual, male flowers in axillary penduncled racemes, female solitary in leaf axils; calyx tube long, cylindrical, dilated, at apex, glandular-pubescent; corolla of 5 white fimbriate petals; stamens 3 in male; in the female ovary inferior, hairy, one-chambered with many ovules; fruit an ovoid or fusiform smooth berry, 2.5 to 7.5 cm long with a long sharp beak, green striped with white when young, orange red when ripe.

Distribution: The plant is found distributed in Bengal, Gujarat, Konkan, Deccan and Kerala in the plains as well as in the lower hills. Also in Sri Lanka, India, tropical Himalaya, Malesia, Polynesia and N.Australia.

Taxonomic note: The two varieties of this species, primarily distinguished by their fruits (small, fusiform, to 7.5 cm long in *paṭōla* and long, cylindric, to about 1 m in *svādupaṭōla*) have been earlier treated as two different species, *T. cucumerina* L. and *T. anguina* L. (Fig. 182) in most of our Floras. Jeffrey (1980) is however, of the opinion that they form different varieties of the same species, namely *T. cucumerina* var. *cucumerina* and var. *anguina*.

Note: Shah and Shah (1967) have studied the detailed pharmacognosy of *Trichosanthes cucumerina*.

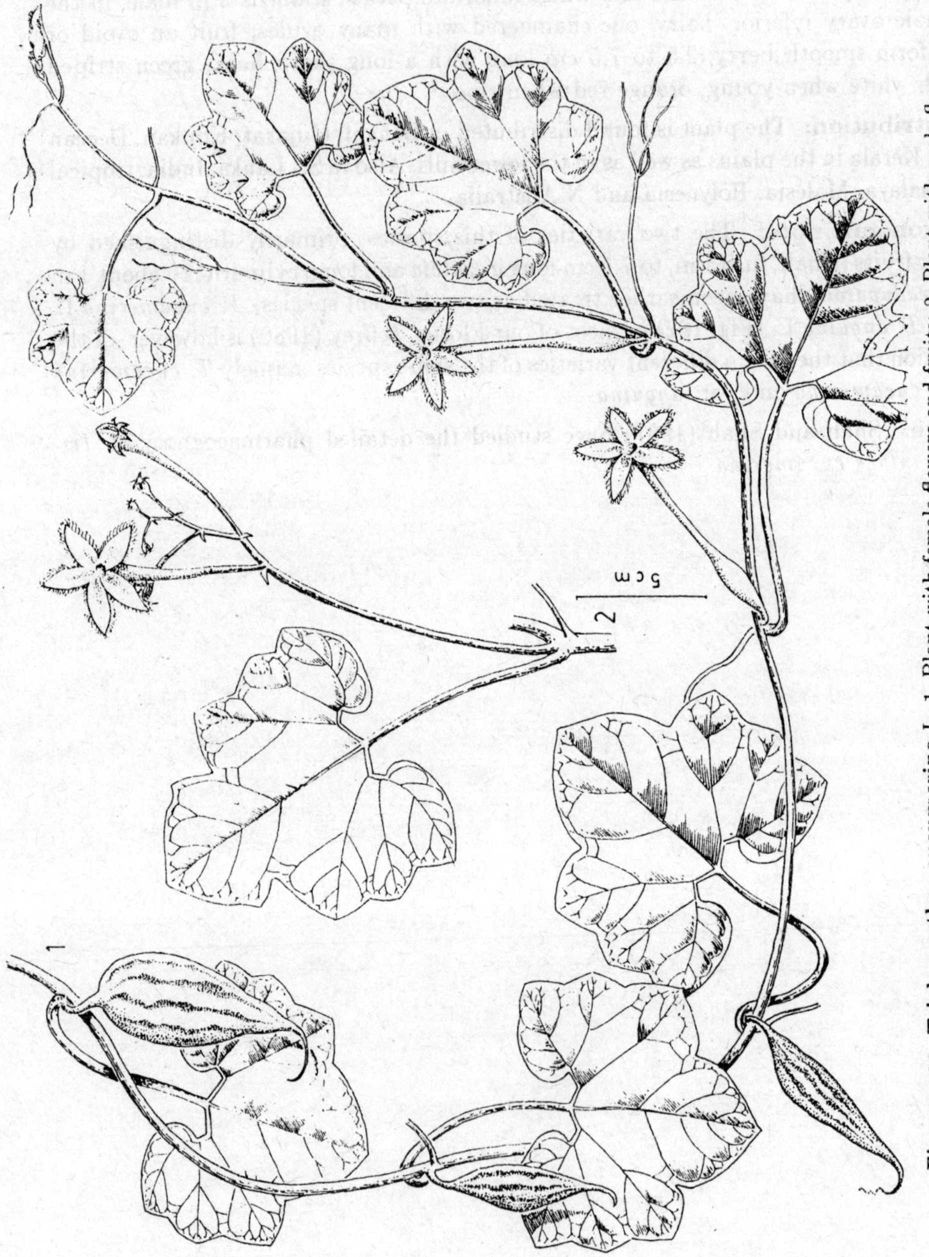

Figure 181: Trichosanthes cucumerina L. 1, Plant with female flowers and fruits; 2, Plant with male flowers.

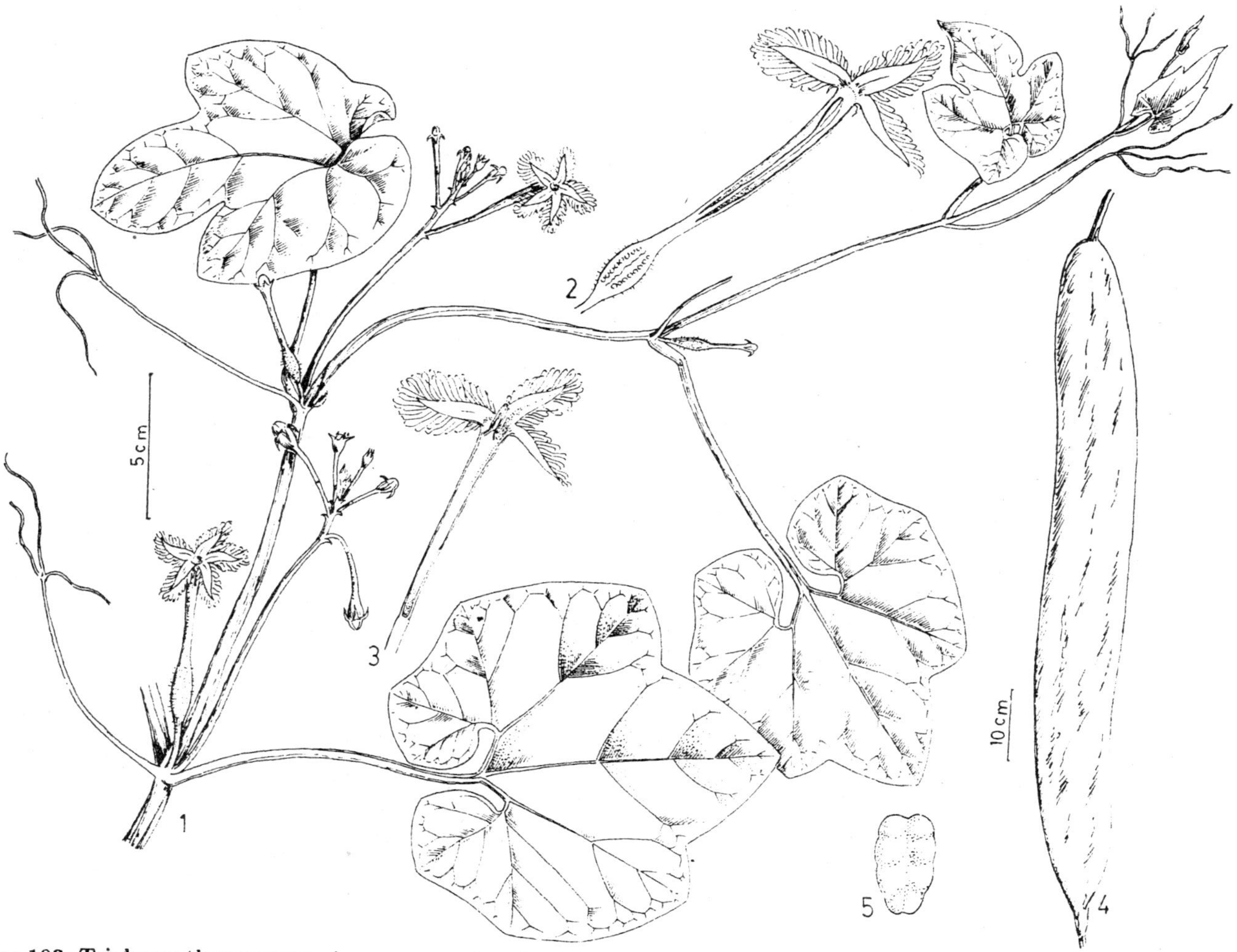

Figure 182: Trichosanthes cucumerina var. **anguina** (L.) Jeffrey. 1, Habit; 2, L.S. of female flower; 3, L.S. of male flower; 4, Fruit; 5, Seed.

PIPPALĪ (Mal. TIPPALI, KĀṬṬUTIPPALI)

Pippali is an important *mēdhya rasāyana* drug that is capable of improving intellect and memory power and also to regain health by dispelling diseases. It is reportedly acrid, hot, light, digestive, appetiser, aphrodisiac and tonic. It cures cough, dyspnoea, ascites, leprosy, diabetes, piles, colic, indigestion, anaemia, thirst and dispels cardiac and splenic disorders, chronic fever, loss of appetite and worm troubles. It rehabilitates vitiated *vāta* and *kapha*. Dried ripe fruits and roots are the officinal parts. The important formulations using the drug are *Abhayāriṣṭaṃ, Drākṣāriṣṭāṃ, Cyavanaprāśaṃ, Pippalyāsavaṃ,* etc.

According to the synonymy, the plant is commonly found in Magadha (*māgadhī*) and Vidēha (*vaidēhī*), both in present day Bihar, growing near streams or other water resources (*upakulyā*) as creepers (*kolā*). The herb has got very pungent fruits (*kaṭubījā, tīkṣṇataṇḍulā*) which are black in colour (*śyāmā, kṛṣṇā*) and are used with condiments while serving liquor (*śauṇḍī*) (cf. Aiyer & Kolammal, 1966. 9: 52)

Piper longum L. (Piperaceae) is the accepted source of the drugs *pippali* and *pippalīmūlaṃ* throughout the country, While *pippali* is the dried ripe fruits, *pippalīmūlaṃ* is the roots of this plant (Mooss, 1976: 99)—See also Rheede, Hort. Malab. 7. t. 14. 1688-*cattutirpali*-.

Piper longum *Linn.* **(Piperaceae)** (Fig. 183)
Chavica roxburghii Miq.

Dioecious creepers or root climbers with fastigate branches; leaves simple, alternate, ovate to oblong, deeply cordate, often oblique at base, acuminate at apex, to 12 × 6 cms; flowers minute on unisexual, axillary, cylindric spikes, green at first, turning yellow later, to 5 cm long, male spikes longer than female; fruits small berries, dark red when ripe and partially sunk in the fleshy axis of the spike.

Distribution: The plant, considered indigenous to the hotter parts of India, is found growing wild in the West Coast as an undergrowth in the evergreen forests of the Western Ghats. It is also occasionally cultivated.

Note: Clinical studies have revealed that *pippali* is very effective in the treatment of bronchial asthma in children (Dahanukar *et al.*, 1984). Anshuman *et al.* (1984) found that *vaṛdhamāna pippali* i.e. *pippali* in increasing dosage is effective in patients with respiratory disorders. Compounds isolated from *Piper longum* were found to have antitubercular activity (Kurup *et al.*, 1979: 166) while dehydropiperonaline from the dried fruits displayed coronary vasodilating activity (Shoj N. *et al.*, 1986).

There is a mention of four types of *pippali* in *Rājanighaṇṭu*, namely *pippali, vanapippali, saiṁhaḷi* and *gajapippali*. Sharma has (1983: 276) equated the former three with *Piper longum, P. sylvaticum* Roxb. and *P. retrofractum* Vahl, respectively. Of these, *P. sylvaticum* is a Himalayan species and *P. retrofractum* is an "indeterminable" taxon, as mentioned by Hooker (Fl. Brit. India 5: 96: 1886). However.

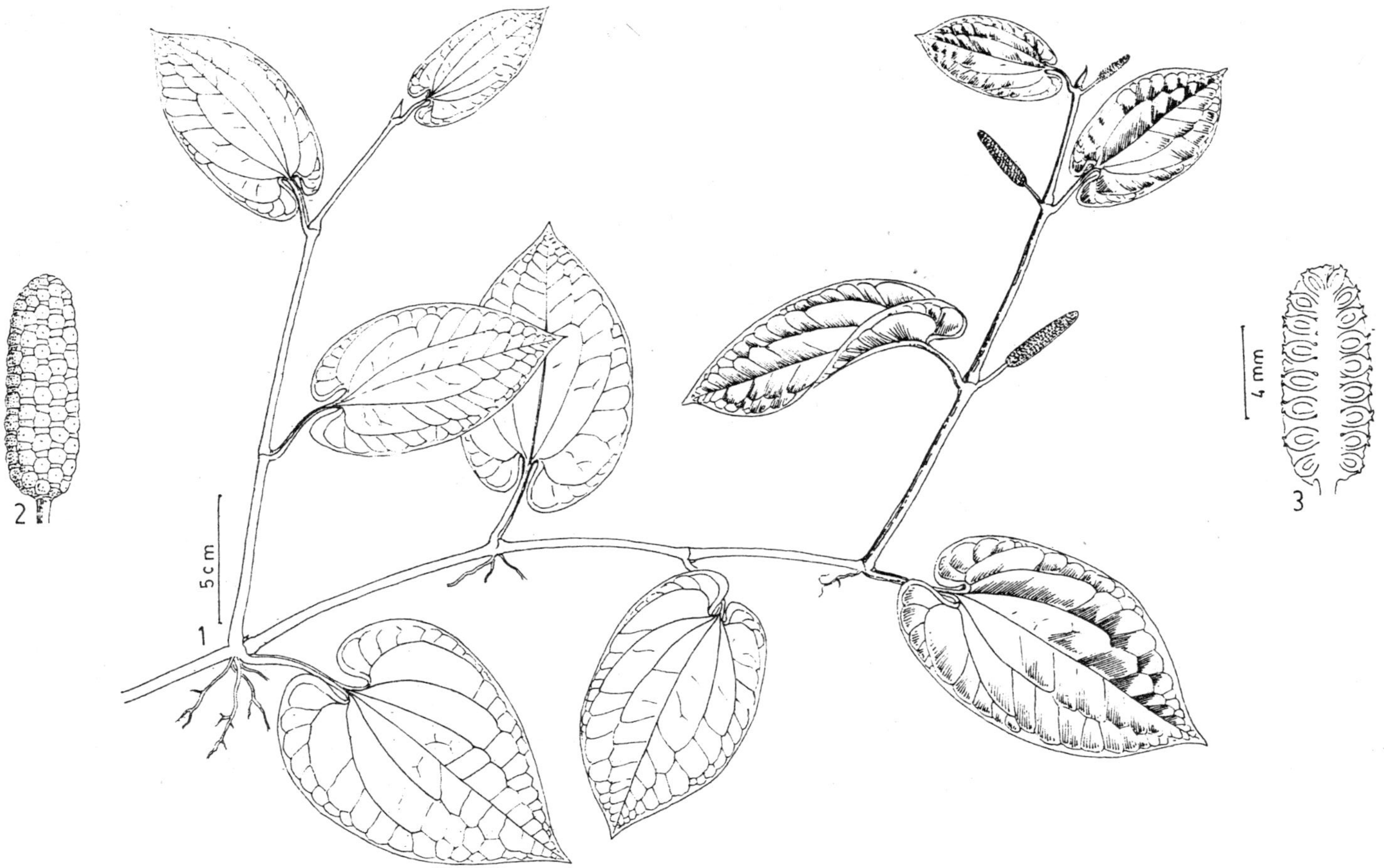

Figure 183: Piper longum L. 1, Habit; 2, Female spike; 3, spike L.S.

Kerala physicians do not make a distinction of the three and *P. longum* is accepted for all. *gajapippali* is considered as a different drug but its identity is highly controversial. According to some it is the fruits of *Piper chaba* Hunt, a species known under cultivation in India and Malaya (Chunekar, 1982: 21; Sharma 1983: 276). But, Kerala physicians equate this species with a different drug, *chavya*. Yet others have accepted the spikes of *Scindapsis officinalis* of Araceae as *gajapippali* (Vaidya, KM. 1936: 181; Nadkarni, 1954: 1117; Chopra *et al.*, 1956: 224; Mooss, 1980: 86). However, our market survey has revealed that *Balanophora fungosa* (Balanophoraceae), a root-parasite which superficially resembles the inflorescence of *Scindapsis officinalis* and chopped stem of *Raphidophora pertusa* (Araceae) are also used as *gajapippali*.

PḶAKṢAḤ (Mal. ITTI)

Pḷakṣaḥ is one of the five ingredients of the group *pañcavalkala* i.e. five barks, the decoction of which is extensively used to clear ulcers and as a douche in leucorrhoea and other vaginal diseases. In scabies affecting children, this decoction is administered externally and internally with satisfactory results. *Pḷakṣaḥ* is acclaimed as cooling, astringent and curative of *raktapitta dōṣās*, ulcers, skin diseases, burning sensation, inflammation and oedema. It is found to have good healing property and is used in preparation of oils and ointments for external application in the treatment of ulcers. (Aiyer & Kolammal, 1957. 3: 101). The stem bark is used to prepare *Uśīrāsavam, Gandhatailam, Nālpāmarādi tailam, Dinēśavalyādi kuḻambu, Pārantyādi tailam, Valiya marmaguḷika* etc.

According to the description in the texts, the tree has few branches (*supārśvaḥ*) and many adventitious roots growing downward (*pḷakṣaḥ*). The term *kamaṇḍalu* probably indicates the habitat near fresh water or it may also refer to the shape of fruit (Aiyer *et al.* 1957. 3: 100).

The botanical source of *pḷakṣaḥ* in Kerala is *Ficus microcarpa* L. of Moraceae, known as *itti* in vernacular. It is also equated with many other species of the genus viz. *Ficus infectoria* Roxb. (cf. Nadkarni, 1954: 551, Kapoor & Mitra, 1979: 67; Chunekar, 1982: 518). *F. arnottiana* Miq., *F. lacor* Buch.-Ham and *F. talboti* King (cf. Nadkarni, 1954: 543, 554; Singh & Chunekar, 1972: 264; Kapoor & Mitra, 1979: 67; Sharma, 1983: 670).

The fact that in Kerala, *Ficus microcarpa* has been the accepted source of the drug since Rheede's time is substantiated by his description and illustration of the tree (Hort.Malab.3: 69–70, t. 55. *"Itty-alu"* 1682.)

Ficus microcarpa *Linn. f.* **(Moraceae)** (Fig. 184)
F. retusa auct. non Linn.

Tree with slender aerial roots; leaves alternate, elliptic or obovate-obtuse, basally 3-nerved, glabrous above, pale beneath, upto 12.5 × 5.5 cms; figs moneocious, axillary or on leafless branches, often paired, sessile, globose 0.7–1 cm across, orange-red when ripe; achenes smooth.

Distribution: Widely distributed throughout India in all districts from sea level to about 4,000 ft and also in Sri Lanka, S. China, Ryuku Isls and New Britain.

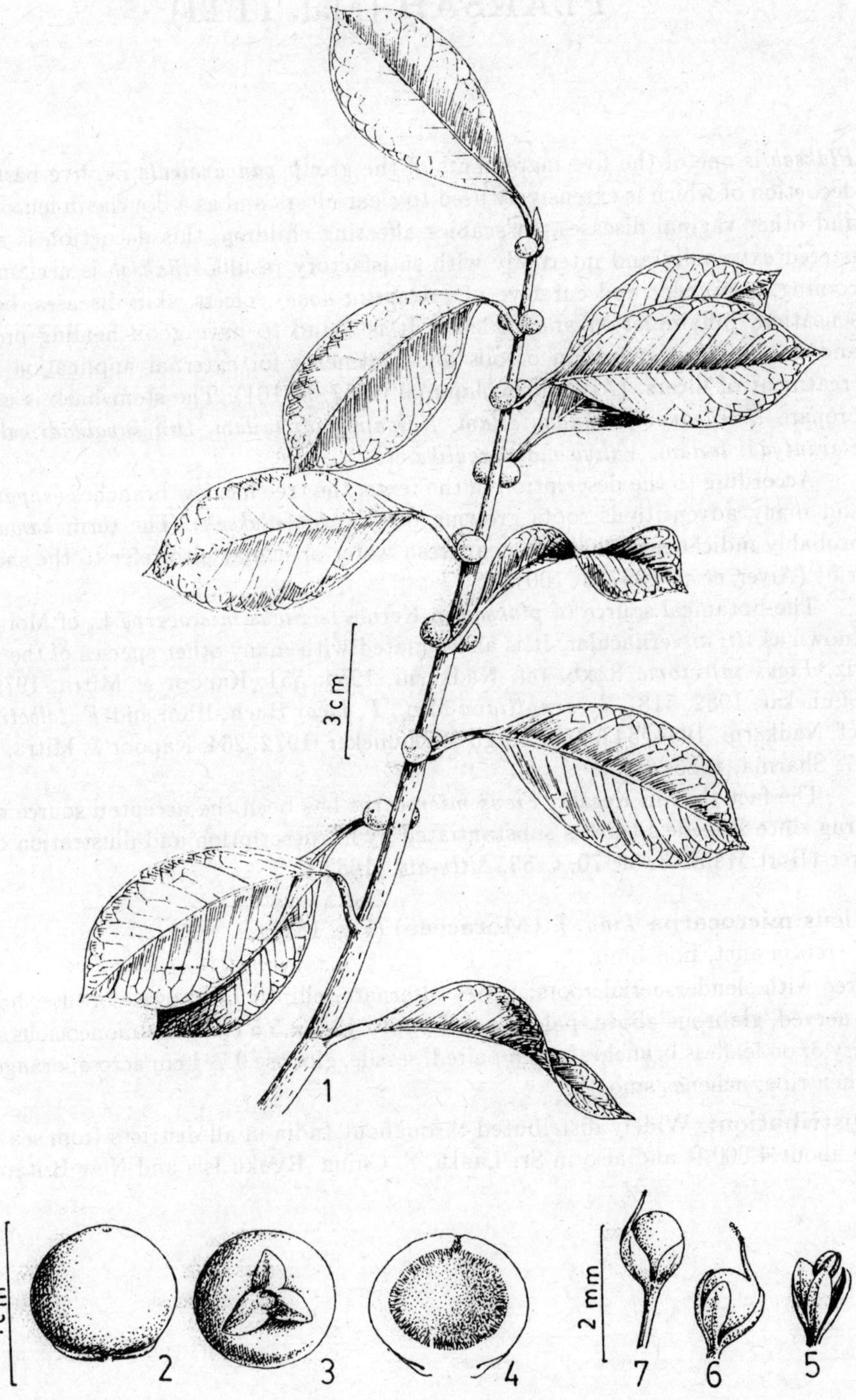

Figure 184: Ficus microcarpa L. f. 1, A branch; 2–3, Figs; 4, Fig L.S.; 5, Male flower; 6, Female flower; 7, Fruit.

PṚASĀRAṆĪ (Mal. PṚASĀRAṆI, TALANĪḶI)

The term *pṛasāraṇī* indicates the spreading habit of the plant. It also indicates the property of the drug of stretching out parts of the body contracted by paralysis. Due to this property, *pṛasāraṇī* is regarded as a specific remedy in rheumatic affections with contraction and stiffness of the joints. The entire plant is used medicinally. It is reported to be heavy, laxative, bitter, astringent, aphrodisiac and hot in action. It overcomes the ill effect of *vāta* and *kapha* and helps in building up the basic tissues of the body. It promotes sexual vigour, increases semen, gives bodily strength and youthful glow and is useful in curing piles and oedema (Aiyer & Kolammal, 1963. 6: 68). The important preparations using the drug are *Pṛasāraṇyādi kaṣāyaṃ*, *Pṛasāraṇyāditailaṃ*, *Pṛabhañjanaṃ kuḻaṁbu*, *Balāriṣṭaṃ* etc.

Several authors have equated this drug with *Paederia foetida* Linn. of Rubiaceae (See Kirtikar & Basu, 1918: 662; Vaidya, K.M. 1936: 372; Nadkarni, 1954: 892; Kurup *et al.*, 1979: 168; Dey, 1980: 122; Chunekar, 1982: 425; Sharma, 1983: 62) and this is probably the plant used as the drug source in North India. According to Ayurvedic formulary of India also, this is the accepted source (Anonymous, 1978a: 252). In Kerala, however, the source of this drug is an altogether different plant, *Merremia tridentata* of Convolvulaceae. There are two subspecies of this species, viz. subsp. *tridentata* and subsp. *hastata*, available here, which can easily be recognised by their foliar characters. However, men of Āyurvēda do not make a distinction of these taxa and use both as *pṛasāraṇi* (See also Rheede, Hort. Malab. 11: 113. t. 55. 1692. *Talanili*).

The two subspecies can be distinguished as follows.

Merremia tridentata (*Linn.*) *Hallier f. ssp.* **tridentata. (Convolvulaceae)** (Fig. 185)

Slender, glabrous, trailing herb; leaves simple, alternate, exstipulate, very short-petioled, oblanceolate-obtuse, mucronate, tridentate at base, to 2.6 x 0.7 cms; flowers creamy yellow in axillary, 1–3 flowered, slender peduncles; calyx of 5 elliptic, subequal, mucronate lobes; corolla campanulate, pale yellow with a pink eye, the limb plicate; stamens 5, epipetalous, filaments filiform, often villous at base; ovary bicarpellary syncarpous, 2–4 chambered, 4-ovuled, style filiform, stigma biglobose; fruit a 2–4 celled globose capsule; seeds trigonous.

Distribution: A pantropical species, found in all the plains districts in various parts of South India.

Merremia tridentata (*Linn.*) *Hall. f. ssp.* **hastata** (*Desv.*) *Oost.* **(Convolvulaceae)**

Slender, twining herb; leaves simple, alternate, very short-petioled, linear or lanceolate, acute or acuminate, at apex, hastate at base, upto 7.5 x 1.2 cms; flowers small, creamy yellow with a dark throat, borne on long, slender, axillary peduncles;

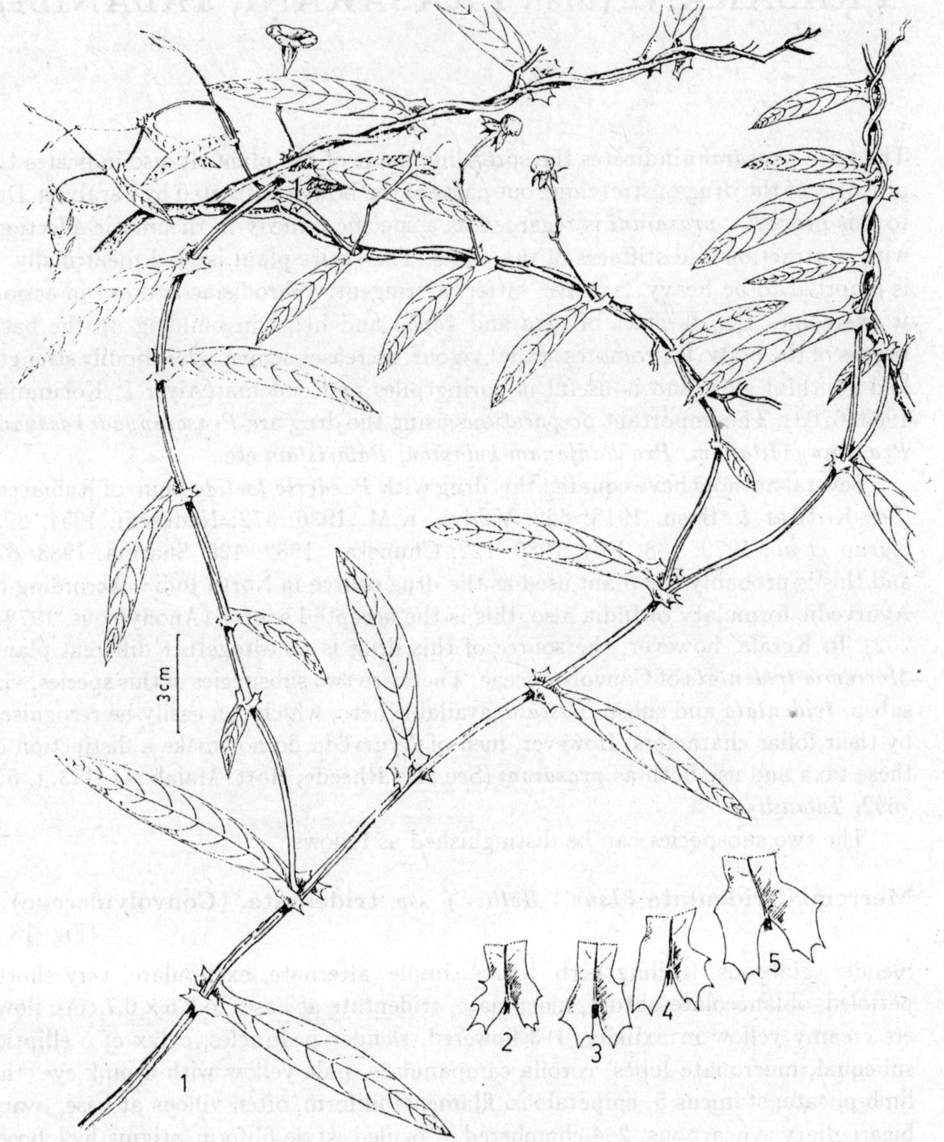

Figure 185: Merremia tridentata (L.) Hall. f. subsp. tridentata. 1, Habit; 2–5, variation in leaf-bases; 6, calyx; 7, seed.

calyx of 5 ovate-acuminate sepals with recurved tips; corolla funnel-shaped, pale yellow with a purple eye, limbs with shallow lobes; stamens 5, filaments epipetalous, free; ovary bicarpellary syncarpous, 2–4 celled, 4-ovuled; fruit an ovoid 2-celled capsule with a thin papery pericarp surrounded by the slightly enlarged sepals; seeds glabrous.

Distribution: Pantropical weedy species found almost throughout peninsular India.

PṚŚNIPAṚṆĪ (Mal. ŌRILA)

Pṛśniparṇī is one of the ten drugs that constitute the *daśamūla* (ten roots) groups. The drug is reported to be a good cardiotonic, useful in the treatment of cardiac disorders. It is hot, sweet, diuretic, laxative and nervine tonic. It overcomes corruption of the three *dōṣās*, burning sensation, fever, cough, difficult breathing, dysentery, thirst and vomiting. It is also useful in *vātarakta*, insanity and ulcers (Kolammal, 1978. 2: 74). Root is the officinal part and it forms an ingredient of formulations like *Daśamūlariṣṭaṃ, Cyavanaprāśaṃ, Dhānvantaraṃ kuḻaṁbu*, etc.

According to the synonymy, *pṛśniparṇī* is a strong-rooted (*anghṛibalā*) plant with long (*dīrghaparṇī*), variegated leaves (*citṛaparṇī, pṛśniparṇī, cakṛaparṇī*) and foxtail-like inflorescence (*krōṣṭuvinnā, sṛgālavinnā, siṁhapucchī*) (cf. Kolammal, 1978. 2: 74).

Some confusion exists regarding the botanical sources of *pṛśniparṇī* and *śāliparṇī* which are mostly used together, due to various common synonyms that are attributed to both. Several publications on Indian matria medica equate *Uraria lagopoides* DC. (Papilionaceae) with *pṛśniparṇī* (Kirtikar & Basu, 1918; 423; Vaidya, 1936: 367; Nadkarni, 1954: 1255; Chopra *et al.*, 1956: 250; Dey 1980: 122). *Uraria picta* Desv. is also considered as the source of the drug by some (Kurup *et al.*, 1979: 169; Anonymous, 1978a: 251; Bapalal Vaidya, 1982: 227; Sharma, 1983: 822). Chunekar (1982: 287), in his commentary on *Bhāvaprakāśa nighaṇṭu*, equates both these plants with *pṛśniparṇī*.

In Kerala, however, *Desmodium gangeticum* DC. of Papilionaceae, known as *ōrila* in Malayalam, is used as the drug source. Other species of *Desmodium* like *D. velutinum* and *D. laxiflorum* are also used in several places in Kerala as the drug source.

The different species can be distinguished as follows.

Desmodium gangeticum (*Linn.*) *DC.* **(Papilionaceae)** (Fig. 186)
Hedysarum gangeticum Linn.

Suberect, diffusely branched under shrub, leaves unifoliolate, alternate; stipulate, leaflet ovate-acute, to 14 × 10 cms; flowers small, pink in terminal elongate raceme; calyx campanulate, hairy outside, with triangular teeth; corolla papilionaceous, exserted; stamens diadelphous; ovary sessile, many ovuled, style filiform, incurved stigma capitate; fruit compressed, moniliform, 6–8 seeded.

Distribution: The plant is distributed throughout India extending from the Himalayas southwards to Kerala, in the plains and as an undergrowth of the semi-deciduous forests. Also found in Tropical Africa, Sri Lanka, S.E.Asia, China, Malesia and Australia.

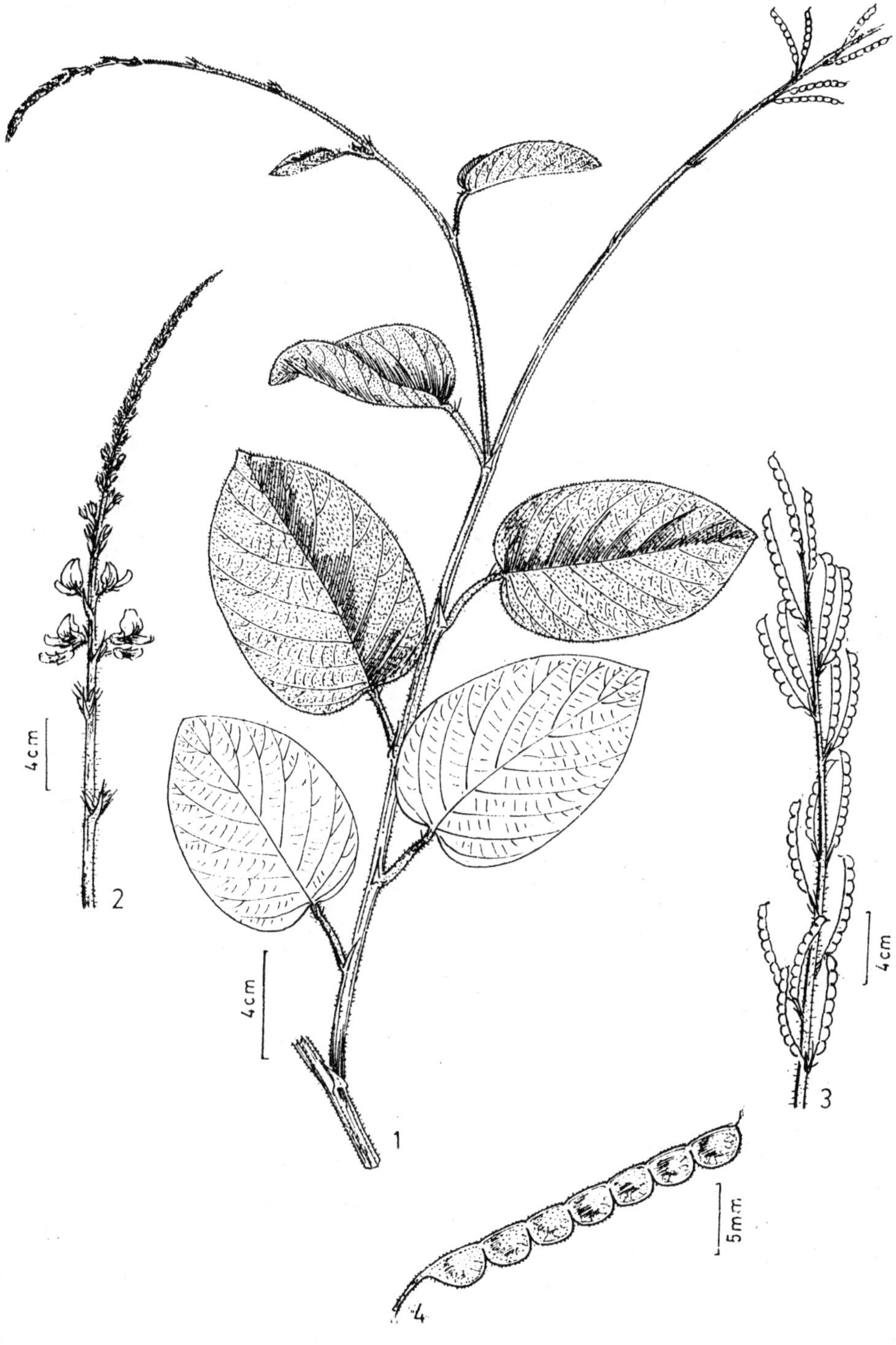

Figure 186: **Desmodium gangeticum** (L.) DC. 1, A branch; 2, Inflorescence; 3, A bunch of pods; 4, A single pod enlarged.

Desmodium velutinum (*Willd.*) *DC.* **(Papilionaceae)** (Fig. 187)
D. latifolium DC.

Much branched undershrubs; branches clothed with fulvous hairy tomentum; leaves unifoliolate, short-petioled, alternate, broadly ovate-acute to roundish, cordate, to 17×11 cms, pubescent above, tomentose below; flowers rose-purple in dense-flowered terminal raceme; pod to 2 cm indented on both margins, densely pubescent, seeds 1 mm across.

Distribution: The plant is distributed throughout South India. It is fairly common in N. Circars, hilly parts of Konkan, Western Ghats and Kerala, in dry open places. Also reported from Africa, Sri Lanka, Burma, Siam, Indo-China and Malesia.

Desmodium laxiflorum *DC.* **(Papilionaceae)** (Fig. 188)
D. diffusum DC.
Hedysarum recurvatum Roxb.

Sub-shrub; branchlets angular and puberulous; leaves alternate, 3-foliolate; leaflets ovate-elliptic acute, terminal leaflet much larger than the laterals, to 10 × 5 cm, puberulous above, adpressed-pubescent below; stipules narrowly triangular; flowers bluish in fascicles on a long slender raceme; calyx 4 lobed, upper lobes connate; corolla papilionaceous, standard ovate or orbicular, wings auriculate at base; stamens (9)+1; stipitate, to 2 cm, margins indented.

Distribution: W. Ghats, Mysore, Coimbatore, Nilgiris and Travancore, upto 3,000 ft. Reported also from Malesia and Formosa.

Note: The pharmacognosy, chemistry and pharmacology of *D. gangeticum* have been discussed by Satyavati *et al.* (1976). Gangetin-a pterocarpanoid isolated from *Desmodium gangeticum* was found to possess antifertility activity (Pillai *et al*. 1981).

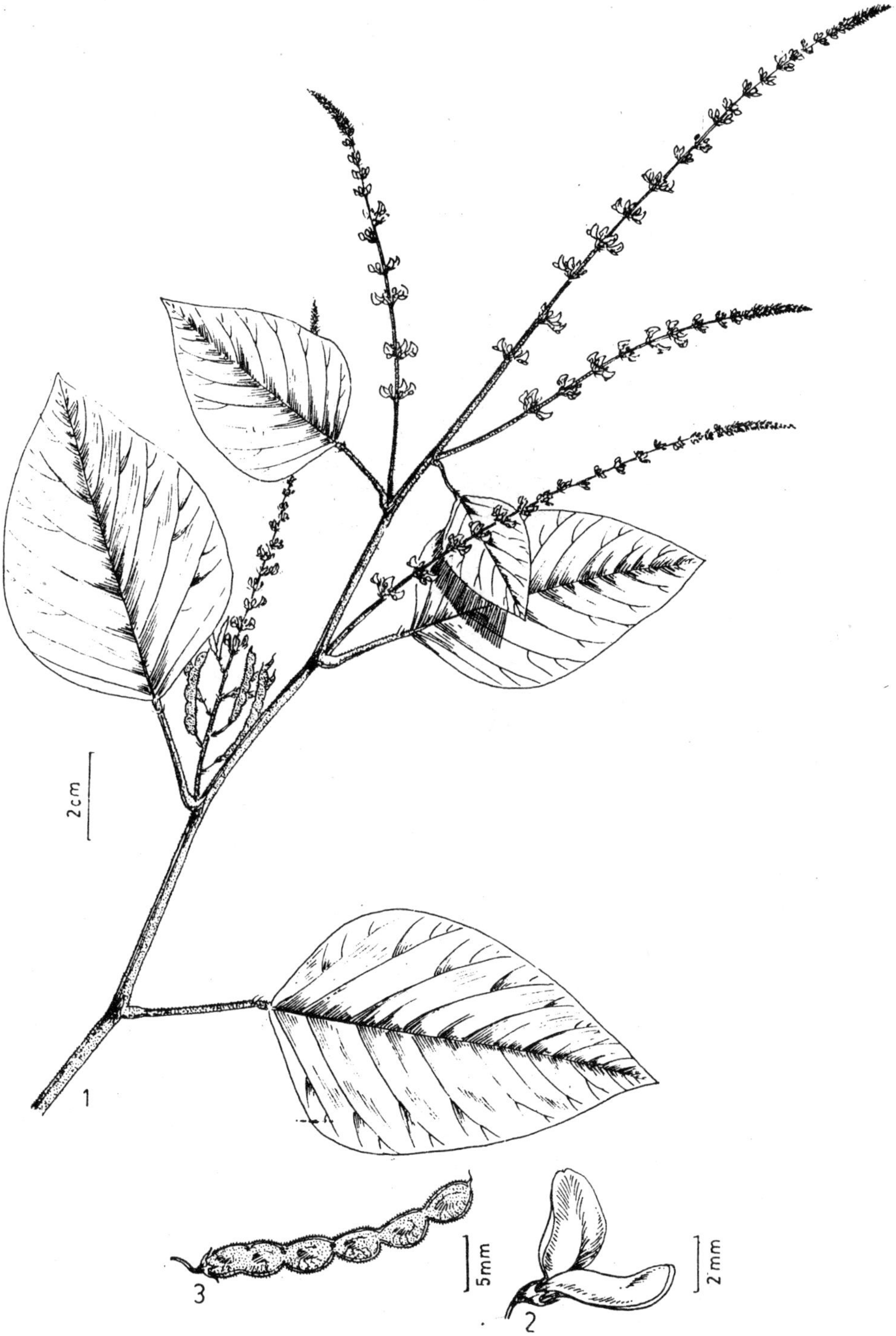

Figure 187: **Desmodium velutinum** (Willd.) DC. 1, A branch; 2, Flower; 3, Pod.

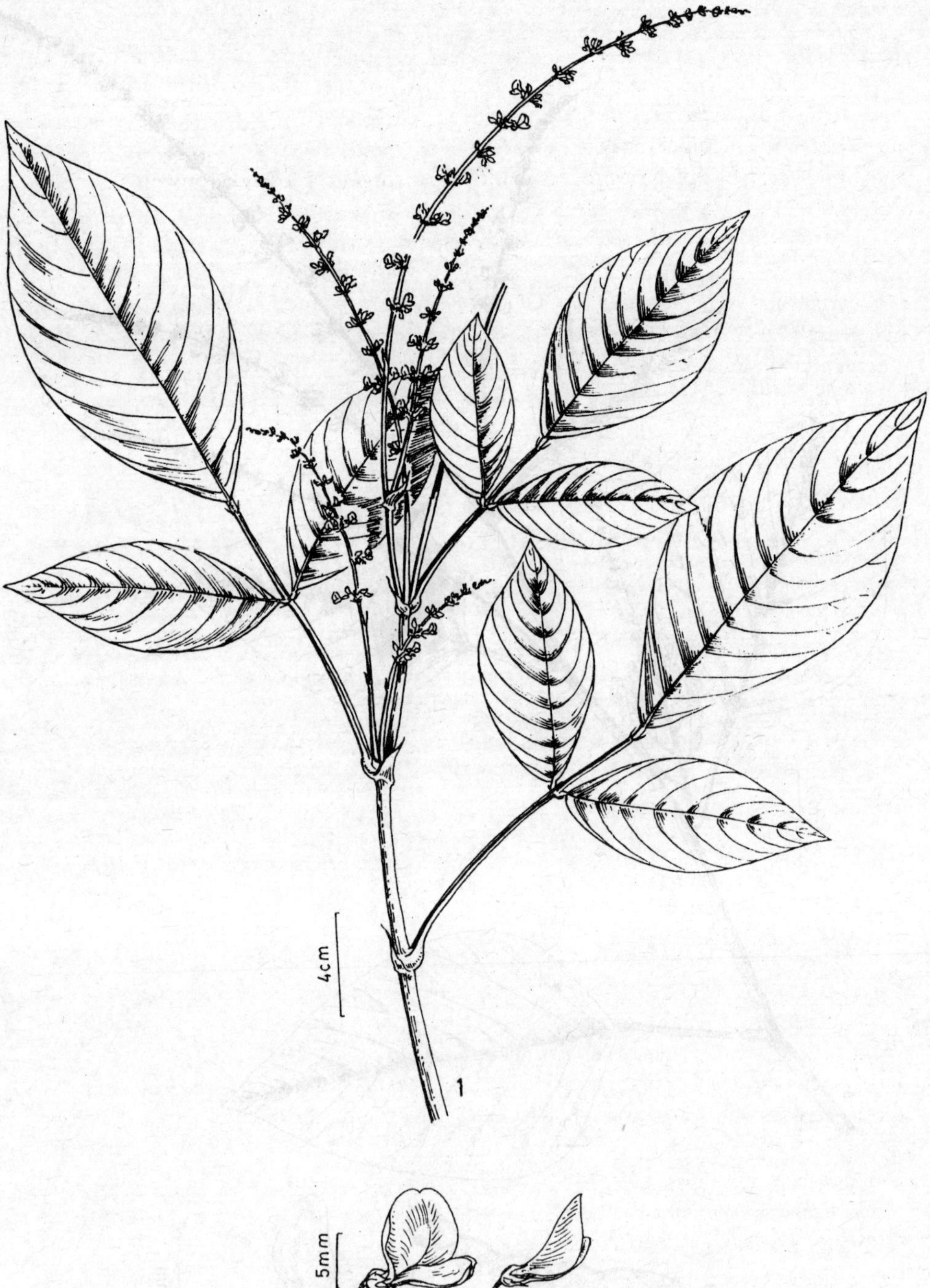

Figure 188: Desmodium laxiflorum DC. 1, A branch; 2–3, Flowers.

PUNAṚNAVĀ (Mal. TAVIḶĀMA, TAḶUTĀMA)

Punarnavā is an important rejuvenative drug used in Āyurvēda and is included in the *Vidāryādi gaṇa* of *Vāgbhaṭa*. It is bitter, astringent, cooling, stomachic, laxative, diuretic, expectorant, antipyretic and cardiotonic. It stimulates the function of heart and kidney and is specific for jaundice, diabetes, general debility, oedema and other diseases caused by morbid *kapha* and *pitta* (Aiyer & Kolammal, 1962, 5: 15). The officinal part is the root and it forms a chief ingredient of several formulations like *Punarnavāsavaṃ, Kumāryāsavaṃ, Dhānvantaraṃ kuḷaṁbu, Cyavanaprāśaṃ, Vastyāmayāntaka ghṛtaṃ* and the like.

Texts indicate that it is a perennial plant (*kaṭhillaḥ, kaṭhillakaḥ, śaśivāṭikā*), growing diffuse on the ground (*vṛścīkaḥ, bhaumaḥ*). The aerial part which flourishes during the rainy season (*vaiśākhī, prāvṛṣēṇyā, varṣābhavaḥ*) die off after season, but revives or sprouts up again next year (*punarnavā*). The aerial parts are often reddish (*raktākhyā, raktakāṇḍā, raktapatrikā, raktavarṣābhū*) and has reddish flowers (*raktapuṣpā*) (Aiyer & Kolammal, 1962. 5: 14).

Āyurvēdic texts mention two varieties of *punarnavā* viz. *raktapunarnavā*, the red variety and *śvētapunarnavā*, the white variety. They give separate synonyms and attribute different properties to them. *Raktapunarnavā* is bitter, acrid, cool and light. It is constipating and overcomes morbid *kapha* and *pitta*. *Śvētapunarnavā* is reported to be hot, bitter and dry. It alleviates morbid *kapha* and is useful in oedema, cough, bronchitis, anaemia, heart diseases and abdominal pain. According to *Bhāvaprakāśa*, it increases digestive power, destroys *kapha* and *vāta*, swelling, ascites, ulcers and inguinal hernea. *Śvētapunarnavā* is also considered specific for rat-bite poison, rabbies and eye diseases (Aiyer & Kolammal, 1962. 5: 15; Chunekar, 1982: 422).

In *Rājanighaṇṭu* a blue variety is also mentioned. But this is not in vogue in practice. In Kerala, only the red and white varieties are accepted. With regard to the identification of the different varieties of *punarnavā*, there is difference of opinion among the Āyurvēdic puṇḍits. Some of them have relied on the pigmentation of the plant body for this. Yet others are of opinion that these two *punarnavās* are to be recognised by the flower colour, *Raktapunarnavā* is invariably equated with *Boerhaavia diffusa* L. (Nyctaginaceae). *Trianthema portulacastrum* L. (Aizoaceae) is regarded as the source of *śvētapunarnavā* by many, probably due to the resemblence of its leaves with that of *Boerhaavia diffusa* (Aiyer & Kolammal, 1962. 5: 23). But this view point has not been accepted by many, because red and white (*rakta* and *śvēta*) forms are seen in both the species. Moreover, Chunekar (1982: 421) considers *punarnavā* and *varṣābhū* as two different drugs, the latter being an exclusively rainy season annual, while the other grows in other seasons, as well. *Trianthema portulacastrum*, being a rainy season annual, is equated with *varṣābhū* and the red and white forms of *Boerhaavia diffusa* with the red and white varieties of *punarnavā* (Bapalal Vaidya; 1982: 200).

Those who hold that the two varieties have to be recognised by their red and white flowers, equate them with different species of *Boerhaavia*. The accepted source of *raktapunarṇavā* is *Boerhaavia diffusa* L. However, Rheede's illustration (7: 105. t. 56, 1688) cited in the protologue of this species, has now been established as *B. repens* Linn. distinguished by its axillary, pedunculate cymes or umbels as against the strictly terminal paniculate inflorescence of the former (See Nicolson *et al.* 1988). But most authors consider these two as conspecific. These are finer botanical details beyond the comprehension of men of traditional medicine. Possibly both these species have been taken for the drug, by men of Āyurvēda.

Śvētapunarṇavā has since been equated with two white-flowered species, *B. erecta* L. (= *B. punarnava* Saha & Krishnamurthy, 1961. See also Sivarjan & Balachandran, 1985) and *Commicarpus verticillatus* (Poir.) Standl. (Anonymous 1978a: 257). However, *B. erecta* is an American weed, seemingly introduced into India rather recently (Nair, 1967) and hence cannot be considered as the original source of the drug.

Kerala physicians very often do not make a distinction between the two varieties in practice and *Boerhaavia diffusa* is invariably used for both, eventhough *Trianthema portulacastrum* is sometimes used as a substitute. The plants can be distinguished as follows.

Boerhaavia diffusa *Linn.* **(Nyctaginaceae)** (Fig. 189)
B. repens Linn.

Diffusely branched, low spreading perennial herb with an elongate fusiform tuberous tap root, branches often reddish coloured; leaves simple, opposite, ovate or oblong-obtuse to nearly suborbicular, in unequal pairs, 2–4 × 2–3.5 cm, thick, green glossy above, silvery white beneath; flowers small, pink on long axillary peduncled umbellate clusters, or in terminal panicles; perianth urceolate or funnel-form, constricted about the middle; stamens 2 or 3; style slender ending in an obtuse peltate stigma; fruits clavate, ribbed, glandular, 1-seeded.

The plant is a very common weed of sandy tracts, waste lands and roadsides of the plains districts, found all over India, especially during rainy season.

Boerhaavia erecta *Linn.* **(Nyctaginaceae)** (Fig. 190)
B. punarnava Saha & Krishnamurthy

Erect or diffuse herb, often reddish; leaves elliptic-ovate or lanceolate, acute in unequal pairs, margins wavy, 1.5–3.5 × 0.7–1.5 cms, thick glabrescent to puberulous; flowers white in slender, axillary and/or terminal panicle; fruits clavate, truncate, glabrous.

Distribution: This pantropical weed is now common along with the Malabar coast especially along the railway embankments and in moist sandy areas.

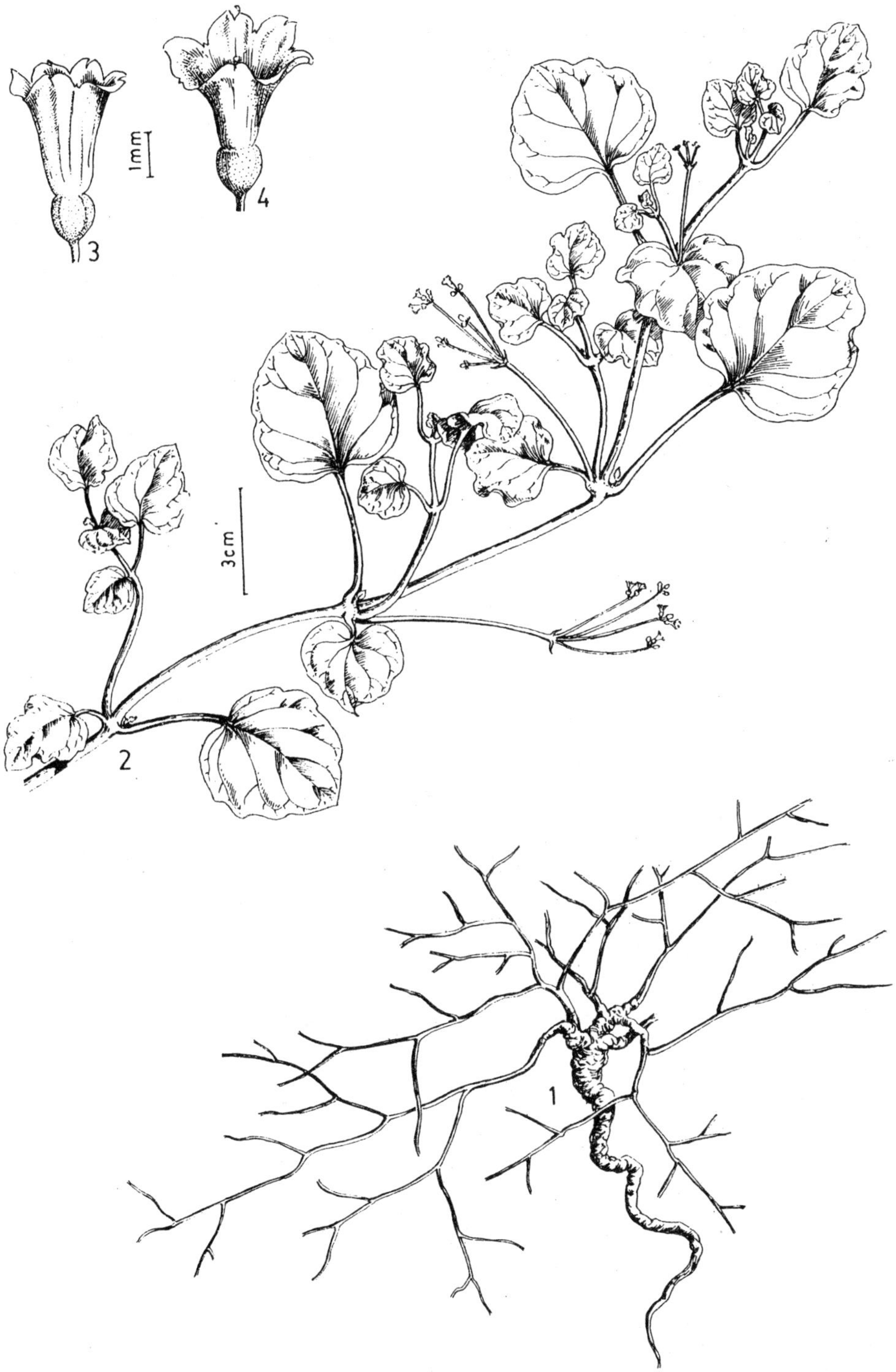

Figure 189: Boerhaavia diffusa L. 1, Habit (diagrammatic); 2, A flowering branch; 3–4, Flowers.

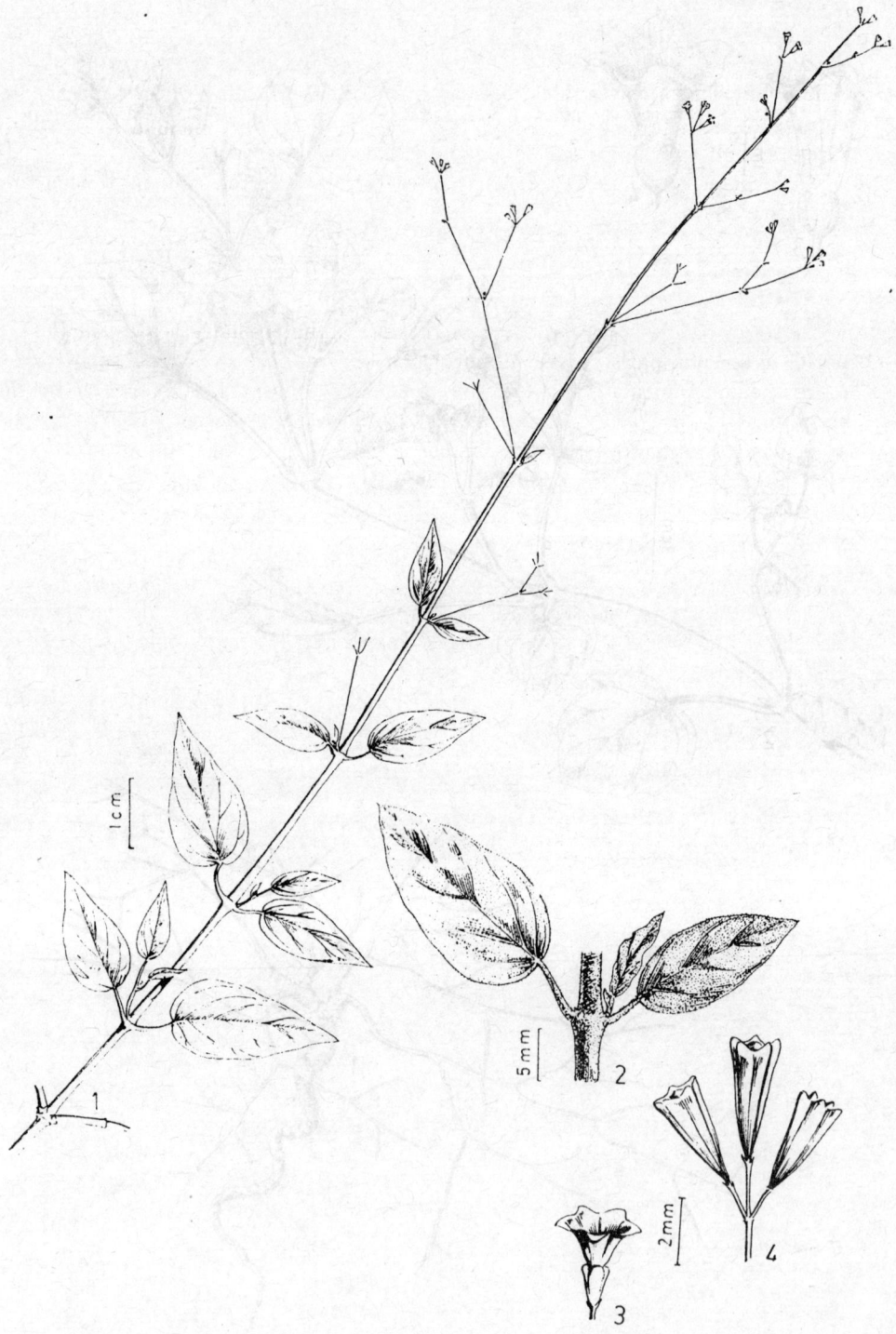

Figure 190: Boerhaavia erecta L. 1, A branch; 2, A node with leaves; 3, Flower; 4, Fruits.

Commicarpus verticillatus (*Poir.*) *Standl.* **(Nyctaginaceae)**
Boerhaavia verticillata Poir.
B. stellata Wt.

A rambling shrub; leaves thick, broadly ovate or suborbicular, obtuse, mucronate, cordate at base upto 6 cm across, glabrous; flowers white in long pedunculate racemes; fruit with large stalked globose glands on the crown, clavate.

The plant grows in dry district, often on black cotton soil, in Deccan and Carnatic.

Trianthema portulacastrum *Linn.* **(Aizoaceae)** (Fig. 191)
T. monogyna Linn.

Prostrate or diffuse succulent herb; stem terete, minutely hairy; leaves simple, opposite in unequal pairs, larger ones orbicular-obovate, 3.5 x 2.5 cms, smaller ones narrow, oblong-apiculate at apex; flowers axillary, solitary, sessile, enclosed in the sheathing leaf-base; calyx 5-lobed; petals 5, pinkish white; stamens 10–15; capsules opercular with many seeds in the chambers and 1–2 in the operculum.

Distribution: A pantropical weed of roadsides, waste lands, fallow rice fields etc. in most plains districts throughout India. It is abundant during the rainy season. Often used as a vegetable.

Note: Clinical studies conducted by Bhalla *et al.*, (1971) prove that *Boerhaavia diffusa* root possesses antiinflammatory and antiarthritic activity. The root extract also showed hypotensive activity in anaesthetized dogs (Ramabhimaiah *et al.*, 1984) and cardiovascular action in rats and cats (Ojewole Jao and Adesina, 1985).

Vohra *et al.*, (1983) found that *Trianthema portulacastrum* exhibits antipyretic, analgesic and anti-inflammatory activities.

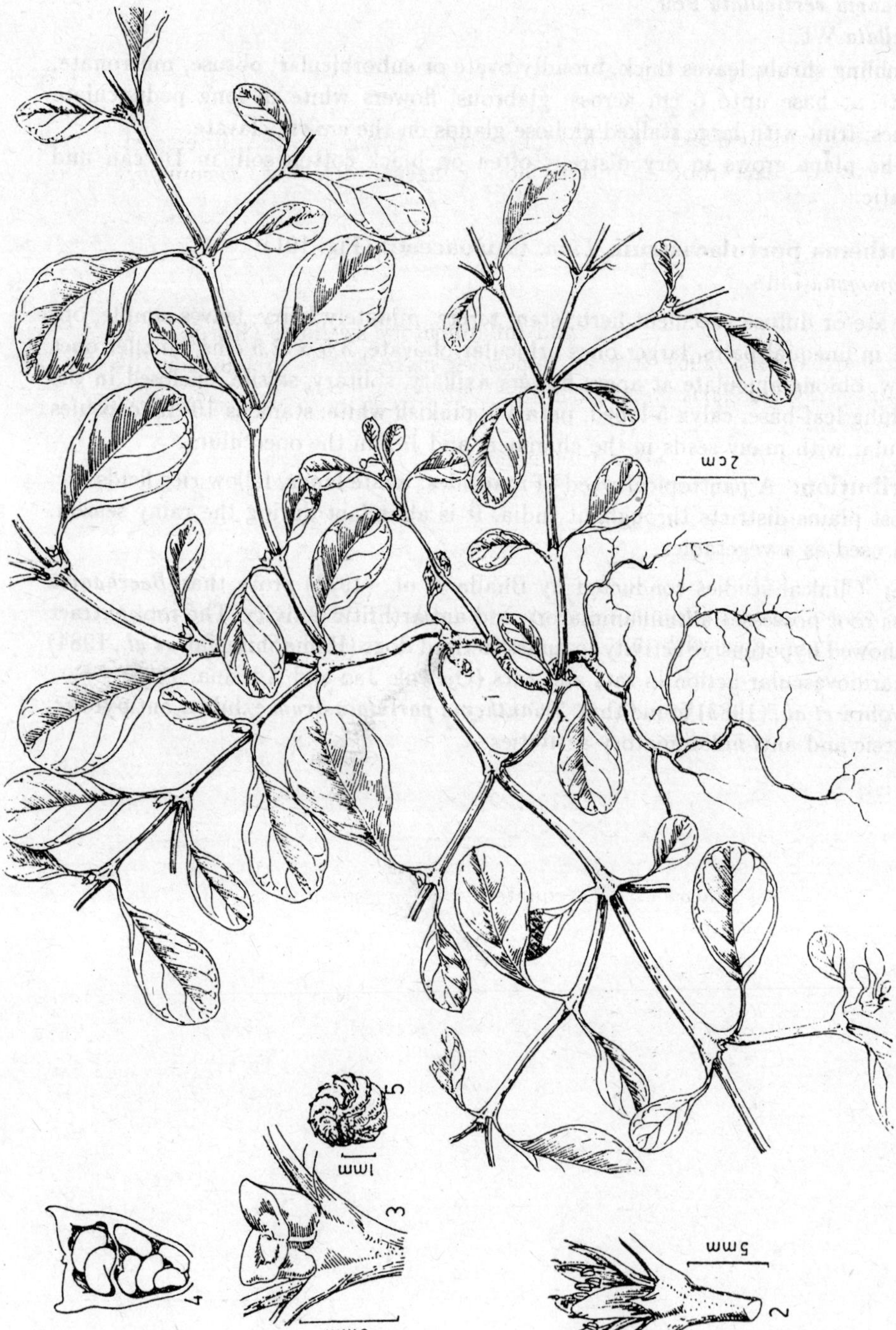

Figure 191: Trianthema portulacastrum L. 1, Habit; 2, Flower; 3, Fruit; 4, Fruit L.S.; 5, Seed.

PUṢKARAMŪLAṂ (Mal. PUṢKARAMŪLAṂ)

Puṣkaramūlaṃ is considered specific for cough, dyspnoea and intercoastal pain (*pārśvaśūla*). The root is bitter, hot, pungent, digestive, carminative, antiinflammatory, aphrodisiac, diuretic and febrifuge. It is reported to cure anaemia, catarrh, coryza, dyspepsia, indigestion, cardiac disorders, skin diseases, oedema and also diseases due to *kapha* and *vāta*. The drug is said to be useful against chronic cough, hiccough, brain affections, dysmenorrhoea and dysuria. A paste of the root is applied to indolent ulcers and inflammatory swellings (Kurup *et al.*, 1979: 173; Sharma, 1983: 296). It is an important ingredient of preparations like *Kumāryāsavaṃ, Daśamūlariṣṭaṃ, Valiya nārāyaṇa tailaṃ, Dhānvantaraṃ ghṛtaṃ* and *Cyavanaprāśaṃ*.

The synonyms attributed to this drug indicate that the plant occurs in Kashmir Himalayas (*kāśmīraṃ*) and that its leaves resemble that of lotus (*padmapatraṃ*). The terms *puṣkaraṃ, pouṣkaraṃ*, etc. refer to its capacity to improve general health and vigour. (cf. Moosad, 1983: 376).

The very few indications given in the texts do not lead us anywhere near a conclusive determination of its plant source. Nor do they fit well with those plants that are currently equated with this drug. To add to the trouble, the very name of the drug is a topic of semantic debate. While some people recognise *puṣkaramūla* (referring to the officinal part i.e. the roots of the plant *puṣkara*) and *puṣkaramulla* (a puṣkar with jasmine (*mulla* in vernacular)—like flowers) as two distinct drugs, the overwhelming opinion among Kerala physicians is that both refer to one and the same drug. Mooss (1981: 45), however, opines that the officinal part, as mentioned in the texts, is not the roots, but some reddish powdẹr on its fruits. Consequently, the plant source of this drug is highly controversial. According to *Bhāvaprakāśa*, it is a variety of drug *kuṣṭ* which has been equated with *Saussurea lappa* C.B. Clarke of Asteraceae and has similar curative properties (cf. Chunekar, 1982: 94). But this view is not accepted by other authors who consider them to be quite different, so much so that both are specifically mentioned in the same formulary.

Most of the works on Indian materia medica equate the drug with the roots of *Inula racemosa* Hook. f. (Asteraceae) (Singh & Chunekar, 1972: 255; Kurup *et al.*, 1979: 173; Kapoor & Mitra, 1979: 67; Dey, 1980: 121; Sharma, 1983: 296; Nesamony, 1985: 364). This plant, restricted to the Kashmir Himalayas, is locally known as *'poshkar'* (Kirtikar & Basu, 1918: 682; Chopra *et al.*, 1956: 141). Others have equated it with a West Himalayan species of *Iris* (Iridaceae), which they call *Iris germanica*, locally called *padmapuṣkara* (See Chunekar, 1982: 95). A perusal of taxonomic literature, however, indicates that *Iris germanica* is an European species and these authors have, in all probability, misidentified the Kashmiri element. In the absence of reliable material, we can only conclude that the plant used in Kashmir is some species of *Iris*.

Kirtikar & Basu (1918: 1260) and Nadkarni (1954: 385) have listed the Sanskrit names *'puṣkara'* and *puṣkaramūla* under *Costus speciosus* (Koenig) Smith belonging to Zingiberaceae. But in Kerala, this plant is used as the source of another drug *caṇḍā* (described elsewhere in this treatise).

The accepted source of *puṣkaramūla* in Kerala is *Coffea travancorensis* Wt. & Arn. (now, *Psilanthus travancorensis*) (Rubiaceae) which was abundant in the Kerala forests in the past, but now very scarce. (See Sivarajan & Balachandran, 1985.) This plant, however, finds no mention in any authentic publication of Indian medicinal plants. But Rheede has portrayed this species under the names *cherumulla* and *katu-mulla* (Hort. Malab. 6: 85. t. 49 & 6: 99 t. 56). Comparative and clinical studies on these plants are still wanting to substantiate their therapeutic prowess. On the other hand, clinical studies conducted on *Inula racemosa* (the powdered root mixed with the powdered oleoresin of *guggulu—Commiphora mukul* of Burseraceae) have proved that it is effective against Ischaemic heart diseases (Sharma *et al.*, 1986).

The three plants involved in the tangle of *puṣkaramūla* can be distinguished as follows.

Inula racemosa *Hook. f.* **(Asteraceae)**

A tall, stout herb, 50 cm–1.5 cm–1.5 m, stem grooved, leaves coriaceous, radical, 20–45 x 12.5–20 cm, elliptic-lanceolate narrowed into a petiole as long, cauline, often deeply lobed at the base, scabrid above, densely tomentone beneath; heads many, racemed, outer involucral bracts linear-acute; ligules slender 1.5 cm; achenes 0.4 cm, glabrous, slender; pappus 0.6 cm; reddish.

Distribution: Himachal Pradesh, Jammu & Kashmir, upto 5000–7000 ft.

Psilanthus travancorensis (*Wt. & Arn.*) *Leroy* **(Rubiaceae)** (Fig. 192)
Coffea travancorensis Wt. & Arn. **(Rubiaceae)**

A bushy shrub about 1.5 m tall, profusely branched; leaves upto 7 × 3.5 cms, broadly elliptic, acute or shortly acuminate, entire, slightly coriaceous, glabrous, shining green above; flowers white, fragrant, in axillary clusters of 3 or 4; calyx small, truncate; corolla tube cylindrical, 1.5 cms long, lobes 5, spreading; fruit didymous, 8 mm across, black when mature; seeds flat, smooth.

Distribution: Western Ghats in Malabar and Travancore, also recorded from Sri Lanka.

Iris germanica *Linn.* **(Iridaceae)**

Perennial herbs; root stock bulbous or creeping, leaves equitant, ensiform; perianth tube long or short, segments large, outer (sepals) largest, stipitate, reflexed, inner (petals) smaller, suberect or reflexed; stamens inserted at the base of the outer segments, anthers linear, basifixed; ovary 3-gonous, style stout, stigma petaloid, arching over the stamens, 2-fid and with a transverse dorsal crest; capsule coriaceous, 3 or 6 ribbed, seeds flat or globose.

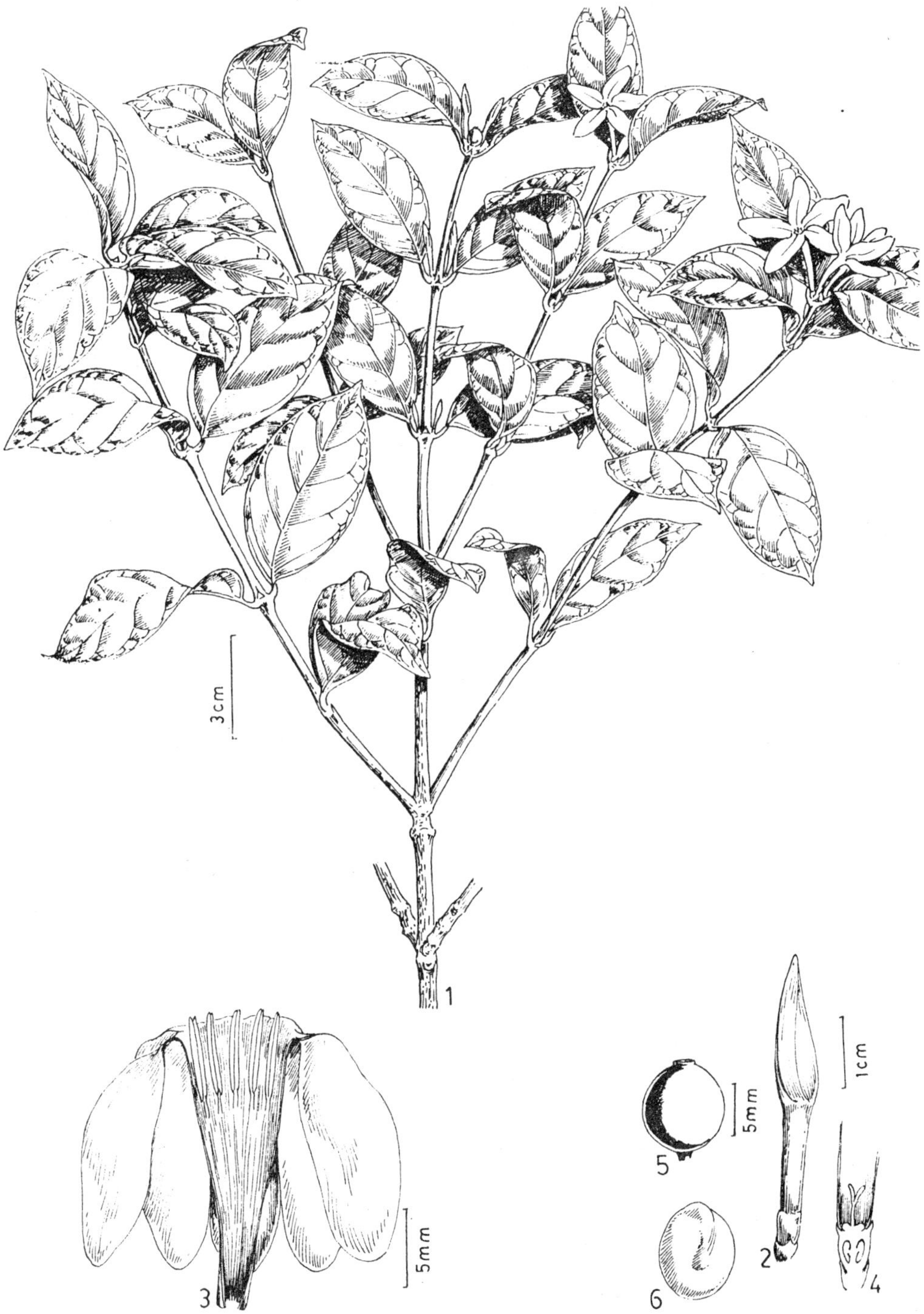

Figure 192: Psilanthus travancorensis (Wt. & Arn.) Leroy. 1, Flowering twig; 2, Flower bud; 3, Corolla opened with stamens; 4, L.S. of ovary; 5, Fruit; 6, Seed.

RAKTACANDANAḤ (Mal. RAKTACANDANAṀ)

As the name indicates, the wood is commonly called the 'red sandal wood'. It is reported to be cooling, antipyretic, antiperiodic, astringent, bitter, diaphoretic and febrifuge and is used in abscesses, boils, eye troubles, headache, haemophilic disorders, inflammation, thirst and vomiting. It purifies blood and cures skin diseases and poisonous affections (Kurup *et al.*, 1979: 174; Sharma, 1983: 718).

Contrary to the appellation *candana* (Sandal wood) in its name, the wood of this plant is odourless and hence the synonym ***kucandana***. The term ***raktacandana*** (rakta = blood red) denotes the red colour of the wood. But for these, there are no useful indications in the ancient texts which would help us in the accurate identification of the drug. Nevertheless, there is little doubt about the botanical source of the drug, which is ***Pterocarpus santalinus*** Linn. of Papilionaceae.

Pterocarpus santalinus *Linn.* **(Papilionaceae)** (Fig. 193)

Tree, leaves 3-foliolate; leaflets to 9 × 8 cms, ovate-orbicular, base obtuse or subcordate, apex emarginate, margin entire; flowers in axillary racemes; calyx tube 4.5 mm, tomentose, lobes ovate; corolla papilionaceous; stamens 10; ovary stipitate, 6 mm; pod narrowly 5 × 4.5 cm.

Distribution: The tree is found mainly in southern India in Deccan, in the hills of Cuddapah, S. Kurnool, N. Arcot and Chinglepet, upto 1,500 ft.

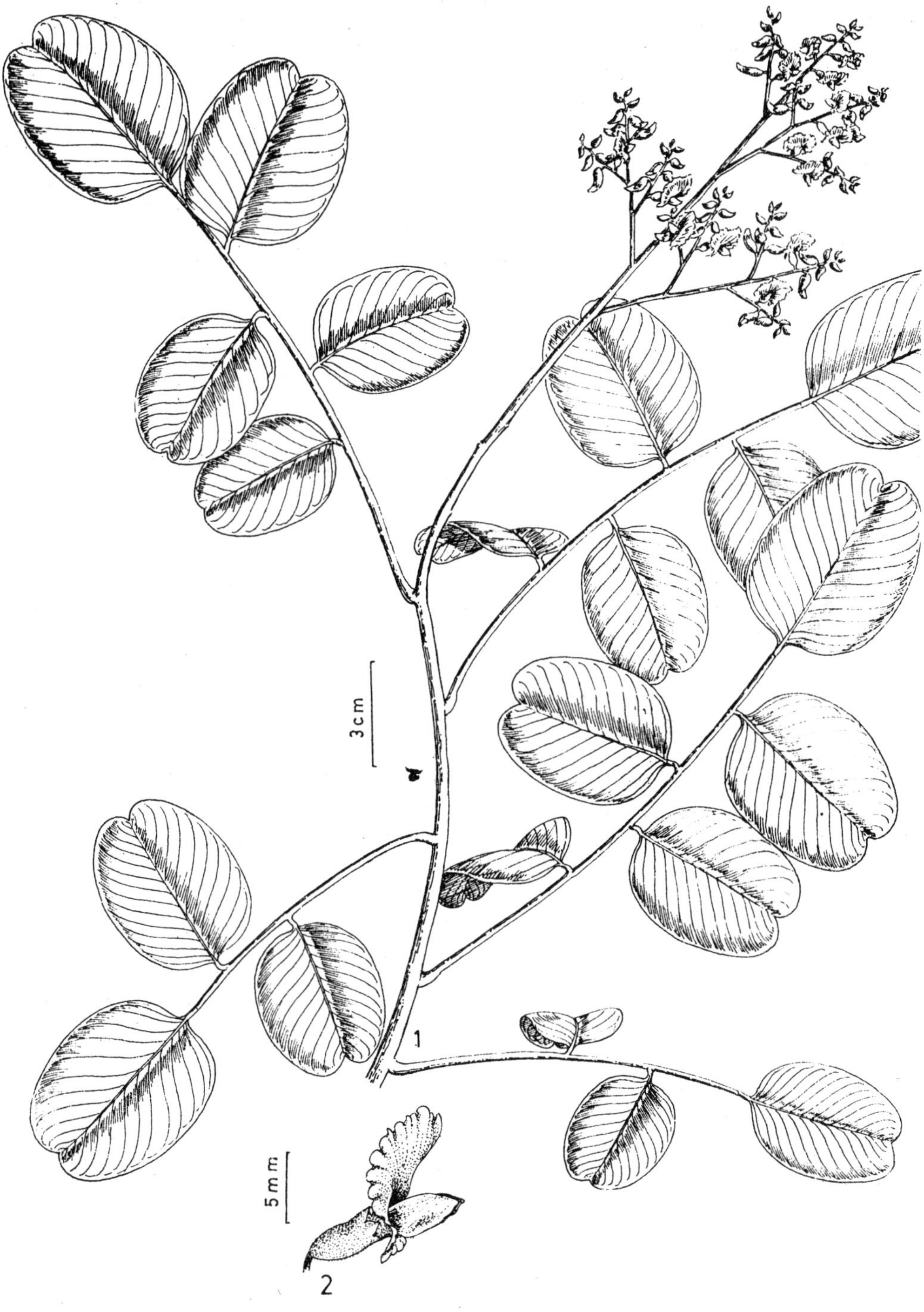

Figure 193: Pterocarpus santalinus L. 1, A flowering branch; 2, Flower.

RĀSNĀ (Mal. ARATTA)

Caraka includes *rāsnā* in the *Vayasthāpana varga*, the group of drugs that are capable of maintaining the youthful vigour and strength. The drug is also a popular remedy for rheumatism, intermitent fevers, dyspepsia, cough, bronchitis, asthma and other respiratory ailments. It is bitter, hot and aromatic and overcomes *kapha* and *vāta*, poison, intestinal and biliary colic. The drug stimulates digestion, purifies blood and improves voice (Chunekar, 1982: 76). The officinal part is the rhizome which forms a major ingredient of preparations like *Rāsnādi kaṣāyaṃ, Rāsnādi cūrṇaṃ, Rāsnādi tailaṃ, Aśvagandhāriṣṭaṃ*, etc.

Except for the mention that the plant has got leaves which resemble those of *ēla* (=*Elettaria cardamomum*) (*ēlāparṇī*) and that it has got fragrant tubers (*sugandhā, suvahā*), the ancient texts do not lend any assistance in finding out the accurate identity of the plant source and consequently, there is great confusion with regard to the identity of the drug.

A number of widely different plants are equated with it by different people. *Nākulī* and *gandhanākulī* are often treated as synonyms of *rāsnā* by some (Moosad, 1983: 351) whereas they are considered different by others. The application of names such as *sugandhā* to more than one drug (homonym), has further deepened the dispute. The name *sugandhā* is a synonym of *rāsnā, gandhanākulī, śāribā* and *nākulī* (Singh & Chunekar, 1972: 219).

Rājanighaṇṭu mentions three types of *rāsnā*, namely *mūlarāsnā, patrarāsnā* and *tṛṇarāsnā*, whereas Caraka, Suśruta and Vāgbhaṭa do not make any mention of such a distinction, nor is it in vogue among practioners of Kerala.

In most of the publications on Indian materia medica, *rāsnā* is equated with an orchid *Vanda tessellata* (Roxb.) Hook ex Don (=*Vanda roxburghii* R.Br.) (Kirtikar & Basu, 1918: 1244; Vaidya, 1936: 478; Nadkarni, 1954: 1263; Chopra *et al.*, 1956: 252; Kurup *et al.*, 1979: 176; Kapoor & Mitra, 1979: 67; Dey, 1980: 128). Some others consider *Pluchea lanceolata* (Asteraceae) as the real source of *rāsnā* (Singh & Chunekar, 1972: 338, Sharma, 1983: 39). This is the *rāsnā* of Punjab and Gujarat (Vaidya Bapalal, 1982: 34). Its roots, when dried under shade, develop a faint aroma and they are being used by the country people in rheumatic conditions (Singh & Chunekar, 1972: 338). But none of them is taken as the drug source in Kerala. Throughout South India it is the aromatic rhizomes of *Alpinia galanga* Sw. (Zingiberaceae) that is accepted as the source of *rāsnā*. As the synonyms *ēlāparṇī* and *sugandhā* suit this plant well, this is believed to be the true *rāsnā* by South Indian physicians. Some authors equate this plant with *kulañjana* or *sugandhavacā* (Nadkarni, 1954: 77: Chopra *et al.*, 1956: 13; Sharma, 1983: 304) giving the Malayalam equivalent of *rāsnā*, namely *aratta*. Ayurvedic formulary of India suggests *Pluchea lanceolata* as the real *rāsnā* and *Alpinia galanga* as a substitute (Anonymous, 1978a: 255).

Studies on the market samples reveal that two types of *rāsnā* are sold in South Indian markets—one with light brown colour and aromatic odour identified as the rhizomes of *Alpinia calcarata*, locally called *pēraratta* and the other less aromatic, *A. galanga*, known as *cittaratta* or *aratta* in vernacular (Nair *et al.*, 1982). The two species that are used as the drug sources in Kerala can be identified as follows.

Alpinia galanga *Sw.* **(Zingiberaceae)** (Fig. 194)

Perennial rhizomatous herb; leafy stem 2–3 mm high; leaves short-petioled oblong-lanceolate, acuminate, to 60 × 10 cm, glabrous; flowers in terminal panicle, about 20 cm long; greenish white; calyx tubular, white, shortly 3 lobed at apex; corolla tubular below with three linear-oblong spreading lobes; fertile stamen 1, anther 2-celled, introrse, lip orbicular-spathulate with reddish veins, ovary glabrous, 3-celled, many ovuled, style filiform ending in subglobose stigma.

Distribution: The plant is seen along the W. Ghats. Often cultivated for its rhizomes.

Note: Itokawa *et al.* (1987) isolated two antitumour principles from *Aplinia galanga*.

Alpinia calcarata *Rosc.* **(Zingiberaceae)** (Fig. 195)

Perennial rhizomatous herb; leafy stem about 1–2.5 m high; leaves linear, lanceolate acuminate, glabrous, upto 40 × 8 cm; flowers white with red lip in terminal panicle about 15 cm long; calyx white tubular, lobed at apex; corolla tube as long as calyx, lateral lobes oblong, apically concave, upper one broader, lebellum variegated with red and yellow, to 3 × 1 cm, margin fimbriate, apex rounded; staminodes teethlike, filament flattened, anther cell apically diverging. Ovary densely pilose, 3-celled, ovules many on axile placenta, stigma subglobose.

Distribution: The plant is common along W. Ghats. Often cultivated in Sri Lanka, Malay Peninsula and China.

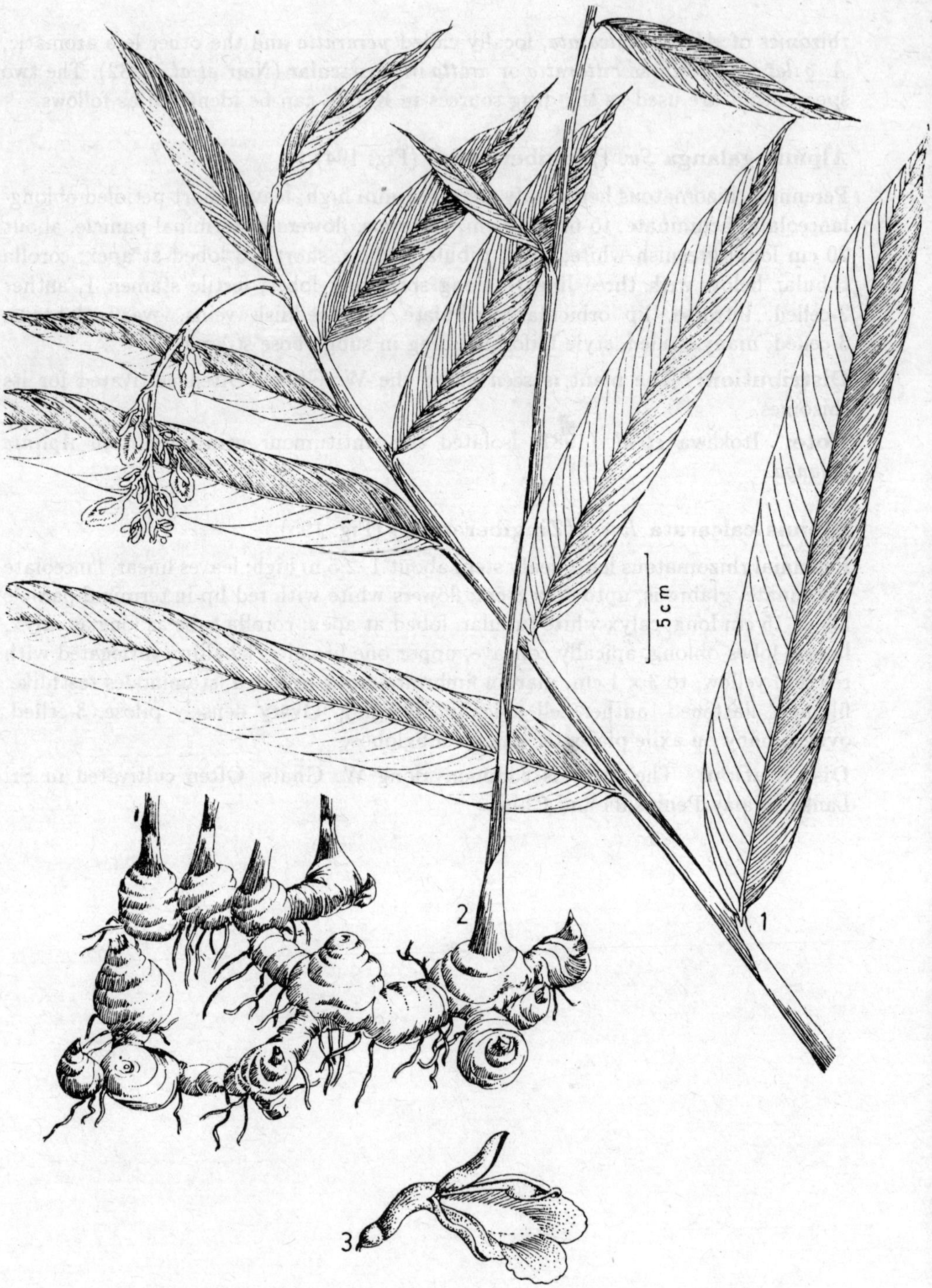

Figure 194: Alpinia galanga Sw. 1, Vegetative shoot with rhizomes; 2, Flowering shoot; 3, Flower.

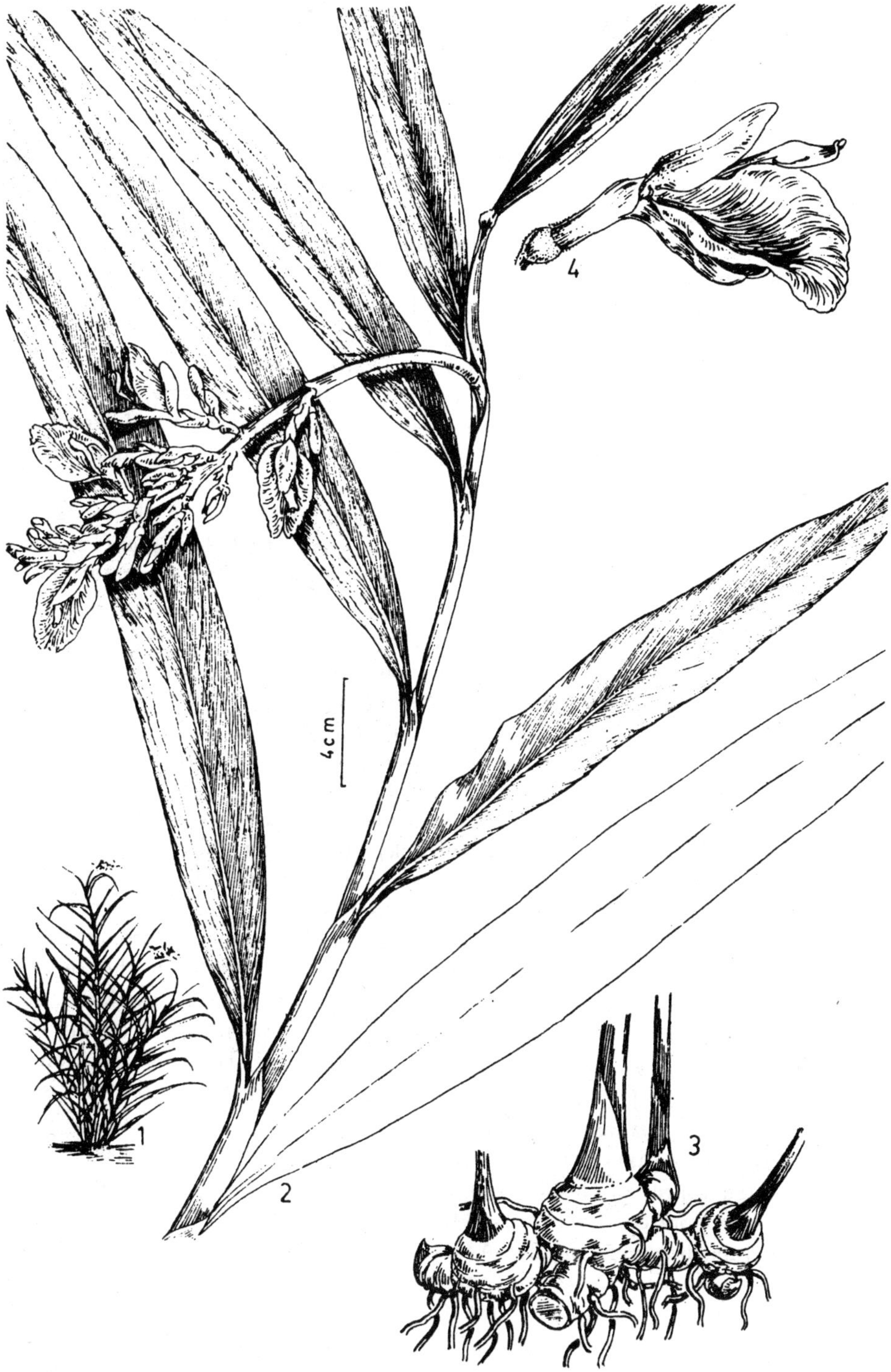

Figure 195: **Alpinia calcarata** Rosc. 1, Habit (diagrammatic); 2, Aerial shoot with inflorescence; 3, Rhizomes; 4, Flower.

SAHACARAḤ (Mal. KARIṀKURUÑÑI)

Sahacara is an important drug in Āyurvēda, widely used against neurological disorders such as paraplegia, sciatica etc. This drug also helps heal ulcers, glandular swellings, poisonous affections, itching, leprosy and other skin diseases, cough, oedema, toothache and gum diseases and to strengthen the nerves. The juice of the leaves purifies blood and semen (Chunekar, 1982: 503; Sharma, 1983: 186). The root, which is the official part, forms a major ingredient of preparations like *Sahacarādi tailaṃ, Sahacarādi kaṣāyaṃ, Valiya Rāsnādi kaṣāyaṃ*, etc.

According to the texts, this is a gregarious shrub (*sahacaraḥ, sahācaraḥ*), having sharp piercing structures like spines (*kuranṭakaḥ, rujākaraḥ*) and occuring in fully exposed habitats like deserts, naked hill tops or the tidal areas along the seacoast (*sairēyaḥ*) (cf. Singh & Chunekar, 1972: 445).

Different varieties of *sahacara* are found mentioned in the texts and their distinction is mainly based on flower colour. *Bhāvaprakāśa nighaṇṭu* mentions four varieties having red, yellow, blue and white flowers giving separate synonyms for each, whereas *Dhanvantarinighaṇṭu* describes only three with yellow, red and blue flowers. These varieties have been equated with different species of plants, mostly of *Barleria*. The red and white flowered varieties are equated with *Barleria cristata*, the yellow flowered with *B. prionitis* and the blue flowered with *B. strigosa* of Acanthaceae (Chunekar, 1982: 502; Sharma, 1983: 185). Many authors do not make a distinction of these varieties and equate *sahacara* with *Barleria prionitis* (Kapoor & Mitra, 1979: 67; Anonymous 1978a: 258).

Kerala physicians, however, recognise two *sairēyakās*—the dark variety or *kariṁkuruññi* (= *kariṁ* = dark or black) which is generally accepted as *'sahacara'* and the white variety i.e. *veṇkuruññi* (*veṇ* = white). They are together called *sairyaka yugmaṃ* (*yugmaṃ* = a pair). Discussions with practitioners have revealed that these two are considered to possess similar therapeutic properties and hence can be used in place of each other. In cases where both the *sairēyakās* are recommended, they usually take the one, which is easily available, double the amount. However, specific mention about *'sairyakayugmaṃ'* in certain formularies in the texts (eg. *Varaṇādi gaṇa* of Vāgbhaṭa) makes this assertion to be of doubtful merit. Of the two varieties, the most commonly used one is the black variety or *kariṁkuruññi*. Perusal of Rheede's Hortus Malabaricus (2: 31–32, t. 20. 1679) reveals that *Ecbolium viride* (Forsk.) Alston (Acanthaceae) had been the accepted source of the drug in Kerala in those days. Some other authors have also corroborated this (Vaidya, 1936: 602; Mooss, 1980: 57). In current practice, in Kerala, however, another Acanthaceous plant, *Nilgirianthus ciliatus* is mainly used as *sahacara*. A scrutiny of the market samples reveals that roots of some other species of the same genus (e.g. *N. heyneanus*, see Santha *et al.*, 1988) are also used as the plant source of this drug. Nair *et al.* (1985) are of opinion that the synonyms like *sahacara* (plants in groups giving bushy appearance and covering large area), *mṛdukaṇṭaka* (soft-spiny nature), *bāṇa* (causing mild pain on touch), *anantā* (continuous propagation of the plant vegetatively), *mṛdukāṇḍa* (soft stem) etc. are all applicable to this genus.

The botanical identity of *śvētasahacara* or *veṇkuruññi* is also disputed. Nadkarni (1954: 174) and Chopra *et al.* (1956: 33) equate this with *Barleria courtallica.* Rheede in his Hortus Malabaricus (2: 33–34, t. 21. 1679) portrays *Justicia betonica* (Acanthaceae) as the source of the drug and this has been accepted by Mooss (1980: 57) also. There are several followers for this point of view, even now. In the northern part of Malabar, practitioners prefer a different Acanthaceous plant, namely *Calacanthus grandiflorus* (= *C. dalzelliana*), also known as *vāḷakuruññi* in vernacular, reportedly because of the similarity of its roots with *vāḷa* i.e. plantain.

The distinguishing features of the various plants used as the source of the drug are as follows.

Nilgirianthus ciliatus (*Nees*) *Bremek.* **(Acanthaceae)** (Fig. 196)
Strobilanthes ciliatus Nees.

Gregarious shrub, often growing in large colonies; stem and leaves dark green; leaves simple, opposite, elliptic-acuminate, serrate, to 17 × 5 cms; flowers pale rose in short, glandular, bracteate, deflexed spikes; calyx lobes 5, lanceolate, acuminate; corolla base cylindric, upper part campanulate, spreading; stamens didynamous; ovary 2-celled with 2 ovules in each; capsule clavate, slightly exserted from the glandular fruiting calyx.

Distribution: The plant is common in W. Ghats, S. Canara to Travancore, in evergreen forests upto 4,000 ft.

Ecbolium viride (*Forsk.*) *Alston* **(Acanthaceae)** (Fig. 197)
E. linneanum Kurz.

Woody undershrub; leaves simple, opposite, elliptic-ovate obtuse or acute, base narrowed down to a short petiole, 11 × 4.5 cms, glabrous green above, pale beneath; flowers greenish blue in terminal spikes; bracts large, green, orbicular or lanceolate; calyx lobes 5, subequal, lanceolate, glandular-pubescent without; corolla tube slender, long, limb distinctly bilabiate, upper lip linear, lower lip spreading, 3-lobed; stamens 2, attached at the base of upper lip, exserted; capsule clavate, compressed; seeds 2, orbicular, tuberculate on curved retinacula.

Distribution: Usually seen in waste places and exposed habitats. Distributed in Sri Lanka, India, Africa and Malaya.

Justicia betonica *Linn.* **(Acanthaceae)** (Fig. 198)

Gregarious tall shrub; leaves simple, opposite, long-petioled, ovate-lanceolate, to 22 × 7 cms, entire to crenate-dentate, glabrous; flowers white speckled with pink in long terminal bracteate spikes; bracts and bracteoles similar, leafy, elliptic to ovate acute, white with green nerves; calyx lobes 5; corolla tube short, limb distinctly bilabiate; stamens 2; clavate; seeds spinulose when wetted.

Distribution: A pantropical species, this is found in all districts in India in waste lands and forest clearings.

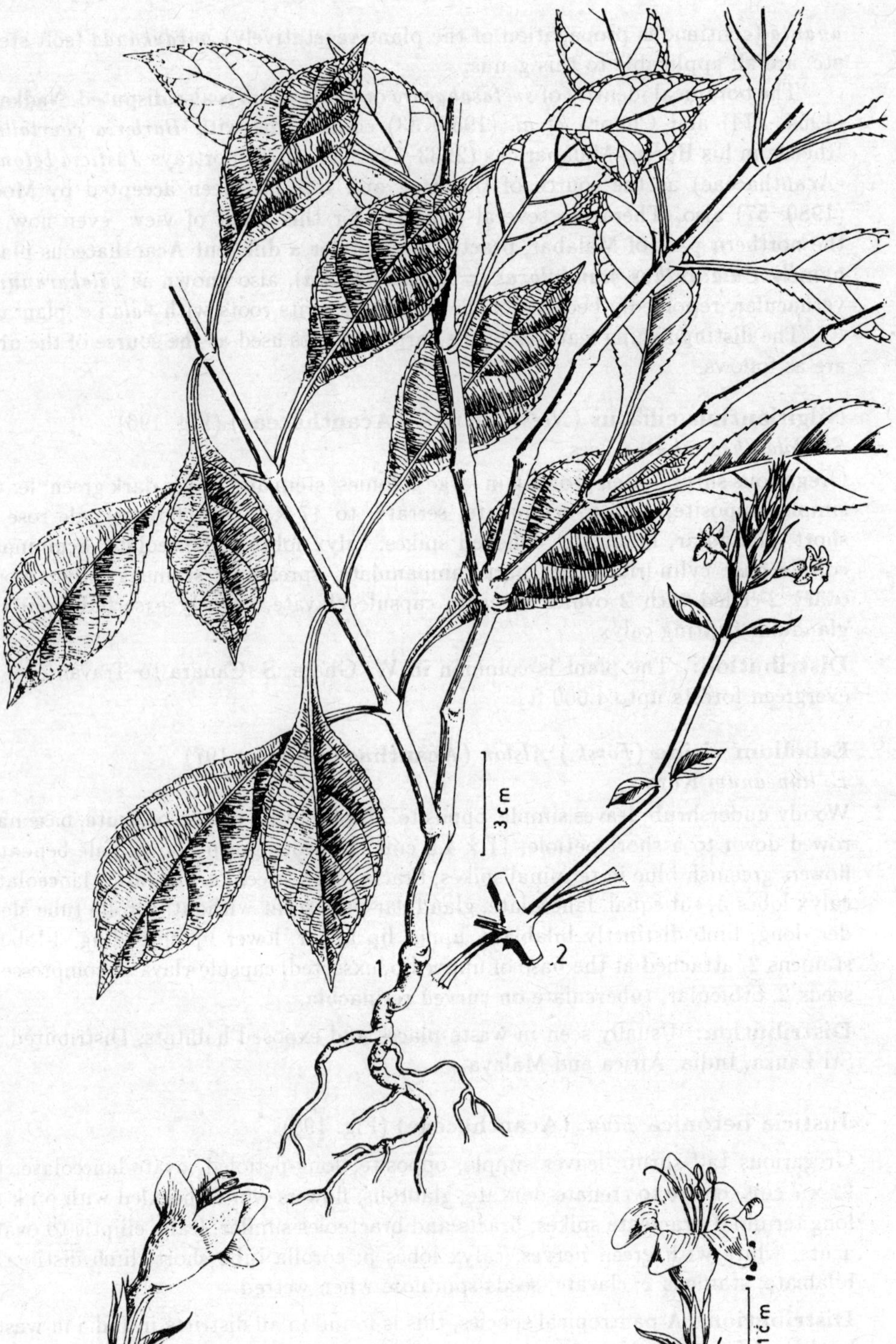

Figure 196: Nilgirianthus ciliatus (Nees) Bremek. 1, Habit; 2, Flowering shoot; 3–4, Flowers.

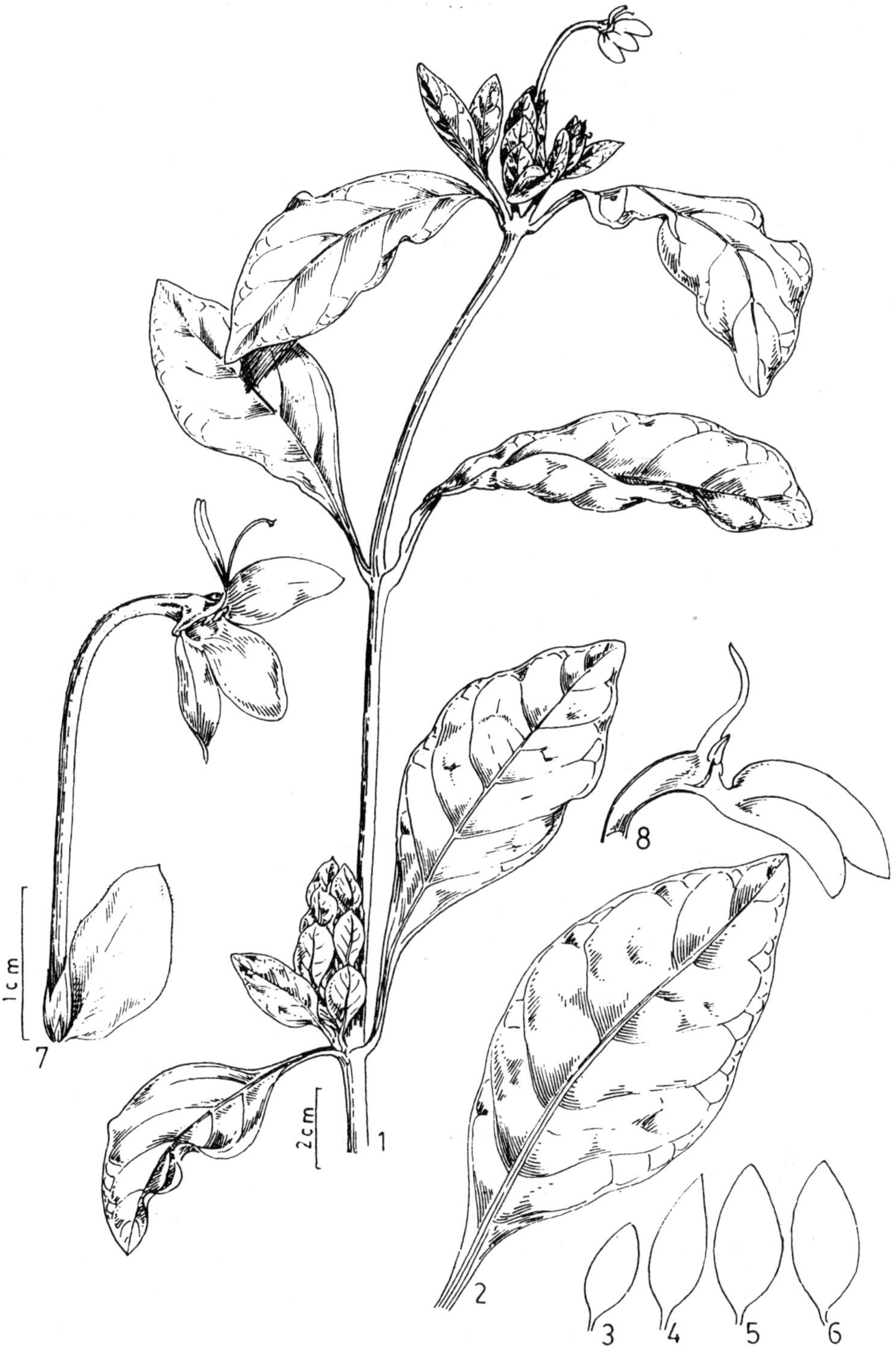

Figure 197: Ecbolium viride (Forsk.) Alston. 1, A branch; 2, Leaf; 3–6, Bracts; 7, Flower; 8, Corolla L.S.

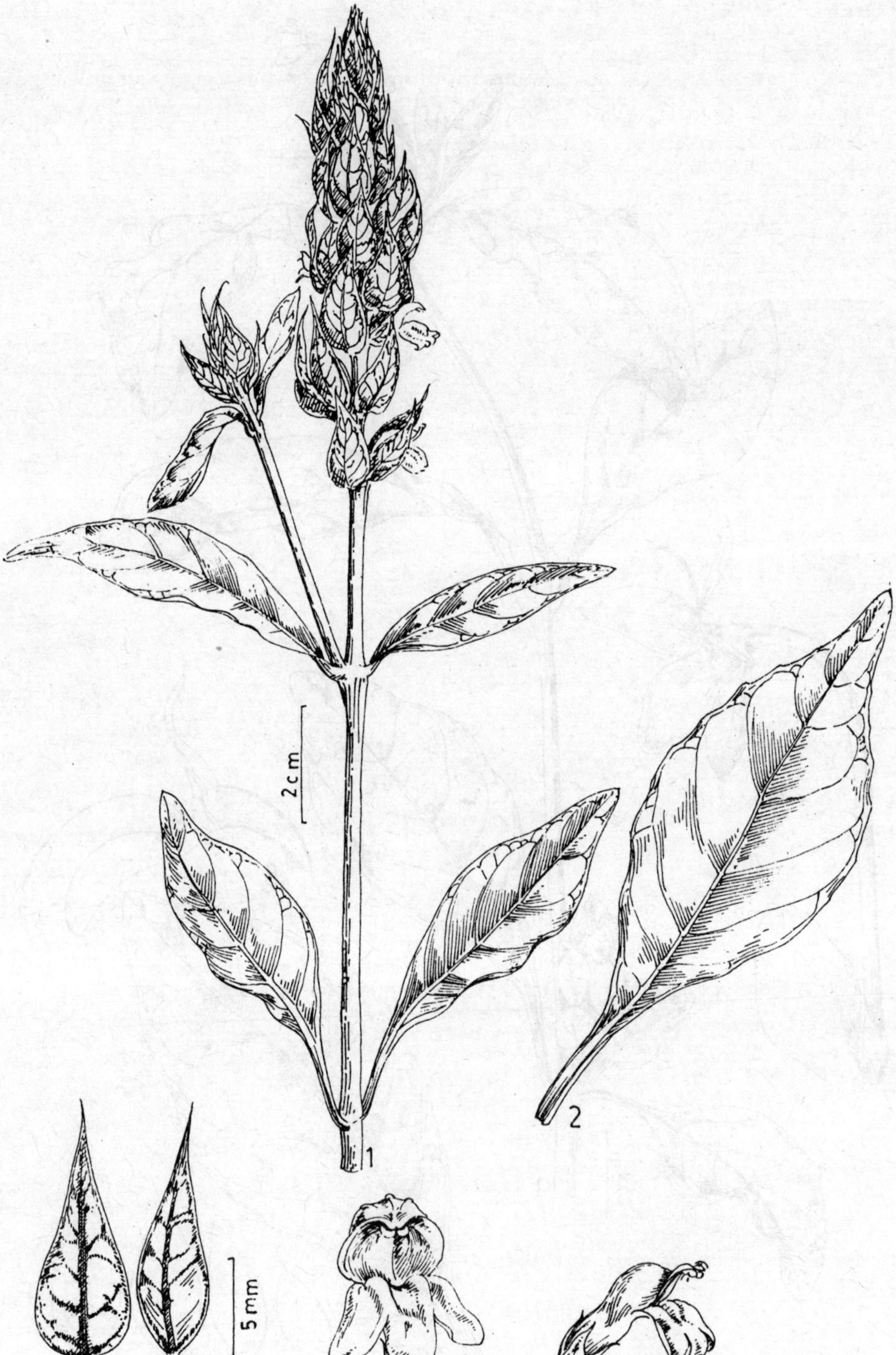

Figure 198: Justicia betonica L. 1, Habit; 2, Leaf; 3–4, Bracts; 5–6, Flowers.

Calacanthus grandiflorus (*Dalz.*) *Radlk.* **(Acanthaceae)** (Fig. 199)
C. dalzelliana Anders.

Profusely branched, gregarious shrub with prominently swollen nodes and obtusely 4 angled stem; leaves simple, opposite, elliptic-lanceolate, acuminate, serrulate, to 26 x 8.5 cms, flowers purple in terminal bracteate spikes; bracts large, ovate, closely inbricating; calyx 5-partite, the lobes unequal, corolla purple, deeply 2-lipped, upper lip narrow, emarginate; lower lip large, shortly 3-lobed, with a yellow central groove; stamens 4, didynamous, filaments connate at base; capsule obovoid, compressed, pubescent, 2-seeded; seeds compressed, hairy, on curved retinacula.

Distribution: The plant is seen in the hills of S. Canara upto 3,000 ft.

Barleria prionitis *Linn.* **(Acanthaceae)** (Fig. 200)

Armed subshrub, with sharp axillary spines; leaves simple, opposite, elliptic, acute or acuminate, entire, 4–12 x 2–6 cm; flowers yellow, solitary in lower axils, spicate above; bracts 2, lanceolate, spine-tipped; calyx lobes 4, spine-tipped; corolla tube 2.5 cm, limb subequally 5-lobed; stamens 2; capsule ovoid, 2-seeded.

Distribution: The plant is found in all plains districts, especially the Deccan and Carnatic, chiefly on waste lands and roadsides. It is also distributed in tropical Africa, tropical Asia, Sri Lanka and Malacca.

Barleria strigosa *Wall.* **(Acanthaceae)**

Woody shrub; leaves ovate, acuminate, long-decurrent on the petiole, glabrate; flowers deep blue in dense, axillary, one-sided spikes; bracts large, ovate-oblong; outer calyx lobes ovate, denticulate, minutely strigose, inner linear-lanceolate, white, hirsute; capsule 4-seeded.

Distribution: The plant grows as a forest undergrowth in N. Circars, Deccan, in Kurnool Nallamalais and Ramdurg in Bellary.

Barleria cristata *Linn.* **(Acanthaceae)** (Fig. 201)

Sub shrubs; leaves elliptic to lanceolate, acute, entire; flowers 1–4 in axillary cymes; bracts lanceolate, serrate-dentate, scabrous; calyx lobes 4, puberulous, spinous ciliate; corolla blue or white, funnel-shaped; limb subequally 5 lobed; capsule oblong, 4 seeded.

Distribution: Common in deciduous forests in all dry plains districts upto about 3,000 ft. Also grown as an ornamental.

Barleria courtallica *Nees* **(Acanthaceae)**

Unarmed shrub; leaves elliptic, obovate or lanceolate, acuminate, glabrous; flowers blue in glandular hairy spikes; bracts linear; calyx lobes 4, thick, glandular-hairy without; corolla tube 3.5 cms, lobes 5, broadly obovate, sparsely hairy; stamens 4; ovary 4-ovuled, style sparsely hairy below, stigma fusiform.

Distribution: The plant is found in evergreen forests in N. Circars, Rampa Hills of Godavari, W. Ghats, in all districts.

Note: Ravisankar *et al.* (1984) and Nair *et al.* (1988) found that ethanol extract and aqueous extract of *Strobilanthes heyneanus* stem possess marked anti-inflammatory effect. *S. ciliatus* is found to be efficaceous in the treatment of hemiplegia (Namboodiri, *et al.* 1985).

Pharmacognostical studies on the root and leaves of *sahacara-Nilgirianthus heyneanus* have been carried out by Santha *et al.* (1988).

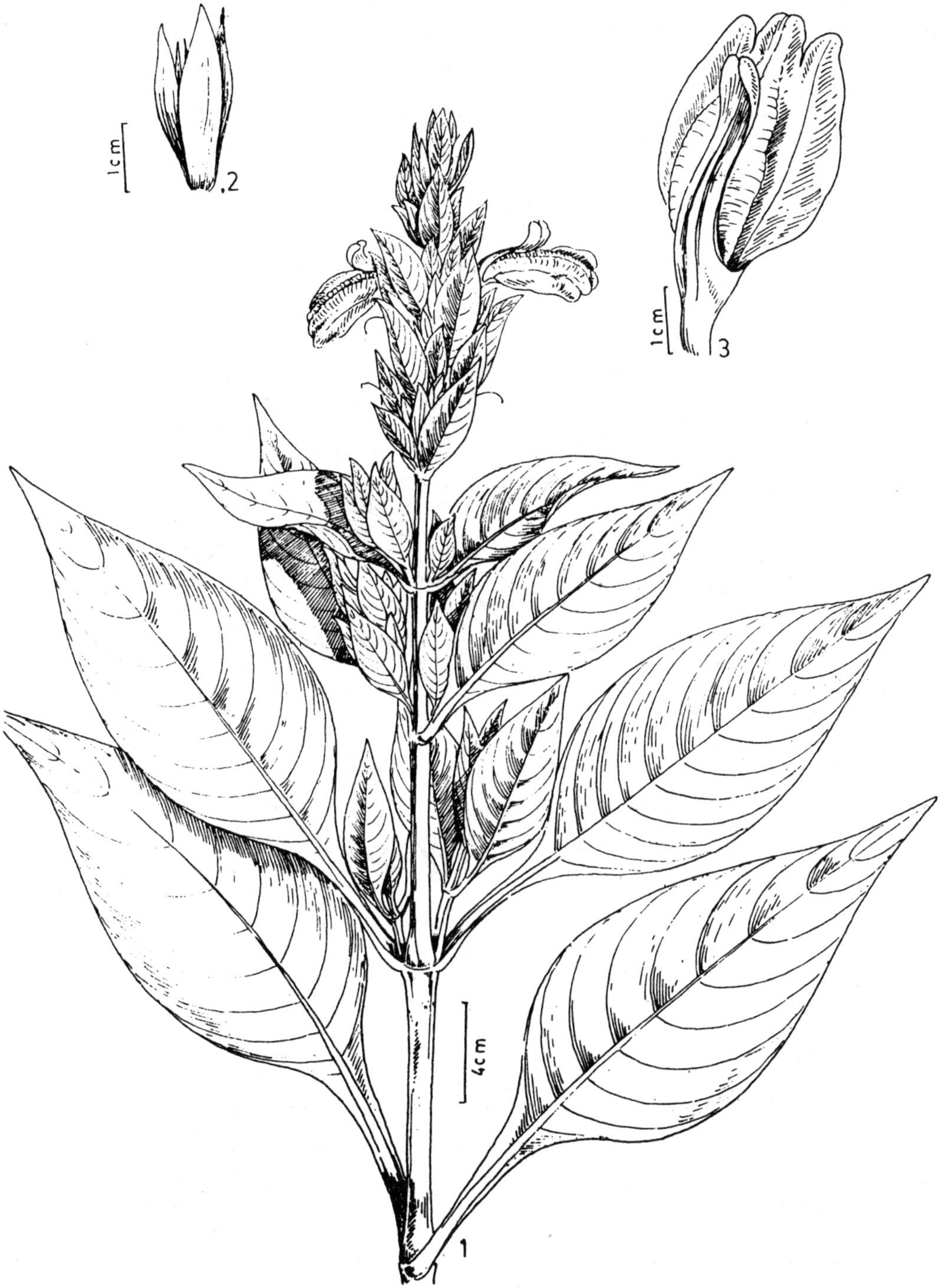

Figure 199: Calacanthus grandiflorus (Dalz.) Radlk. 1, A Flowering branch; 2, Calyx; 3, Corolla.

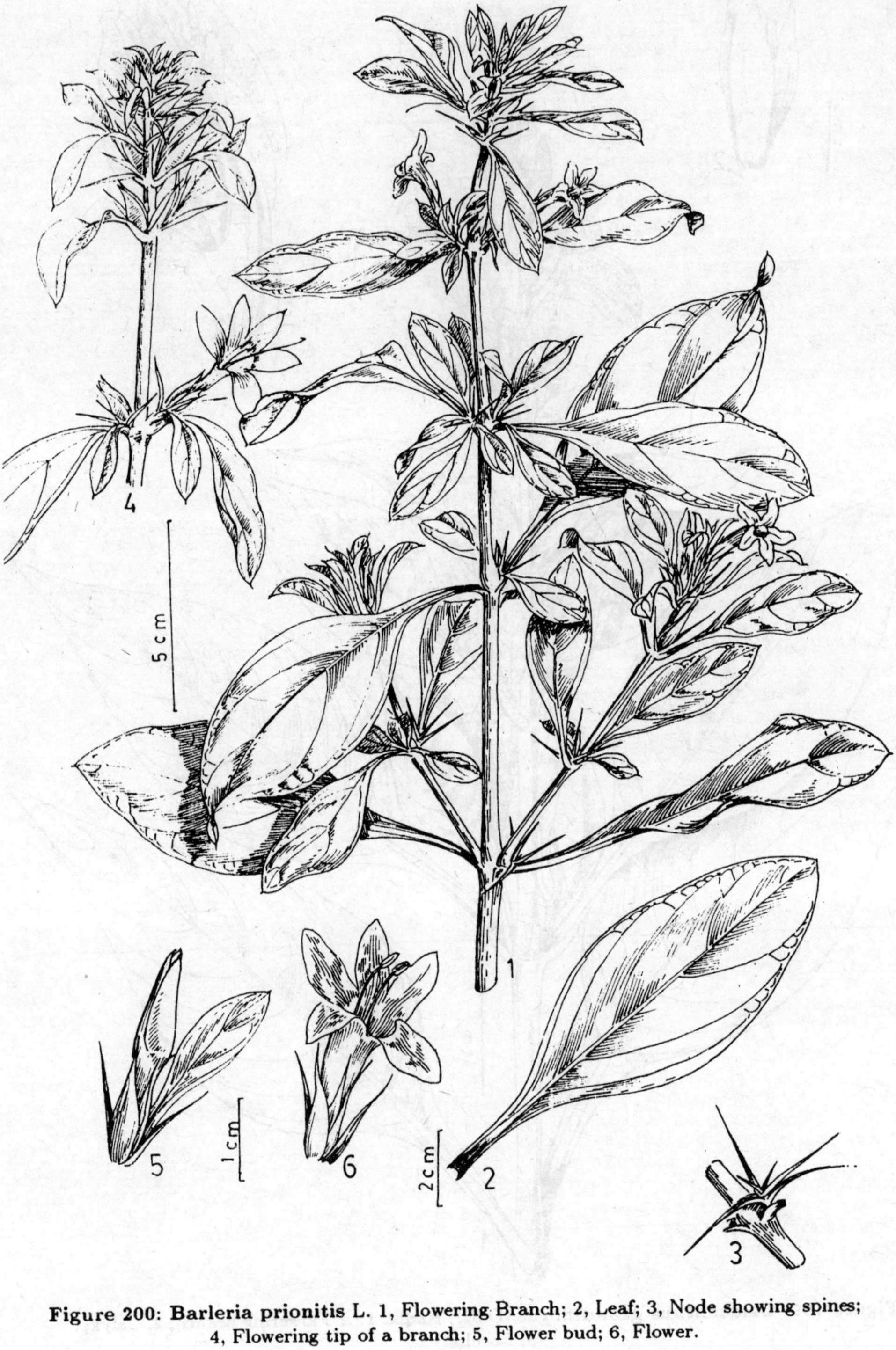

Figure 200: Barleria prionitis L. 1, Flowering Branch; 2, Leaf; 3, Node showing spines; 4, Flowering tip of a branch; 5, Flower bud; 6, Flower.

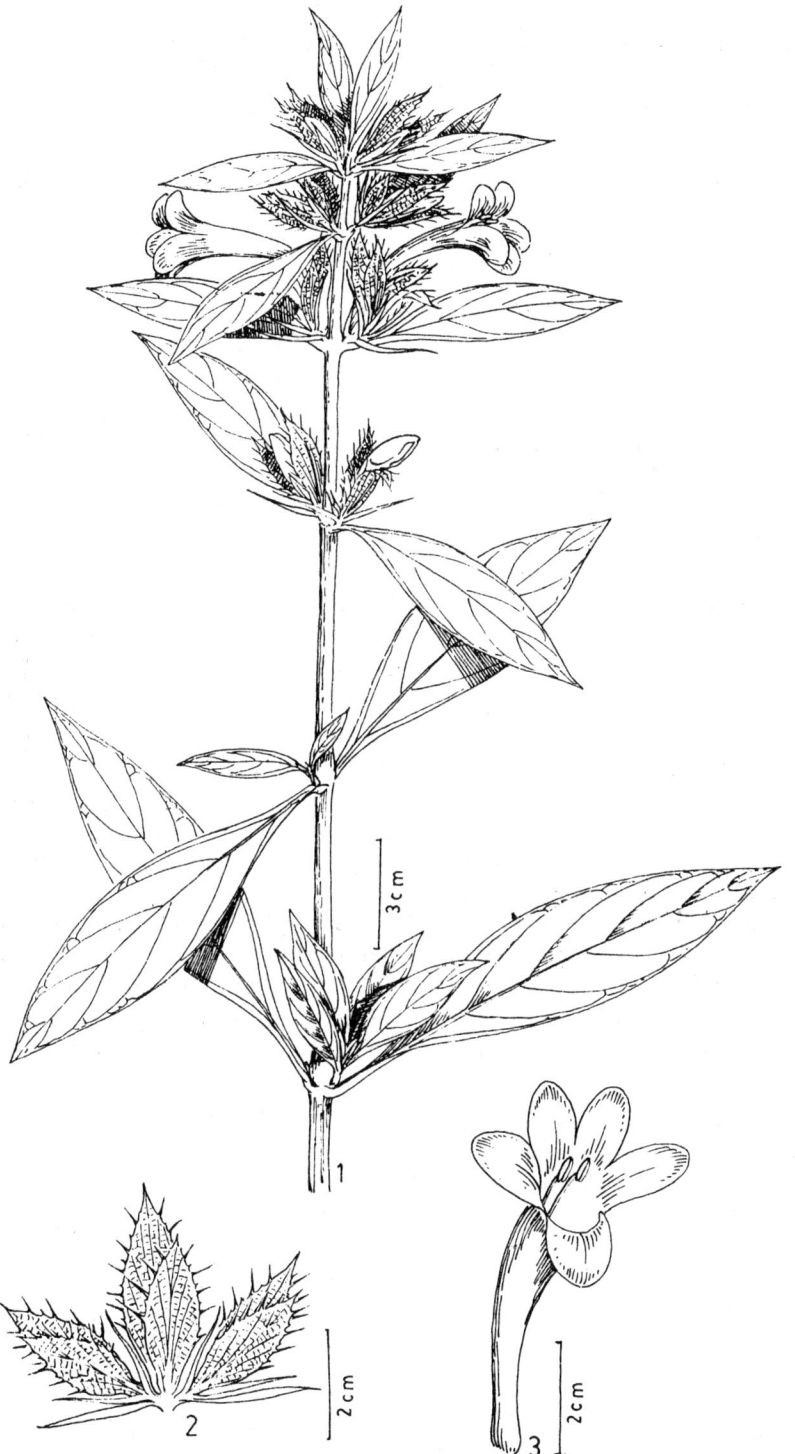

Figure 201: Barleria cristata L. 1, Flowering branch; 2, Bracts; 3, Corolla.

SAHADĒVĪ (Mal. PŪVĀṀKUṚUNTAL)

This is one of the ten auspicious herbs that constitute the group *Daśapuṣpa*. The entire plant is considered very beneficial in fever (*jvaraharā*). It is febrifuge, diaphoretic, alterative and purifies the blood, bile and semen. It subdues mental distraction (*cētōvikāraghnī*) and bestows happiness and beauty (*maṅgalyā* and *kānti*) to women. According to *Yogāmṛtaṃ*, it is a specific for leucorrhoea (*astisṛāvaṃ*) and excessive bleeding. It is also used in chronic skin diseases, dysuria, bladder stones, piles, worms and haematological disorders. The whole plant is a remedy for spasm of the bladder and strangury. The juice of the plant is good for the eyes. Flowers are administered in conjuctivitis. The drug is also used in scorpion sting. (Nadkarni, 1954: 1270; Aiyer & Kolammal, 1963. 6: 10, Sharma, 1983: 691).

Sahadēvī is sometimes treated as a synonym for *mahābalā* (cf. Chunekar, 1982: 369). But most authors consider it as a separate drug and equate it with *Vernonia cinerea* (Linn.) Less. of Asteraceae (cf. Kirtikar & Basu, 1918: 669; Nadkarni, 1954: 1270; Chopra *et al.*, 1956: 254; Kapoor & Mitra, 1979: 67; Sharma, 1983: 690). In Kerala, the plant is known as *pūvāṁkuṛuntal*. Rheede also describes the plant under the same name (Hort. Malab. 10: 127, t. 64. 1690).

Vernonia cinerea (*Linn.*) *Less.* **(Asteraceae)** (Fig. 202)
Conyza cinerea Linn.

Erect, hispid herb; leaves simple, alternate, exstipulate, very variable in shape and size, the basal ones larger, the upper smaller, broadly elliptic or lanceolate, obtuse, or acute, margin entire or irregularly toothed, 2.5–5 × 1.8–3.6 cms, more or less pubescent on both sides; heads pinkish violet in lax terminal corymbose panicles, homogamous; flowers bisexual; involucral bracts linear-lanceolate, awned, silky on the back; pappus of 2 series of long white hairs, the outer shorter and setose; corolla tubular, 5-lobed; stamens 5, epipetalous, anthers syngenesious; ovary inferior, unilocular with one basal ovule, style arms hairy; achenes 5-angled, adpressed hairy.

Distribution: The plant is found distributed throughout India in all plains districts and also in tropical Asia, Africa, Austria and New Zealand. It is a very common weed of the roadsides, open forests and garden lands.

Note: Dey and Das (1985) have studied the detailed pharmacognosy of *Vernonia cinerea*.

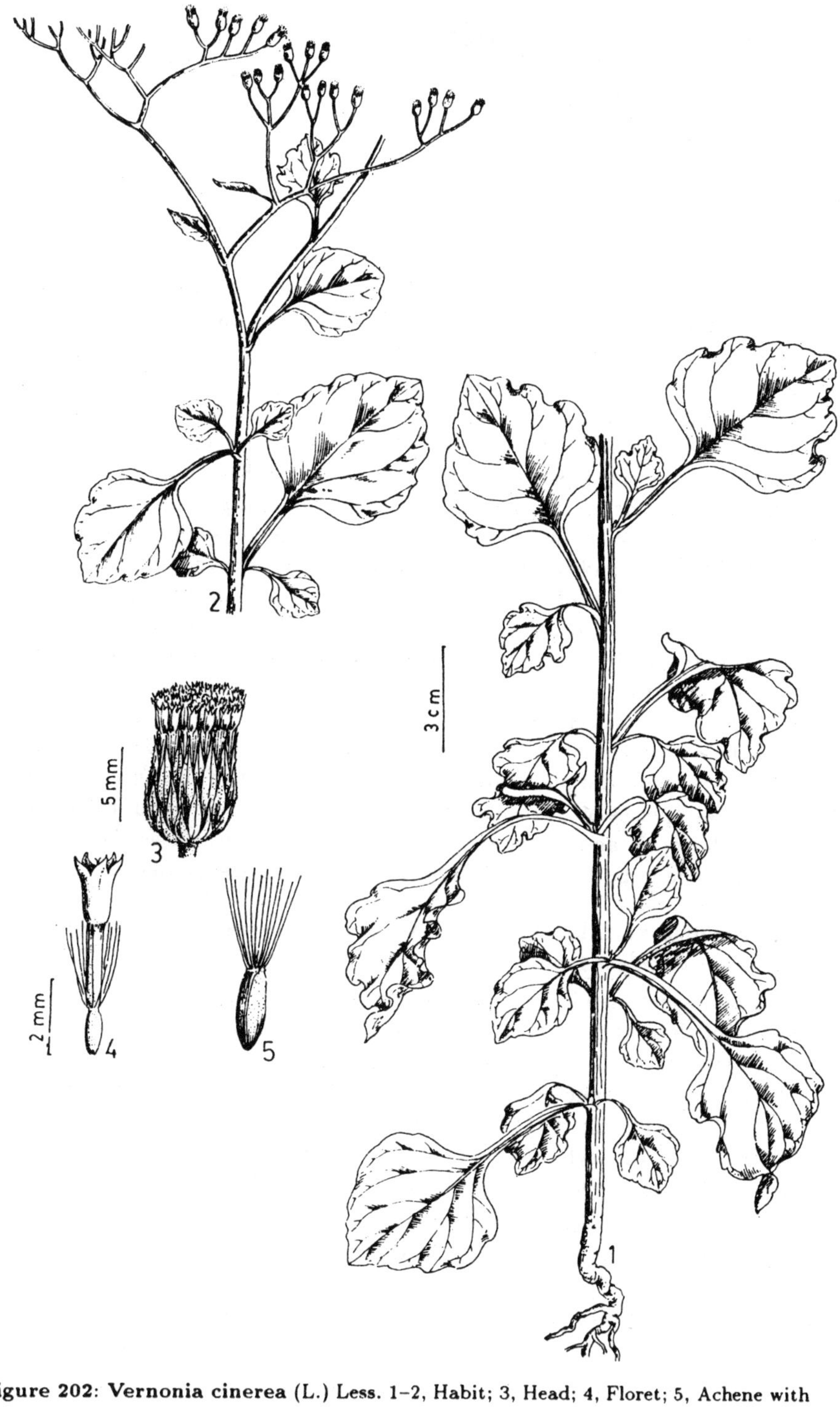

Figure 202: **Vernonia cinerea** (L.) Less. 1–2, Habit; 3, Head; 4, Floret; 5, Achene with pappus.

ŚĀLIPAṚṆĪ (Mal. MŪVILA)

Śāliparṇī and *pṛśniparṇī* are two important constituents of the *daśamūla* group and are together called *aṁśumatīdvayaṃ* (*pṛśniparṇī* is described elsewhere). *Śāliparṇī* is bitter, hot, tonic, aphrodisiac and promoter of body tissues. It is strength-giving and overcomes intermittent fever, *vāta*, urinary diseases, tumours, oedema, burning sensation, difficult breathing and toxic conditions (Kolammal, 1978. 2: 70). Root is the officinal part and it forms an ingredient of preparations like *Daśamūlāriṣṭaṃ, Agastyarasāyanaṃ, Aṇutailaṃ, Valiya pañcagavyaghṛtaṃ*, etc.

The texts describe the plant as a perennial (*sthirā*) shrub with long branches (*dīṛghāṅgī*) and long, single root (*dīṛghamūlā, ēkamūlā*). The plant smells like *vidāri* (*vidārigandhā*) and is yellowish in colour (*pītinī*) (cf. Kolammal, 1978. 2: 69). Interestingly enough, the most popularly accepted name *śāliparṇī* is a matter of semantic debate. While most of the people accept the name as such, meaning having long leaves like those of paddy, and support it with another synonym *vṛīhiparṇikā* (*vṛihi* = paddy, *parṇa* = leaf), some others have come up with the idea that the name is actually *sālaparṇī* (= having leaves like those of Sāl-*Shorea robusta*). None of the plants equated with this drug at present, has paddy-like leaves. Roughly, they are more similar to those of Sāl, but then this does not go well with the synonyms like *dīṛghaparṇī* and *vṛīhiparṇikā*.

In the current practice, there is wide-ranging difference of opinion among men of Āyurvēda, as to the plant source of this drug. Most of the publications equate it with the two species of *Uraria* viz. *U. lagapodioides* and *U. picta*. Kerala physicians, however, have, by and large, accepted *Pseudarthria viscida* as the source plant of this drug. The important characters of these plants are as follows.

Pseudarthria viscida (*Linn.*) *W. & A.* **(Papilionaceae)** (Fig. 203)
Hedysarum viscidum Linn.

Viscid-pubescent, semierect, perennial undershrubs with slender branches; leaves 3-foliolate, alternate, stipulate; leaflets ovate-rhomboid, acute, to 8× 8 cm, laterals obliquely ovate-acute or rhombiform, subcoriaceous; flowers small, pinkish white in long terminal branched racemes; calyx 2-lipped, campanulate, hairy outside, 4-toothed; corolla exserted, papilionaceous; stamens diadelphous; ovary subsessile with many ovules, style incurved, stigma capitate; fruit densely viscid-hairy, flat, linear-oblong, one-celled legume; seeds 4–6, compressed.

Distribution: All districts of southern India from Godavari southwards, as an undergrowth in damp forests. Also reported from Sri Lanka and Timor.

Uraria lagapodioides (*Linn.*) **Desv. (Papilionaceae)** (Fig. 204)

Trailing perennial undershrub; stem caespitose, woody, pubescent; leaves 1 or 3 foliolate, leaflets ovate-obtuse, rounded, at base, mucronate at apex, glabrous above, finely downy below; flowers in dense short racemes; bracts subpersistent, distinctly

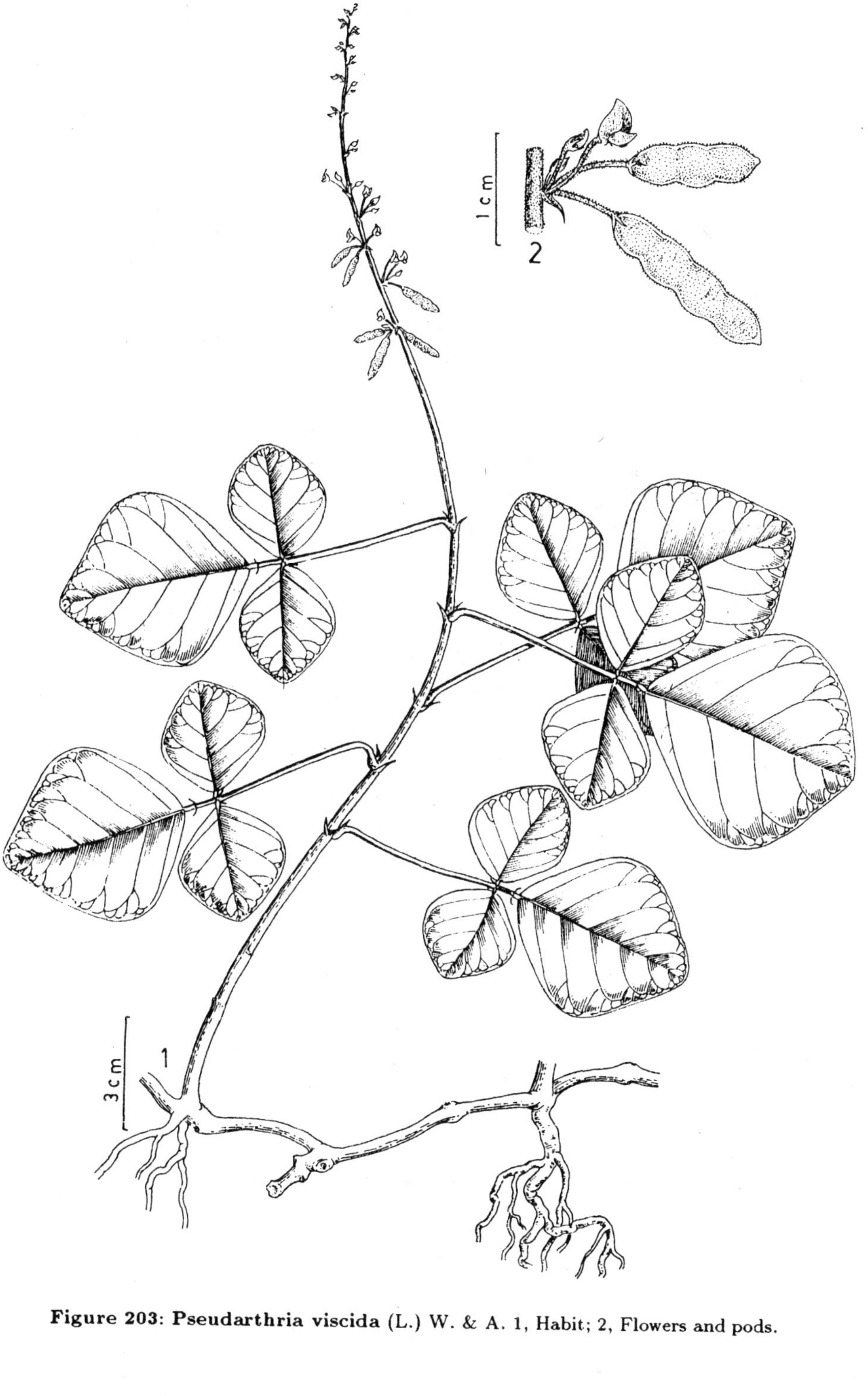

Figure 203: Pseudarthria viscida (L.) W. & A. 1, Habit; 2, Flowers and pods.

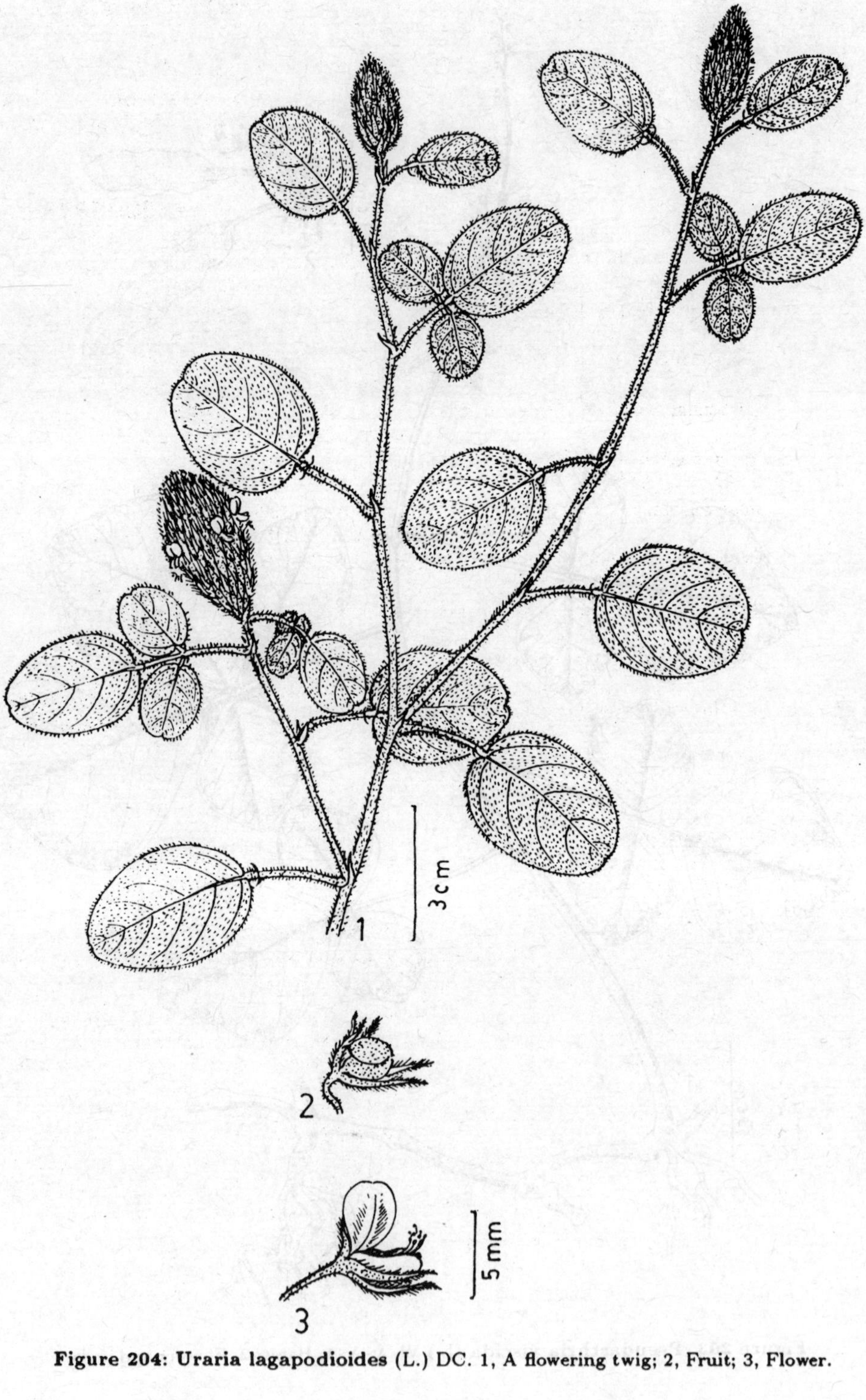

Figure 204: Uraria lagapodioides (L.) DC. 1, A flowering twig; 2, Fruit; 3, Flower.

ciliated; lower teeth of calyx very long, the upper very small; corolla papilionaceous, scarcely exserted; stamens diadelphous; ovary sessile or shortly stalked; pod a lomentum of 2 joints.

Distribution: W. Ghats, E. Slopes of the Pulney hills.

Uraria picta *Desv.* **(Papilionaceae)** (Fig. 205)

Erect undershrub; upper leaves 4–6, rarely 9-foliolate, leaflets linear-oblong, obtuse, mucronate at apex, to 19 x 2 cms, white-clowded above, rigidly sub-coriaceous, pubescent below; flowers purple in dense cylindrical racemes; bracts scarious, deciduous, not distinctly ciliated; calyx teeth subulate-lanceolate, lower twice the length of the upper, plumose; corolla papilionaceous, slightly exserted; lomentum of 3–6 joints.

Distribution: N. Circars, in the Sal Forests of Ganjam.

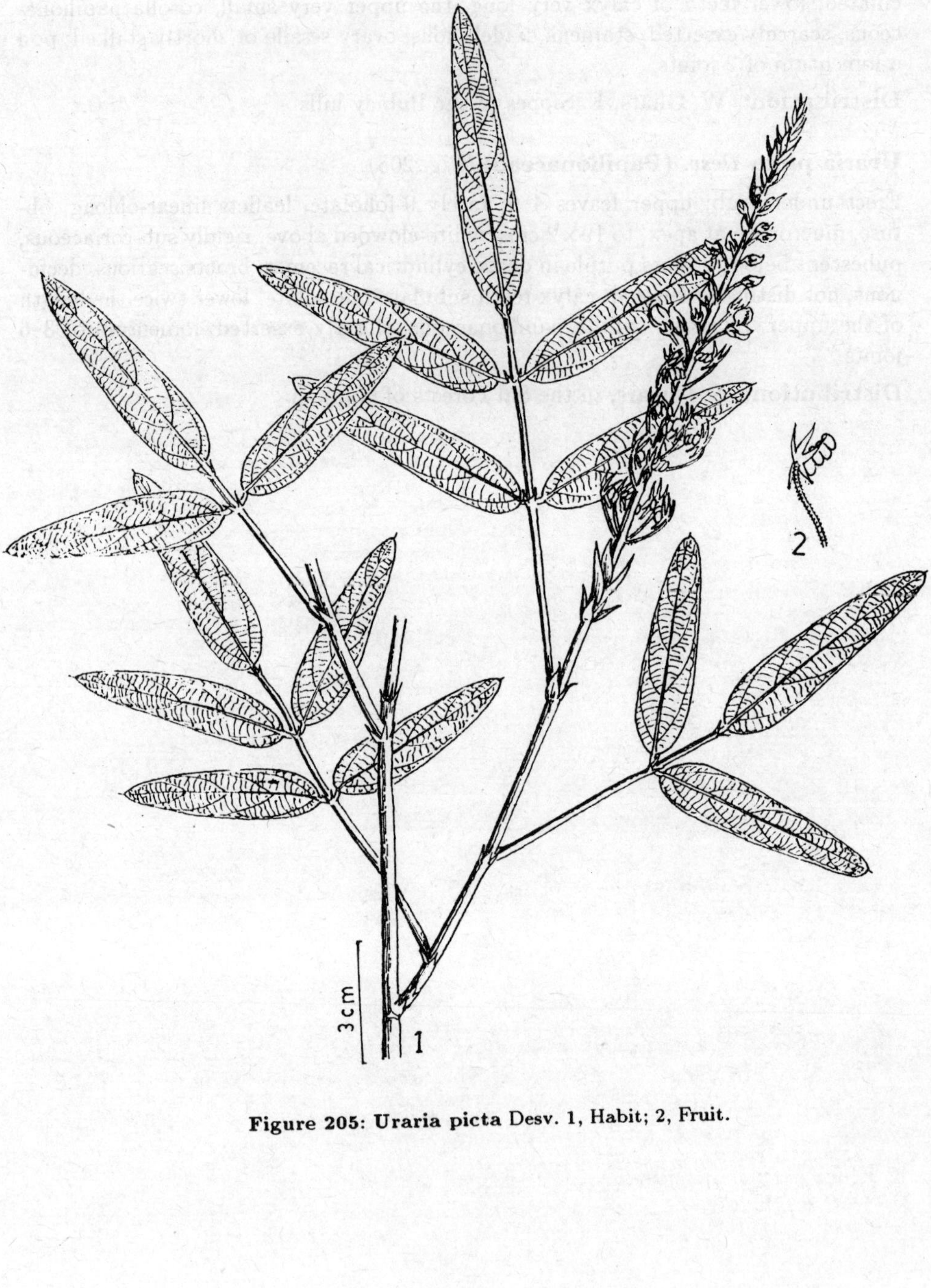

Figure 205: Uraria picta Desv. 1, Habit; 2, Fruit.

ŚAṆAPUṢPĪ (Mal. KILUKILUPPA)

This is an ingredient of preparations like *Nirguṇḍyādi guḷika* and *Nirguṇḍyādi ghṛtaṃ*. The whole plant is used medicinally. It is light, bitter, astringent, acrid and overcomes morbid *kapha* and *pitta*. Root causes vomiting. Leaves are useful in diarrhoea, dysentery and bleeding disorders. Leaf paste is applied to swellings, leprosy and other skin diseases. Paste of the seeds cures ulcers (Sharma, 1983: 393).

The synonyms *ghaṇṭā, ghaṇṭāravā*, etc. indicate the sound producing property of the fruits (Moosad, 1983: 345). The Malayalam name *kilukiluppa* also implies the same meaning which is rather common to several species of *Crotalaria* (Papilionaceae). Most of the authors equate the drug with *Crotalaria verrucosa* Linn. (Vaidya, 1936: 546; Nadkarni, 1954: 394; Chunekar, 1982: 430; Sharma, 1983: 392). Some others consider *Crotalaria juncea* as the drug source (Anonymous, 1978a: 20; Kapoor & Mitra, 1979: 68). In practice, different species of *Crotalaria* like *C. pallida, C. juncea, C. retusa* and *C. verrucosa* are being used as *kilukiluppa*. Rheede describes *C. juncea* and *C. retusa* under the vernacular name *tandale-cotti* (Hort. Malab. 9: 47, t. 26. 1689; 9: 45–46, t. 25. 1689) and *C. verrucosa* as *pee-tandale-cotti* (Hort. Malab. 9: 43, 6. 29. 1689).

The various species can be identified as follows:

Crotalaria pallida *Aiton* **(Papilionaceae)** (Fig. 206)
C. mucronata Desv.
C. striata DC.

Subshrub; leaves alternate, long-petioled, trifoliolate, leaflets obovate, obtuse-rotund, middle one larger, 6.5 × 3.8 cms, base cuneate, subacute, margin entire, glaucous below; flowers yellow in terminal racemes; calyx tube short, appressed pubescent, lobes lanceolate-acuminate; corolla yellow striped with red; stamens 10, united in a staminal sheath, 5 with long filaments and ovoid anthers, 5 with short filaments and oblong anthers; ovary densely pubescent, many ovuled, style curved, pubescent on the inner side; pod oblong, 4 × 0.7 cm, glabrescent; seeds many.

Distribution: Western peninsular India. Native in central and tropical America, now introduced in tropical Africa, Asia and Malesia and Queensland.

Crotalaria juncea *Linn.* **(Papilionaceae)** (Fig. 207)

Erect, densely hispid shrub; leaves simple, alternate, oblong-elliptic, obtuse, mucronate, 3–6 × 0.8–1.5 cms, soft-tomentose on either side; flowers large, bright yellow in terminal, hispid racemes; calyx tube sericeous, lobes lanceolate, narrow, unequal; corolla papilionaceous; staminal sheath 4 mm; ovary sessile, villous, style curved, pubescent on the inner side; pod sessile, oblong, terete, 3 × 1 cm, pubescent.

Distribution: Probably a native of India, now common in most tropical countries. Wild in the Circar hills and W. Ghats.

Crotalaria retusa *Linn.* **(Papilionaceae)** (Fig. 208)

Sub shrubs; leaves simple, alternate, oblanceolate, obtuse-retuse, 3–6 × 1.5–2 cm, glabrous above, glaucous beneath, base attenuate, margin entire; flowers bright yellow in terminal racemes; calyx tube appressed puberulous, lobes lanceolate; corolla papilionaceous; staminal sheath 8 mm; ovary glabrous, style curved, pubescent; pod shortly stipitate, oblong, terete, 4.5 × 1.5 cm glabrous.

Distribution: Probably a native in S.E. Asia, now pantropical. In India it is seen in all districts in fields and waste places.

Crotalaria verrucosa *Linn.* **(Papilionaceae)** (Fig. 209)

Subshrubs; stem and branches angular, appressed pubescent; leaves simple, alternate, ovate or rhomboid-deltoid, obtuse, 7.5 cms, base attenuate, margin entire; stipules large, auriculate; flowers blue, large in terminal racemes; calyx tube pubescent, lobes elongate, lanceolate; staminal sheath 6 mm; ovary stipitate, appressed pubescent, style geniculate, pubescent on the inner side; pod oblong, terete, 4 × 1 cm, sparsely pubescent.

Distribution: Pantropical weed of unknown origin. In India it is found in almost all districts in waste places, gardens and fields.

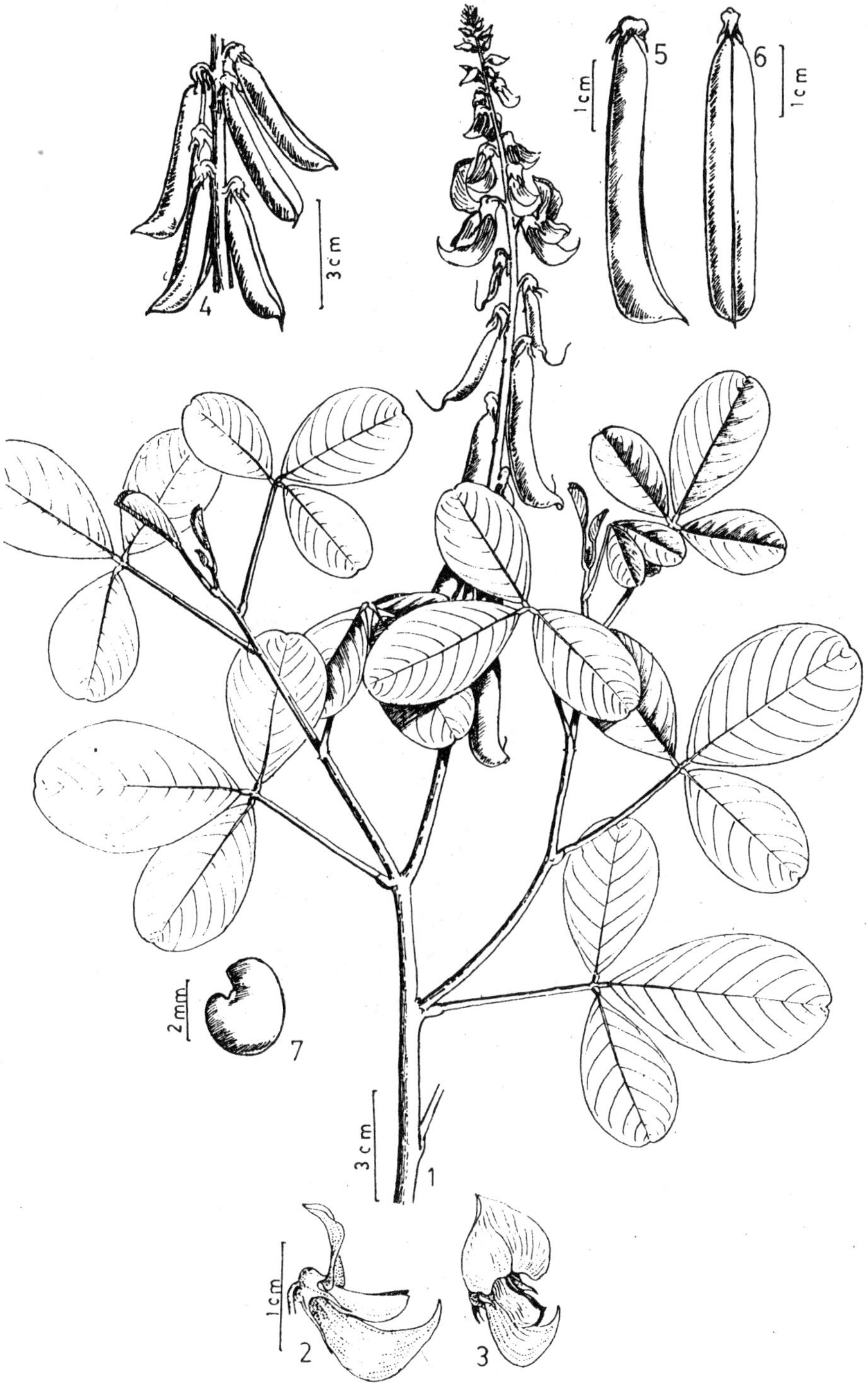

Figure 206: **Crotalaria pallida** Ait. 1, Flowering branch; 2–3, Flowers; 4, Bunch of pods; 5–6, Pods enlarged; 7, Seed.

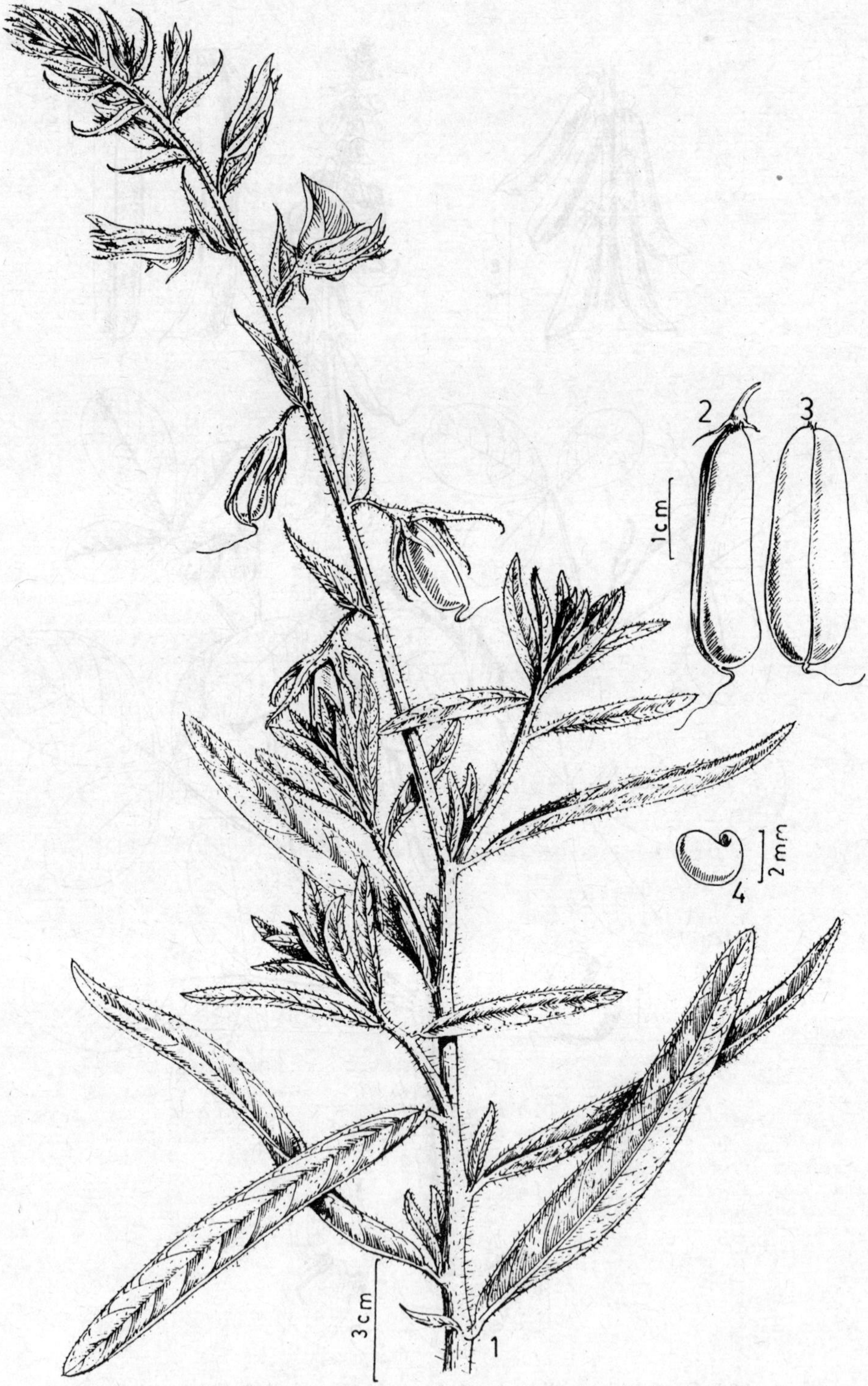

Figure 207: Crotalaria juncea L. 1, Flowering twig; 2–3, Pods; 4, Seed.

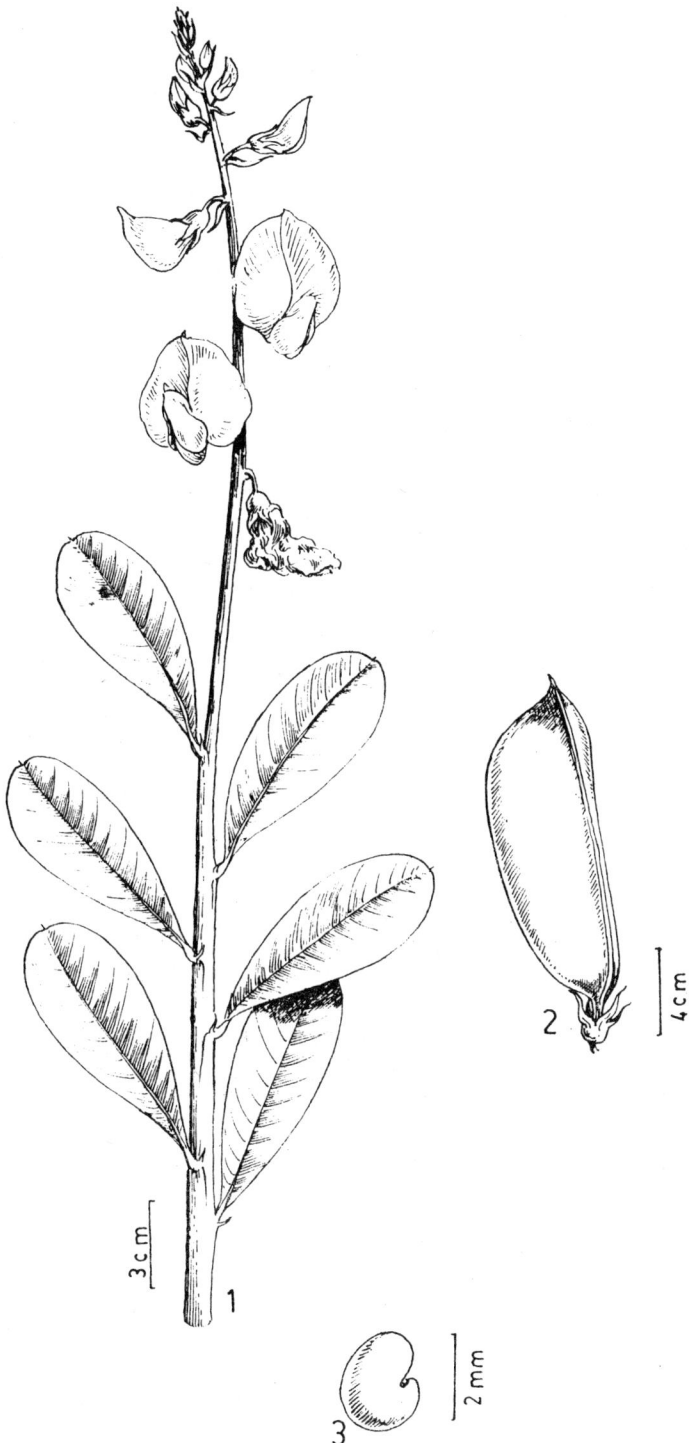

Figure 208: **Crotalaria retusa** L. 1, Flowering branch; 2, Pod; 3, Seed.

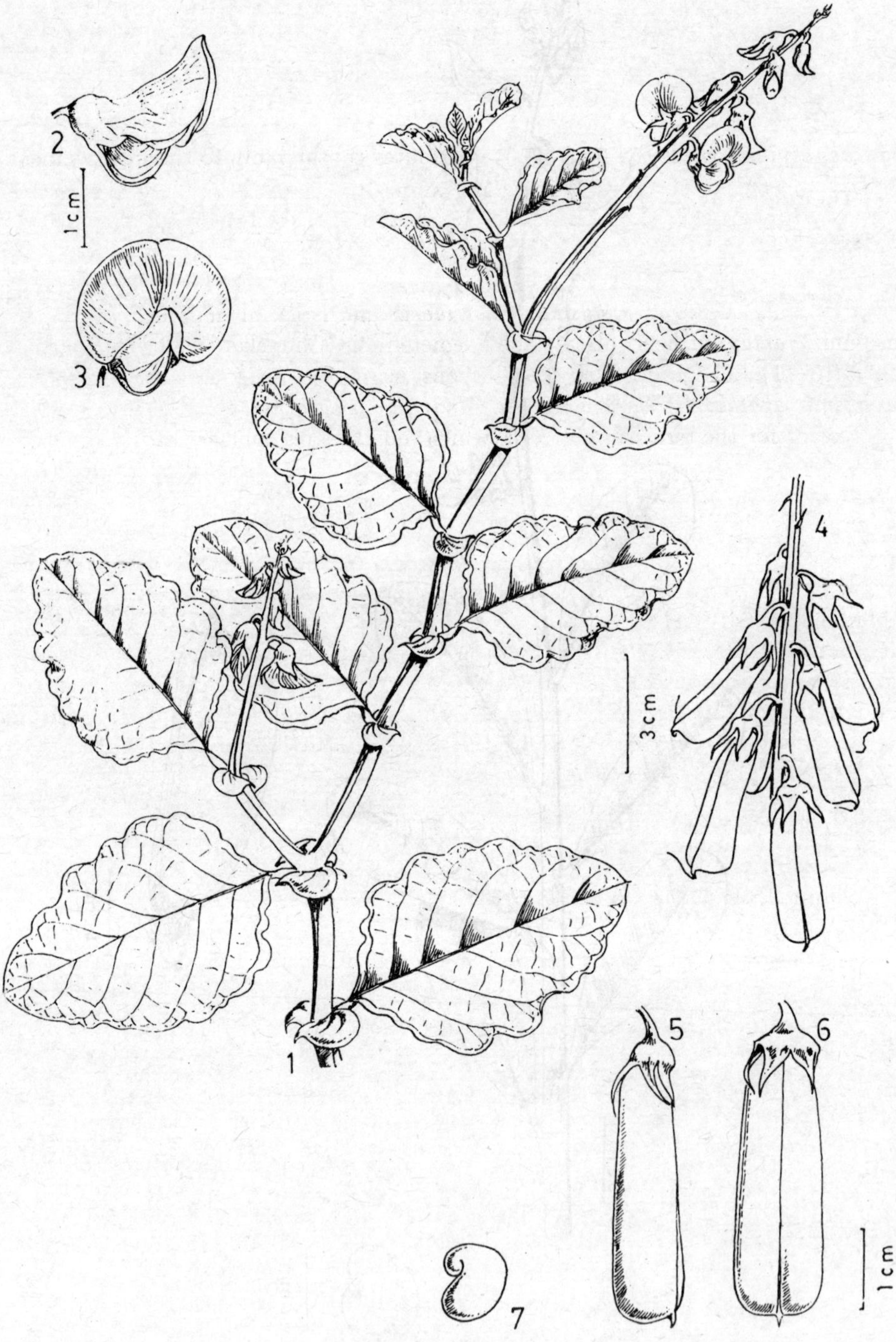

Figure 209: Crotalaria verrucosa L. 1, Flowering twig; 2–3, Flowers; 4, Bunch of pods; 5–6, Pods enlarged; 7, Seed.

ŚAṄKHAPUṢPĪ (Mal. ŚAṄKHUPUṢPAṂ)

Śaṅkhapuṣpī is a *mēdhya* drug which contributes considerably to the improvement of the memory power and intellect. The whole plant is medicinal. It is astringent, hot, aphrodisiac, rejuvenating and a nervine tonic. It improves strength, digestive power, complexion, voice and cures intestinal worms, animal poisoning, skin diseases, cough, dyspnoea, diabetes, dysuria and uterine disorder. The drug also cures diseases due to the morbidity of *tridōṣās* and is useful in epilepsy, insanity, insomnia, *raktapitta*, heart disease and haemetemesis (Chunekar, 1982: 455; Sharma, 1983: 10–11). The important formulations using the drug are *Brāhmīghṛtaṃ, Mānasmitṛavaṭakaṃ, Miśṛakasnēhaṃ, Mañjiṣṭhādi kaṣāyaṃ*, etc.

Except for the term *śaṅkhapuṣpī*, which indicates resemblence of its flowers to that of a conch-shell, the synonyms do not give any clue in identifying the plant.

There seems to be a lot of confusion in equating the terms *viṣṇukṛāntā, śaṅkhapuṣpī, aparājitā, girikarṇī*, etc. to their respective botanical sources. These are considered as synonyms by some and as different drugs by others according to traditional usage or the interpretation of the verses in ancient texts (Aiyer & Kolammal, 1964. 8: 11).

In most of the works, *viṣṇukṛāntā* is treated as a variety of *śaṅkhapuṣpī Rājanighaṇṭu* considers it as the blue flowered variety of *śaṅkhapuṣpī* (also see Vaidya, 1936: 543; Chunekar, 1982: 454), while *Bhāvaprakāśa Nighaṇṭu* treats it as a synonym of *aparājitā*. In practice, in Kerala, *viṣṇukṛāntā* is treated as a separate drug known by the same local name i.e. *viṣṇukṛānti* and *Evolvulus alsinoides* (Convolvulaceae) is used as the drug source (see also Rheede, Hort. Malab. 11: 131–132. t. 64. 1692 *'vistnu-clandi'*). *Aparājitā* is equated with the blue and white flowered varieties of *Clitoria ternatea* of Papilionaceae (Nadkarni, 1954: 354; Aiyer & Kolammal, 1964. 8: 11; Chunekar, 1982: 342), locally called *'śaṅkhupuṣpaṃ'* (see also Rheede, Hort. Malab. 8: 69–70. t. 38. 1688 *'Schanga-cuspi'*).

The botanical identity of *śaṅkhapuṣpī* is highly controversial. While some authors equate it with *Canscora decussata* of Gentianaceae (Vaidya, 1936: 543; Kapoor & Mitra, 1979: 68), others consider *Convolvulus pluricaulis* (Convolvulaceae) as the source plant (Singh & Chunekar, 1972: 385; Anonymous, 1978a: 256; Dey, 1980: 138; Chunekar, 1982: 454; Sharma, 1983: 9). The latter is extensively used as *śaṅkhapuṣpī* in North India. Due to the application of the synonym *viṣṇukṛānti* to this drug, some people accept *Evolvulus alsinoides* as the source plant of *śaṅkhapuṣpī* (Chunekar, 1982: 454; Vaidya Bapalal, 1982: 229). However, Kerala physicians do not descriminate between *aparājitā* and *śaṅkhapuṣpī* and use *Clitoria ternatea* (Papilionaceae) in place of both. Mooss (1976: 47) opines that the purgative action of *śaṅkhapuṣpī*, combined with its property of being a good nervine tonic in mental disorders, is clearly evinced in *Clitoria ternatea*. The synonyms like *śaṅkhapuṣpī, vanamālini* etc. fit into this taxon well (Nair *et al.*, 1982).

The various plant sources can be distinguished as follows.

1. Clitoria ternatea *Linn.* **(Papilionaceae)** (Fig. 210)

Twining shrub with slender, terete, appressed tomentose branches and branchlets; leaves alternate; stipulate, imparipinnate; leaflets 5 to 7, ovate or elliptic-obtuse, entire, upto 5.6 × 3.7 cms, glabrous; flowers large, conch-shell shaped, blue or white, axillary, solitary; bracts small, persistent; bracteoles large, foliaceous, roundish, persistent; calyx gamosepalous, tubular, 5-cleft, teeth lanceolate, the upper two subconnate; corolla papilionaceous; stamens diadelphous; ovary monocarpellary, stipitate, many ovuled, style elongate, incurved, bearded along the inner side; pod linear-oblong, flat, 10.5 × 1 cms, sharply beaked, appressed hairy; seeds 6–10, compressed.

Distribution: The plant is probably a native of S. America but is now naturalised all over the tropical parts of India. It is found wild growing over hedges and thickets and also cultivated in gardens as an ornamental.

Canscora decussata *Schultes* & *Schultes f.* **(Gentianaceae)** (Fig. 211)

Herb; stem narrowly 4-winged; leaves elliptic-lanceolate, 2–3 × 1–1.5 cm, 3-nerved, base rounded to acute, apex acute; flowers white in axillary or terminal dichasial cymes; pedicel winged, 1 cm, bracts lanceolate; calyx lobes 4, winged; corolla tube 7 mm, lobes 4, oblong-obtuse; stamens 4, inserted on the corolla tube; ovary 1-celled,many ovuled, style filiform, stigma 2-fid, recurved, hispidulous; capsule obscurely 2-valved; seeds angular.

Distribution: The plant is seen in all plains districts and upto 3,000 ft in the hills. It is distributed in Sri Lanka, tropical Africa and S.E. Asia.

Convolvulus pluricaulis *Chois.* **(Convolvulaceae)**

Herb with woody root-stock; stem slender, wiry, thinly hairy; leaves subsessile, radical, more spathulate, short-petioled; flowers 1–3 axillary, pedicelled; bracts linear, small; sepals narrowly linear-lanceolate, sparsely hairy; corolla wide, funnel-shaped, pale rose; stamens included, filaments unequal; ovary glabrous, 2-celled; fruit a globose capsule.

Distribution: The plant is found in the plains of Hindustan and Bihar.

Note: *Convolvulus pluricaulis* has been found to be effective in reducing the different types of stress including psychological, chemical and traumatic (Prasad *et al.*, 1974). The drug also exhibits significant antianxiety activity (Singh & Mehta, 1977, Koushik and Singh, 1982), tranquilising effect and anti-thyroid property (Gupta *et al.*, 1981).

Singh *et al.* (1988) have studied the pharmacognosy, phytochemistry, pharmacology and clinical aspects of the four plants used as *śaṅkhapuṣpi* in different places. i.e. *Convolvulus pluricaulis, Evolvulus alsinoides, Canscora decussata* and *Clitoria ternatea.*

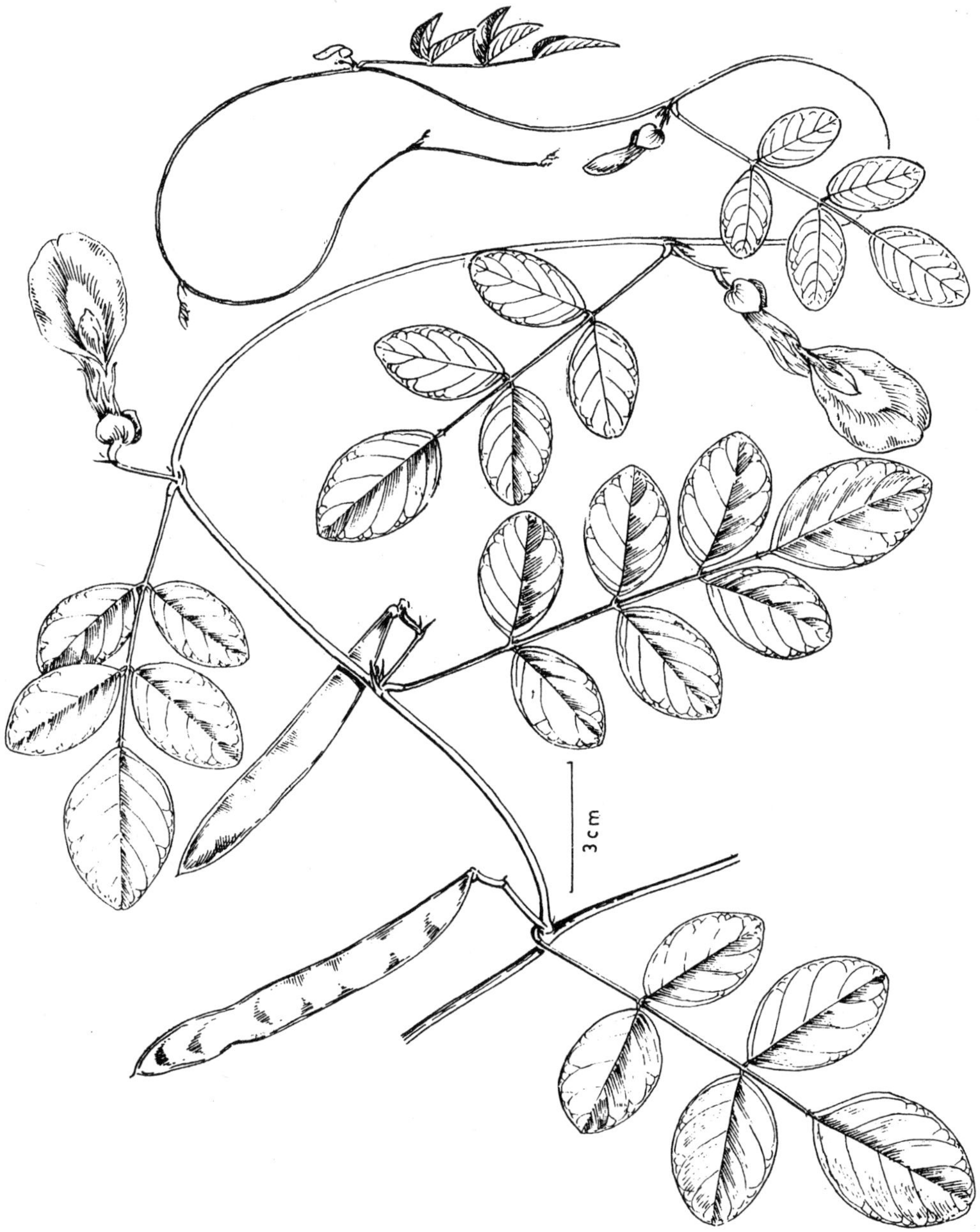

Figure 210: Clitoria ternatea L.

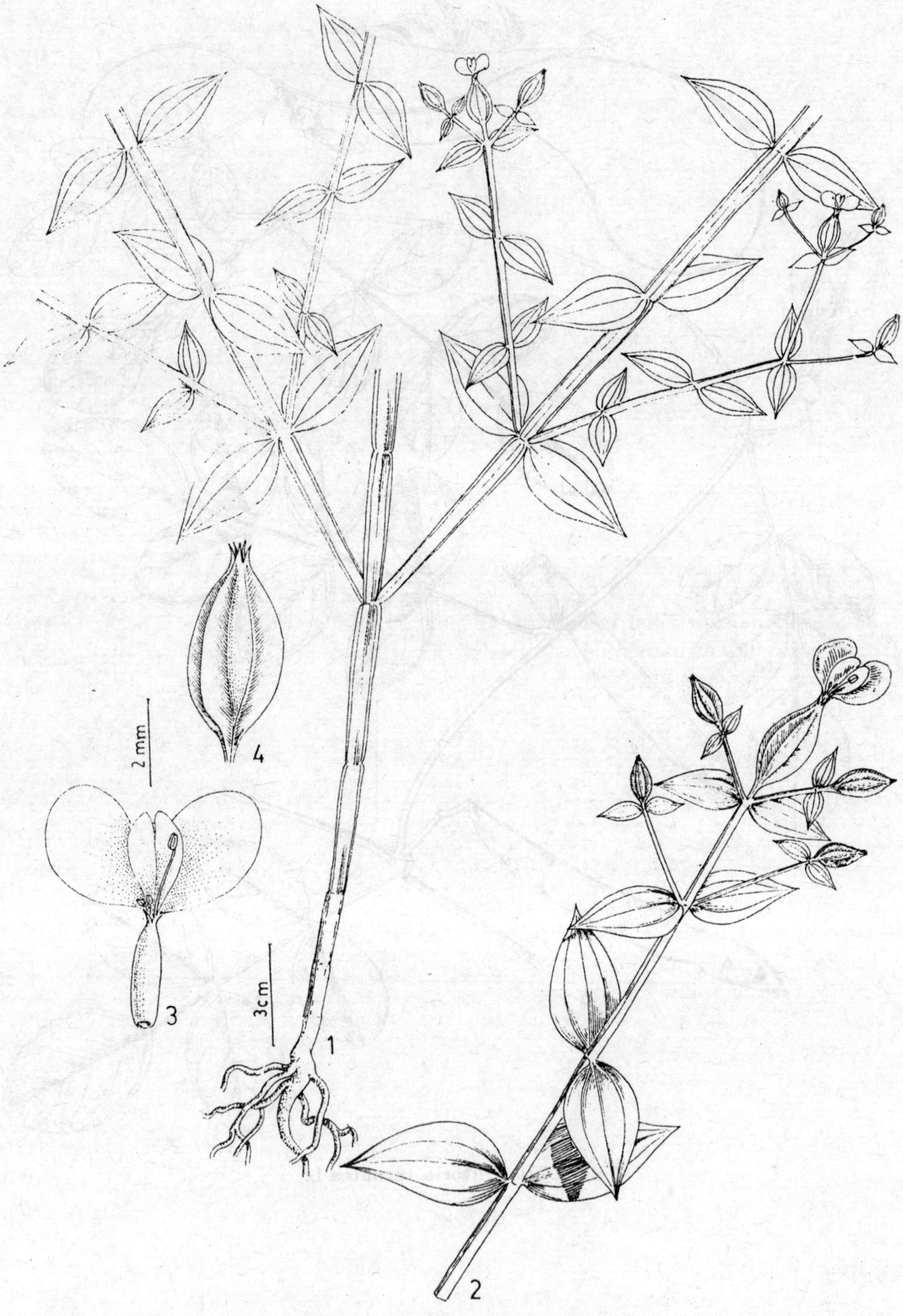

Figure 211: Canscora decussata Sch. & Sch. f. 1, Habit; 2, Flowering shoot; 3, Corolla with stamens; 4, Calyx with enclosed fruit.

ŚARAḤ (Mal. AMA)

The drug is light, cooling, sweet, galactagogue and aphrodisiac. It is used in the morbid conditions of *tṛidōṣās*, thirst, dysuria, blood diseases like *raktapitta*, erysipelas, leucorrhoea, piles and eye diseases (Sharma, 1983: 638). Root is the officinal part. *Sukumāraṃ lēhaṃ, Sukumāraṃ kaṣāyaṃ* and *Sukumāra ghṛtaṃ* are some of the formulations using the drug.

Saccharum arundinaceum Retz. (Poaceae), known as *ama* in vernacular, is the drug source. Some people equate it with *Saccharum munja* Roxb. (now *S. bengalense* Retz.) (See Singh & Chunekar, 1972: 391; Anonymous, 1978a: 257; Sharma, 1983: 637.) However, in practice in Kerala, *Arundo donax* Linn. (Poaceae) is also found used in many places as the drug source.

Saccharum arundinaceum *Retz.* **(Poaceae)** (Fig. 212)
Erianthus arundinaceus (Retz.) Jeswiet.

Perennial tufted grass, 3–6 metres tall, erect from a stout root-stock; culm jointed and leafy; leaves 90–150 × 5.8 cms, linear lanceolate, acuminate, sheath beared at mouth; ligule short, hairy; panicles 30–60 cms long, erect, clothed with soft silky hairs; spikelets in pairs, one sessile and the other pedicelled, pale green, violet or brownish; glumes white; villous, except the upper one of the sessile spikelet; palea quadrate.

Distribution: Throughout the plains and low hills of India, Ceylon and Burma; wild relative of *S. officinarum*, this runs wild and is used only for medicinal purposes.

Arundo donax *Linn.* **(Poaceae)** (Fig. 213)

Tall stout perennial grass; stem creeping below; leaves 30–60 cms long, linear-lanceolate, rounded or cordate and amplexicaul, glabrous; ligule a ridge of hairs, panicles large, decompound, silky hairy; spikelets oblong, 3-flowered, green or yellowish; rachilla jointed below each floret, glabrous; glumes subequal, oblong lanceolate, 3 nerved; lemma lanceolate, long-pilose without at base, 3-nerved, nerves apically produced as aristae; palea 2-keeled, densely ciliate on keels; anthers 3.

Distribution: Mediterranian region eastwards to Burma; N. Africa, India, Pakistan, introduced into many parts of the world. In India, it is seen in most districts except the W. Coast, upto 2,000 ft.

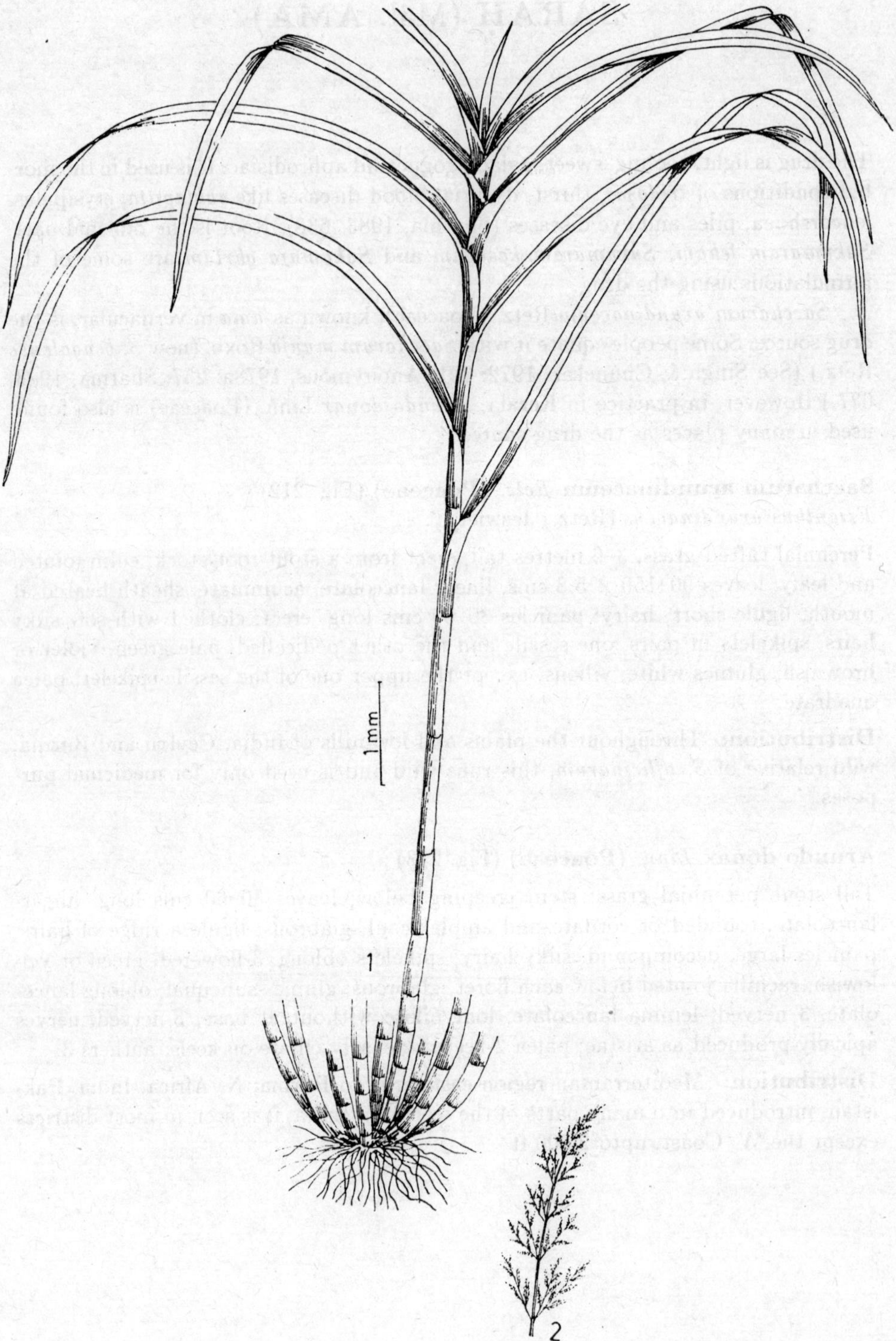

Figure 212: Saccharum arundinaceum Retz. 1, Vegetative shoot; 2, Portion of inflorescence.

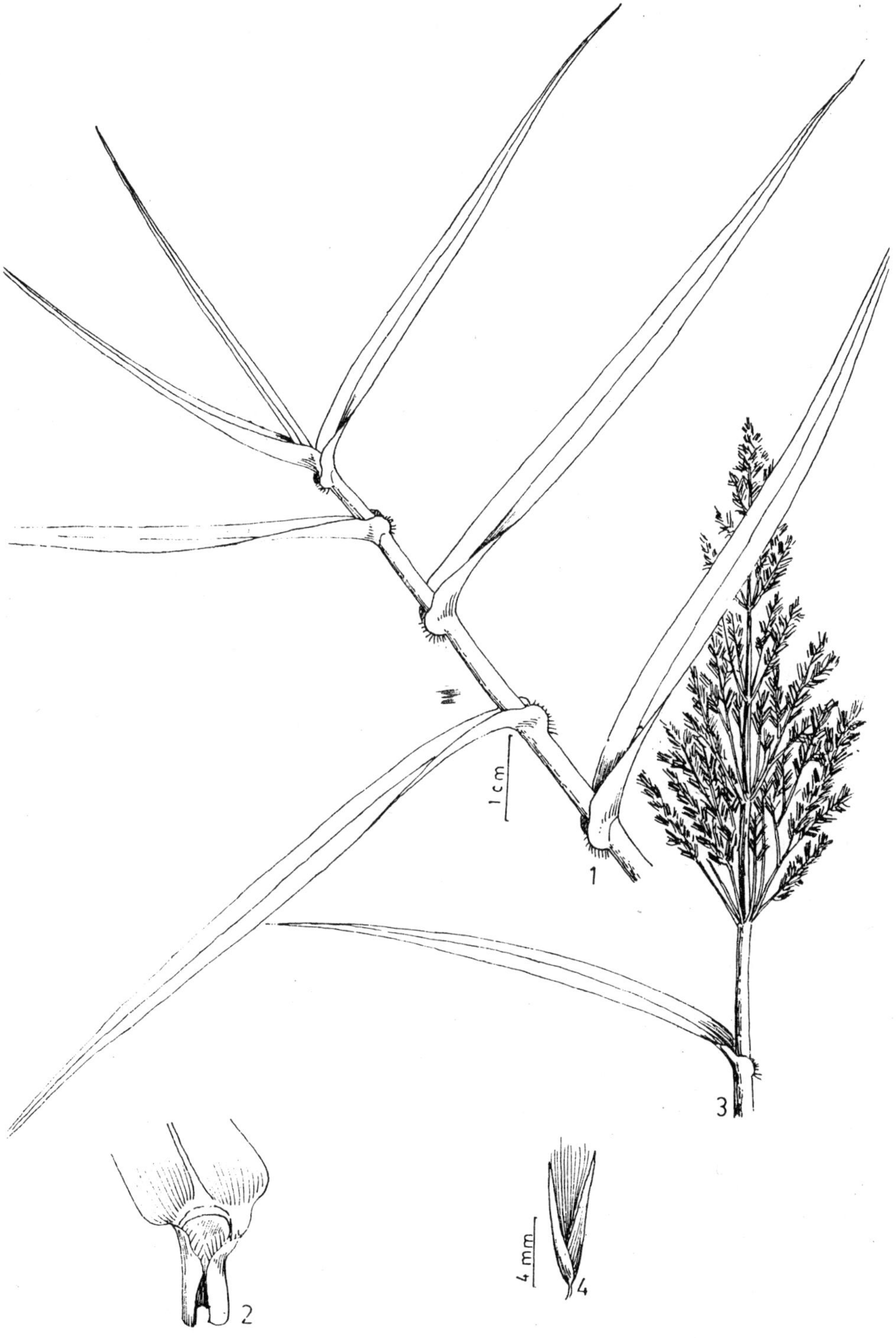

Figure 213: **Arundo donax** L. 1, Vegetative shoot; 2, Leaf sheath; 3, Inflorescence; 4, Floret.

ŚARAPUṄKHAḤ (Mal. KOḶIÑÑIL)

The drug is considered to be highly beneficial in inflammation and enlargement of spleen and liver and hence the name *plīhaśatru, plīhāri*, etc. (*plīha* = spleen). Roots and sometimes the whole plant are used in medicine. It is bitter, astringent, acrid, anthelmintic, antipyretic, diuretic and laxative. It cures cough, asthma, fever, ulcers, gulma, poisonous affections, leprosy and other skin diseases. The drug purifies blood and overcomes diseases due to morbid *kapha* and *vāta*. The root is very efficaceous against hydrocele, dyspepsia, chronic diarrhoea and obstinate colic. Seeds are employed as an anthelmintic for children (Nadkarni, 1954: 562; Sharma, 1983: 555). The drug enters into the composition of preparations like *Āragvadhādi kaṣāyaṃ, Vīratarādi kaṣāyaṃ, Grahaṇyāntaka ghṛtaṃ*, etc.

According to the description in the texts, the plant resembles *nīlivṛkṣa* (*nīlīvṛkṣākṛti*) i.e. *Indigofera tinctoria* of Papilionaceae.

Two varieties of *śarapuṅkha* are found mentioned in classical Āyurvēdic literature viz. *śarapuṅkha* or *raktaśarapuṅkha* and *śvētaśarapuṅkha*. Opinions vary as to how these two are to be recognised. Some consider that flower colour is the diagnostic feature and equate the *raktaśarapuṅkha* with the red or purple flowered *Tephrosia purpurea* (Papilionaceae). *'svetaśarapuṅkha'*, has however, been equated with the white flowered form of *Tephrosia procumbens* Buch.-Ham. and *T. candida* DC. by some (Sharma,1983:554) while the white flowered, *T. purpurea* form *albiflora* Paul & Gupta has been accepted as the source plant by Gupta (1988). But others are of opinion that the names only refer to the colouration of the plant as a whole and equate the *śvētaśarapuṅkha* with *T. villosa* Pers., a plant with dense whitish tomentum on the stem (See Raghunathan & Mitra, 1982: 38; Chunekar, 1982: 408). *Kāṇṭhapuṅkha*, another variety mentioned in *Rājanighaṇṭu* has been equated with *T. spinosa* Pers. (Sharma, 1983: 555).

This varietal distinction is not observed by Kerala physicians and only *T. purpurea*, locally called *koḷiññil* is used as the drug source. Rheede's description and illustration of this plant under the name *Colinil* (Hort. Malab. 1: 103–104, 6. 55. 1678) is ample testimony for the fact that this has been in use in Kerala, since long.

Tephrosia purpurea (*Linn.*) *Pers.* **(Papilionaceae)** (Fig. 214)
Cracca purpurea Linn.

Much branched undershrubs, leaves pinnate, leaflets elliptic or oblanceolate, mucronate, 2 × 0.7 cms with numerous, closely parallel veins; flowers small, reddish or purple in axillary or terminal racemes; calyx tube campanulate, lobes subequal; corolla papilionaceous; stamens 9, anthers 2-celled; ovary linear, sessile, many ovuled, style incurved, flattened, stigma terminal; pods falcate, compressed, glabrous, dehiscing by both sutures; seeds 4–6, ovoid, glabrous.

Distribution: The plant is common in all plains districts in waste lands and along roadsides. It is distributed in India, Burma and Malesia.

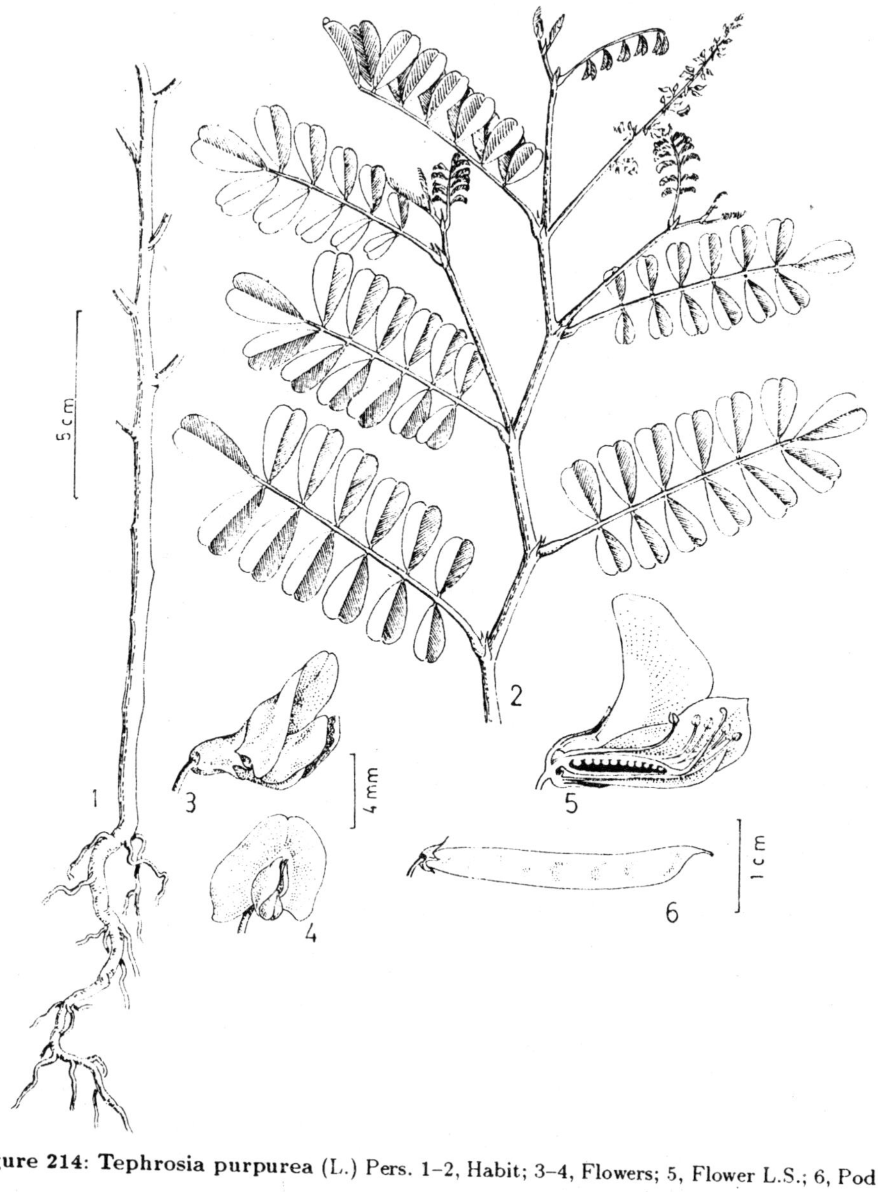

Figure 214: **Tephrosia purpurea** (L.) Pers. 1–2, Habit; 3–4, Flowers; 5, Flower L.S.; 6, Pod.

Note: The pharmacognostic and pharmacological work done on *T. purpurea* have been discussed by Raghunathan & Mitra (1982: 939–954). Clinical studies have demonstrated its roots to be effective against inflammations of tonsil and adenoids (Karnick & Pathak, 1983). Leaf extract exhibits dose dependent hypotensive activity (Rao, 1984) and seed extract lowers blood glucose levels considerably. (Rahman *et al.*, 1985).

ŚĀRIBĀ (Mal. NANNĀṚI, NAṚUNĪṆṬI)

Śāribā, a well known drug of Āyurvēdic materia medica, has been in wide use since ancient times. The tuberous root is reputed for its cooling and blood purifying action and is hence used to make refreshing drinks. The root is also alterative, aphrodisiac, refringerant, diuretic and tonic. It overcomes vitiated *vāta, pitta* and ***kapha*** and cures dyspepsia, deficient digestive power, dysentery, cough, bronchitis, leucorrhoea, uterine haemorrhage, dysuria and blood diseases. The drug is useful in skin diseases, fever, thirst, vomiting, poisoning, chronic rheumatism, anaemia and debility (Aiyer, 1951. 14: Kurup *et al.*, 1979: 184; Sharma, 1983: 799). The important formulations using the drug are *Śāribādyāsavaṃ, Piṇḍatailaṃ, Vidāryādi lēhaṃ, Drākṣādi kaṣāyaṃ, Jātyādi ghṛtaṃ*, etc.

The synonyms indicate that the plant is a laticiferous (*gōpī, gōpavallī, gōpavadhu, gōpakanyā*), slender vine (*kṛśōdarī, latā*), having long, fragrant root (*anantamūlā, candanā*). The Āyurvēdic texts mention two varieties of *śāribā*, viz. a *kṛṣṇa* or black variety and a *śvēta* or white variety (Aiyer, 1951: 13) which together constitute the pair, *śāribādvayaṃ*.

Regarding the botanical identity, the white variety or *śvētaśāribā* is unanimously identified as *Hemidesmus indicus* Linn. (Asclepiadaceae), locally known as *nannāṛi* or *naṛunīṇṭi* by all the authors (see also Rheede, Hort. Malab. 10: 67–68, t. 34. 1690). Two plants, namely, *Ichnocarpus frutescens* (Apocynaceae), known as *pāl-vaḷḷi* in vernacular (Rheede, Hort. Malab. 9: 19, t. 12. 1689) and *Cryptolepis buchanani* (Asclepiadaceae) (Rheede calls it *Kāṭupālvaḷḷi* Hort. Malab. 9: 17–18, t. 11. 1689), are equated with the black variety or *kṛṣṅaśāribā* (see Chunekar, 1982: 427; Sharma, 1983: 798). Ayurvedic formulary of India accepts *Hemedesmus indicus* and *Cryptolepis buchanani* as the white and black varieties respectively (Anonymous, 1978a: 257, 246). In practice, in Kerala, *Ichnocarpus frutescens* and *H. indicus* are commonly used as the two constituents of *śāribādvayaṃ*.

The studies on the market samples made by Togunashi *et al.* (1978) found that in Kerala, Tamil Nadu and Karnataka, the aromatic tuberous roots of another Asclepiadaceae plant, *Decalepis hamiltonii* are sold as the source of *śāribā*. As the chemical constituents of this plant are found to be similar to that of *Hemidesmus indicus*, the authors are of opinion that this plant can be used as a new source of *śāribā*. Besides, as *kṛṣṇasāribā* and *śvētaśāribā* are grouped under aromatic drugs in Āyurvēda, the roots of *Decalepis hamiltonii* form a better substitute for *śāribā* than *Ichnocarpus frutescens* and *Cryptolepis buchanani*, the roots of which do not have aroma. The authors identify *Hemidesmus indicus* as *kṛṣṇaśāribā* as the roots are blackish in colour and *Decalepis hamiltonii* as *śvētaśāribā*, the roots being brownish white in colour. A comparison of the pharmacognostical characters of the roots of *D. hamiltonii* and *H. indicus* have been made by Nayar *et al.* (1978). The macro and microscopical characters, physical constants, fluorescence characters and chemical constituents, of these four different taxa have been compared by Nayar (1979) and Wahi *et al.* (1979).

The identifying features of the various plant sources are described below:

Hemidesmus indicus (*Linn.*) *R. Br.* **(Asclepiadaceae)** (Fig. 215)
Periploca indica Linn.

Twining under shrub, with many slender wiry laticiferous branches; leaves simple, opposite or whorld, linear, lanceolate to elliptic-oblong, apiculate, acute or obtuse; 9.5 × 1 cm, entire, leathery, shiny, dark green above, paler beneath; flowers greenish yellow or greenish purple in subsessile axillary fascicles; calyx deeply 5-lobed, glandular within; corolla 5-partite, lobes thick, ovate-oblong, rugose within; corona single, corolline; stamens 5, connivent around styles, filaments incurved, distinct, pollinial bags spherical, closely appressed to the brownish caudicle; ovaries conic, stigma flat, circular; follicles terete, gradually narrowed, abruptly acuminate; seeds oblong, flattened, ventrally ridged, coma brownish white.

Distribution: The plant is found throughout India and Sri Lanka.

Ichnocarpus frutescens (*Linn.*) *R. Br.* **(Apocynaceae)** (Fig. 216)
Apocynum frutescens Linn.

Extensively branched, evergreen, woody twiner, tender parts rusty-pubescent; leaves simple, short-petioled, oblong or elliptic-obovate, 3–7 × 1.5–3.5 cm, subcoriaceous, base acute to attenuate, apex obtuse to acutely apiculate; flowers cream in axillary and terminal paniculate cymes; calyx cupular, lobes 5, subequal, ovate, alternating with 5 glandular scales; corolla salver-shaped, lobes 5, villous within, undulate; stamens 5, attached below the middle, included, anthers sagitate, shortly spurred, connivent around stigma; ovaries 2, partly connate, ovules many; fruit of 2 slender, cylindric follicles; seeds linear, crowned with silky hairs.

Distribution: Distributed throughout India in all districts in the plains and lower hills. Also reported from Sri Lanka, S.E. Asia and Australia.

Cryptolepis buchanani *Roemer & Schultes* **(Asclepiadaceae)** (Fig. 217)
Nerium reticulatum Roxb.

Large, much-branched climber; leaves simple, opposite, oblong to elliptic, obtusely acuminate, 8–15 × 5–7 cm, glabrous green above, pale, whitish beneath; flowers creamy white in lax, few-flowered axillary cymes, calyx lobes 5, ovate-lanceolate, acute; corolla lobes 5, oblong-lanceolate acute; stamens 5, attached near the base of the corolla tube, filaments subconnate, anthers short, pollen masses cohering in pairs; ovary of 2 carpels; fruit of 2 divaricate, follicular mericarps.

Distribution: Peninsula. In India it is seen in N. Circars, Deccan, Carnatic and W. Coast, in deciduous forests and in hedges.

Decalepis hamiltonii *Wight & Arn.* **(Asclepiadaceae)**

Glabrous twining shrub; branchlets terete with swollen, winged nodes; leaves simple, opposite, entire, ovate or elliptic-obovate, 2.5–7 × 1.5–5 cm, subcoriaceous, base attenuate to truncate, apex subacute to obtuse; flowers small, creamy white in axillary branched cymes; calyx lobes oblong, tinged with brown; corolla campanulate, lobes spreading, villous within; stamens 5, connivent; pollinial bags closely adherent, fla-

caudicle indistinct; corona double, staminal, outer scale-like, truncate, inner flat, adhering to gynostegium; ovaries subglobose; follicle oblong or lanceolate, cylindric; seeds ovate, tipped with long, white, silky coma.

Distribution: Peninsula. The plant occurs in Deccan, Horsleykonda, at 4,500 ft, Madamapalle in Chittoor at 3,000 ft, hills of N. Coimbatore, Carnatic, Veligonda hills of Nellore, Kambakam hills of Cingleput, W. Ghats, Anamalais.

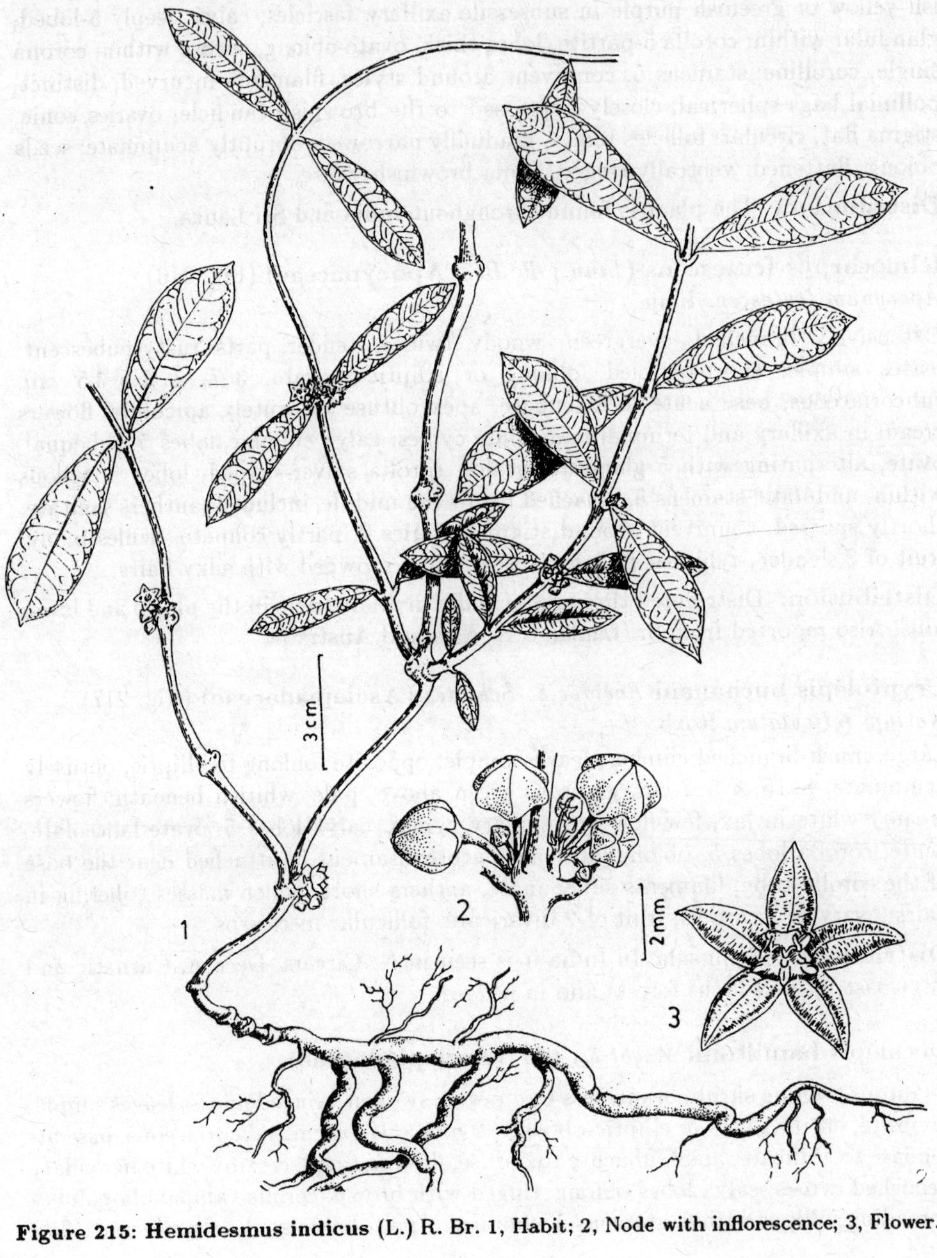

Figure 215: Hemidesmus indicus (L.) R. Br. 1, Habit; 2, Node with inflorescence; 3, Flower.

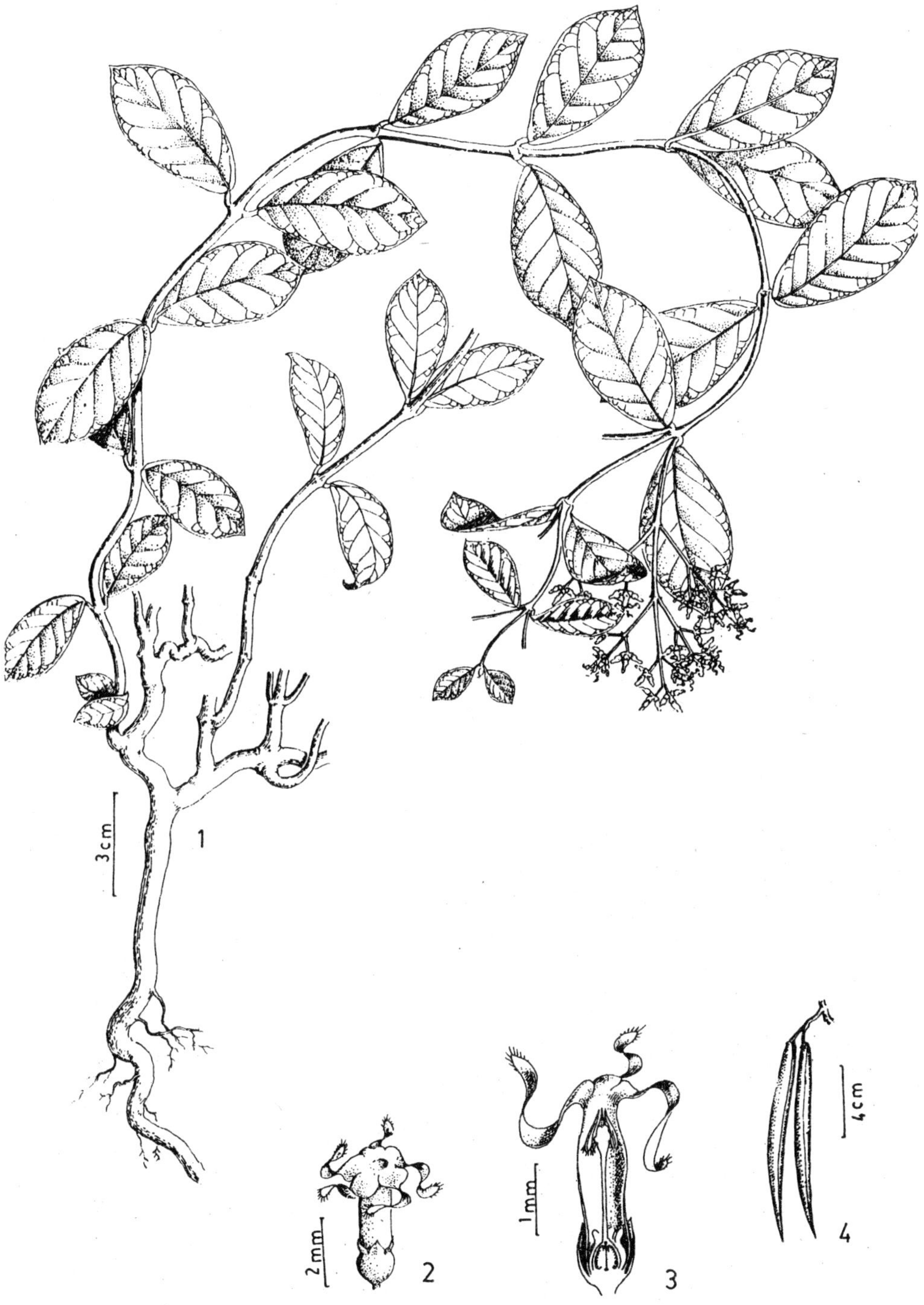

Figure 216: **Ichnocarpus frutescens** (L.) R. Br. 1, Habit; 2, Flower; 3, Flower L.S.; 4, **Fruits**.

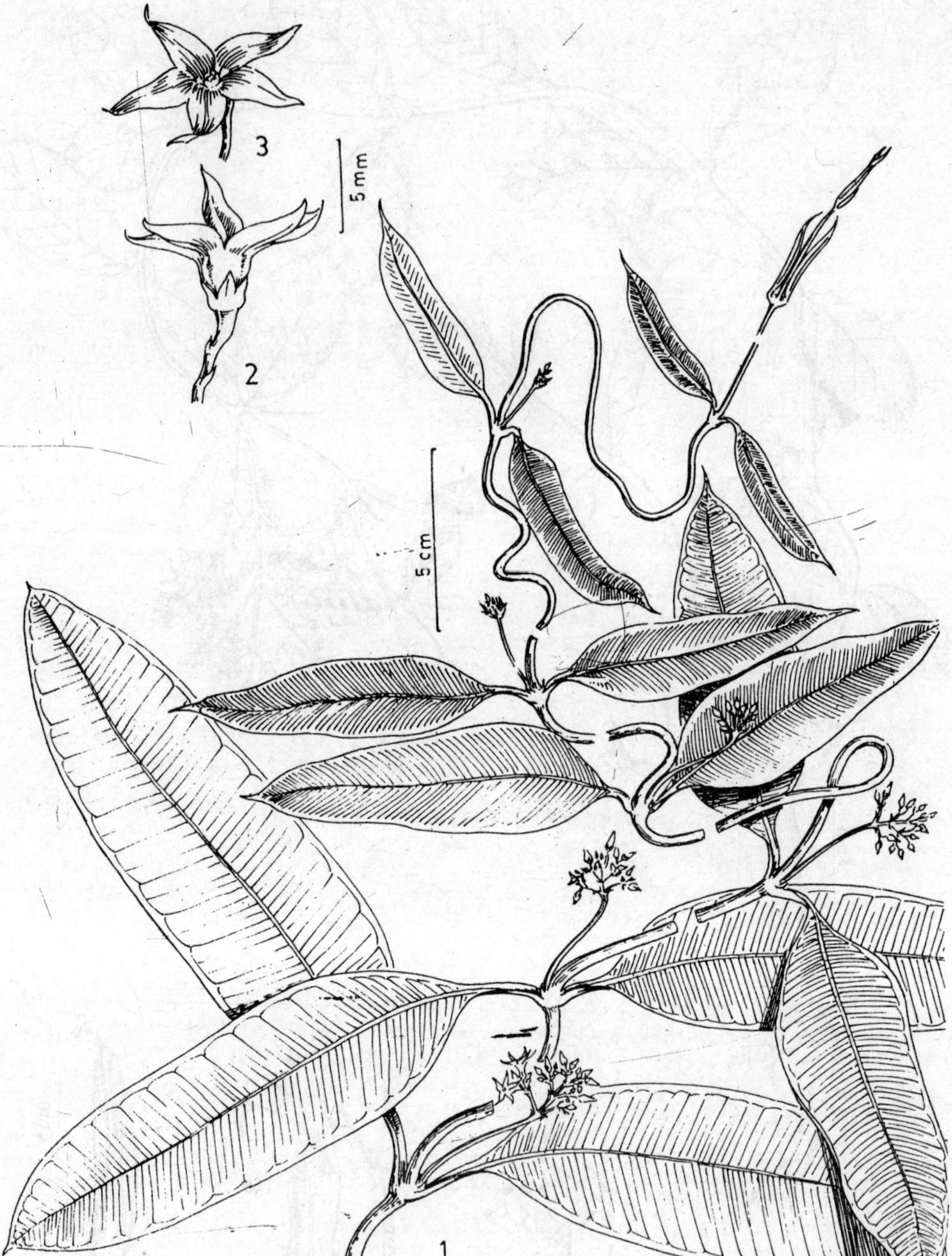

Figure 217: Cryptolepis buchanani R. & S. 1, Habit; 2–3, Flowers.

SAṚPAGANDHĀ (Mal. AMALPORI)

Sarpagandhā is probably one of the important contributions of ancient Indian medicine to the world health care system. It has great demand in the international market, eversince it was found to be efficacious in treating hypertension. The alkaloid reserpin present in the roots of this plant, has been proved to be an effective remedy against hypertension. Āyurvēdic texts also describe its sedative and hypnotic action. *Sarpagandhā* root is reported to be hot, bitter, acrid, anthelmintic, cardiodepressent and digestive and is used in insanity, insomnia, epilepsy, dyspepsia, painful affections of the bowel, intestinal worms, sexual aggression, snake bites etc. The drug has been effectively tried in cases of high blood pressure, insanity and schizophrenia. Decoction of the root is reported to be useful to increase uterine contractions and to promote expulsion of the foetus (Nadkarni, 1954: 1053; Kurup *et al.*, 1979: 185). The drug is an important ingredient of preparations like *Sarpagandhādi guḷika, Sarpagandhā cūrṇaṃ, Nirguṇḍyādi ghṛtaṃ*, etc.

Among the ancient seers, only Suśrutha has mentioned the drug *sarpagandhā* in the treatment of mental diseases (cf. Chunekar, 1982: 83) *Bhāvaprakāśa nighaṇṭu* describes it under the name *nākuli*. It mentions two types of this drug *nākuli* and *gandhanākuli*, distinguished from each other on the basis of aroma, the former being equated with *Rauvolfia serpentina* (Apocynaceae) and the latter with *Aristolochia indica* (Aristolochiaceae). Other names attributed to *nākuli* by Suśrutha are *sarpagandhā, sarpasugandhā* and *sugandhā* (Singh & Chunekar, 1972: 219).

In Kerala, however, *Rauvolfia serpentina* is used as the source of *sarpagandhā* which is known as *amalpori* in vernacular. *Aristolochia indica* is accepted as a different drug viz. *īśvari*, locally called *karaḷayaṃ*, specifically indicated for the treatment of snake-bite and is discussed elsewhere.

Rauvolfia serpentina (*Linn.*) *Benth. ex. Kurz.* **(Apocynaceae)** (Fig. 218)

Glabrous shrub; leaves in whorls of 3, oblong or lanceolate, acuminate, upto 16.8 × 5.5 cm; flowers white with pale purple stalks in terminal or axillary sub capitate cymes; fruiting pedicels and calyx red; corolla tube slender, 2.5 cm long, dilated a little above the middle; lobes white; stamens 5, included in the corolla tube; ovary of 2 free carpels; fruit drupaceous, ovoid, green when young, purplish black when mature.

Distribution: This species, distributed widely in Indo Malesia, was once upon a time very common in the plains and slopes of Kerala. But indescriminate extraction of this drug, especially for the international market, has now rendered it extremely rare and vulnerable. Rheede describes the plant under the name *Tsjovanna-amalpodi* (Hort. Malab. 9: 15. t. 10. 1689).

Note: Ajmaloon, a drug from *Rauvolfia serpentina* had been found to be highly effective for the treatment of hypertension (Arora *et al.*, 1987).

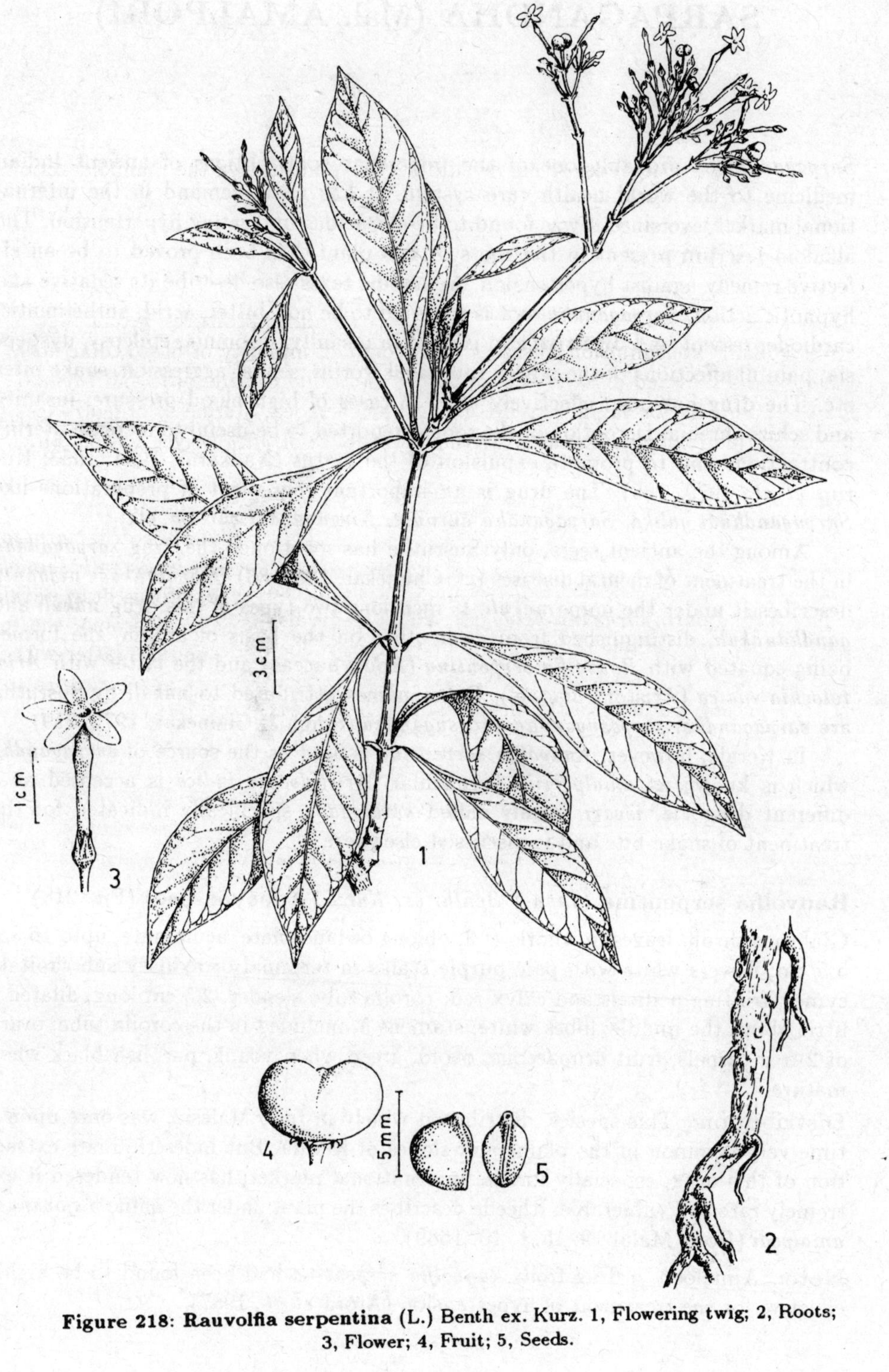

Figure 218: Rauvolfia serpentina (L.) Benth ex. Kurz. 1, Flowering twig; 2, Roots; 3, Flower; 4, Fruit; 5, Seeds.

ŚATĀVARĪ (Mal. ŚATĀVARI)

Ancient works like Ṛgvēda, Atharvavēda etc., have mentioned the manifold action of the drug which is indicated by the synonyms *śatavīrya* and *daśavīrya*. Men of Āyurvēda consider it as a powerful *rasāyana* drug capable of improving memory power, intelligence, and physical strength and maintaining youthfulness. *Śatāvari* is sweet and bitter in taste, tonic, aphrodisiac, galaclagogue, roborant, diuretic, antidysenteric and demulcent. It increases breast milk, promotes sexual vigour, cures swelling, consumption, diseases on account of impurity of blood, diarrhoea, piles, eye diseases and diseases caused by the morbidity of *vāta, pitta* and *kapha*. It is a good remedy for vaginal discharges like leucorrhoea, uterine disorders, excess of bleeding and colic pain caused by the discordance of *pitta* (Aiyer & Kolammal, 1963. 6: 48; Kurup *et al.*, 1979: 194; Nesamony, 1985: 469). The tuberous roots form an important ingredient of preparations like *Śatāvariguḷaṃ*, *Sahacarādi kuḷaṁbu*, *Rāsnādi kaṣāyaṃ*, *Dhātṛyādi ghṛtaṃ* etc.

According to the synonyms given in the texts, the plant has several roots (*śatamūlī, śatapādī*) which are intertwined (*jaṭāmūlā*) and with which the plant is anchored (*indīvarī, nārāyaṇī, śatāvarī*). These terms also indicate that it is an efficaceous tonic, acceptable to hundreds. The plant produces several tillers (*bahusutā*) and minute leaves (*sūkṣmapatṛā*) (Aiyer & Kolammal, 1963. 6: 48).

The accepted source of the drug, namely *Asparagus racemosus* Willd. of Liliaceae, agrees with the description given in the texts, especially in the presence of many long, tuberous roots and small leaf like cladodes. Rheede has described the plant under the name *Schada-Veli-Kelangu* (Hort. Malab. 10: 19–20, t. 10. 1690).

Nighaṇṭus mention another bigger type of *śatāvari* called *mahāśatāvari*. This is equated with *Asparagus sarmentosus* (Chunekar, 1982: 392). This species, however, is characterised by solitary cladodes and is not used. In practice, *A. racemosus* is the one widely used throughout India.

Asparagus racemosus *Willd.* **(Liliaceae)** (Fig. 219)

Extensively branched, rambling, spiny shrub with a stout root-stock bearing numerous, long, fusiform, tuberous roots; leaves reduced to minute spinescent structures subtending the leaflike cladodes which are falcate, slightly compressed and channelled beneath, borne in axillary clusters of 2–6; flowers white, strong-scented in solitary or fasciled racemes; pedicels slender; bracts scarious; perianth six-partite, segments, oblong, reflexed and connivent below; stamens 6, filaments free, opposite to the perianth segments, anthers 2-celled; ovary trigonous, three chambered, style short, columnar ending in three recurved stigmatic lobes; fruits globose berries.

Distribution: The plant is found throughout tropical and subtropical India, in all districts. Also distributed in Africa, through S. Asia to China, S. Malaysia and N. Australia.

Note: According to the texts, *śatāvari* is a reputed drug for peptic ulcer (*pariṇāmaśūla*). Singh and Singh (1980) and Kishore *et al.* (1980) have demonstrated that it is a good cure for duodinal ulcer. Detailed pharmacognostic investigations of the drug have been carried out by Karnick & Joshi (1986).

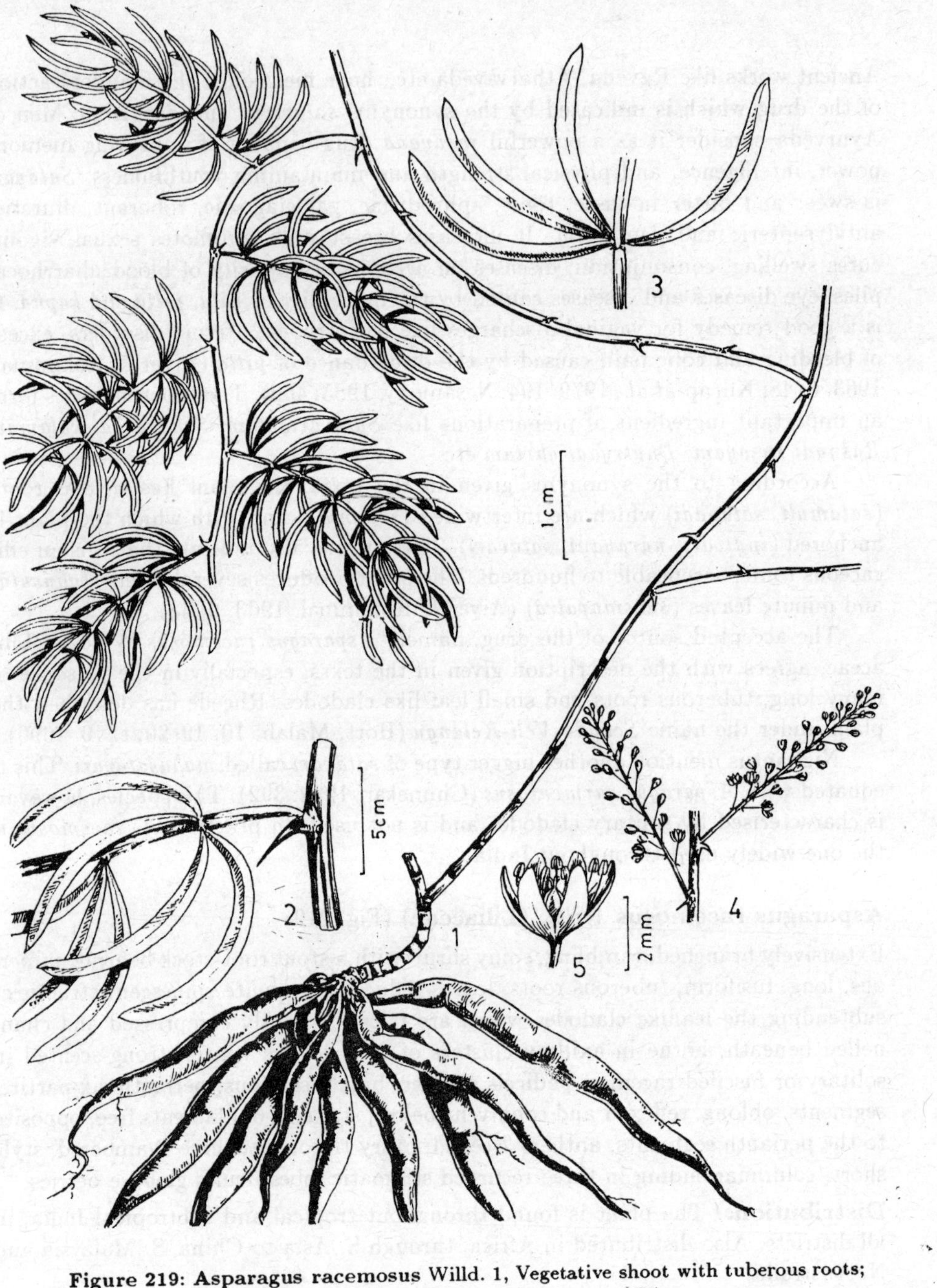

Figure 219: Asparagus racemosus Willd. 1, Vegetative shoot with tuberous roots; 2–3, Cladodes enlarged; 4, Inflorescence; 5, Flower.

ŚAṬHĀṀBAṢṬHĪ (Mal. PANICCAKAṂ)

Paniccakaṃ is a common prickly climber along the plains and hills of south western India, possessing distinctly sour leaves, often used for preparation of chutneys. The leaves are also the source of the drug *śaṭhāṁbaṣṭhi*. This drug, one of the five acid-drugs *(pañcāmḷa)*, is a major constituent of the *Pañcāṁḷatailaṃ*, an oil preparation for body-anointing, *Annabhēdi sindūraṃ* and *Abhṛaṃ* (101). The leaves are sour, astringent, anti-inflammatory and anthelmintic. They are reported to improve digestion and are useful in swellings, intestinal worms, dyspepsia and eye diseases. The roots are cooling, diuretic and anti-inflammatory and are used in burning sensation, swellings and kidney disorders (Anonymous, 1959. 5: 89).

The drug is not found mentioned in the classical Āyurvēdic texts, but is widely used in Kerala. *Hibiscus hispidissimus* (Malvaceae), locally called *paniccakaṃ*, is the accepted source of the drug here.

Hibiscus hispidissimus *Griff.* **(Malvaceae)** (Fig. 220)
H. furcatus Roxb. ex DC.
H. aculeatus Roxb.

Rambling shrub with recurved prickles; leaves digitately 3–5 lobed, apically lanceolate, crenate-serrate, 3–5 × 1–3.5 cm, prickly on the midveins beneath; flower solitary, bright yellow with a dark purple eye; epicalyx segments 8–12, each 2-lobed, calyx lobes 5, lanceolate; petals 5; stamens united to form the staminal tube; capsule globose, 1.5 × 1 cm, bristly hairy, beaked; seeds 3-gonous, warty, glandular.

Distribution: South western India in plains and hills in waste lands. Also reported from Sri Lanka, tropical and S. Africa, and Asia.

Taxonomic notes: The names *H. furcatus* and *H. aculeatus*, have been misapplied to the Indian taxon. Pradeep and Sivarajan (1991) have now set the records straight and the correct name of this Indian Species in *H. hispidissimus* Griffith.

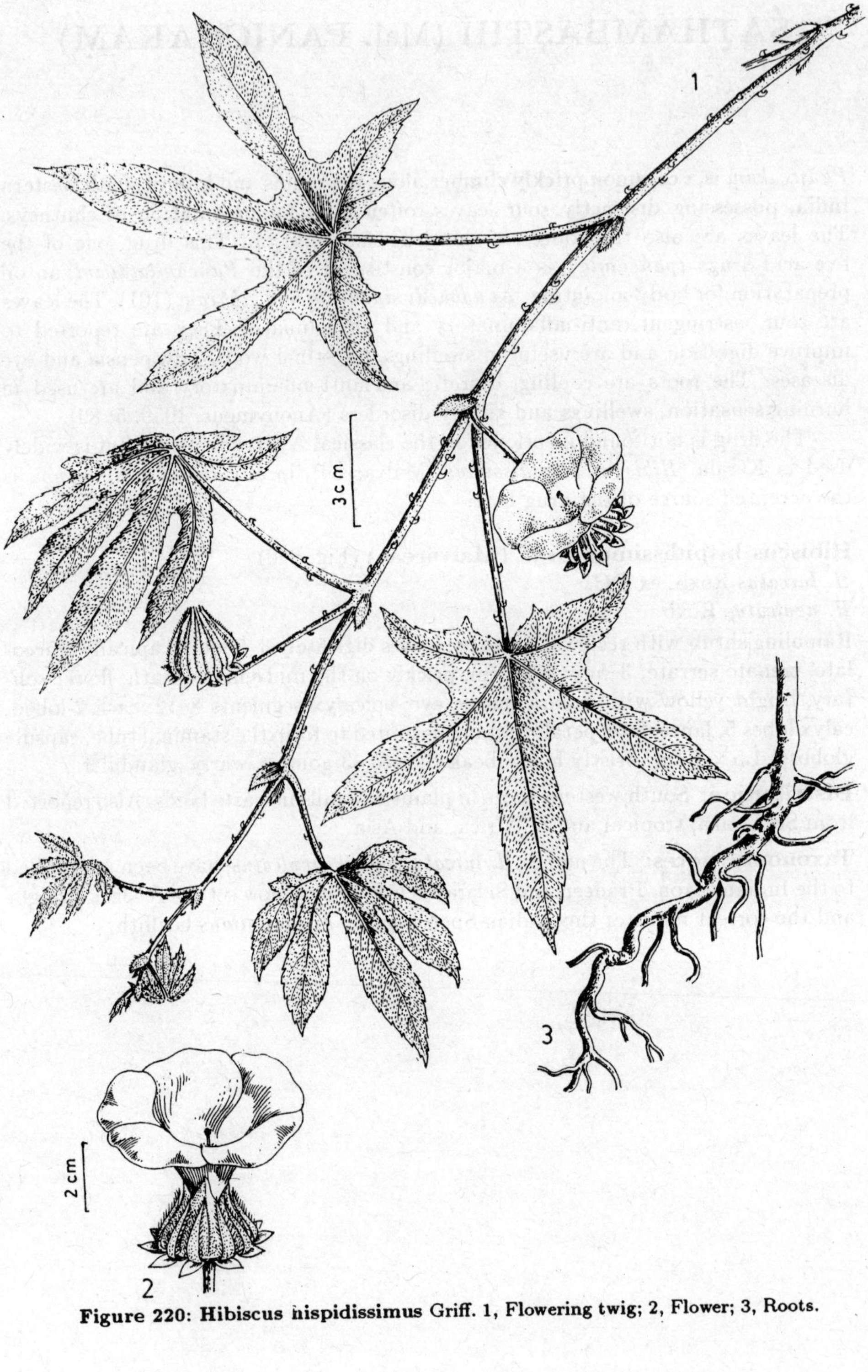

Figure 220: Hibiscus hispidissimus Griff. 1, Flowering twig; 2, Flower; 3, Roots.

ŚIGRU (Mal. MURIṄṄA)

Acrid, hot, sweet and light (*Bhāvapṛakāśa*), this drug is capable of reinstating the balance of humours, disturbed by morbid *vāta* and *kapha*. It improves appetite and digestion, promotes semen and is good for heart and eye problems. It has also been recommended against worms, abscesses, swellings, enlargement of cervical glands, spleen, thyroid, phantom tumour, ulcers, obesity and poisonous affections. Roots, leaves and seeds are used in medicines. Root and root bark are abortifacient and applied externally, cure inflammatory swellings. An infusion of the roots is recommended for asthma, gout, lumbago, rheumatism and inflammation. Fresh roots cure intermittent fever, paralytic problems, epilepsy and hysteria. It is used as a valuable rubefacient externally in bites of rabid animals. Fresh leaf juice mixed with honey is used as an eyedrop in eye diseases and in fainting fits due to nervous debility, spasmodic affections of the bowels, hysteria, etc. Leaves are galactagogue and promote breast milk secretion and are used as a vegetable. Poultice of leaves is a good cure for glandular swellings. Seeds, known as *śvētamaricaṃ* are recommended for eye diseases and poisonous affections (Nadkarni, 1954: 814; Aiyer & Kolammal, 1960. 4: 23; Nesamony, 1985: 426).

Ancient texts reveal that the source plant of this drug is a vegetable (*upadaṁśa-kṣamaḥ*), and it has got pungent roots (*daṁśamūla*), thick bark (*bahuḷatwak*) and leaves with many leaflets (*bahuḷadaḷaḥ*). The name *śigru* is indicative of its ability to cure diseases due to morbidity of *kapha* (cf. Aiyer & Kolammal, 1960. 4: 21; Moosad, 1983: 292).

However, there is a little bit of confusion as to the accurate identity of the plant source, especially with regard to the different varieties of *śigru* mentioned in the texts. *Dhanvantarinighaṇṭu* and *Bhāvaprakāśa* recognise two types: *śvētaśigru* (*śvēta* = white) and *raktaśigru* (*rakta* = red). The author of *Rājanighaṇṭu,* however, mentions a third variety, *nīlaśigru* (*nīla* = blue), in addition to the two mentioned above. *Abhidhānamañjari* also recognises three varieties, but designates them differently, as *śigru, madhuśigru* and *śvētaśigru*, which are called *muriṅṅa, kāṭṭumuriṅṅa* (*kāṭṭu* = wild) and *pūlamuriṅṅa* respectively in the vernacular.

Moringa oleifera (Moringaceae), commonly cultivated throughout India for its leaves, flowers and fruits which are used as vegetables, is the most widely accepted source of *śigru*. With white or creamy white flowers, this has been often equated with the *śvētaśigru* by many and *M. concanensis* with yellow flowers streaked with red, with *raktaśigru* or *madhuśigru*. The identity of *nīlaśigru* however, still remains uncertain (see Aiyer & Kolammal, 1960. 4: 19; Mooss, 1976: 88).

On the practical side, physicians and pharmacists do not make a distinction between these varieties. *M. concanensis*, easily distinguishable from *M. oleifera* by its 2-pinnate leaves and emarginate leaflets (decompound leaves and obtuse or rounded leaflets in the latter) is an occasional species found in the deciduous forests of Peninsular India to Rajasthan. In contrast, *M. oleifera* is widely available and hence, this is the species adopted as the source plant of the drug in the area of present study. (See also Rheede, Hort. Malab. 6: 19–20, t. 11. 1686, *Mouringou.*)

Moringa oleifera *Lam.* **(Moringaceae)** (Fig. 221)
M. pterygosperma Gaertner

Small or medium sized trees; leaves alternate, decompound, rachis articulate at base; leaflets small, elliptic to obovate, obtuse, 2.5 × 1.5 cms, green above, paler beneath; flowers white in axillary or terminal panicles; calyx 5-partite, segments petaloid, unequal, reflexed; petals 5, free, linear-spathulate, unequal; stamens 10, in two series; ovary tricarpellary, stipitate with numerous ovules; fruit an elongate, pendulous, cylindrical, longitudinally ribbed, loculicidal capsule, 35–50 cms long; seeds trigonous, broadly winged on the angles.

Distribution: Widely cultivated all over India and many other tropical countries.

Note: Clinical studies have shown that the stem bark produces significant relief in patients suffering from difficult micturition or *mūtrakṛchṛa* (Shaw & Jana, 1982). The abortifacient activity of *M. oleifera* leaves has been demonstrated by Seth *et al.* (1988).

Moringa concanensis *Nimmo ex. Dalz.* **&** *Gibson* **(Moringaceae)**

Very similar to *M. oleifera* in habit; leaves bipinnate; leaflets 4–6 pairs, broadly elliptic or suborbicular, retuse or emarginate at apex, 1–3 × 1–2 cms, glaucous below; flowers in lax, axillary panicles, pedicelled, irregular, yellow streaked with red; calyx segments white, oblong, reflexed; petals yellow veined with red, oblong or spathulate; stamens 5 fertile, with 4–5 alternating staminodes, filaments hairy at base; ovary tricarpellary, stipitate, tomentose, one chambered with many ovules on parietal placenta; fruit an elongate, beaked, three valved loculicidal capsule, 60 × 1.5 cm; seeds, 3-angled, broadly winged.

Distribution: Peninsular India, Rajasthan and also in Pakistan.

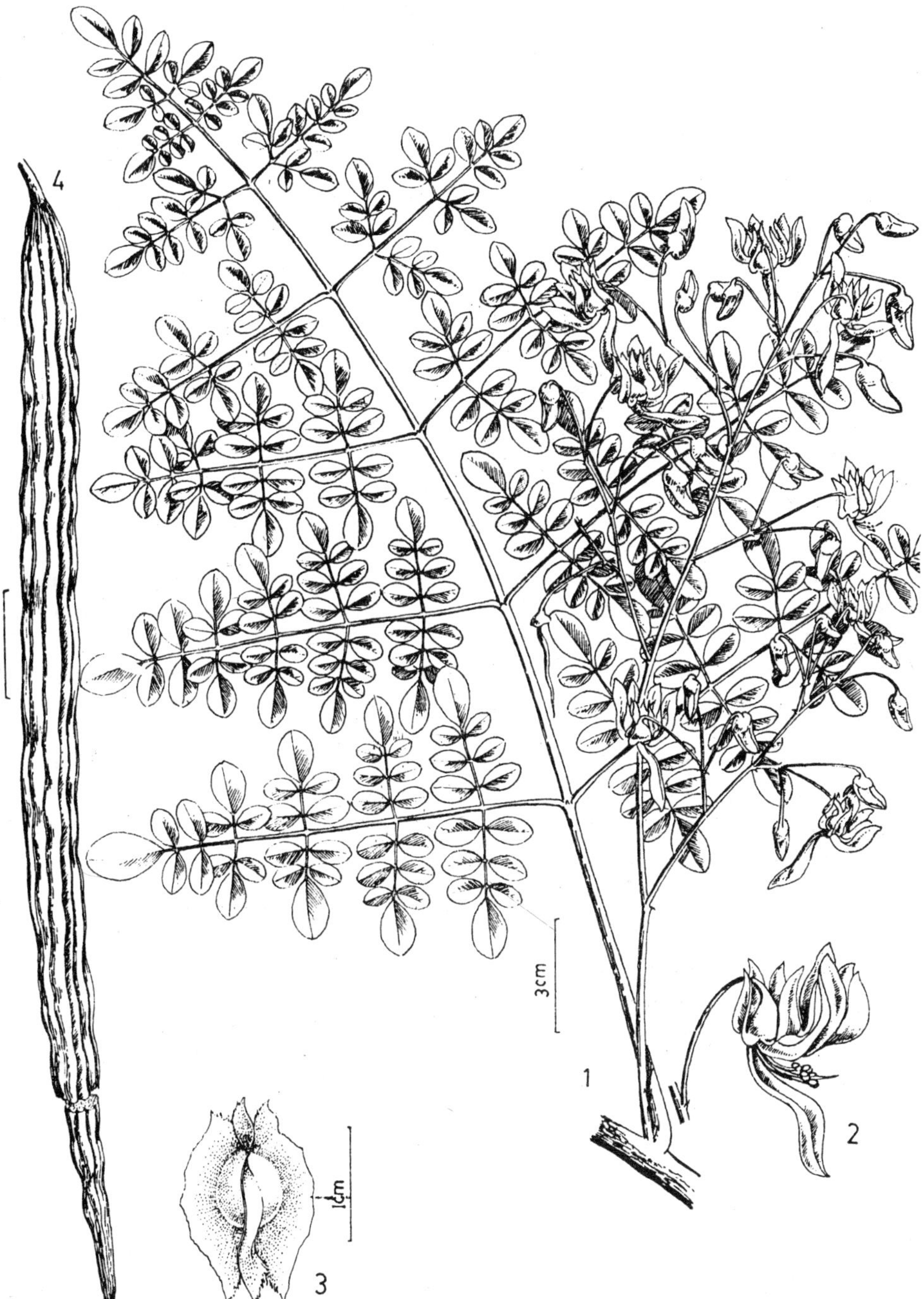

Figure 221: Moringa oleifera Lam. 1, A leaf with axillary inflorescence; 2, Flower; 3, Seed; 4, Fruit.

SNUHĪ (Mal. ILAKKAḶḶI)

Men of Āyurvēda include the drug in the group of purgatives. The stem with the milky latex is the officinal part. The milky juice is bitter, expectorant, locally rubefacient, digestive, stomachic, abortifacient and cures earache, liver and spleen enlargement, asthma, colic, cutaneous affections, dropsy, dyspepsia, flatulence, intermittent fever, jaundice, leprosy, rheumatism and insect bites. The juice is externally applied to remove warts and similar excrescences, ulcers, scabies and glandular swellings to prevent suppuration (Nadkarni, 1954: 525, Dey 1980: 140).

Caraka mentions two varieties of *snuhi*, differentiated on the basis of their spines viz. one which is less spiny called *alpakaṇṭaka* and the other having profuse spines called *bahukaṇṭaka*. The second variety is considered therapeutically more active (Singh & Chunekar, 1972: 459; Sharma, 1983: 431).

Although there are about half a dozen dendroid Euphorbias like *E. neriifolia* L., *E. nivulia* Buch.-Ham; *E. antiquorum* Linn., *E. trigona* Haw., *E. royleana* Boiss etc. in use under this name, *E. neriifolia* Linn. (Euphorbiaceae) is the one most commonly equated with *snuhi* by most of the authors. (Kirtikar & Basu, 1918: 1127; Nadkarni, 1954: 524; Chopra *et al.*, 1956: 114; Kapoor & Mitra, 1979: 68: Dey 1980: 140; Chunekar, 1982: 308; Sharma, 1983: 430). In Kerala also the plant source of *snuhi* is *E. neriifolia* (See Mooss, 1980: 9). However, this species is closely similar to and is often confused with another closely allied species, *E. nivulia*. In fact, Rheede's illustration (Hort. Malab. 2: 83–84. t. 43. 1679) of *E. nivulia* as the source of this drug, is ample testimony for the fact that both the species have been in use in Kerala, since long. These two taxa can however be, easily distinguished as follows:

Stem cylindrical .... *E. nivulia*
Stem 5-angled .... *E. neriifolia*

Euphorbia nivulia *Buch.-Ham.* **(Euphorbiaceae)** (Fig. 222)

Armed deciduous trees; branches cylindric with pairs of straight spines inserted on flat corky bases arranged in vertical rows; leaves alternate, subsucculent, oblanceolate-obtuse, base cuneate, upto 28 × 7.5 cm, lateral nerves obscure; cyathia paired in lax cymes in the axils of fallen leaves; involucre broadly cupular, coriaceous, glands 5, oblong, thick. Male florets roughly in 5 groups of 8 each with sterile florets, bracteolate; female single, laterally pendulous; ovary 3 × 5 mm, style short, branched from above the middle, erect, stigma broad; capsule 0.5 cm across; seeds 4, angular, smooth.

Distribution: The plant is commonly run wild in waste lands, especially in arid parts of southern India. Sometimes cultivated as hedges.

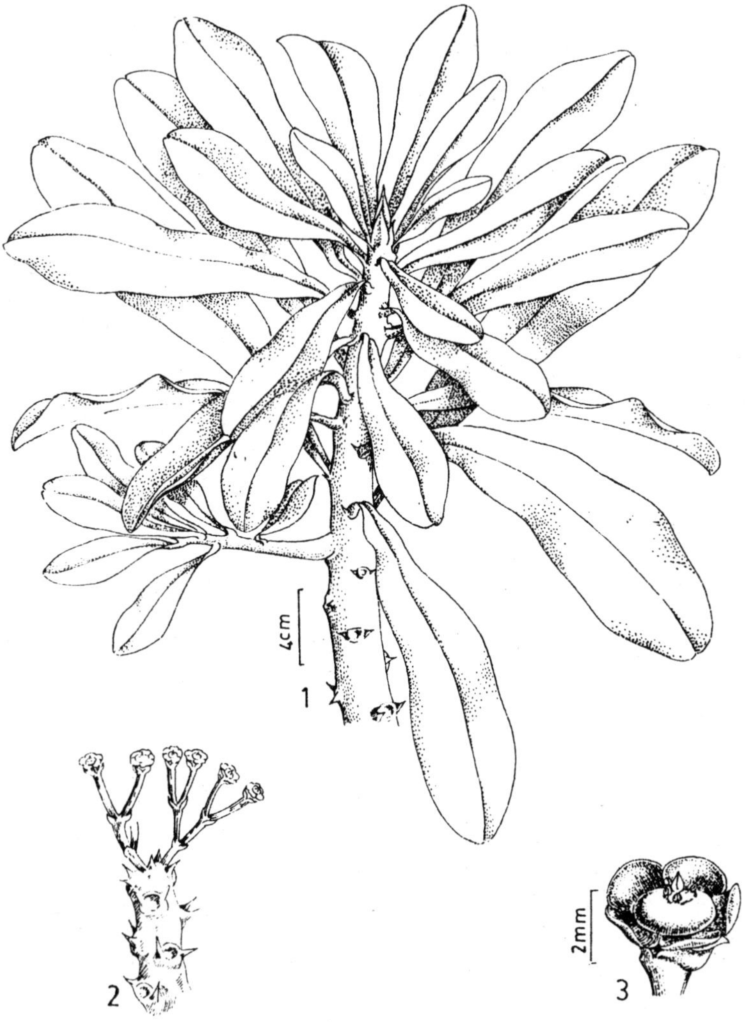

Figure 222: **Euphorbia nivulia** Buch.-Ham. 1, Habit; 2, Inflorescence; 3, A cyathium.

Euphorbia neriifolia *Linn.* (Euphorbiaceae)

Small trees; branches more or less 5-angled with pairs of short spines on small corky bases arranged in spiral lines; leaves shortly acute. Other characters as in *E. nivulia*.

Distribution: In most parts of India, especially in arid regions. Occassionally grown on hedges.

Note: Studies conducted by Lahon *et al.* (1979) on guinea pigs have shown that the alcoholic extract obtained from the fresh stem of *E. neriifolia* has significant local anaesthetic activity.

SPṚKKĀ (Mal. KARIṀTUṀPA)

This is one of the eighteen drugs that constitute the *Surasādi gaṇa* of Vāgbhaṭa. *Spṛkkā* is reported to be cooling, aromatic, bitter and aphrodisiac. It cures all the three *dōṣās*, itching, leprosy, poison, thirst, indigestion, fever and haematological disorders. Infusion of the plant is useful in affections of the stomach and bowels. Juice of leaves is administered in cases of infantile catarrh, cough, colic, dyspepsia and fever caused by teething. Decoction of the plant is an excellent fomentation for rheumatic joints (Nadkarni, 1954: 114; Chunekar, 1982: 265). Roots form an ingredient of formulations like *Surasādi tailaṃ, Pāṭhādi guḷika, Nirguṇḍyādi ghṛtaṃ, Nirguṇḍyādi guḷika*, etc.

This drug, described as aromatic and having crooked flowers by Ḍalhaṇa, has been equated with *Anisomeles malabarica* of Lamiaceae (Kirtikar & Basu, 1918: 1040; Nadkarni, 1954: 114; Chopra *et al.*, 1956: 19; Mooss, 1980: 79; Chunekar, 1982: 265; Vaidya Bapalal, 1982: 193). But, in practice, in Kerala *Adenosma indiana* of Scrophulariaceae is mainly used as the source of the drug. That this has been used as the drug source for long in Kerala, is testified by Rheede's description of this species under the local name *Carim-tumba* (Hort. Malab. 10: 185. t. 93. 1690).

Anisomeles malabarica (*Linn.*) *R. Br. ex Sims* **(Lamiaceae)** (Fig. 223)
Nepeta malabarica Linn.

Aromatic sub-shrub; stem and branches softly white tomentose and obtusely tetragonous; leaves simple, opposite, thick, lanceolate-acute, 12.5 × 3.5 cms, margin serrate, scented, pale green above, white tomentose below; flowers pale purple in terminal whorls of short, densely wooly spikes; calyx 5, gamosepalous, white woolly outside; corolla 2-lipped, upper lip short, white villous without, lower lip spreading, 3-lobed, pilose; stamens 4, didynamous, exserted; ovary 4-partite, style slender, bifid; fruit of 4 nutlets.

Distribution: The plant is distributed in S. Carnatic, from Madras southwards to S. Travancore, West to the E. foot of the ghats. And also in Mauritius, continental S.E. Asia, tropical Australia and Malesia.

Note: Pharmacognosy of *Anisomeles malabarica* has been studied by Kannabiran & Krishnamurthy (1972), and Brinda *et al.* (1981). It has been found to contain essential oil and diterpenoids which possess anti-cancer properties (Brinda *et al.*, 1984).

Adenosma indiana (*Lour.*) *Merr.* **(Scrophulariaceae)** (Fig. 224)
Manulea indiana Lour.
Adenosma bilabiatum (Roxb.) Merr.
Adenosma capitatum Benth.

Erect villous herb; leaves simple, opposite or whorled, ovate to ovate-oblong, coarsely crenate, upto 5 × 2.5 cms; flowers small, bluish violet in dense terminal heads; sepals 5, unequal, lanceolate, hairy outside; corolla gamopetalous, bilabiate; stamens 4, filaments hairy at base; ovary 2-celled, many ovuled; capsule avoid; seeds scabrous.

Distribution: A common weed in open grass lands and in upland cultivations. It is found in W. Coast, W. Ghats, S. Canara to Travancore in rice fields.

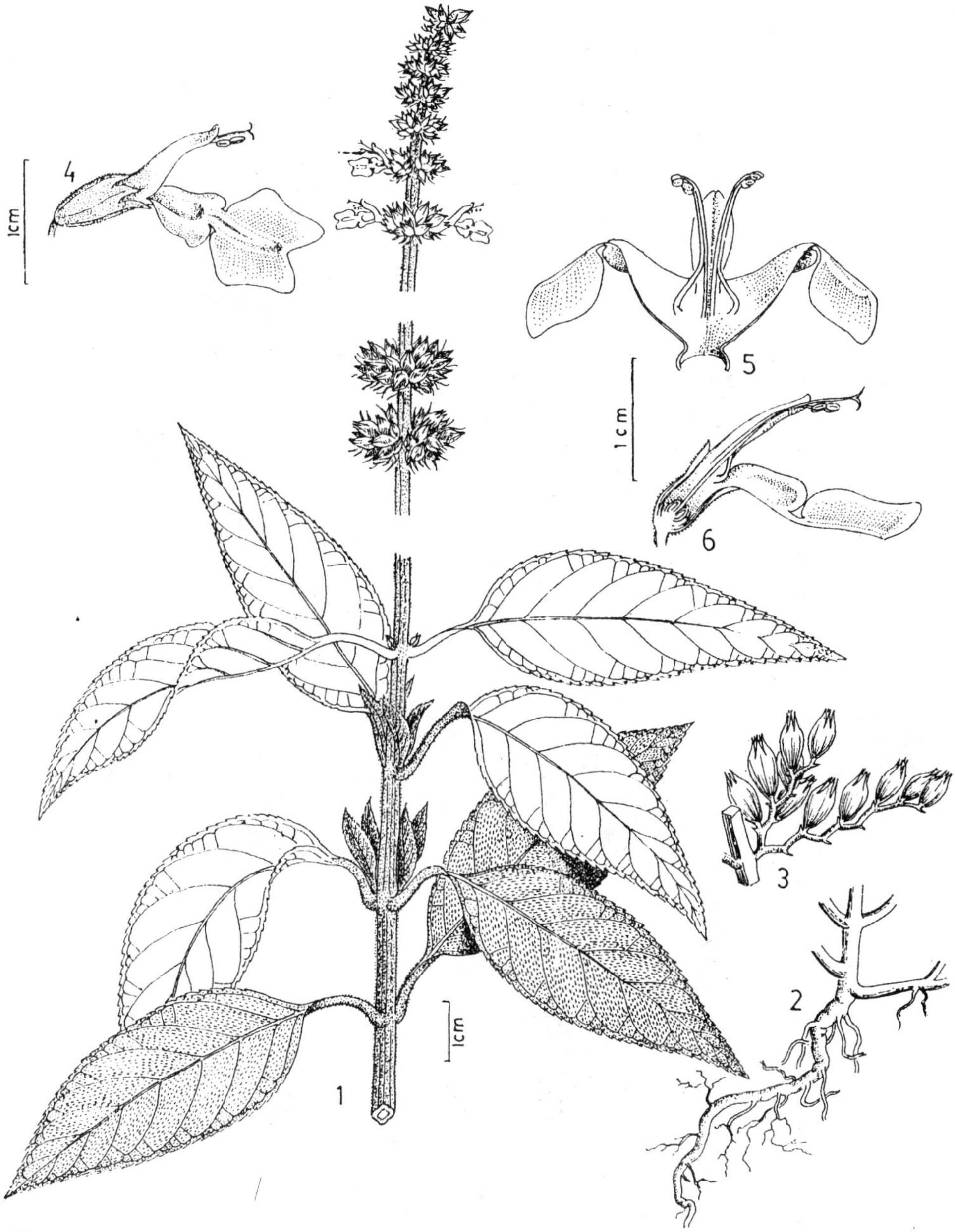

Figure 223: Anisomeles malabarica (L.) R. Br. ex Sims. 1, Flowering branch; 2, Roots; 3, A portion of inflorescence; 4, Flower; 5, Corolla opened with stamens; 6, Flower L.S.

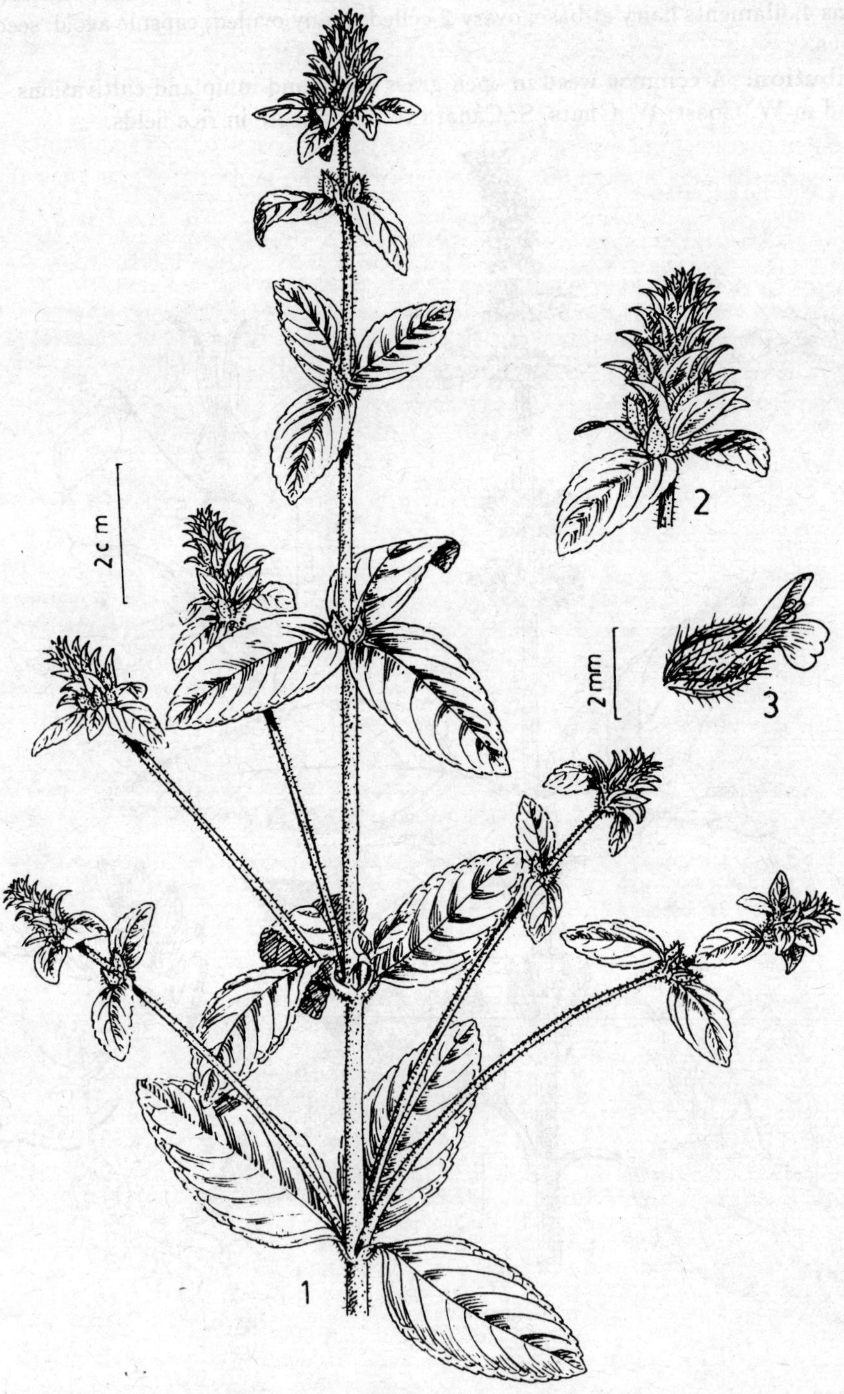

Figure 224: Adenosma indiana (Lour.) Merr. 1, Habit; 2, Inflorescence; 3, Flower.

ŚUKAKANDAḤ (Mal. KARUVIKKIḶAṄṄU)

This is an ingredient of *Valiya marmaguḷika*. The tuberous root is the officinal part. It is reported to be a stimulant and a purgative and is prescribed in gonorrhoea, dysuria and spermatorrhoea. Juice of the leaves is used as a soothing application to the skin inflamed by marking nut (*Semecarpus anacardium* Linn.) allergy (Nadkarni, 1954: 1307; Anonymous, 1962: 335).

There is no mention about this drug in early Āyurvēdic texts. In Kerala *Solena amplexicaulis* (Lam.) Gandhi (= *Solena heterophylla* Lour.) (Cucurbitaceae), locally called *karuvivaḷḷi* or *karuvikkiḷaṅṅu* is being used as the drug source (See also Rheede, Hort. Malab. 8: 51, t. 26. 1688) *Karivi-valli*.

Solena amplexicaulis (*Lam.*) *Gandhi* **(Cucurbitaceae)** (Fig. 225)
Bryonia amplexicaulis Lam.
Solena heterophylla (Lour.) Cogn.
Melothria heterophylla Lour.

Vine; leaves sessile, ovate, 3–5 angled or lobed, 4.5–8 × 4–6 cm, scabrid, base cordate, margin minutely denticulate, apex obtuse-retuse, apiculate; tendril simple; flowers white, unisexual, male flowers in umbellate racemes; calyx tube glabrous, lobes 5, triangular; corolla campanulate, petals 5, oblong-ovate, pubescent without; stamens 3, filaments free, 3-lobed, female flowers solitary; sepals and petals as in male; ovary oblong, apically tapering, style with an annular disc at the base, stigma 3-lobed, papillose, fruit ovoid, 1.5 × 1 cm, apically beaked, smooth.

Distribution: Tropical Asia, Malesia and Australia. In India, this is common in waste lands, twining over bushes and thickets.

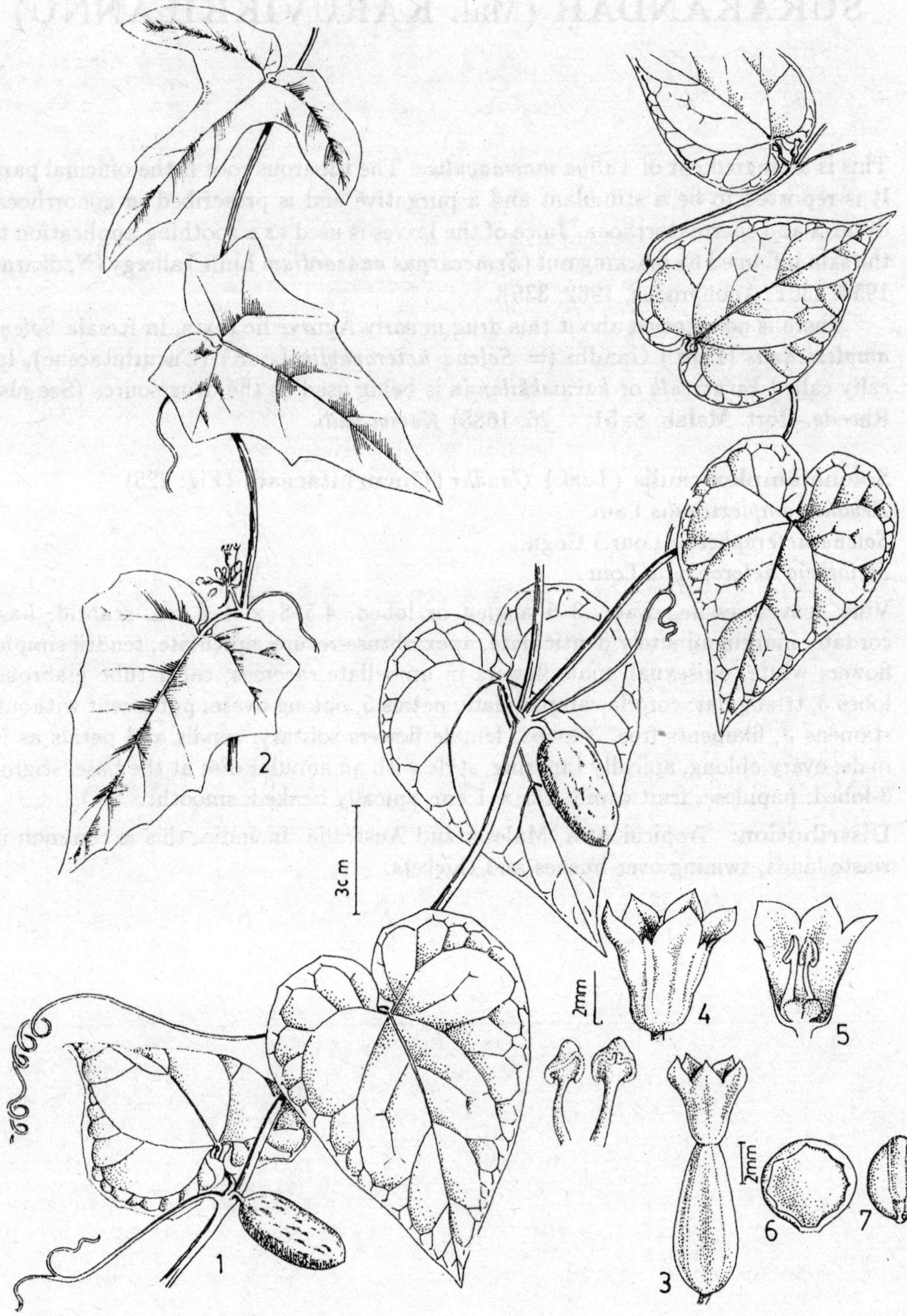

Figure 225: Solena amplexicaulis (Lam.) Gandhi. 1–2, Habit; 3, Female flower; 4, Male flower; 5, Male flower L.S.; 6–7, Seeds.

SUNIṢAṆṆAḤ (Mal. NĪRĀRAL)

According to the texts, the drug is sweet, astringent, cooling, constipating, digestive and diuretic. It promotes appetite, overcomes the three dosas - *vāta, pitta* and *kapha*—excess fat, fever, diabetes, leprosy and other skin diseases. The drug induces sleep and is used in mental and nervous disorders. It is an aphrodisiac, it purifies blood and cures cough, haematological diseases, dyspepsia, piles and poisons. (Chunekar, 1982: 674; Sharma, 1983: 535). The entire plant is used medicinally. The important preparations using the drug are *Dravavarṭi, Valiya Vārāhyādi ghṛtaṃ, Abhṛaṃ* (*101*), etc.

Classical texts describe this plant as a vegetable (*śāka*), always growing in the vicinity of water (*'jalānvitē dēśē'*) and as having four leaflets (*catuṣpatṛī, caturdalaḥ*), which resemble those of *cāṛṅgēri*, i.e. *Oxalis corniculata* (Vaidya Bapalal, 1982: 212). This has been universally accepted as belonging to the genus *Marsilea* (Marsileaceae) and the ancient descriptions compare well with this plant. However, most of the authors have described it under the name *M. quadrifolia*, the taxonomy of which is in some confusion. In a recent paper, Bharadwaja (1980) has concluded that the Indian specimens have wrongly been identified as *M. quadrifolia*. The Indian specimens belong to *M. minuta* with which some authors have equated this drug (Singh & Chunekar, 1972: 436; Chunekar, 1982: 674; Sharma, 1983: 535).

However, there are two varieties of this species found in India var. *minuta* with entire leaf margins and var. *indica* with dentate leaf margins. Men of Āyurvēda do not make any distinction between these varieties and both are taken as the source of the drug.

Marsilea minuta *Linn.* **(Marsileaceae)** (Fig. 226)
M. quadrifolia auct., non Linn.

A creeping herb with long, slender rhizomes; leaves alternate, in two rows on the rhizome; petiole long, slender, with the four obovate-retuse, glabrous leaflets at the tip, arranged in a whorl. Flowers absent. Fructifications (sporocarps) produced during summer, dark brown, hard and bean-shaped with two unequal horns.

Distribution: This plant is an emergent aquatic fern very commonly found in wet or flooded low lands in most parts of India.

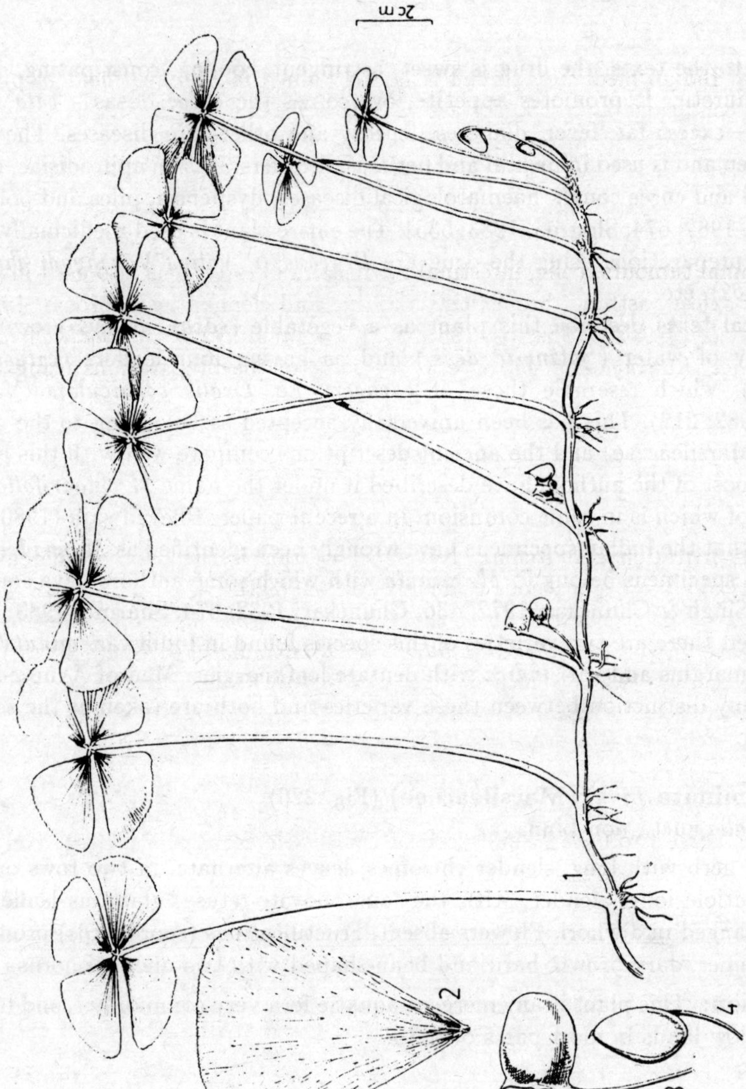

Figure 226: Marsilea minuta L. 1, Habit; 2, Leaflet enlarged; 3–4, Capsules.

SŪRAṆAḤ (Mal. CĒNA)

In traditional Indian medicine, *sūraṇa* is highly valued in the treatment of piles, haemophilic conditions and skin diseases. Due to the restorative properties, the tubers are used as a wholesome vegetable and as a diet during illness and convalescence.

The tuber is irritant, acrid, astringent, carminative and anthelmintic. It improves appetite and digestion, alleviates *kapha* and *vāta* and is very useful in curing piles, abdominal tumours, colic, intestinal worms and obesity. It is also used in enlargement of spleen, asthma, bronchitis, vomiting and elephantiasis (Mooss, 1978: 38; Kurup *et al.*, 1979: 206; Sharma, 1983: 532). *Sūraṇādi lēhaṃ, Sūraṇādi ghṛtaṃ, Laśuna ghṛtaṃ, Kāṅkāyanaṃ guḷika*, etc. are some of the preparations using the drug.

The synonyms given in the texts indicate only the properties of the drug.

Āyurvēdic treatises mention two types of *sūraṇa*, the wild type called *vanasūraṇa* and the cultivated form. Compared to the cultivated edible variety, *vanasūraṇa* has reddish white tubers with abundant calcium oxalate crystals causing great irritation and itching. Nevertheless, this is the one considered to be therapeutically more efficaceous (Chunekar, 1982: 693).

Most of the authors have equated this drug with *Amorphophalus campanulatus* Decne (now known as *A. paeoniifolius* var. *campanulatus* (Decne) Sivad.) of Araceae (See Vaidya, 1936: 621; Kurup *et al.*, 1979: 206; Kapoor & Mitra, 1979: 68; Chunekar, 1982: 693; Sharma, 1983: 532) Ayurvedic Formulary of India (Anonymous, 1978a: 258) has also corroborated this. However, this is the commonly cultivated, edible form which is widely used as a vegetable. The wild form, often with a prickly aerial shoot, is a distinct variety of the species, viz. *A. paeoniifolius* var. *paeoniifolius.* These two have been described by Rheede as *'Schena'* (Hort. Malab. 11: 35–36. t. 18. 1692) and *Mulenschena* (Hort. Malab. 11: 37. t. 19. 1692) respectively. He also describes *Katu-schena*—the wild form of *Schena* (Hort. Malab. 11: 41. t. 21. 1692), but attributes the name for another plant, *Tacca leontopetaloides* (Linn.) Kuntze (Taccaceae) which is often misidentified as an aroid.

Of these, the current practitioners prefer *A. paeoniifolius* var. *paeoniifolius.* However, faced with an increasing scarcity of this, they are now taking the cultivated elephant-foot-yam also i.e. *A. paeoniifolius* var. *campanulatus. Tacca leontopetaloides*, being a very scarce species with very small tubers, is seldom found to be in use now (see also Sivarajan & Balachandran, 1987b).

Amorphophalus paeoniifolius (*Dennst.*) *Nicolson* **(Araceae)**
var. **paeoniifolius:**
Arum paeoniifolium Dennst.

Tuberous, stout herb, 1–1.5 m high with an underground corm to 22 cm diameter; leaf solitary, large, 3-partite, appearing long after the flowers, petiole to 1.2 m long, mottled and often muricate; lamina highly pinnately lobed, 30–60 cm long;

inflorescence short-peduncled, but elongating in fruit, spathe broadly campanulate, to 25 × 28 cm, narrow below and spreading above, outside light green with whitish patches, inside dark purple with a yellowish base; spadix stout and sessile, to 40 cm long; pistillate flowers below, light purplish with elongate styles; stigma reniform to 2–3 lobed; male flowers reduced; stamens cream yellow; berries to 1.5 cm long.

The plant is seen wild in the upland areas, but now scarce.

Amorphophalus paeoniifolius *var.* **campanulatus** (*Decne.*) *Sivad.* **(Araceae)** (Fig. 227)

A. campanulatus Decne.

A. dubius Blume

This plant is similar to the var. *paeoniifolius* but the two can be distinguished as follows:

1. Petiole usually purplish brown with light pinkish blotches, strongly muricate, leaflet bases strongly decurrent; appendix longer than broad; style 2X the ovary length; stigma usually 2 lobed; fruit commonly set .... var. *paeoniifolius*
1. Petiole usually greenish white with blotches, smooth but sometimes roughish; leaflet bases not decurrent; appendix broader than long; style 3–4X the ovary length; stigma usually 3-lobed; fruit rarely set .... var. *campanulatus*.

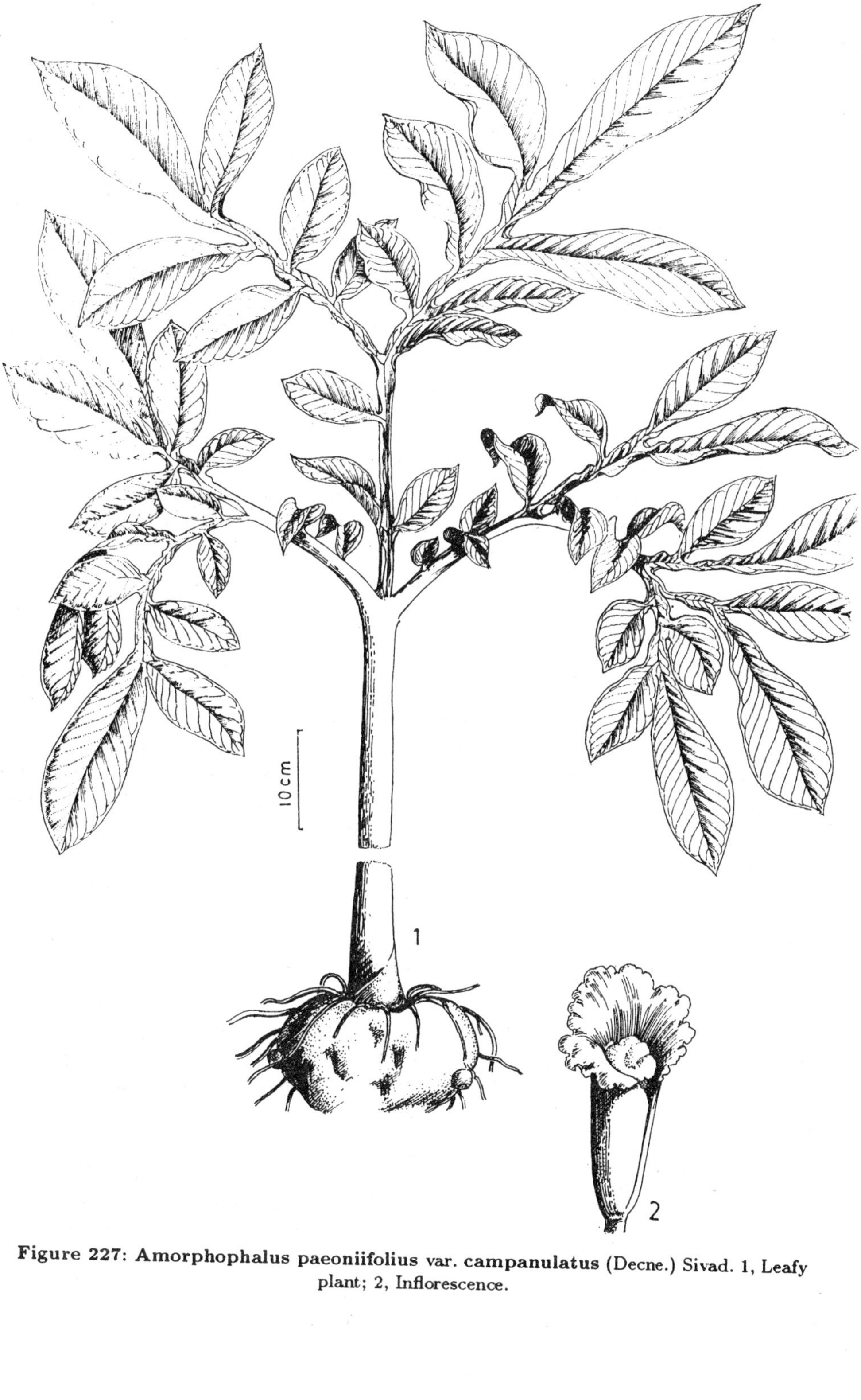

Figure 227: Amorphophalus paeoniifolius var. campanulatus (Decne.) Sivad. 1, Leafy plant; 2, Inflorescence.

SVARṆAKṢĪRĪ (Mal. PONNUṀMATTU)

This herb, which abounds in golden yellow juice as the name indicates, is reportedly light, bitter, alterative, aperient, astringent, anthelmintic and tonic and rehabilitates morbid *kapha* and *pitta*. It cures rheumatism, constipation, dysentery, colic and other intestinal affections. The golden yellow exudate is a remedy for blisters, indolent ulcers, leprosy and other cutaneous affections. Seeds are useful in cough, catarrhal affections of the throat and pulmonary mucous membrane and asthma. Oil from seeds is applied externally to ulcers, herpetic eruptions and other skin diseases (Nadkarni, 1954: 135; Sharma, 1983: 425).

The identity of the plant source is controversial. From the texts, one can only deduce that it is an alpine species (*himāvatī, haimavatī*) with acrid leaves (*kaṭuparṇī*) and abounding in golden yellow exudate (*svarṇakṣīrī, kāñcanakṣīrī, hēmakṣīrī*).

Suśrutha mentions two varieties of *kāñcanakṣīri*. Singh & Chunekar (1972: 462) equate them with *Garcinia morella* Desv. (Clusiaceae) and *Euphorbia thomsoniana* (Euphorbiaceae). Ḍalhaṇa, the commentator of *Suśruthasaṁhita* while commenting on this drug, refers to the term *'kaṅkuṣṭa'* which is the dried solidified yellow latex of *Garcinia morella*, commonly known as 'gum gamboge'. But, in practice, this is used as a different drug by men of Āyurvēda (Bapalal Vaidya, 1982: 224). Sharma (1983: 426) has concluded that the original plant source of this drug should have been *Euphorbia thomsoniana*. The fact that this is a high-altitude plant seen along the Tibetan Himalayas and Ḍalhaṇa's description of this plant as having leaves similar to those of *śāriba* (= *Hemidesmus indicus*), seem to fit rather well with this species. The local name *'hiyāvali'* in Ḍalhaṇa's commentary also agrees with its current Kashmiri name *'hirvi'* and it has profuse golden yellow latex (Vaidya Bapalal, 1982: 222–223).

Inspite of the fact that it does not agree well with the synonyms, in practice, *Argemone mexicana* of Papaveraceae is being used as the drug source (Nadkarni, 1954: 134; Kapoor & Mitra, 1979: 72; Dey 1980: 143; Chunekar 1982: 76; Sharma, 1983: 424; Nesamony, 1985: 84). The Ayurvedic Formulary of India, while mentioning *Euphorbia thomsoniana* as the original source of the drug, suggests *Argemone mexicana* as a suitable substitute (Anonymous, 1978a: 258). In any case, there is little chance of the latter being the original source of the drug, because this Mexican native has been introduced into India rather late. However, this must have been chosen as a matter of practical convenience by our physicians because of its abundance in our waste lands in contrast to the non-availability of *E. thomsoniana* in the plains.

Argemone mexicana *Linn.* **(Papaveraceae)** (Fig. 228)

Erect, glaucous, prickly annual herb; leaves alternate, sessile, 9–11 × 4–5.5 cm, oblong or obovate, sinuately pinnatified, margin spinulose, dentate, pale green variegated with white; flowers yellow, solitary, terminal; sepals 3, cohering in a cup; petals 6, elliptic-obtuse or obovate; stamens numerous, ovary 1-celled, ovules many

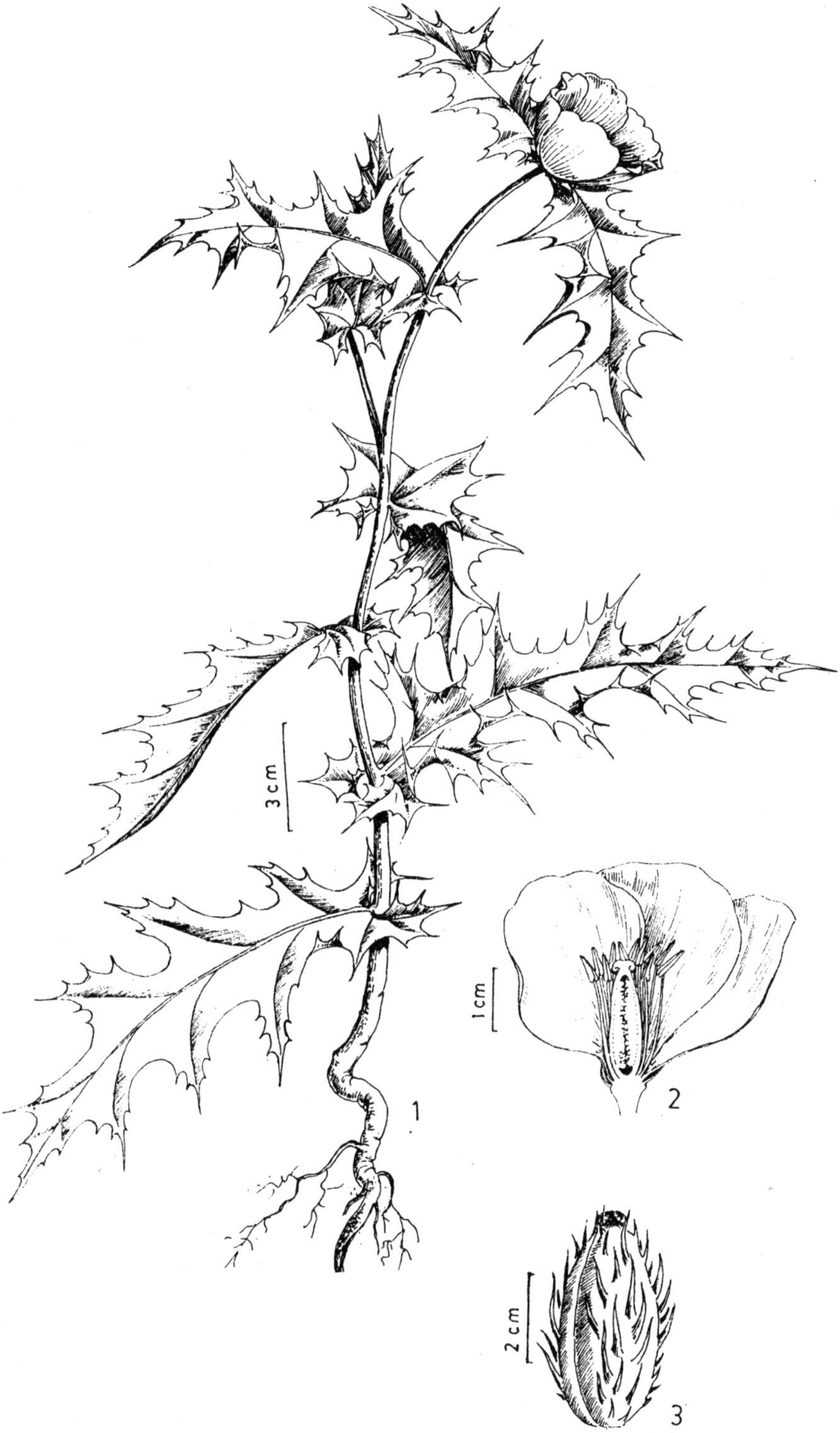

Figure 228: **Argemone mexicana** L. 1, Habit; 2, Flower L.S.; 3, Capsule.

on parietal placentae, stigma subsessile, 5-lobed; capsule ovoid or oblong, spinous; seeds many, pitted.

Distribution: A native of Mexico, now widely naturalised in the tropics, this is now a common weed along roadsides, waste places and fallow fields in all districts.

Garcinia morella (*Gaertn.*) *Desv.* **(Clusiaceae)** (Fig. 229)

Moderate-sized tree; leaves obovate or oblanceolate, acuminate, base tapered, coriaceous, midrib prominent, lateral nerves slender, parallel; flowers sessile in the axils of leaves or fallen leaves; male flowers 2–3 together, females usually solitary; sepals 4, greenish white, elliptic, concave; petals 4, white to pink, rather fleshy, veined, broadly elliptic, concave. Male flower: Stamens monadelphous, filaments connate into a central column with the apical part free, anthers red. Female flowers: ovary greenish, globose, 4 celled, style absent, stigma peltate; fruit globose, smooth, yellowish, upto 2.5 cm diam, apex crowned by the flat, tuberculate stigma; seeds kidney shaped, laterally compressed.

Distribution: The plant is distributed throughout southern India. It is seen in W. Ghats from S. Canara and Mysore to Travancore, upto 3,000 ft.

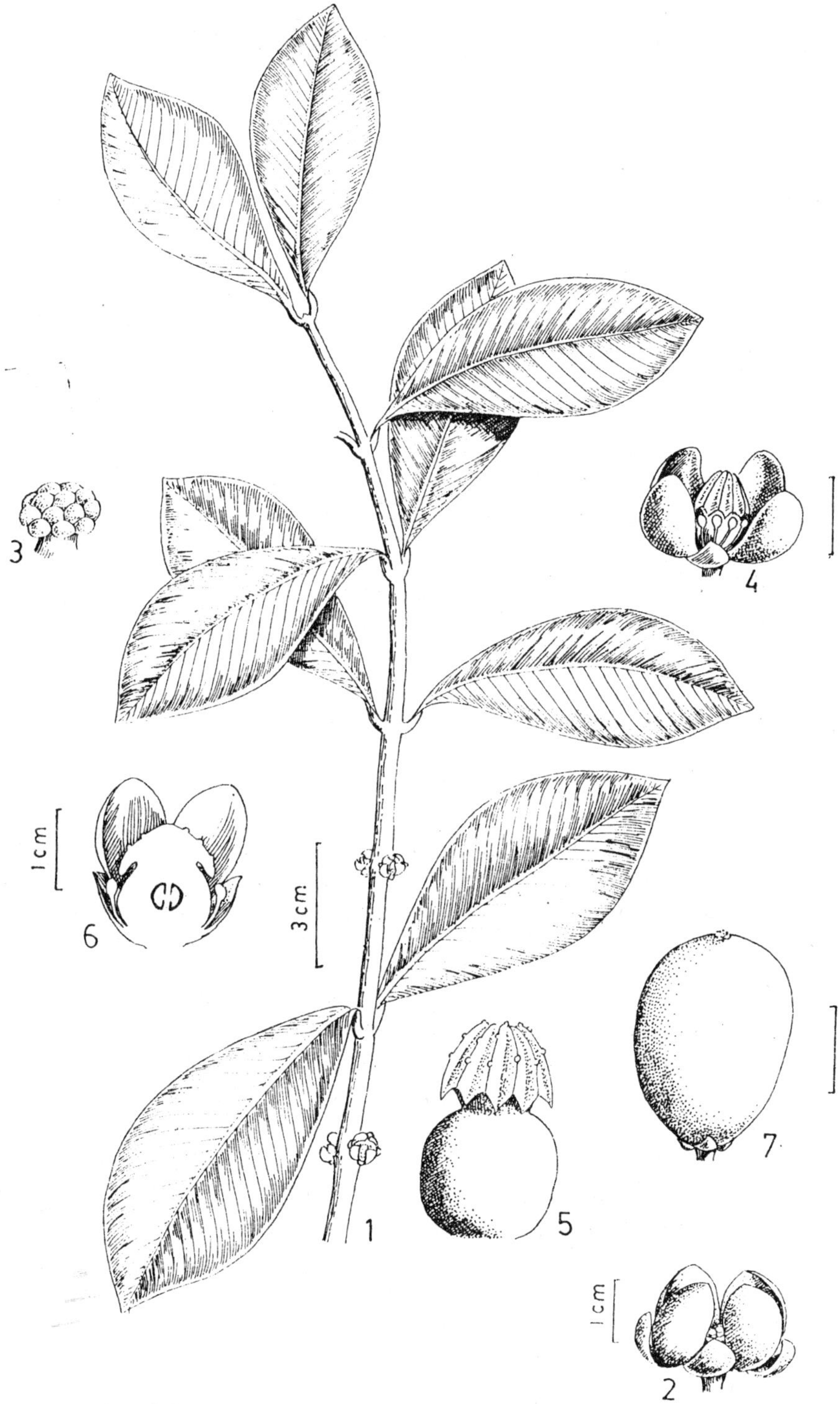

Figure 229: **Garcinia morella** (Gaertn.) Desv. 1, Flowering twig; 2, Male flower; 3, Stamens; 4, Female flower; 5, Pistil; 6, Female flower L.S.; 7, Fruit.

ŚYŌNĀKAḤ (Mal. PALAKAPPAYYĀNI)

The drug is an ingredient of the well known *daśamūla* (ten roots) group. It is reported to be bitter, hot, astringent, carminative, diuretic, stomachic, aphrodisiac and strength-giving. It stimulates digestion, cures fever, cough and other respiratory disorders caused by the derangement of the three *dōṣās—vāta, pitta* and *kapha* and is useful in diarrhoea, dysentery, abdominal pain, thirst, vomiting, anorexia, rheumatism, worms, leprosy and other skin diseases, oedema and urinogenital disorders. Root is the officinal part. The tender fruit is also reported to cure morbid *vāta* and *kapha*, improve digestion, promote taste and destroy *gulma* (gas tumour), piles and worms (Kolammal, 1978. 2: 29, Kurup *et al.*, 1979: 205). The drug enters into the composition of preparations like *Daśamūlariṣṭaṃ, Dhānvantaraṃ kaṣāyaṃ, Dhānvantaraṃ kuḻaṁbu, Cyavanaprāśaṃ*, etc.

According to the synonymy, the plant has long stalk (rachis) (*dīrghavṛntaḥ*) which is warty like a peacock's leg (*mayūrajaṅgha*). Its flower buds look like the beak of a parrot (*śukanāsaḥ*), fruits are long and broad like a scabbard (*pṛthuśiṃbaḥ*) and the seeds have thin silky membraneous wings (*patrōṛṇaṃ*) (Kolammal, 1978. 2: 28). The description agrees well with *Oroxylum indicum* (Linn.) Vent (Bignoniaceae), locally called *palakappayyāni* which is the accepted source of the drug throughout Kerala (see also Rheede, Hort. Malab. 1: 77. 78a, t. 43. 1678).

Oroxylum indicum (*Linn.*) *Vent.* **(Bignoniaceae)** (Fig. 230)
Bignonia indica Linn.

Trees; leaves large, opposite, bipinnate; rachis stout, cylindric, warty; leaflets unequal, broadly elliptic-acuminate, entire, 16 × 9 cms, glabrous, dark green above, paler beneath; flowers large, pale purple, in long terminal racemes; calyx large, leathery, oblong, campanulate, truncate, obscurely toothed, persistent; corolla large, fleshy, subcampanulate, tube short, limb somewhat two-lipped and 5-lobed, lobes crumpled in bud and thickly covered with papillose hairs on both sides; stamens 5, filaments free, unequal, inserted near the base of the tube, woolly at base, anthers 2-celled; ovary subsessile, glabrous, oblong, 2-celled with many ovules in each cell; fruit large, woody, broadly linear, compressed capsule, to 80 × 10 cm; seeds thin, flat, hyaline winged.

Distribution: The plant is fairly common throughout India from the Himalayas southwards to Konkan, Malabar, the Ghats and Coromandal. It is found in moist places of the deciduous forest and in evergreen forests in Travancore, upto 2,000 ft.

Note: The pharmacognostical studies of the root bark and stem bark have been carried out by Prakash and Prasad (1969b). The root bark of *Oroxylum indicum* has been found to be effective in the treatment of amoebic dysentery (Anonymous, 1973).

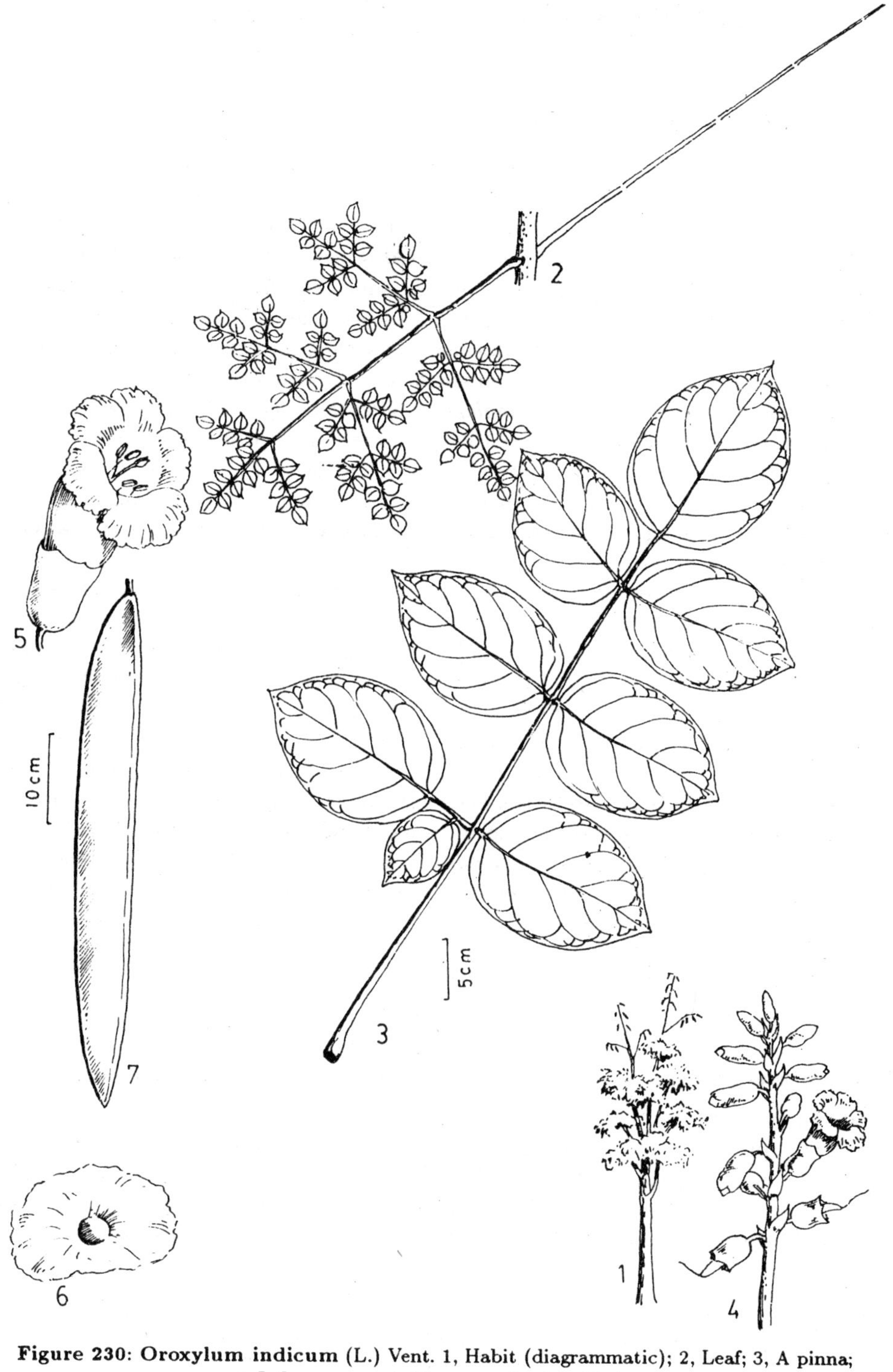

Figure 230: Oroxylum indicum (L.) Vent. 1, Habit (diagrammatic); 2, Leaf; 3, A pinna; 4, Inflorescence; 5, Flower; 6, Seed; 7, Fruit.

TĀMALAKĪ (Mal. KĪḺĀṚNELLI)

The drug is highly reputed as a single drug remedy in the treatment of jaundice in traditional medicine. The whole plant is medicinal. It is diuretic, carminative, styptic, astringent, cooling and febrifuge. It is used in chronic dysentery, dyspepsia, cough, indigestion, diabetes, urinary tract diseases and skin eruptions. Whole plant pounded, is used as a poultice for ulcers, sores, swellings and skin affections (Nadkarni, 1954: 948; Kurup *et al.*, 1979: 37). In practice, it is mainly used for the treatment of jaundice. The important formulations using the drug are *Ceṁparutyādi tailaṃ, Madhuyaṣṭyādi tailaṃ, Amṛtapṛāśaghṛtaṃ, Cyavanapṛāśalēhaṃ*, etc.

Tāmalaki is a close relative of *āmalaki* (*Phyllanthus emblica*), growing close to the ground (*bhūmyāmalakī, bhūdhātṛī*) having many small leaves (*bahupatṛā*) and fruits (*bahuphalā*). The term *bahuvīryā* indicates the several potencies of the drug (cf. Moosad, 1983: 361). Both *āmalaki* and *bhūmyāmalaki* belong to the same family (Euphorbiaceae) and have many features in common, but the former is a tree while the latter is a small herb.

Most of the treatises on Āyurvēdic herbs wrongly identify the drug as *Phyllanthus niruri* Linn. of Euphorbiaceae (cf. Kirtikar & Basu, 1918: 1143; Vaidya K.M., 1936: 255; Nadkarni, 1954; 947; Chopra *et al.*, 1956: 191; Kapoor & Mitra, 1979: 60; Chunekar, 1982: 460). According to the Āyurvēdic Formulary of India also, this is the accepted source of the drug (Anonymous, 1978a: 248). But taxonomic studies done on this genus by Prof. Webster of California University reveal that *Phyllanthus niruri* is an American species. The Indian material assigned to *P. niruri* Linn. by Hooker (1887) has been subsequently identified to be *P. fraternus* Webster and consequently some authors have equated *tāmalaki* with the latter (Kurup *et al.*, 1979: 37; Sharma, 1983: 640; Nesamony, 1985: 170). But this species is not commonly available in Kerala. Our studies have revealed that two closely related species, *P. amarus* and *P. airy-shawii* (*P. debilis*) which are very common here, are used by Kerala physicians as the source of this drug (see Sivarajan & Balachandran, 1983).

These two species can be distinguished as follows.

Phyllanthus amarus *Schum. & Thonn.* **(Euphorbiaceae)** (Fig. 231)

Erect, annual herb; stem terete; cataphylls obovate, obtuse or retuse; leaves closely arranged, upto 1.5 × 0.6 cm, obtuse or retuse at apex; flowers yellowish green in minute cymules, pendant from the axils of leaves. Male flowers: tepals 5 to 6, obovate; stamens 3, filaments connate. Female flowers: tepals much shorter than the capsule; ovary minute, styles 3; capsule oblate, smooth; seeds 6, blackish, concentrically striate.

Distribution: This species is a native of America and is now a circumtropical weed. It is common in cultivated fields, gardens and waste places in Kerala.

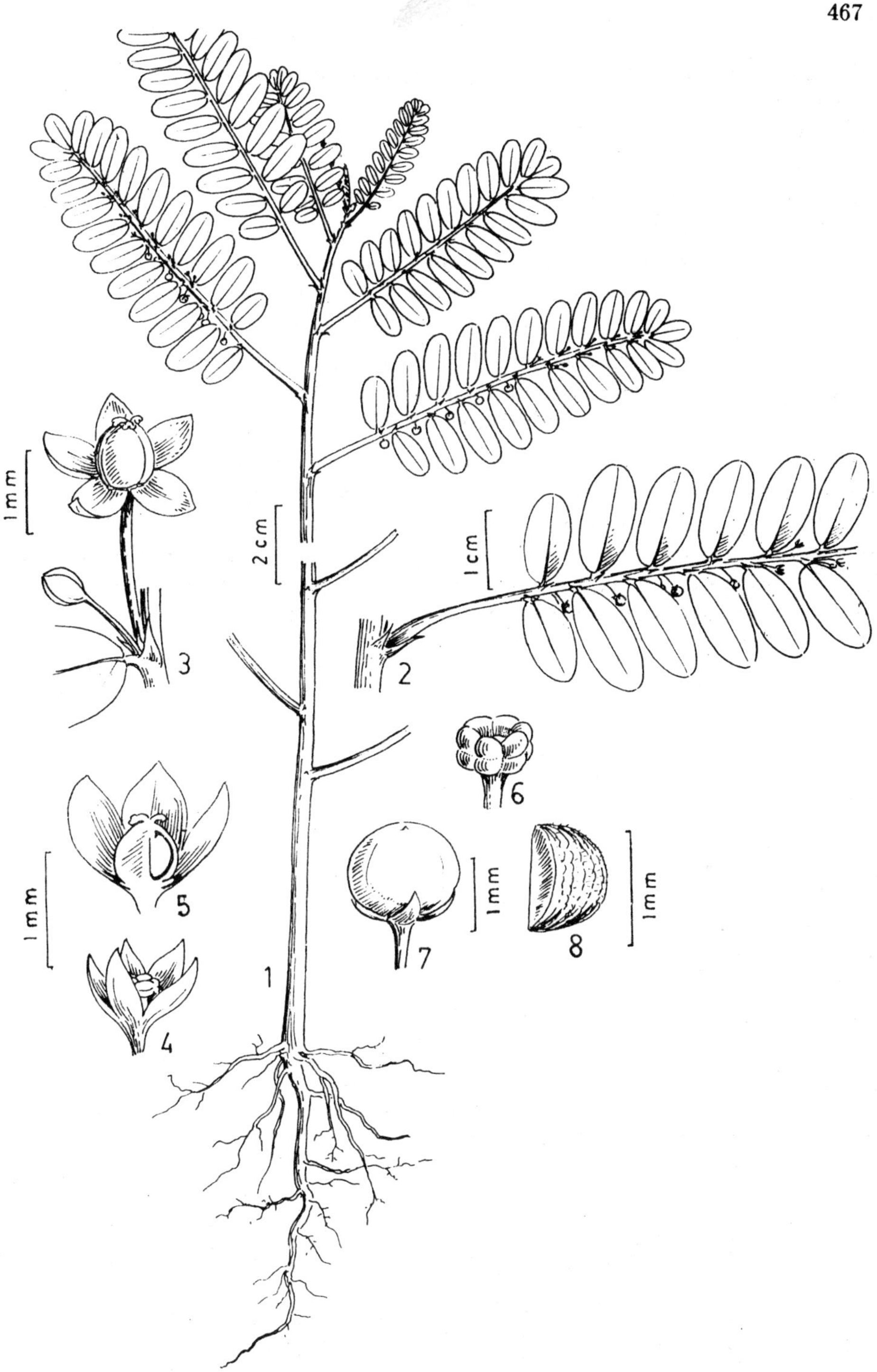

Figure 231: **Phyllanthus amarus** Schum. & Thonn. 1, Habit; 2, Short-shoot from the axil of a cataphyll; 3, Female Flower; 4, Male flower 5, Female flower L.S.; 6, Stamens in male flower; 7, Fruit; 8, Seed.

Phyllanthus airy-shawii *Brunal & Roux* **(Euphorbiaceae)** (Fig. 232)
Phyllanthus debilis Klein ex Willd.

Erect, delicate herbs, the younger parts of the stem angular; cataphylls upto 2 × 0.4 cm, narrowly oblong or elliptic, obtuse or subacute; leaves 1.2 × 0.4 cm, alternate, distant, elliptic to oblong, acute, or obtuse; flowers in short axillary cymules. Male flowers: tepals 5 to 6, obovate; stamens 3, filaments connate throughout. Female flowers: tepals almost same as in male; ovary subglobose with a lobed disc at its base, styles 3, spreading, each one again 2-lobed; capsule smooth, 6-valved; fruiting perianth as long as the capsule; seeds 6, blackish, striate.

Distribution: This species is probably a native of South India and Sri Lanka and is now naturalised in Indonesia, Pacific Islands and West Indies. In Kerala it is a very common weed in gardens, cultivated fields and elsewhere.

Note: *Bhūmyāmalaki (Phyllanthus niruri* Linn.) is found to be very effective in the treatment of infective hepatitis in children (Dixit & Achar, 1983). The diuretic activity of *P. niruri* had been clinically tried by Vimaladevi *et al.* (1986). One cannot be sure about the identity of the plants used here in these studies, (as this name has been wrongly applied to Indian taxa) unless and until one sees them. It could be any of the species of *Phyllanthus* mentioned earlier.

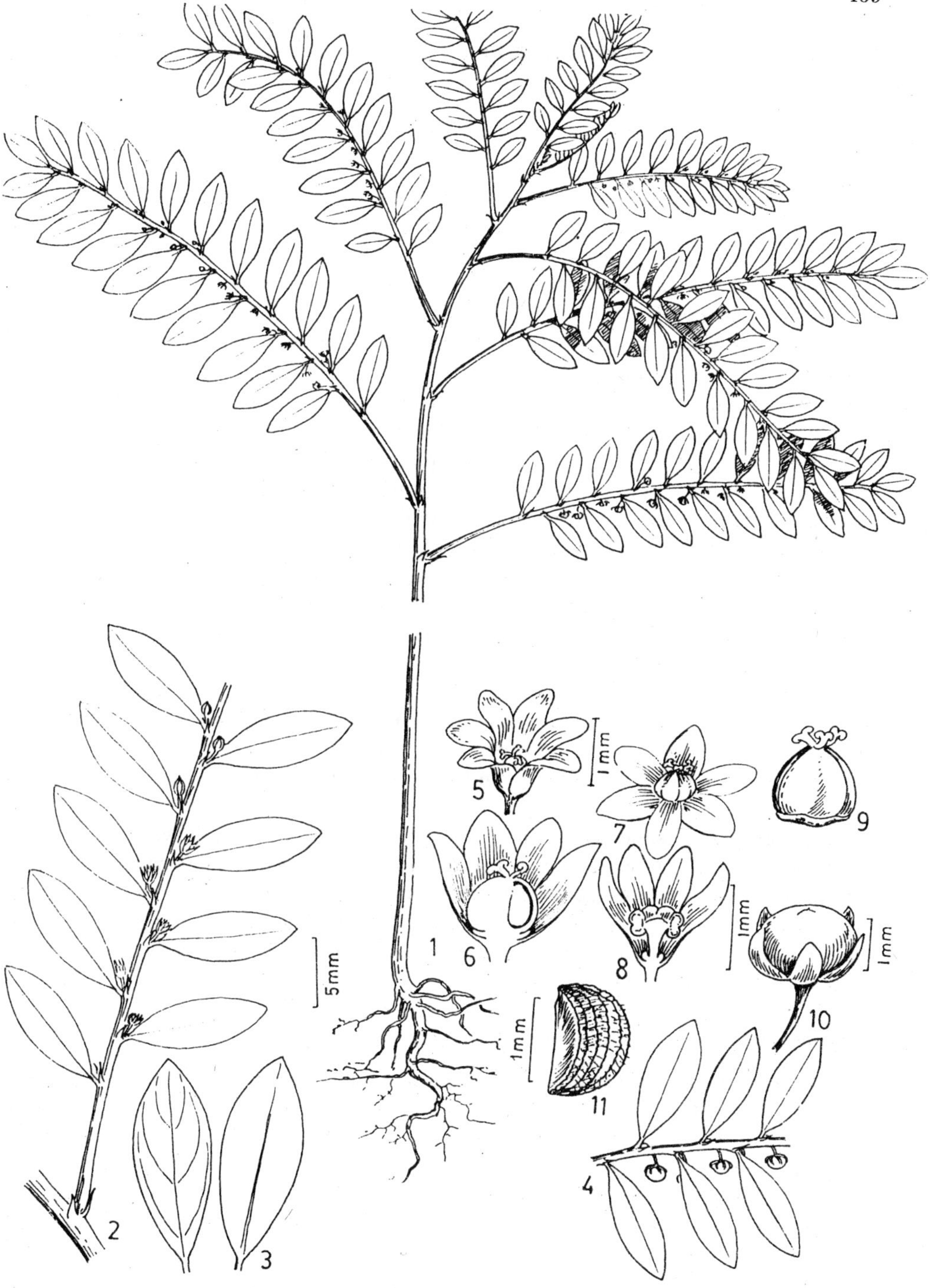

Figure 232: Phyllanthus airy-shawii Brunal & Roux. 1, Habit; 2, Short-shoot and the subtending cataphyll; 3, Leaves; 4, a portion of short-shoot enlarged; 5,7, Female flowers; 6, Female flower L.S.; 8, Male flower L.S.; 9, Pistil; 10, Fruit; 11, Seed.

TĀṀBŪLAḤ (Mal. VEṬṬILA)

Betel-chewing is an ancient custom among people of the Indian subcontinent. Of the four components, betel leaf (lime, tobacco and betel-nut are the others) is the most important. Betel leaf, locally called *veṭṭila* is extensively cultivated in certain parts of southern India, mostly to cater to this need. However, this is also used in Indian medicine. It is hot, acrid, bitter, astringent, aromatic, carminative, stimulant, aphrodisiac and antiseptic. It improves digestion, clears voice, gives good strength and cures dyspepsia, worms, fever, phantom tumour, flatulence and all diseases caused by the morbidity of *vāta* and *kapha.* The leaf juice is given internally in cough, dyspnoea, deranged phlegm and indigestion in children. Warm leaves smeared with oil form a valuable application to the chest in cases of cough, bronchitis and difficulty of breathing during infancy and childhood. A paste of the leaves in hot water taken internally cures filariasis. Roots are used to produce sterility in women (Nadkarni, 1954: 961; Aiyer & Kolammal, 1966. 9: 77; Sharma, 1983: 210). Chiefly the leaves and occasionally the roots and stem are used in medicine. The important preparations using the drug are *Tāṁbūla lēhaṃ, Āraṇyatuḷasyādi* coconut oil, *Rasasindūraṃ, Ākārakarabhādi guḷika*, etc.

The synonyms *nāgavallī, nāgavallarī, pātāḷavāsinī*, etc. bestow this plant with a celestial hallow. It is believed that the plant bestows '*maṅgaḷa*' or good fortune (*bhadrā, amṛtā, kāmadā*) to the users. Due to its invigorating nature in sexual enjoyments (*kāmajananī, āmōdajananī, rañjinī*), it is said that *tāṃbūlī* should not be used by widows, celibates and ascetics (Aiyer & Kolammal, 1966. 9: 77–78).

According to some texts, there are seven kinds of betel leaves viz. *śrīvāṭi, aṁḷavāṭi, sātasā, saptaśirā, aṁḷasarā, paṭulikā* and *hvēsaṇīyā*, differing slightly in shape and efficacy according to the soil in which they are grown. There are, indeed, different cultivated forms of betel, but nevertheless, all of them belong to *Piper betle* Linn. (Piperaceae), known as *veṭṭila koḍi* in vernacular. (See also Rheede, Hort. Malab. 7: 29, t. 15. 1688, Beetla codi.)

Piper betle *Linn.* **(Piperaceae)** (Fig. 233)

Diocious perennial, root-climber; stem purplish and puberulous; leaves simple, alternate, long petioled, broadly ovate-cordate or obliquely elliptic, entire, glabrous, to 8–16 × 5–10 cms, acuminate; flowers small, unisexual, arranged closely on leaf-opposed, long-peduncled, pendulous spikes, male spikes narrow upto 15 cms, female spikes cylindrical, to 12 cms; flowers minute, bracteate, unisexual, perianth (zero) 0; stamens 2 in male; in female ovary unilocular with a single ovule, stigma sessile, 3–6 lobed; fruits ovoid or globose berries.

Distribution: The plant is considered indigenous to Malaya, Java etc. but widely cultivated throughout the hotter and damper parts of India.

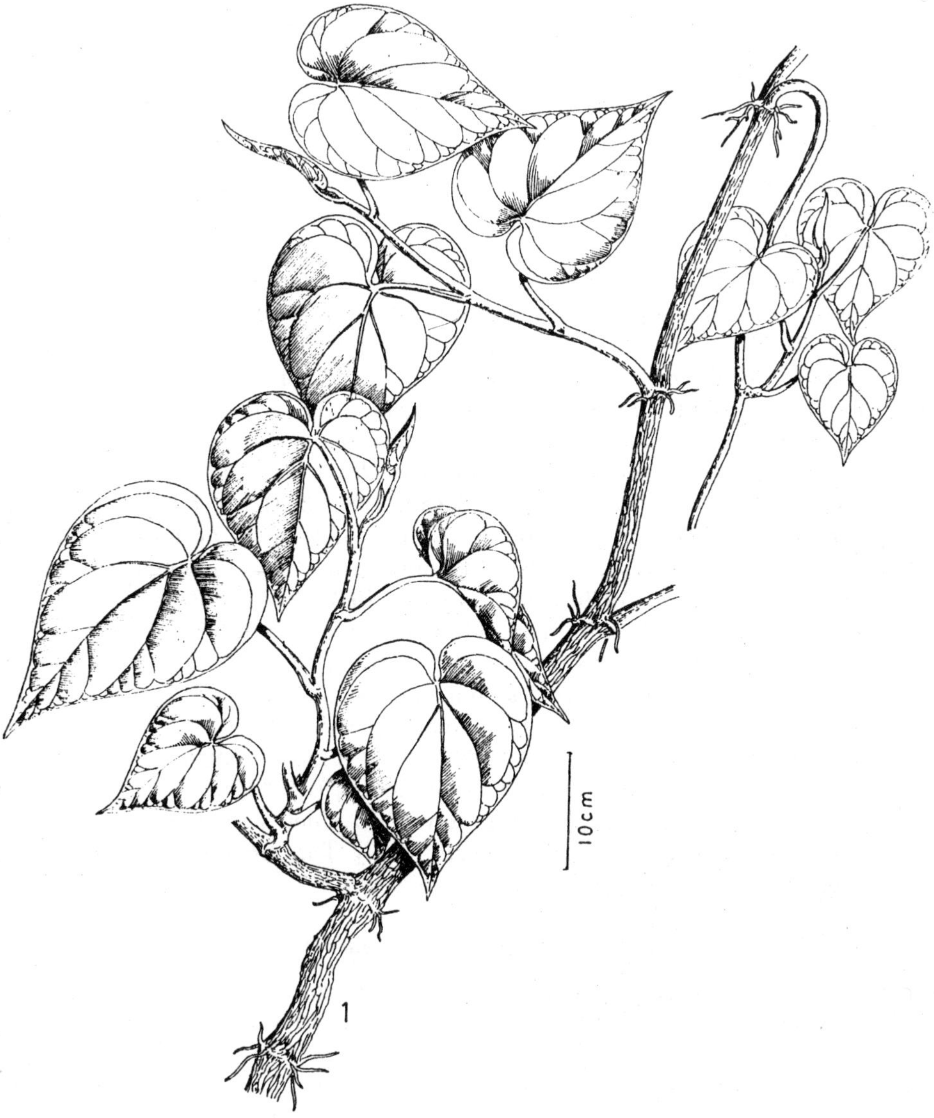

Figure 233: Piper betle L.

Note: The antifertility effect of betel-leaf stalk has been studied by Tewari *et al.* (1970).

TAṆḌULĪYAḤ
(Mal. MUḶḶANCĪRA, CEṚUCĪRA)

This comes under the *śākavarga* or leafy vegetable group. The drug is reported to be light, cooling, acrid, carminative, diuretic and laxative. It promotes appetite, improves digestion and cures diseases caused by the morbidity of *pitta* and *kapha*. It is also used against burning sensation, dyspepsia, haemophilic conditions, urinary tract diseases and poisonous affections. The whole plant is medicinal (Kurup *et al.*, 1979: 216; Chunekar, 1982: 666). Kerala physicians recognise two varieties of *taṇḍulīya*, locally called *muḷḷancīra* and *ceṛucīra* respectively. The former (the whole plant) is used to prepare *Kanmadabhasmaṃ*. The roots of the latter form an ingredient in formulations like *Śatāvaryādi kaṣāyaṃ, Aśōkāriṣṭaṃ*, etc.

This drug, which looks like small spinach (*alpamāriṣa*) and having small seeds resembling broken rice (*taṇḍulīya*) (Moosad, 1983: 368) has been equated with *Amaranthus spinosus* Linn. (Amaranthaceae) by most of the authors (see Kirtikar & Basu, 1918: 1057; Vaidya, 1936: 250; Chopra *et al.*, 1956: 15; Singh & Chunekar, 1972: 174; Kurup *et al.*, 1979: 216; Chunekar, 1982: 666). In Kerala, this is used under the name *muḷḷancīra*. Nadkarni (1954: 91) and Chopra *et al.* (1956: 15) have mentioned *Amaranthus viridis* Linn. as the source of the drug *taṇḍulīya*. In Kerala, this plant, as well as *Celosia argentea* Linn. of the same family, are used as the source of *ceṛucīra*. Rheede has attributed the name *Tsjeria belutta adecamanyen* to *Celosia argentea* (Hort. Malab. 10: 77. t. 39. 1690). This is most likely a mistake because: (i) Such a name is not in use anywhere in Kerala. (ii) *Adecamanyen* and *Belutta adecamanyen* used by Kerala physicians have been widely accepted as *Sphaeranthus indicus* and *S. africanus* (Asteraceae) respectively. They are discussed elsewhere in this text.

Amaranthus spinosus *Linn.* **(Amaranthaceae)** (Fig. 234)

Erect herb with axillary spines; leaves long-petioled, ovate to lanceolate, acute or obtuse, glabrous, 3.9 × 2.4 cm; flowers polygamous, minute, green in axillary clusters or in terminal paniculate spikes; bracts and bracteoles narrowly ovate-lanceolate. Male: Tepals 5, unequal with prominant midrib; stamens 5, anthers oblong, sagitate. Female: Tepals 5, (sub.) equal; styles 2; utricle circumscissible; seeds shining.

Distribution: A very common weed in waste places, fields, gardens and road sides in all plains districts. A native of America, this is now distributed through the warmer regions of the world.

Amaranthus viridis *Linn.* **(Amaranthaceae)** (Fig. 235)
A. gracilis Desf.

Erect or diffuse herb; leaves ovate to lanceolate, entire or undulate, 3.8 × 2.5 cms; flowers polygamous, green in slender terminal or axillary interrupted paniculate spikes; bracts and bracteoles ovate-lanceolate with prominent midvein. Male: Tepals

3, oblong-lanceolate or obovate, shortly excurrent; stamens 3, free. Female: Tepals as in male; styles 2; utricle rugose, brownish; seeds black.

A very common weed in waste places and along roadsides in all plains districts.

Distribution: Pantropical.

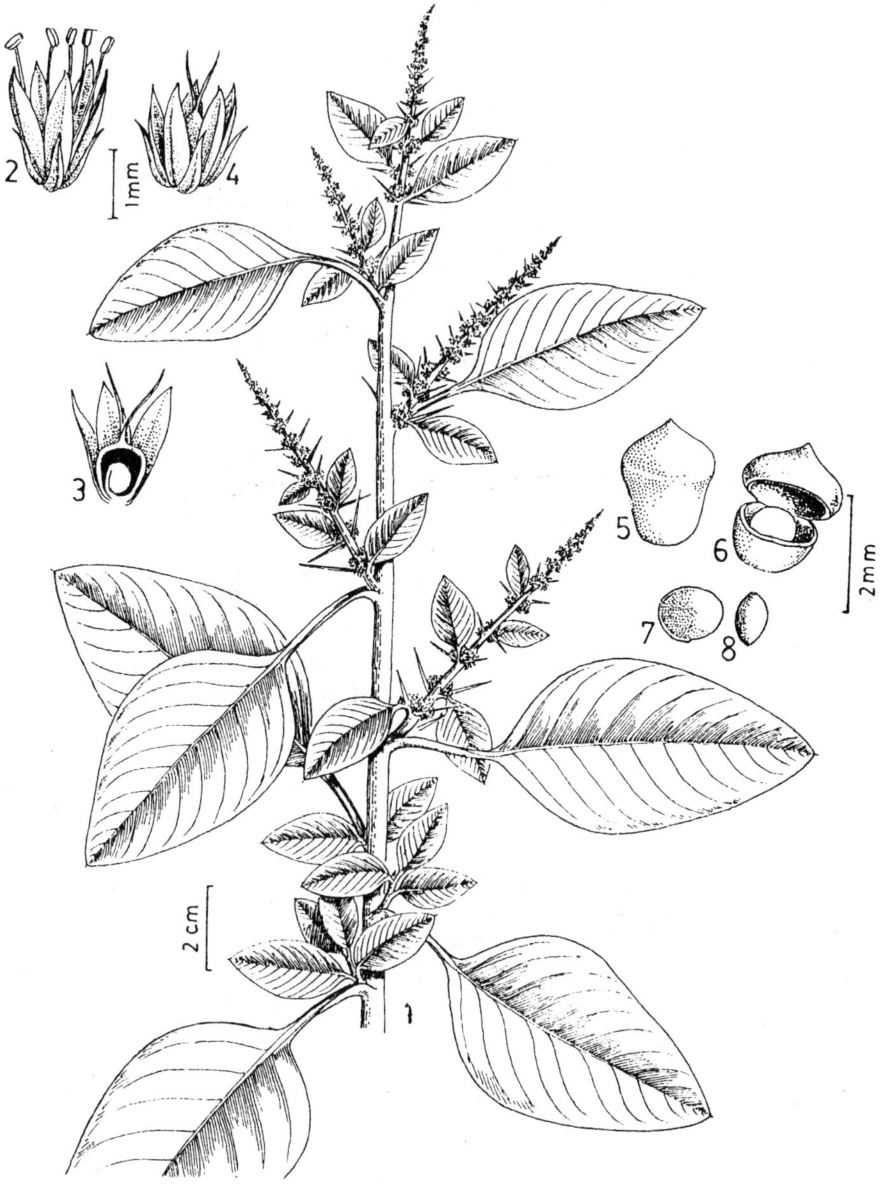

Figure 234: Amaranthus spinosus L. 1, A branch; 2, Male flower; 3, Female flower L.S.; 4, Female flower; 5, Fruit; 6, Dehisced fruit; 7–8, Seed.

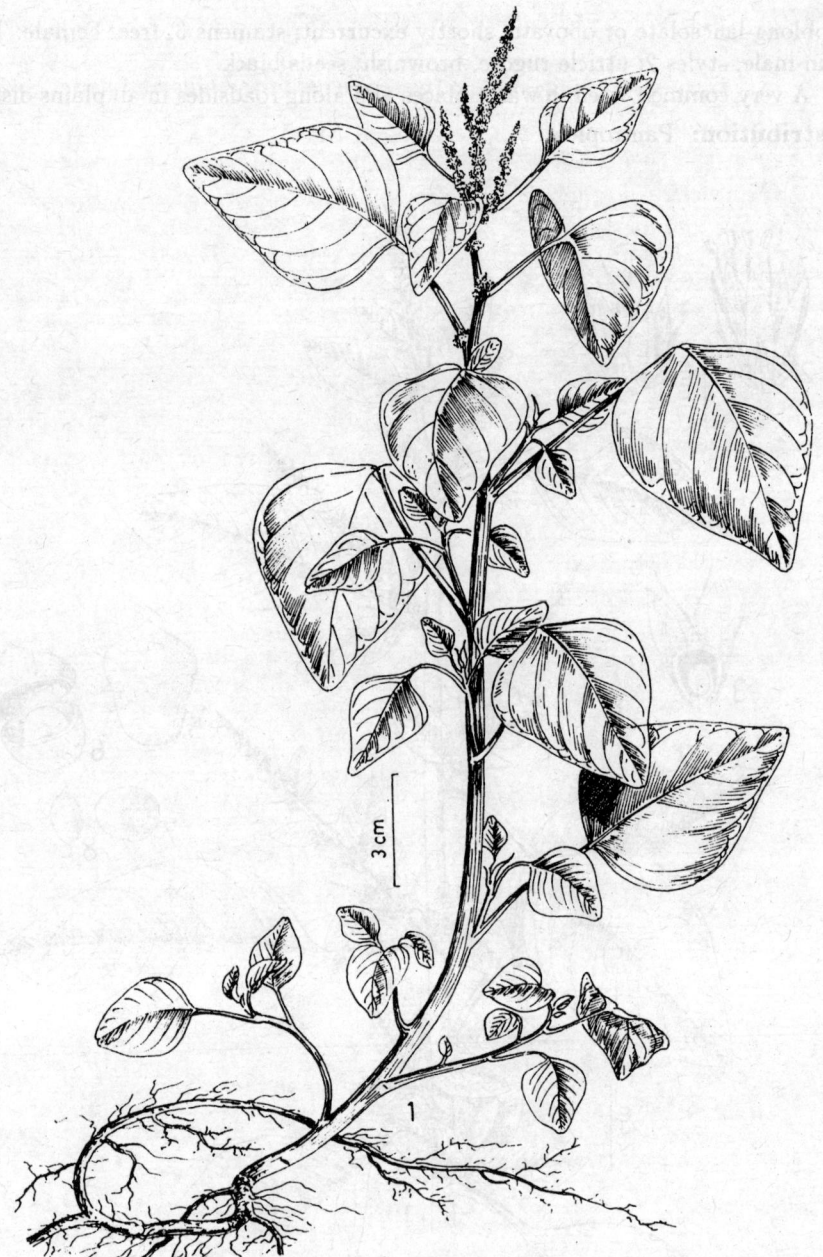

Figure 235: Amaranthus viridis L.

Celosia argentea *Linn.* **(Amaranthaceae)** (Fig. 236)

Erect herb; leaves alternate, elliptic to lanceolate, acute or acuminate, entire above, 7–13 × 0.5–1 cm; flowers bisexual, pink or white in terminal elongated spikes; bracteoles oblanceolate, curved, persistent, midrib excurrent, aristate. Tepals 5, chaffy, broadly ovate-lanceolate, hyaline, 1-nerved; stamens 5; utricle globose; seeds black, shining.

A weed in waste lands and cultivated fields in the hills and plains.

Distribution: Pantropical.

Note: Alcoholic extract of *Celosia argentea* showed good antilithiatic activity by preventing stone formation and also removed the artificially introduced urinary stones in experimental rats (Dubey *et al.*, 1982).

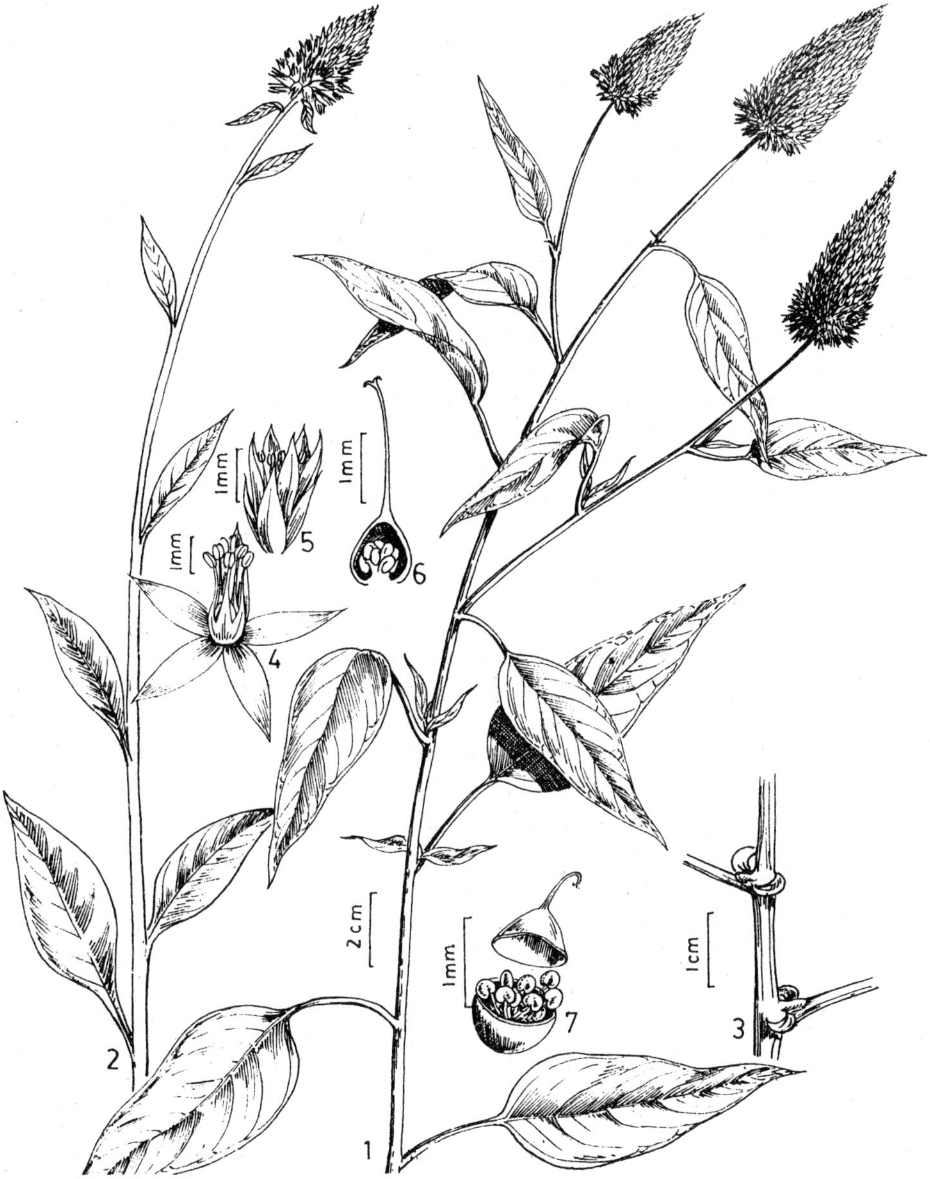

Figure 236: Celosia argentea L. 1–2, Flowering branches; 3, Node; 4–5, Flowers; 6, Ovary L.S.; 7, Dehisced fruit.

TINIŚAḤ (Mal. TOṬUKĀRA)

This is one of the twenty three drugs that constitute the *Asanādi gaṇa* of Vāgbhaṭa which cures leucoderma and other skin diseases, morbid ***kapha***, worms, anaemia, diabetes and disorders due to deranged fat (Mooss, 1980: 51). ***Tiniśa*** is light, cooling, astringent and tonic and is useful in the vitiated conditions of ***kapha*** and ***pitta***, ulcers, inflammatory swellings, leprosy, leucoderma and general ebility. It also cures diabetes, thirst, blood diseases, dysentery and diarrhoea. The bark and the heart wood are used medicinally (Chunekar, 1982: 548; Sharma, 1983: 676). The drug forms an ingredient of *Ayaskṛti.*

The synonyms are indicative of only the nature of wood i.e. it is light, strong (*citṛakṛt*) and long lasting (***tiniśa***) and is used to make chariots (***syandana, nēmi, rathadru***). (cf. Moosad, 1983: 290). All these clearly point out that the drug source is a tree. Most of the authors equate the drug with ***Ougenia dalbergioides*** of Papilionaceae (Kirtikar & Basu, 1918: 427; Vaidya, K.M. 1936: 262; Nadkarni, 1954: 890; Chopra *et al.*, 1956: 183; Chunekar, 1982: 546; Sharma, 1983: 676). Kerala commentators, however, equate ***tiniśa*** with ***toṭukāra***, even though, it does not go well with the synonyms. Our field studies have revealed that ***Melastoma malabathricum*** and ***Osbeckia aspera*** of Melastomataceae are the main sources of this drug in Kerala. These two plants can be identified as follows.

Melastoma malabathricum *Linn.* **(Melastomataceae)** (Fig. 237)
Melastoma royenii Blume

Much branched shrubs covered with appressed scales; leaves simple, opposite, elliptic-acute, 8–14 × 2–4.5 cms, prominently 3-veined from base; flowers large, mauve-coloured, in few flowered terminal cymes; calyx tube campanulate, covered with strigose hairs, lobes 5, ovate-triangular; petals 5, violet, broadly orbicular; stamens 10, dimorphic; ovary ovoid, more or less adnate to the calyx tube, ovules numerous; fruit an ovoid capsule, irregularly dehiscing.

Distribution: The plant grows in wet places in peninsular India ana in S.E. Asia.

Osbeckia aspera (*Linn.*) *Blume* **(Melastomataceae)**
Osbeckia wightiana Benth. ex Wight & Arn.

Much branched shrub; stem and branches reddish with short appressed bristles; leaves simple, opposite, elliptic-acute, to 7 × 2 cms, 3–5 veined from base, adpressed hairy on both surfaces; flowers showy, dark purple, in terminal panicles; calyx tube urceolate, covered with bulbous-based bristles, lobes 5; petals 5, broadly obovate-obtuse; stamens 10, all alike; ovary 5-celled covered, with soft bristles; fruit a capsule.

Distribution: W. Ghats, in the Nilgiri, Anamalai and Pulney Hills, at 4,000–7,000 ft, often in rocky place.

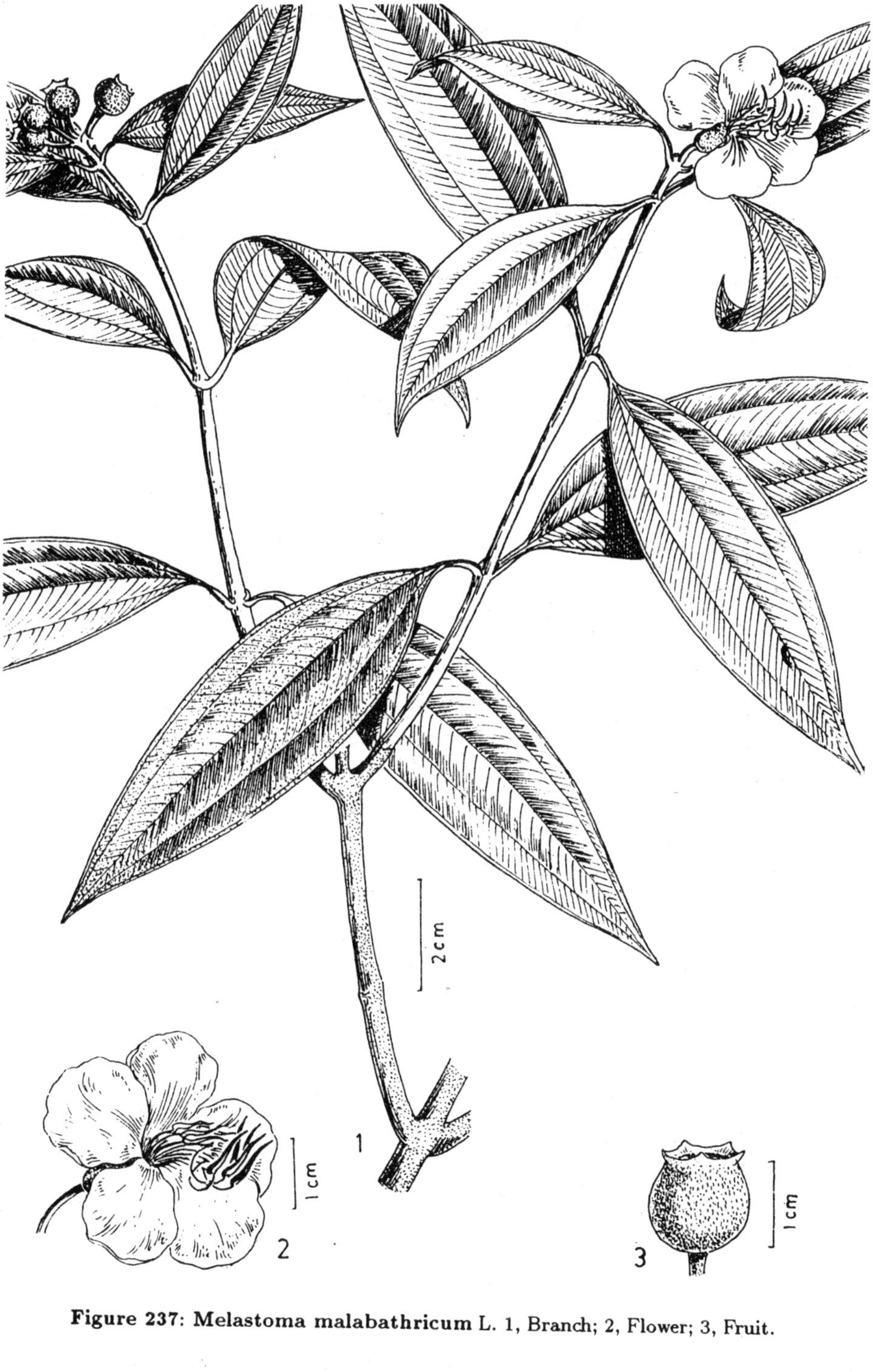

Figure 237: **Melastoma malabathricum** L. 1, Branch; 2, Flower; 3, Fruit.

TṚIKŌŚAKĪ (Mal. MUKKĀLPĪRAṂ)

The drug is an ingredient of *Mānasamitṛa vaṭakaṃ*. The whole plant is used medicinally. It is reported to have expectorant properties and it is prescribed against chronic diseases with cough as a predominant system. The tender shoots and bitter leaves are used as a gentle aperient and are used in vertigo and biliousness. The root relieves toothache. A decoction of the root is given in flatulence (Nadkarni, 1954: 820; Anonymous, 1962. 6: 336).

There is little reference about this drug in the texts. Kerala physicians equate this drug with the Malayalam name *mukkālpīraṃ* and use *Mukia maderaspatana* (Cucurbitaceae) as the drug source.

Mukia maderaspatana (*Linn.*) *M. Roemer* **(Cucurbitaceae)** (Fig. 238)
Mukia scabrella (L. f.) Arn.
Melothria maderaspatana (Linn.) Cogn.

Slender, scabrous climber; tendrils simple, opposite to the leaves; leaves simple, alternate, long-petioled, 3–5 angled, 7–9 × 7–9 cms, scabrid above, hispid below, base cordate, margin denticulate, apex acute to acuminate; flowers small, yellow, unisexual in axillary cymes; calyx tube villous, lobes linear; corolla yellow, petals ovate, villous without; stamens 3, anthers oblong; ovary villous; fruit an ovoid berry, 1 × 0.8 cm, green when young and red when ripe.

Distribution: Distributed in Africa, India, China, Taiwan, Malesia, Australia, New Zealand. In India it is seen in most districts of the Deccan, Carnatic and lower hills of W. Ghats.

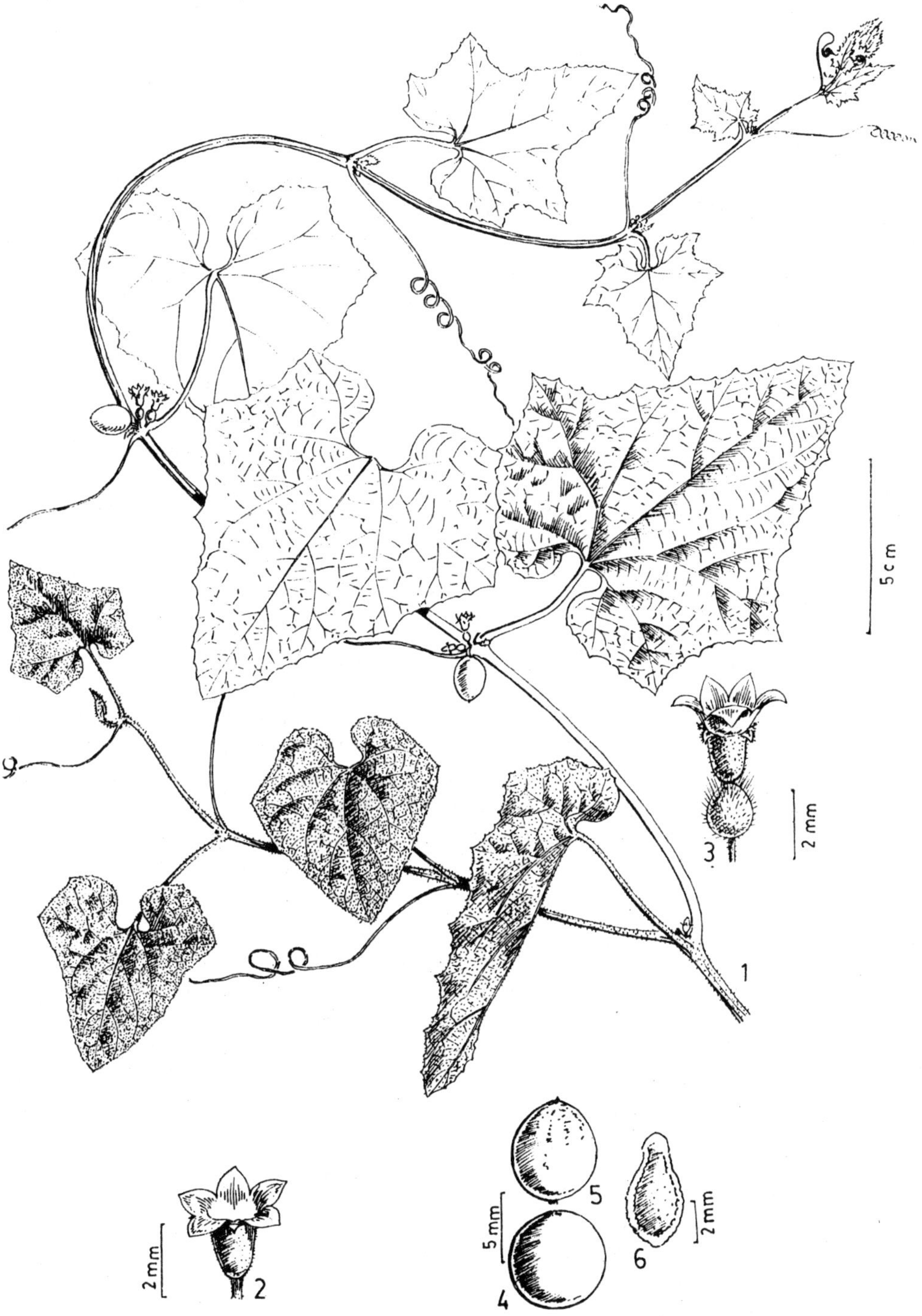

Figure 238: **Mukia maderaspatana** (L.) M. Roem. 1, Habit; 2, Male flower; 3, Female flower; 4–5, Fruit; 6, Seed.

TṚIVṚT (Mal. TṚIKŌLPAKKONNA)

The drug *tṛivṛt*, also known as *tṛivṛta* and *tṛipuṭā* (indicative of probably the three layered bark) is an efficacious drug. It has found its ways to European market since early times, through Arabs, as is obvious from Garcia da Ortás (1563: 430–446) writings. In Malabar, it was then used as a specific (often mixed with ginger) against various kinds of inflammations. A composite of all the six rasās (*sarvānubhūti*), this can cure all the three *dōṣās* (due to morbid *vāta, pitta* and *kapha*) and hence is also named as *'tṛibhaṇḍi'*. Men of Āyurvēda have classified it among purgative drugs (*rēcana, saraḷa*). Root and rootbark are cathartic, purgative and are particularly useful in rheumatic and paralytic affections (Nadkarni, 1954: 692). It is light, bitter and acrid and is reported to be beneficial also in general anasarca, skin diseases, consumption, dropsy, eye diseases, fever, oedema and hepatic and haemophilic disorders. The powder of rootbark is used as a purgative in cases of constipation, piles, jaundice, etc. Traditionally, it is administered against dropsy due to heart, kidney or liver diseases (Kurup *et al.*, 1979: 219; Nesamony, 1985: 295). The drug is an important ingredient of formulations like *Tṛivṛllēhaṃ, Avipatti cūṛṇaṃ, Āragvadhāriṣṭaṃ* and *Kaiśōragulguluvaṭakaṃ*.

Caraka has recognised two varieties of *tṛivṛt*, namely the red (*aruṇa*) and the black (*śyāma*), presumably recognised on the basis of colouration of roots (Sharma, 1983: 420), while Suśruta has mentioned yet another variety, *Mahātṛivṛt* or *mahāśyāmā* (cf. Singh & Chunekar, 1972: 197). *Bhāvapṛakāśa*, however, refers to the two varieties as white (*śvēta*) and black (*śyāmā*). While the white variety is a moderate cathartic, the black one is said to be more powerful and drastic in action, causing vomiting and fainting (cf. Chunekar, 1982: 398).

Market survey of the drug has revealed that two varieties—black and white—are available. The black variety which is preferred by physicians are the roots of *Operculina turpethum* of Convolvulaceae. The roots of this plant are blackish in colour. The white variety sold in the market has been found to be the decorticated roots of *Marsdenia tenacissima* of Asclepiadaceae. But unlike the account given by *Bhāvamiśra*, this does not have any purgative property and hence does not seem to be the actual source of the drug. Moreover, this is one of the several disputed plant sources of a different drug, *mūṛvā* (Vaidya Bapalal, 1982: 128; Sharma, 1983: 420) (see description under *Mūṛva*).

Mahātṛivṛt does not exist in practice. In Kerala, the adopted plant source of *tṛivṛt* is *Operculina turpethum*.

Operculina turpethum (*Linn.*) *A. Silva Manso* **(Convolvulaceae)** (Fig. 239)
Convolvulus turpethum Linn.
Ipomoea turpethum (Linn.) R. Br.
Merremia turpethum (Linn.) G.L. Shaw & R.G. Bhat

Large climbing shrub; stem 4-angled, winged; leaves simple, alternate, broadly ovate to cordate, obtuse at apex, 8–12 × 7–13 cms, puberulous; flowers showy, creamy

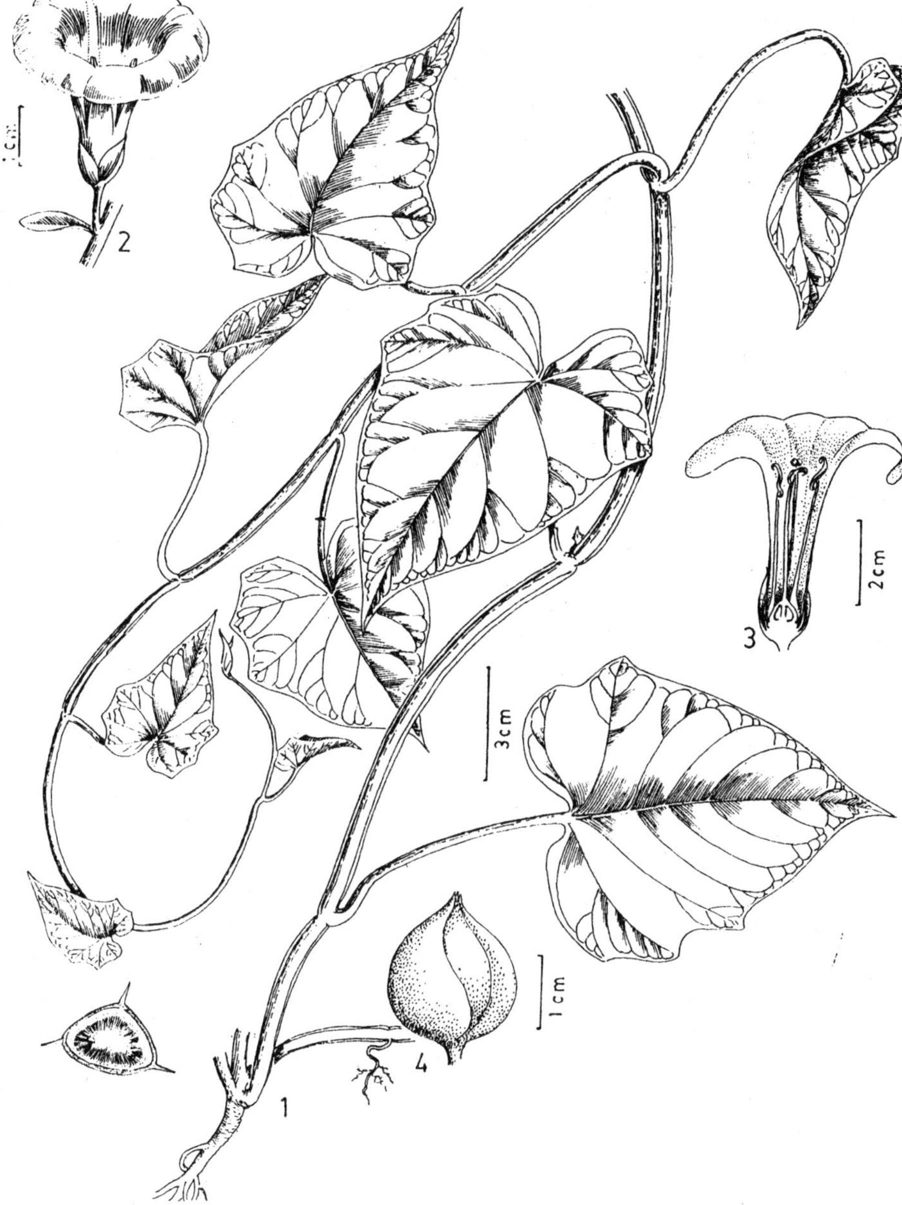

Figure 239: Operculina turpethum (L.) Manso. 1, Habit; 2, Flower; 3, Flower L.S.; 4, Fruit.

white in axillary, long-peduncled, lax, corymbose cymes; bracts large, oblong; calyx lobes unequal, persistent, puberulous without; corolla funnel form, stamens 5; ovary globose; capsule circumscissile, enclosed in the enlarged, woody calyx lobes; seeds 4, black, smooth.

Distribution: Widespread in Old World tropics from E. Africa to N. Australia, this plant is common in Godavari, occasionally found in N. Circars, Deccan and Carnatic to S. Travancore.

Note: The aqueous extract of *O. turpethum* roots has been found to be very potent against acute inflammation in albino rats (Khare *et al.*, 1982).

TŪKAḤ (Mal. TĀṚTĀVAL)

This is one of the twenty one drugs that constitute the *Vīratarādi* or *Vēllantarādi gaṇa* of Vāgbhaṭa which helps restore morbid *vāta* and cures vesical calculus, dysuria and anuria (Mooss, 1980: 63). Whole plant is medicinal. It is acrid, sweet, astringent, stomachic, antibilious, antirheumatic and tonic and is useful in bilious and rheumatic affections, indigestion, flatulence and general debility. The drug enters into the composition of preparations like *Traikaṇṭaka ghṛtaṃ*, *Vastyāmayāntaka ghṛtaṃ*, *Vīratarādi kaṣāyaṃ*, etc.

There is very little mention about this drug in the Āyurvēdic literature. Parameśwara has equated *tūka* with *tāṛtāval* of the Kerala Physicians (cf. Mooss, 1980: 63). *Spermacoce articularis* of Rubiaceae is the accepted source of the drug. But, another closely related species *Spermacoce hispida* is also used in some parts of Kerala (see Rheede, Hort. Malab. 9: 149. t. 76. 1689. *Tardavel*).

Spermacoce articularis *L. f.* **(Rubiaceae)** (Fig. 240:5–10)
Borreria articularis (L. f.) F.N. Will.

Hispid, trailing herb; stem sharply 4-angled, appressed hairy; leaves simple, opposite, short-petioled, elliptic-obovate to lanceolate, acute, to 3 × 1.2 cm, scabrous; flowers pink in axillary clusters; calyx tube hairy, lobes 4; corolla long, funnel-shaped; stamens 4, attached to the throat of the corolla tube; ovary 2-celled, style filiform, stigma capitate; capsule of 2 pyrenes, 2-seeded; seed with longitudinal ventral groove.

Distribution: A common weed growing in all sorts of habitats, almost everywhere in plains in India. Also reported from tropical Africa and Southeast Asia.

Spermacoce hispida *Linn.* **(Rubiaceae)** (Fig. 240:1–4)
Borreria hispida (Linn.) Schuman.

Erect or diffuse hispid herb; stem terete, pilose; leaves simple, opposite decussate, ovate or elliptic-acute, 2 × 0.9 cms, margin flexuous; flowers pink or pale purple in axillary few-flowered clusters; calyx tube united with the ovary, lobes 5, lanceolate acute, hispid; corolla 7 mm long, turbinate, campanulate, lobes 4, oblong-acute; stamens 4, attached to the throat of the tube; capsule globose, 2-seeded; seed with a longitudinal ventral groove.

Distribution: Peninsular India extending to Orissa and Bengal on the eastern coast.

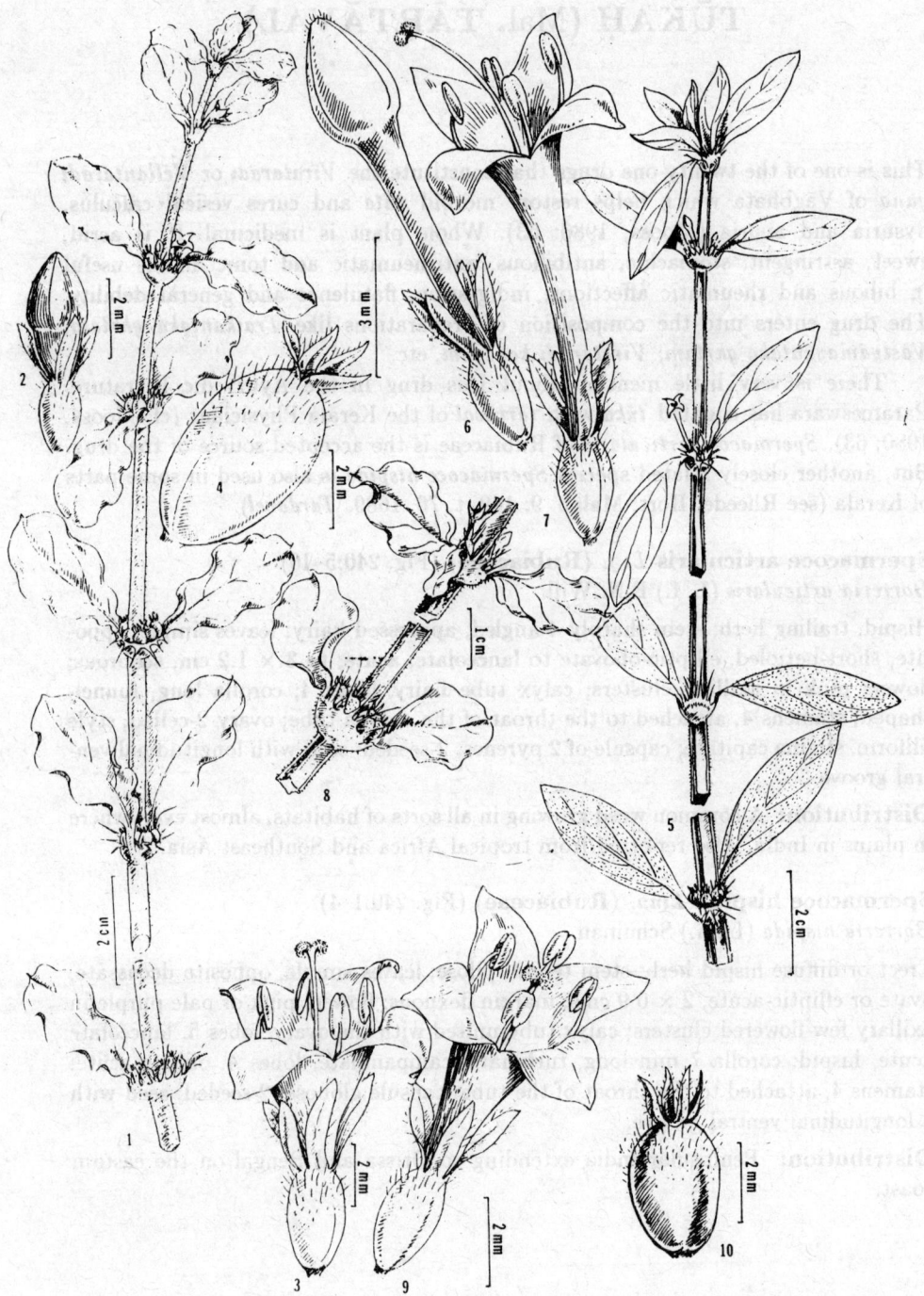

Figure 240: 1–4, **Spermacoce hispida** L. 1, Flowering branch; 2, Flower bud; 3, Open flowers; 4, Fruit.
5–10, **Spermacoce articularis** L.f. 5,8, Habit; 6, Flower bud; 7,9, Open flowers; 10, Fruit.

TUḶASĪ (Mal. TUḶASI, KṚṢṆATUḶASI)

Tuḷasi, often called the 'sacred basil' has been widely used in religious rites by Hindus, since vēdic times. Even now, virtually, every Indian home has a tuḷasi-plot right in front of it and people usually start their daily chores after worshipping it. Besides, it has been a veritable drug, used as a house-hold remedy for a variety of ailments.

Tuḷasi is aromatic, carminative, antipyretic, diaphoretic and expectorant. Leaves, flowers and occasionally the whole plant are used in medicine. Leaf juice is a domestic remedy for infantile cough, cold, bronchitis, catarrh, dysentery and diarrhoea. Infusion of leaves is given in malaria, as a stomachic in gastric diseases of children and in hepatic affections. It improves appetite, afflictions of the ear, destroys intestinal worms and cures skin diseases such as itches, ringworm, leprosy, ulcers and poisonous affections. In Āyurvēda *tuḷasi* is widely used as a specific for all kinds of fevers (Nadkarni, 1954: 865; Kurup *et al.*, 1979: 220; Mooss, 1980: 79). It forms an ingredient of preparations like *Tuḷasyādi tailaṃ, Mānasamitravaṭakaṃ, Śītajvarāri kaṣāyaṃ, Vilvādi guḷika, Balātailaṃ*, etc.

Āyurvēdic texts mention two varieties of the drug, namely the white variety (*śukḷatuḷasi*) and the dark variety (*kṛṣṇatuḷasi*) which are reported to have similar therapeutic properties. (Chunekar, 1982: 509), but the dark variety is preferred in medicine. These are equated with the white and black varieties of *Ocimum tenuiflorum* Linn. of Lamiaceae, throughout the country. (See also Rheede, Hort. Malab. 10: 169, t. 85. 1690. *Nala-tirtava*).

Ocimum tenuiflorum *Linn.* **(Lamiaceae)** (Fig. 241)
O. sanctum Linn.
Erect, much-branched, strongly aromatic subshrub, clothed with spreading hairs; stem and foliage green or dark purple; leaves simple, opposite, elliptic to oblong obtuse or acute, serrate, 2–5.55 × 1–2.8 cms, softly pubescent on both sides; flowers small, purplish, in terminal thyrsoid panicles; calyx purplish, 2-lipped, pubescent, upper lip orbicular, reflexed, lower lip 4-lobed; corolla 2-lipped; stamens 4, didynamous, filaments purple, anthers yellow; nutlets ellipsoid, smooth, mucilaginous when wetted.

Distribution: The plant is seen in all plains districts, mostly grown in home-yards. The plant also occurs in S.W. Sri Lanka, Bangladesh, Burma, China, Thailand and Malesia.

Note: *Tuḷasi* has been found to be very effective in the treatment of viral encephalitis (Das *et al.*, 1983) and tropical pulmonary eosinophilia in children (Sharma *et al.*, 1987b). Its antispasmodic and antiasthmatic activity have been studied by Sharma (1983).

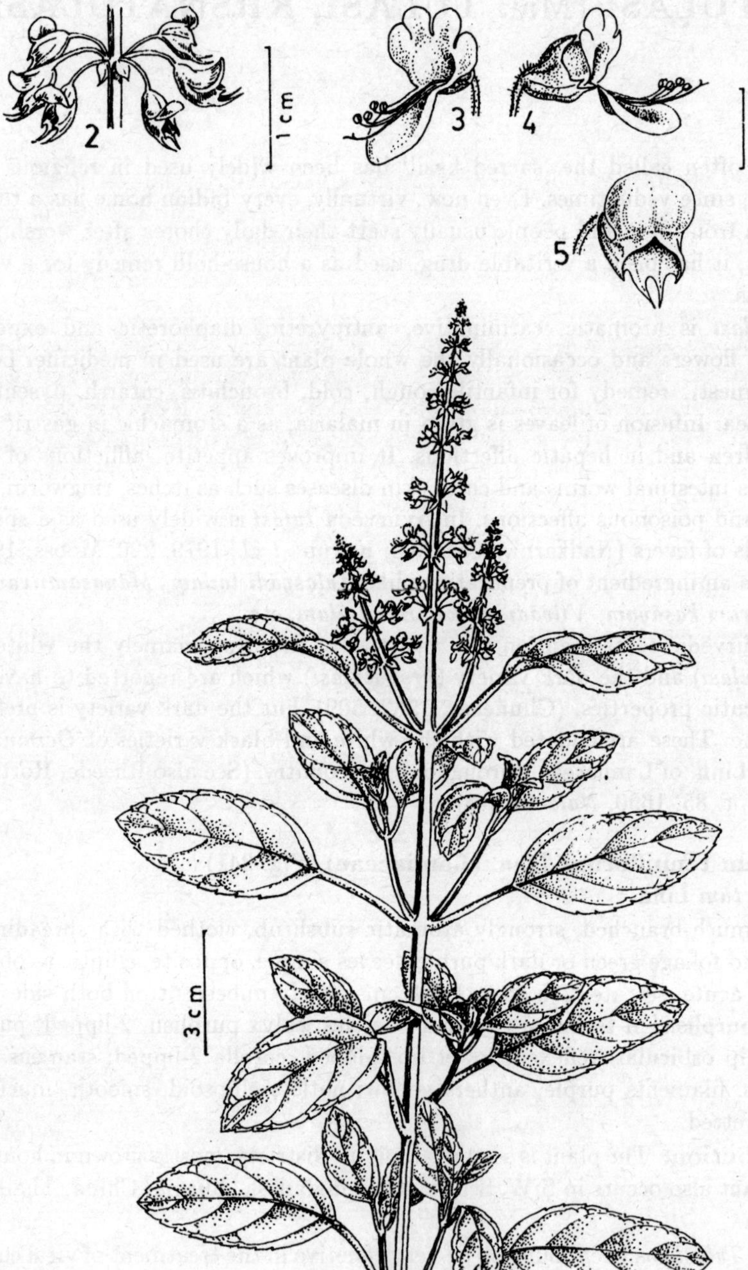

Figure 241: Ocimum tenuiflorum L. **1, A branch; 2, A portion of the inflorescence; 3–4, Flowers; 5, Calyx.**

UDUṀBARAḤ (Mal. ATTI)

This is one of the four *kṣīrivṛkṣās* (trees having milky latex) that constitute the group *nālpāmaraṃ*. The barks of these trees are reputed.for healing ulcers, skin diseases, poisons and vaginal diseases. *Uduṁbaraḥ* is astringent, antiseptic, cooling and highly efficacious in threatened abortions, gonorrhoea, menorrhagia, leucorrhoea, urinary diseases, haemorrhage, skin diseases and ulcers. It promotes complexion, overcomes *pitta, kapha* and *vātarakta*, burning sensation and thirst. Decoction of the bark is useful as an ablution for various forms of skin diseases and ulcers and its paste in inflammatory swellings and boils. The unripe fruits are astringent, sweet, carminative, digestive, stomachic and are useful in diarrhoea, dyspepsia, dysentery, haemorrhage and menorrhagia. The ripe fruits are sweet, cooling and are used in haemoptysis, thirst and vomiting (Nadkarni, 1954: 548–549; Aiyer *et al.*, 1957. 3: 94; Mooss, 1976: 70). Bark and figs are used in medicine. *Nālpāmarādi* coconut oil, *Candanāsavaṃ, Valiya Arimēdastailaṃ, Dinēśavalyādi kuḷaṁbu, Abhṛabhasmaṃ, Valiya candanādi tailaṃ*, etc. are some important preparations using the drug.

This sacrificial tree (*yajñīyaḥ, yajña-yōgyaḥ*) which is considered sacred (*pavitṛakaḥ*), has golden coloured exudate (*hēmadugdhaḥ*) and black bark (*kāḷaskandhaḥ*). The name *jantūphalaḥ* indicates the presence of insects in the fruits (Aiyer *et al.*, 1957. 3: 93).

Ficus racemosa Linn. (Moraceae), known as *atti* in vernacular, is the accepted source of the drug. Rheede describes and portrays this under the name *Attialu* (Hort. Malab. 1: 43–44, t. 25. 1678).

Ficus racemosa *Linn.* **(Moraceae)** (Fig. 242)
Ficus glomerata Roxb.

Evergreen trees; leaves simple, alternate, elliptic-oblong or ovate - lanceolate, entire, glabrous, 3-veined from base, upto 17 × 5.5 cm; figs subglobose, dense tomentose, 1.5–2.5 cm across, on bracteolate, tubercled and warted branchlets clustered on the trunk and older branches, dull reddish when ripe; staminate flowers sessile and situated near the opening of the receptacle, female flowers in the centre and gall flowers found intermixed with male flowers; perianth shortly cupular, tepals 3–5, ovate-lanceolate, scarious, lacerate acute; stamens 2, exserted, filaments connate below; ovary sessile or shortly stalked, style to 3 mm; gall flowers similar, long-stalked, style short; achenes lenticular, obscurely keeled.

Distribution: The tree is distributed all over India, but more common in the outer and sub Himalayan tracts, Rajaputana, Assam, Bengal, Central, Western and Southern India. It grows from sea level to an elevation of about 6,000 ft. in evergreen forests and along the banks of streams in deciduous forests. Also found in Sri Lanka, Pakistan, S. China to New Guinea & Queensland.

Note: Clinical studies conducted by Patel & Vasavada (1985) reveal that the aqueous extract of *F. racemosa* bark possesses remarkable antiulcer activity against

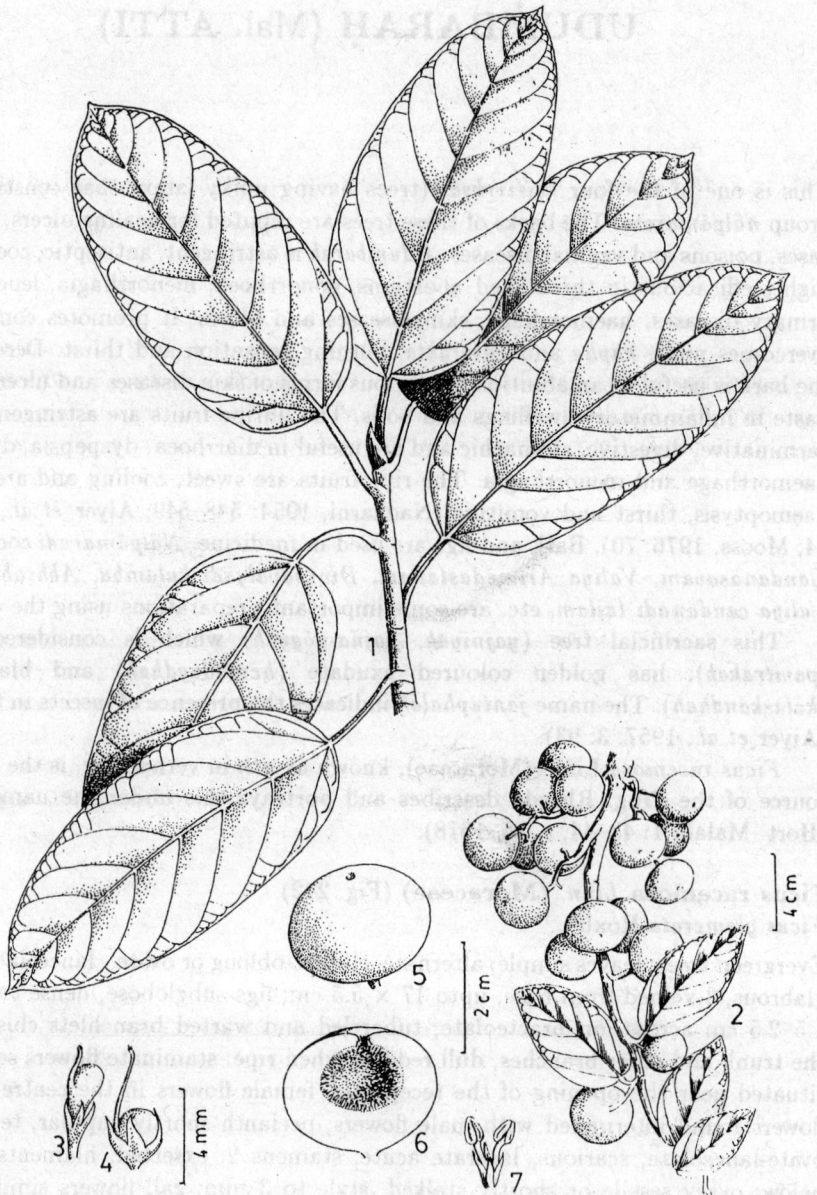

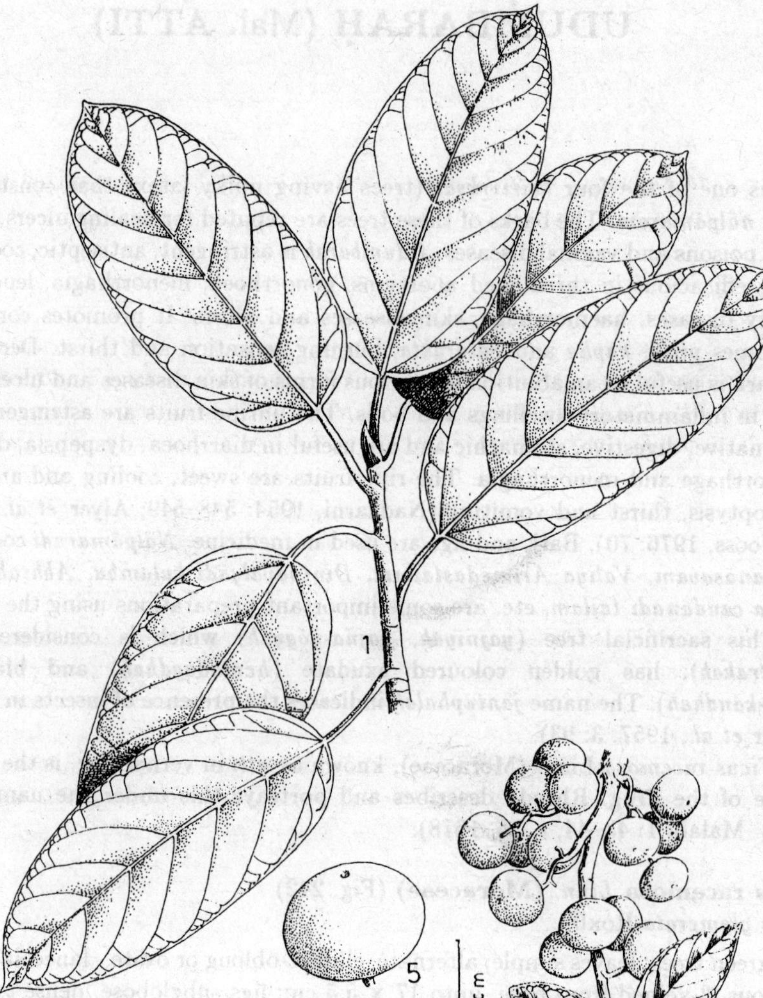

Figure 242: Ficus racemosa L. 1, A vegetative branch; 2, Flowering shoot; 3–4, Female flowers; 5, Fig; 6, Fig L.S.; 7, Male flower.

acute gastric ulcers in animals. It was also found to inhibit acid secretion and to stimulate the gastric juice.

UPŌDIKĀ (Mal. VAŚAḶACCĪRA)

Upōdika (or *upōdaka*) is considered as a specific for burns. Leaf juice mixed with butter is a soothing and cooling application for burns and scalds. It is cooling, diuretic and a mild laxative. It is easily digested and makes a wholesome vegetable. Leaf paste is applied to boils, ulcers and abscesses to hasten suppuration. Juice of leaves together with sugarcandy is useful in catarrhal affections of children and is administered with great benefit in gonorrhoea and balanitis. It overcomes vitiated *vāta* and *pitta*, promotes sleep, helps easy delivery, improves strength and semen and cures *raktapitta* (Nadkarni, 1954: 178; Chunekar, 1982: 665). It is an ingredient of *Sukhapṛasavada ghṛtaṃ*.

The texts do not provide us with any unequivocal description which could help in the identification of the plant source. *Basella alba* Linn. of Basellaceae, locally called *vaśaḷa* or *vaśaḷaccīra* is the accepted source of the drug. (See Nadkarni, 1954: 177; Chopra *et al.*, 1956: 34; Mooss, 1976: 24; Chunekar, 1982: 665). Rheede also describes and portrays the plant under the same vernacular name *vaśala* (Hort. Malab. 7: 45, t. 24. 1688). Two varieties, one with reddish stems and petioles and the other with greenish stem are seen commonly. Both belong to the same species *Basella alba* Linn. However, some species of *Ludwigia* (Onagraceae) (*L. octovalvis, L. peruviana* and *L. hyssopifolia*) and *Portulaca oleracea* (Portulacaceae) are also found occasionally used for this drug, by some practitioners. This seems to be unauthorised substitutes because, these plants are locally known by different vernacular names in Kerala.

The various plant sources can be identified as follows.

Basella alba *Linn.* **(Basellaceae)** (Fig. 243)
B. rubra Linn.

Succulent twiners; green or red; leaves simple, alternate, broadly ovate, acute, cordate at base, entire, glabrous, upto 13 × 10 cms; flowers small, pinkish white in short, axillary spikes; bract ovate, truncate-rounded, acute; bracteoles 2, partly connate with perianth, ovate-concave, acute; perianth urceolate, 5-lobed; stamens 5, inserted below the lobes, filaments basally dilated, anthers oblong; ovary globose; fruit subglobose, purple when mature.

Distribution: Probably a native of tropical Asia and Africa, the plant is now widely cultivated in India as a pot-herb.

Ludwigia hyssopifolia (*Don*) *Exell* **(Onagraceae)** (Fig. 244)
Jussiaea hyssopifolia Don
J. linifolia Vahl
Fissendocarpa linifolia (Vahl) *Bennet*

Erect, glabrous, branched herbs or undershrubs; stem angled and narrowly winged; leaves simple, alternate, elliptic to lanceolate, acute, entire, to 6 × 1.6 cms; flowers small, yellow, axillary, solitary, sessile; calyx tube 1 cm, lobes 4, persistent; petals 4, free; stamens 8; ovary inferior, ovules many; capsule linear, terete, 2–2.5 cm long; seeds many, dimorphic.

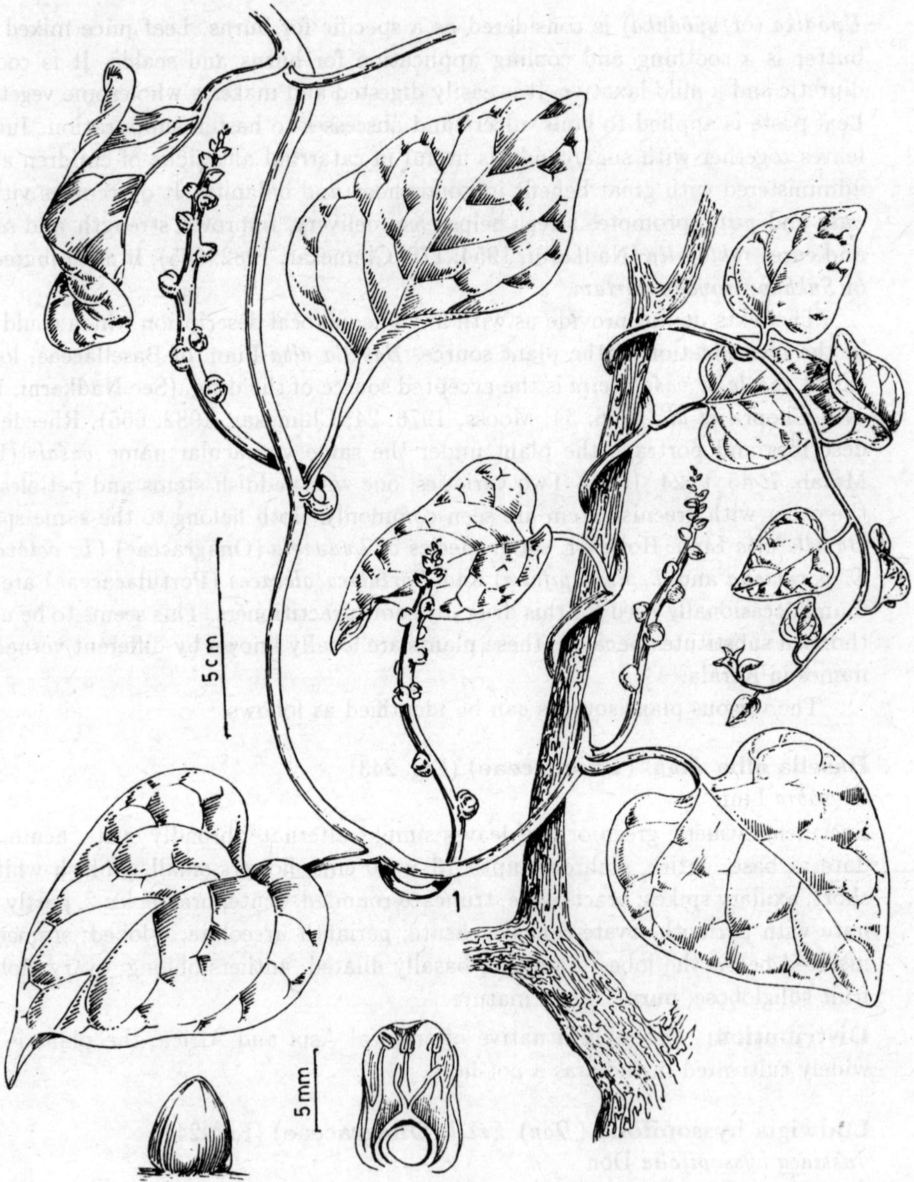

Figure 243: Basella alba L. 1, Habit; 2, Flower; 3, Flower L.S.

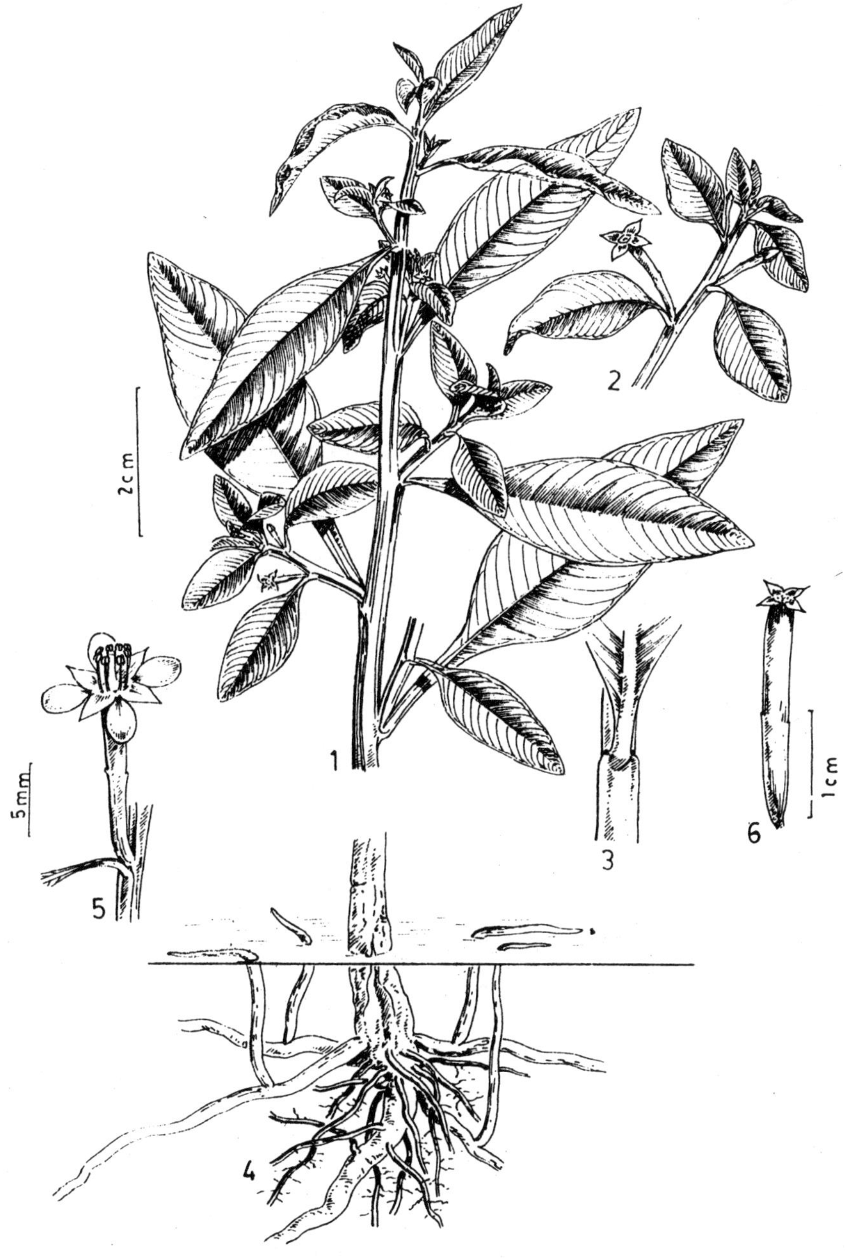

Figure 244: Ludwigia hyssopifolia (Don) Exell. 1,2,4 Habit; 3, Winged petiole; 5, Flower; 6, Fruit.

Distribution: The plant is common in marshy fields and on the banks of fresh water ponds and streams upto 3,000 ft. in Peninsular India. Also reported from tropical Africa, continental S.E. Asia, throughout Malesia to Micronesia and N. Australia.

Ludwigia octovalvis (*Jacq.*) *Raven* **(Onagraceae)** (Fig. 245)
Oenothera octovalvis Jacq.
Jussiaea suffruticosa Linn.

Dense-tomentose sub shrub; stem ridged; leaves elliptic to lanceolate, acute, entire, 7.5 × 1.8 cms adpressed pubescent; flowers axillary, solitary, large, yellow; calyx tube 2 cm, pubescent, lobes 4, lanceolate; petals 4, obovate; stamens 8; ovary 2 cm, 4-celled, ovules many; capsule terete, 8-ridged, adpressed tomentose, about 4 cm long; seeds many.

Distribution: The plant is found throughout the tropics of the world, between C 32°N and 30°S.

Ludwigia octovalvis is locally known as *kāṭṭukarayāmpu* (see also Rheede. Hort. Malab. 2: 97, t. 50. 1679).

Ludwigia peruviana (*Linn.*) *H. Hara* **(Onagraceae)**
Jussiaea peruviana Linn.

Subshrub; branchlets hirsute; leaves broadly oblong-lanceolate or elliptic-acute, 6–13 × 1.5–3 cm, chartaceous, hirsute, base attenuate, margin entire; flowers yellow, 4 cm across; calyx tube 1.5 cm, hirsute, lobes 4, lanceolate; petals 4, golden yellow, obovate-suborbicular, base cuneate, apex rotund; stamens 8, anthers oblong; ovary 4-celled, ovules many, stule 1 mm, stigma elongate; capsule oblong, 2 × 0.8 cm, 4-sided, 4-ribbed, thin walled; seeds ellipsoid, multiseriate.

Distribution: A native of the New World, from S. E. United States throughout S. America, introduced and naturalised elsewhere.

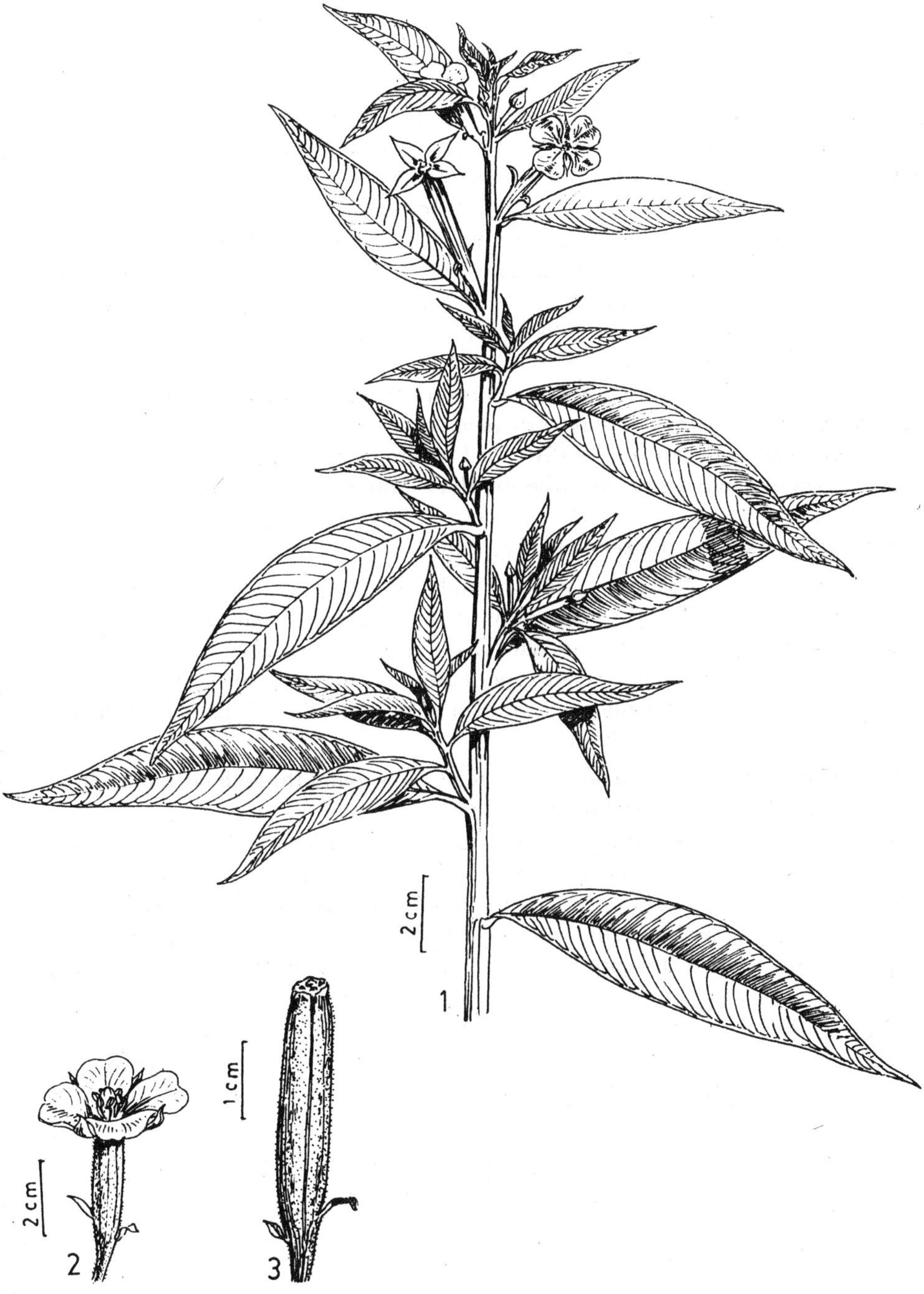

Figure 245: **Ludwigia octovalvis** (Jacq.) Raven. 1, Flowering branch; 2, Flower; 3, Fruit.

VACĀ (Mal. VAYAṀPU)

Vacā is an important *mēdhya* drug, capable of improving memory power and intellect. The officinal part, i.e. rhizome, is strong-smelling (*ugra-gandhā*), acrid and bitter. It is reportedly useful in improving digestion, clearing speech (*vacā*) and curing diarrhoea, dysentery, abdominal obstruction and colic. It is also useful in infantile fever, cough, bronchitis and asthma. The drug is reported to ward off evil spirits (*bhūta*) and to cure hysteria, insanity and chronic rheumatic complaints. Administering a paste of the rhizome in ghee to infants, is one of the first post-natal rituals of Indian mothers. This is believed to contribute to the proper development of intellect of the infant (Nadkarni, 1954: 37; Aiyer *et al.*, 1957: 44; Mooss, 1976: 9). The rhizome is an ingredient of preparations like *Vacāditailaṃ, Ayaskṛti, Koṁpañcādi guḷika, Valiya rāsnādi kaṣāyaṃ*, etc.

Acorus calamus (Araceae), locally called *vayaṁpu* is the accepted source of the drug throughout the country (see Rheede, Hort. Malab. 11: 99, t. 48. 1692).

Acorus calamus *Linn.* **(Araceae)** (Fig. 246)

Strongly aromatic, marsh herb; leaves simple, alternate, distichous, closely arranged, 80 – 1.2 cms, linear to narrowly ensiform, glossy bright green, acute at tip and amplexicaul at base; flowers pale green, fragrant, arranged compactly on a sessile, cylindric, short, stumpy spadix; perianth segments 6, scaly; stamens 6, filaments linear, flat, anthers reniform; ovary superior, conical, 2–3 chambered, many ovuled; fruit a 3-celled fleshy capsule.

Distribution: The plant is a native of Europe. Now found throughout India under cultivation as well as in the wild state.

Note: Pharmacognostic studies of the rhizomes of *Acorus calamus* have been carried out by Dey and Das (1980). The drug has been found to be effective in the treatment of bronchial asthma (Prakash, 1981). The hypocholesterolaemic effect of *Acorus calamus* has been clinically tried by Arora *et al.* (1986). Boyuan and Yaoyuan (1986) studied the anticarcinogenic action of the drug.

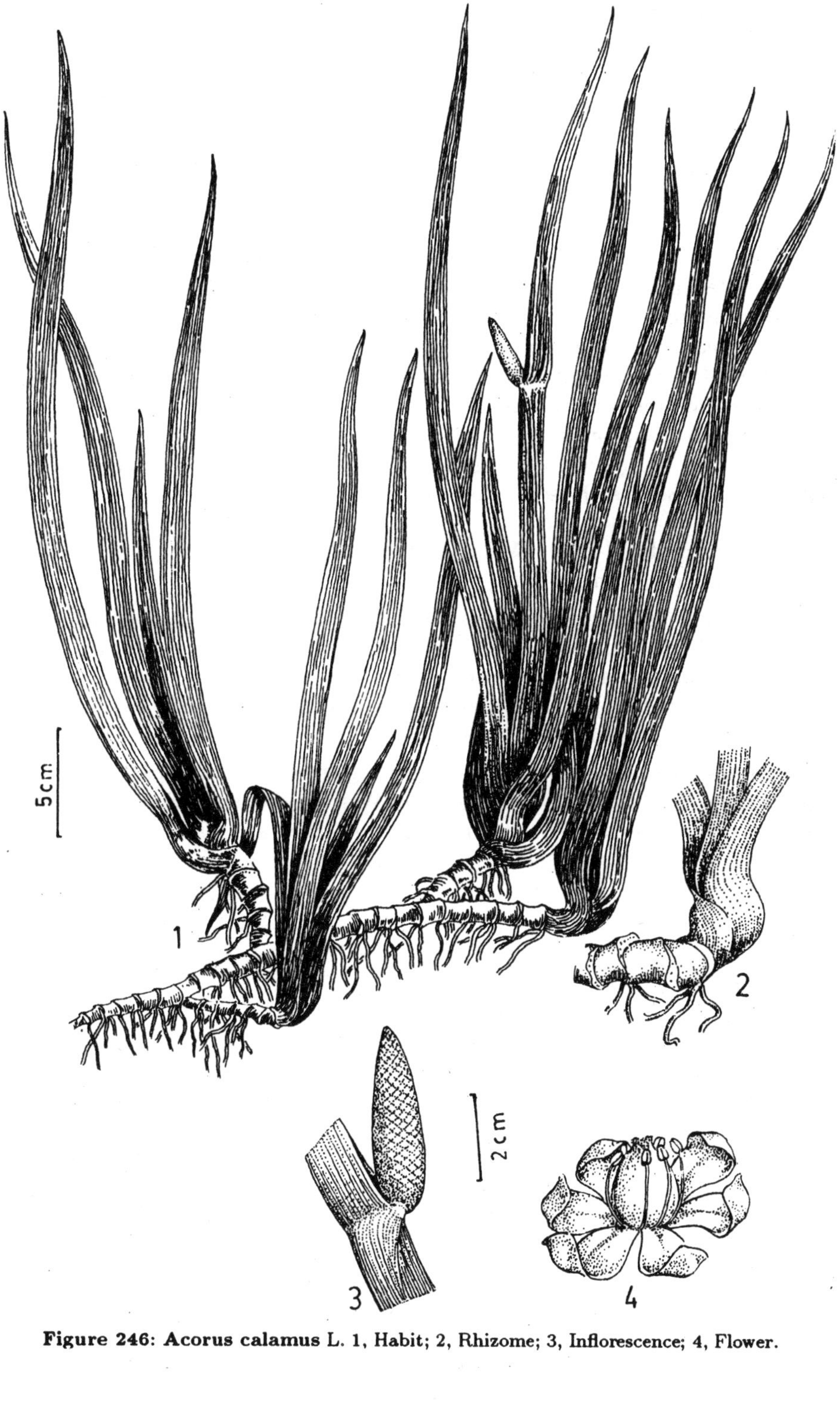

Figure 246: Acorus calamus L. 1, Habit; 2, Rhizome; 3, Inflorescence; 4, Flower.

VAJṚAVALLĪ (Mal. CAṄṄALAṀPARAṆṬA)

The plant is also called *'asthisaṁdhāni'* because of its ability to rejoin broken bones. A paste of the stem is plastered over the fracture and swellings by the traditional healers. The entire plant is used medicinally. It is light, sweet, hot, alterative, carminative, anthelmintic, aphrodisiac, stomachic and overcomes morbidity of *kapha* and *vāta*, gastrointestinal disorders and irregular menstruation. The drug is also useful in dyspepsia, indigestion, piles, worms, asthma and *vātarakta*. Juice of the stem is used as an ear and nasal drop in case of otorrhoea and epistaxis respectively (Nadkarni, 1954: 1284; Kurup *et al.*, 1979: 20; Sharma, 1983: 828; Nesamony, 1985: 227). It enters into the composition of preparations like *Valiya ciñcādi lēhaṃ, Pathyā-punarṇavādi kaṣāyaṃ*, etc.

The accepted source of the drug throughout India is *Cissus quadrangularis* Linn. (Vitaceae) (See also Rheede, Hort. Malab. 7: 77. t. 41. 1688).

Cissus quadrangularis *Linn.* **(Vitaceae)** (Fig. 247)
Vitis quadrangularis (Linn.) Wallich ex Wight

A rambling shrub, climbing over bushes; stem thick, fleshy, quadrangular, glabrous, constricted at the nodes; leaves simple, alternate, thick-coriaceous, broadly ovate to suborbicular, obtuse, margin serrate, 6.5 × 8 cms, tendrils leaf-opposed; flowers small, in leaf-opposed umbellate cymes, calyx cup-shaped, obscurely lobed; petals greenish yellow, red tipped, berry globose.

Distribution: The plant is common in drier regions of N. Circars, Deccan, Carnatic, extending West to the lower E. slopes of Western Ghats and South to S. Travancore. It is also widespread in the drier parts of Africa and Arabia.

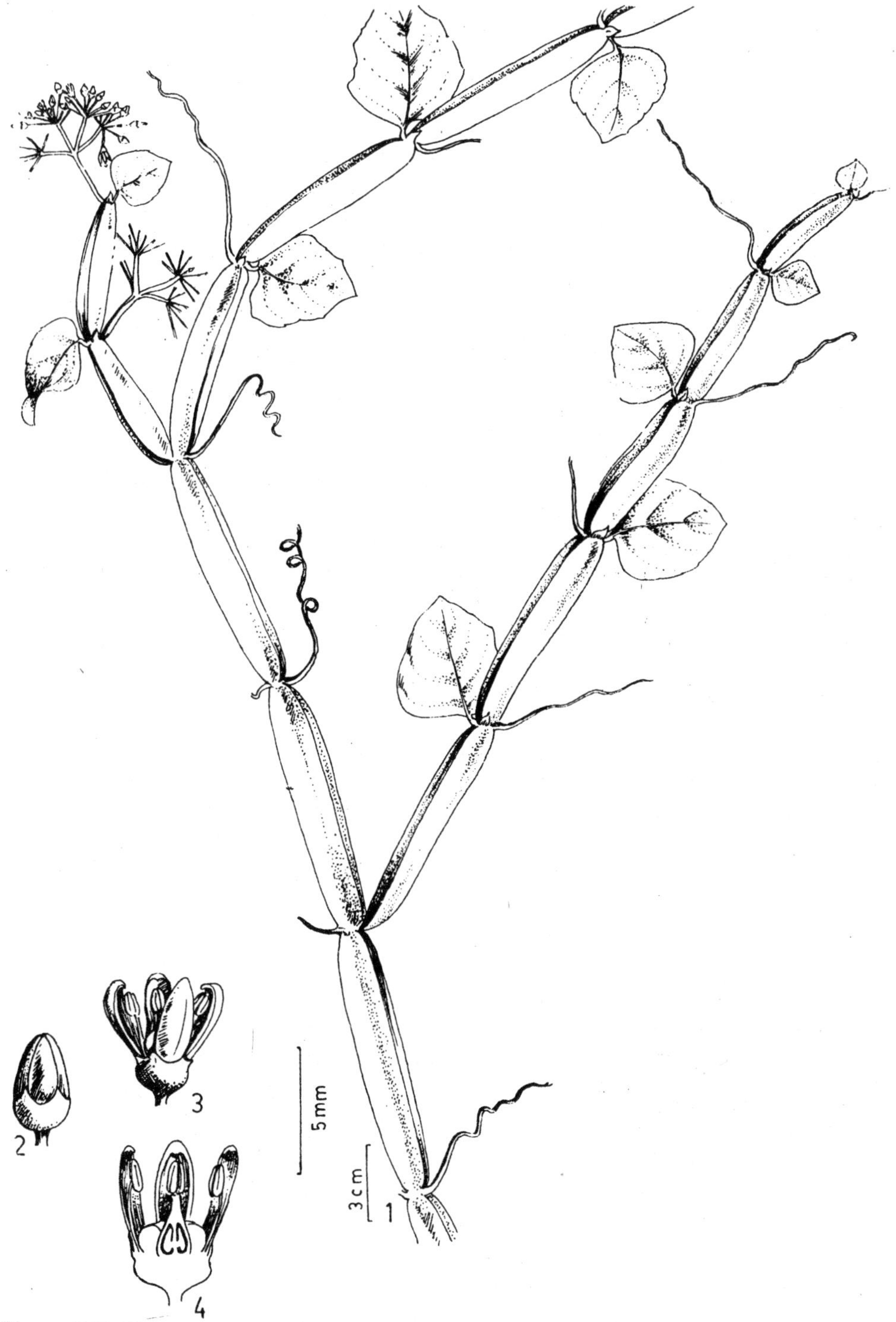

Figure 247: Cissus quadrangularis L. 1, Habit; 2, Flower bud; 3, Open flower; 4, Flower L.S.

VĀḶAKAḤ (Mal. IRUVĒLI)

According to Bhāvapṛakāśanighaṇṭu, this drug, also known as *hṛībēra* and *bāḷaṃ*, is cooling, light, carminative and tonic and cures dyspepsia, indigestion, dysentery, vomiting, thirst, fever, dermatitis, ulcers and bleeding disorders (Chunekar, 1982: 237). The entire plant is used in medicine. *Gandhatailaṃ* and *Ēlāditailaṃ* are some of the preparations using the drug.

Most of the authors equate the drug with *Pavonia odorata* Willd. of Malvaceae (see Kirtikar & Basu 1918: 179; Vaidya K.M., 1936: 517; Nadkarni, 1954: 925; Chopra *et al.*, 1956: 187; Kapoor & Mitra, 1979: 63; Chunekar, 1982: 237). In Kerala, the accepted source of this drug has never been this plant, but certain species of *Coleus* (Lamiaceae) There are two or three species involved. Most of it is derived from *Coleus vettiveroides* (see Anonymous, 1978a: 259; Mooss, 1980: 108). This species, cultivated in the sandy loam on the river banks in some areas of Tamil Nadu, is called *kuṟuveṛ* or *veṭṭivēṛ* in Tamil and has fragrant roots. But the shoots and leaves are rather little odorous compared to *C. zeylanicus* which is also used as the plant source of this drug. The latter, a native of Ceylon, has been known as *Iruweriya* in Kerala folk-medicine since long, (see Nair et al., 1986).

The various plants equated with the drug can be identified as follows.

Coleus zeylanicus (*Benth.*) *Cramer* **(Lamiaceae)**
Plectranthus zeylanicus Benth.

Profusely branched, semi-succulent, strongly aromatic; soft-tomentose herb with fibrous roots; leaves simple, opposite, slightly fleshy, broadly orbicular, retuse or emarginate at apex, rounded or truncate at base, margin crenate-serrate, surface bullate, upto 13 × 13 cms, flowers small, blue or purplish, in terminal thyrsiform panicles; calyx 2-lipped, glandular; corolla 2-lipped, upper lip 4-lobed, lower entire, boat-shaped; stamens 4, didynamous, filaments connate below; ovary 4-lobed; style slender, stigma 2-fid.

Distribution: A native of Ceylon, known only under cultivation in Kerala.

Coleus vettiveroides *Jacob* **(Lamiaceae)**

Succulent, odourous herb with straw-coloured roots; stems and branches quadrangular; leaves broadly ovate with dentate margin, glandular hairy; flowers blue in terminal racemes. Floral and fruit characters as in *C. zeylanicus.*

Distribution: The plant is seen under cultivation in Tanjore, Madras and Tinnevelly districts of Madras on river banks and sandy loams.

Pavonia odorata *Willd.* **(Malvaceae)** (Fig. 248)

Erect, glandular-pubescent, herb; leaves simple, alternate, long-petioled, roundish-ovate, cordate at base, slightly 3–5 lobed, 6 × 6 cm stellately hairy on both surfaces; flowers pinkish, solitary, axillary, long-pedicelled, with an involucre of 10–12 distinct linear bracteoles, each about 8–10 mm, hairy; calyx gamosepalous, 5-lobed above; petals 5, obovate-obtuse, connate and adnate to the staminal tube at base; stamens many, united to form a staminal column; pistil 5-carpellary syncarpous, ovary 5-celled, each 1-ovuled, style long with 10 stylar branches, ending in capitate stigmas.

Distribution: The plant is common in central and southern India in waste places and deciduous forests. Also found in Burma, Sri Lanka and Tropical E. Africa.

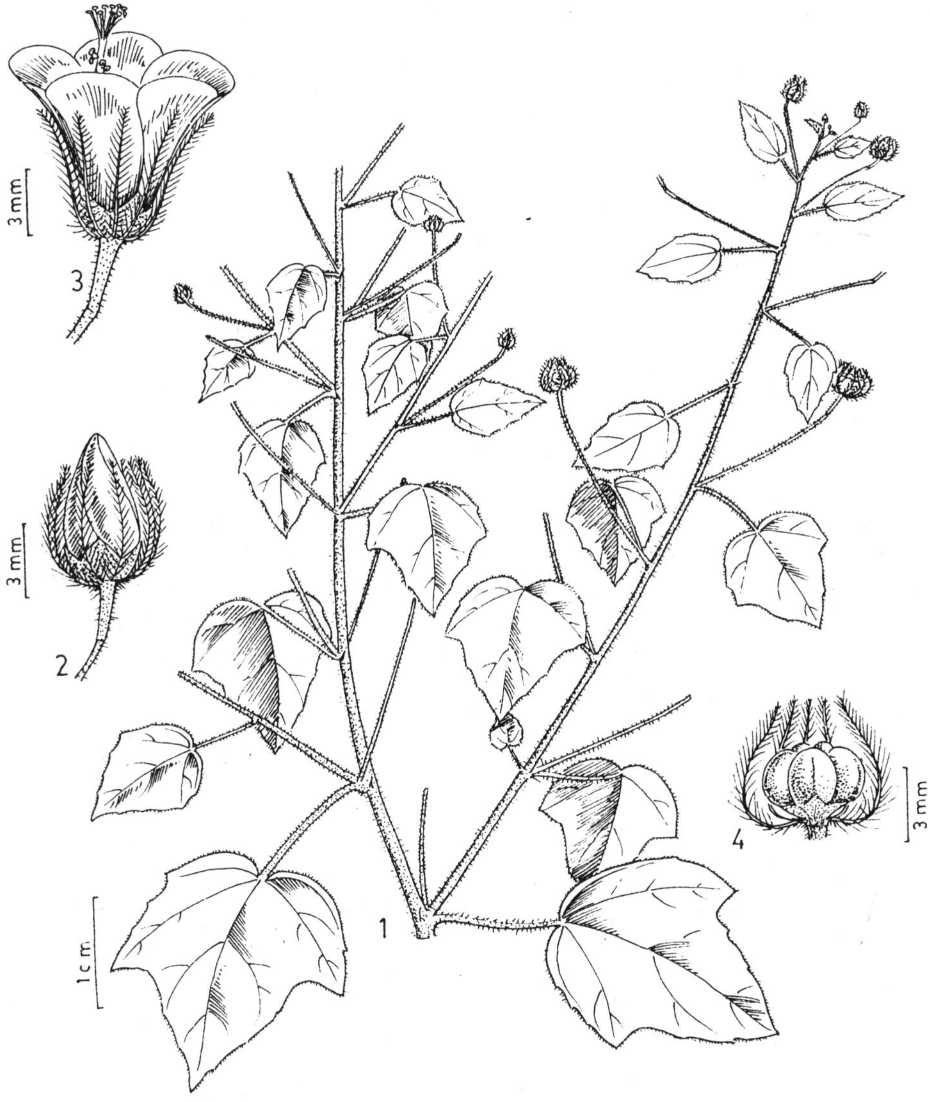

Figure 248: Pavonia odorata Willd. 1, Habit; 2, Flower bud; 3, Open flower; 4, Fruit.

VARUṆAḤ (Mal. NĪṚMĀTAḶAṂ)

This is an important component of the *Varaṇādi gaṇa* of Vāgbhaṭa, a group of seventeen drugs, which alleviates morbid *kapha,* obesity, weakness of the digestive fire, paraplegia (*āḍhya-vāta*), headache, *gulma* and *vidradhi* (malignant tumour) (Mooss, 1980: 57). *Varuṇa* is astringent, bitter, acrid, anthelmintic, carminative, diuretic, laxative and stomachic. It improves digestive power, purifies blood and cures arthritis, internal abscesses, dysuria, calculus, headache, certain heart diseases like angina pectoris and vaginismus. The drug is also useful in bladder and uterine affections and enlargement of the abdominal viscera. A decoction made out of the bark is a good remedy for renal calculus and hence the name *aśmarighna.* Bark and leaves form a good external application for painful rheumatic swellings (Aiyer & Kolammal, 1966. 9: 122; Dey, 1980: 158). *Varuṇādi kaṣāyaṃ, Pṛabhañjanaṃ kuḻaṁbu, Candrapṛabhā guḷika, Dhānvantaraṃ ghṛtaṃ,* etc. are some of the preparations using the drug.

According to the description in the texts, the tree has abundant green foliage (*ūrumāṇaḥ*) and beautiful white flowers which resemble peacocks' tail (*baṛhapuṣpaḥ*) and bitter shoots (*tiktaśākaḥ*) (Aiyer & Kolammal, 1966. 9: 121).

Species of the genus *Crataeva* (Capparaceae), are the sources of this drug through out the country. There are two taxa, *C. magna* and *C. adansonii* subsp. *odora* in India. They can be easily distinguished by their foliage characters (in other features they are closely similar). Despite that most authors have equated the drug with the former, it has been found that the latter is also being used by Kerala practitioners. Rheede (Hort. Malab. 3:49–50. t. 42. 1682) has, however, attributed the name *'Nirvala'* to this, possibly inadvertently, because *'nīṛvāḷa,* in Ayurvedic parlance, is an altogether different drug derived from *Croton tiglium* of Euphorbiaceae.

Crataeva magna (*Lour.*) *DC.* **(Capparaceae)** (Fig. 249)
Capparis magna Lour.
Crataeva nurvala Buch.-Ham.
C. religiosa auct., non Forst.f.

Moderate-sized deciduous tree; leaves alternate, exstipulate, long-petioled, trifoliolate; leaflets lanceolate with gradually tapering tips, 15 × 4.2 cms, glabrous above, glaucous beneath, laterals oblique at base; flowers white in terminal corymbose panicles; pedicels long; sepals 4, small, petaloid; petals 4, long-clawed, obovate-obtuse; stamens many, inserted on the margin of the disc adnate to the base of the gynophore. filaments purplish; ovary ovoid, one celled, many-ovuled, on a long gynophore; berries ovoid.

Distribution: The plant is found in almost all districts of India, Burma, China, Indochina and Malesia. Here it grows mostly along the banks of streams or rivers.

Crataeva adansonii *DC. subsp.* **odora** (*Buch.-Ham.*) *Jacobs* **(Capparaceae)**
C. odora Buch.-Ham.
C. religiosa var. *roxburghii* (R. Br.) Hook. f. & Thoms.

Deciduous trees, very similar to *C. nurvala* but can be distinguished by its ovate-lanceolate abruptly acuminate leaves.

Distribution: Occasionally found in the hills and plains of Southern India.

Note: Pharmacognosy of this drug has been discussed in detail by Raghunathan & Mitra (1982). Clinical trials have revealed significantly anti-inflammatory activity for its bark (Das *et al.*, 1974) and that it is efficaceous in urinary disorders (Kumar *et al.*, 1982; Deshpande *et al.*, 1982).

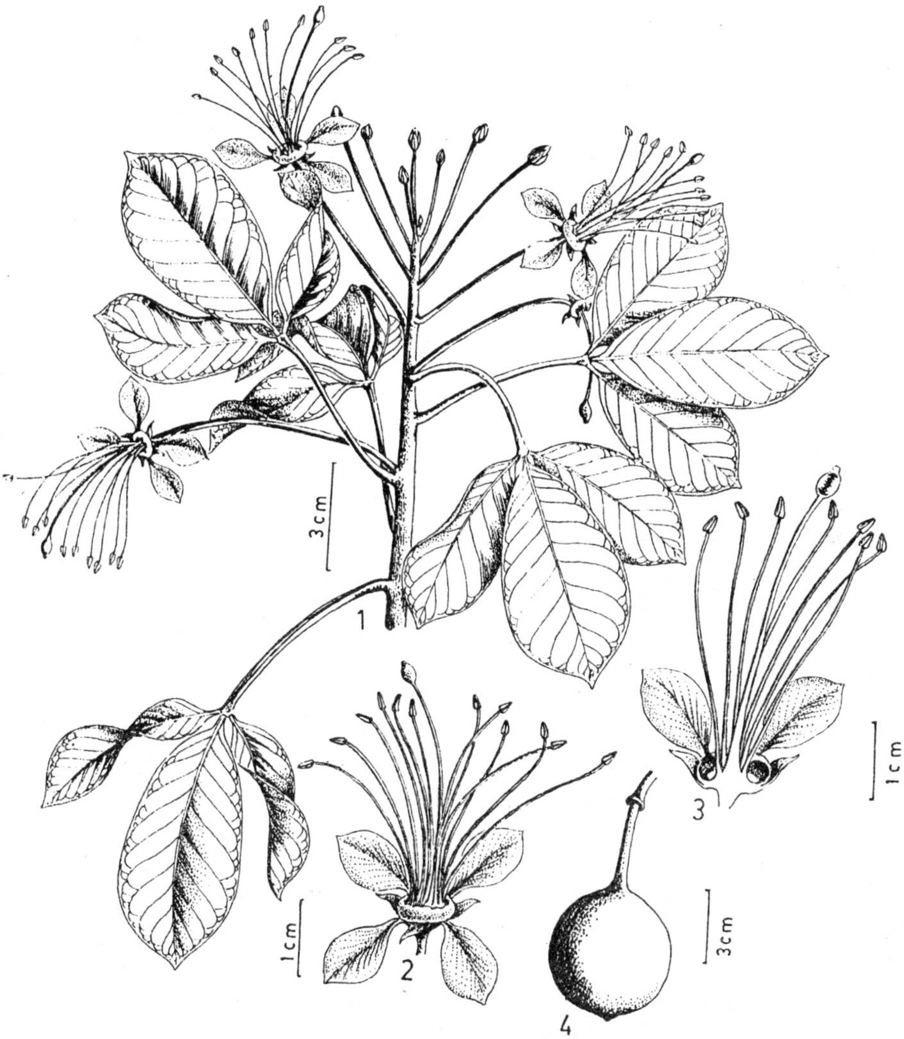

Figure 249: Crataeva adansonii subsp. **odora** (Buch,-Ham.) Jacobs. 1, Flowering branch; 2, Flower; 3, Flower L.S.; 4, Fruit.

VĀŚĀ (Mal. ĀṬALŌṬAKAṂ)

Vāśā has been a reputed remedy for cough, bronchitis, asthma and other respiratory disorders due to its expectorant action. The juice of the leaves relieves cough by its soothening action on the nerves and by liquefying the sputum which makes expectoration easier. It is reported to be bitter, astringent, antispasmodic and alterative and cures vomiting, thirst, fever, dermatosis, jaundice, phthisis, haematemesis and diseases due to the morbidity of *kapha* and *pitta*. The leaf juice is especially used in anaemia and haemorrhage, in traditional medicine. Flowers and leaves are considered efficacious against rheumatic, painful swellings and form a good application to scabies and other skin complaints. (Nadkarni, 1954: 42, Aiyer & Kolammal, 1963: 7. 54; Kurup *et al.*, 1979: 227). The drug forms an ingredient of preparations like *Vāśāriṣṭaṃ, Valiya rāsnādi kaṣāyaṃ, Cyavanaprāśaṃ, Gulgulutiktakaṃ ghṛtaṃ*, etc.

Of the various synonyms attributed to this drug, only a few like *siṁhikā, siṁhāsyaḥ*, and *siṁhaparṇaḥ* (which probably refers to the shape of the open flower resembling the mouth of a lion) give some idea about the morphological features. Other synonyms are only indicative of the strong therapeutic properties of the drug. The drug is described as one earnestly desired by the patients (*vāśā, vāsakaḥ, vāsikā*), on account of its excellent medicinal properties and as one showering nectar (*vṛṣa*) which probably indicates the capacity to overcome diseases and thus enable to remain youthful. (cf. Aiyer & Kolammal, 1963. 7: 54).

Though the Sanskrit synonyms do not give any useful indication as to the identity of the actual plant source, there is no confusion with regard to the source of the drug. *Adhatoda zeylanica* of Acanthaceae is the one which is most commonly equated with the drug. Kerala physicians, however, recognise two varieties of *vāśā*, locally known as *āṭalōṭakaṃ* which is seen growing wild almost throughout India and '*ciṫṫāṭalōṭakaṃ*, which is known only under cultivation. The latter is so called because of its smaller stature, smaller leaves and flowers. Consequently, most of the recent authors on Ayurvedic Materia Medica have considered them as two different species and have equated the former with *Adhatoda zeylanica* (=*A. vasica*) and the latter with *A. beddomei* respectively. There is no doubt as far as *A. zeylanica* is concerned. But, we had doubts about the identity of *ciṫṫāṭalōṭakaṃ*, because, in the first place, *A. beddomei* has been known to be a very rare and endangered species for quite some time (Henry *et al.*, 1978). After an exhaustive floristic survey of the southern Western Ghats, a team of scientists from the National Beaureau of Plant Genetic Resources, Trissur, could not locate this plant in the area (Amalraj *et al.*, 1991).

Now we have got specimens of *ciṫṫāṭalōṭakaṃ* compared with authentic specimens of *A. beddomei* at Kew. They differed substantially. *A. zeylanica*, being a widely distributed species, is somewhat variable and our *ciṫṫāṭalōṭakaṃ* is nothing more than a form of *A. zeylanica* itself.

Adhatoda zeylanica *Medicus* **(Acanthaceae)** (Fig. 250)
Justicia adhatoda Linn.
Adhatoda vasica Nees.

Profusely branched, evergreen shrub, branchlets grey-pubescent; leaves simple, opposite, short-petioled, elliptic-lanceolate acuminate, entire, prominently veined, upto 20 × 8 cms, dark green above, paler beneath; flowers white in axillary, bracteate spikes; bracts large, deccussate, leafy, ovate; calyx deeply 5-lobed, lobes lanceolate, equal, corolla bilabiate, white, tube short, throat villous; stamens 2, attached at the throat of the tube, exserted; filaments villous below, anthers oblong, 2-celled; ovary 4-ovuled, stigma minutely 2-fid; capsule clavate, stalked below, compressed; seeds orbicular, compressed.

Distribution: The plant runs wild in most parts of India and is also frequently cultivated as a hedge plant. Distributed also in subtropical Himalaya, Indo-China and Malaya.

Note: Recent studies have shown that *vāśā* is effective against *amḷapitta* (non-ulcer dyspepsia) (Chaturvedi *et al.*, 1981, 1983) and pyorrhoea (Doshi *et al.*, 1983). Vasicine and Vasicinone extracted from *Adhatoda zeylanica* are good for asthmatic bronchitis due to their bronchodilatory activity (Shah *et al.*, 1987) and hence is used widely in preparing cough syrups like glycodin, while Gupta *et al.* (1978) have found vasicine to be an abortifacient during his trials in animals.

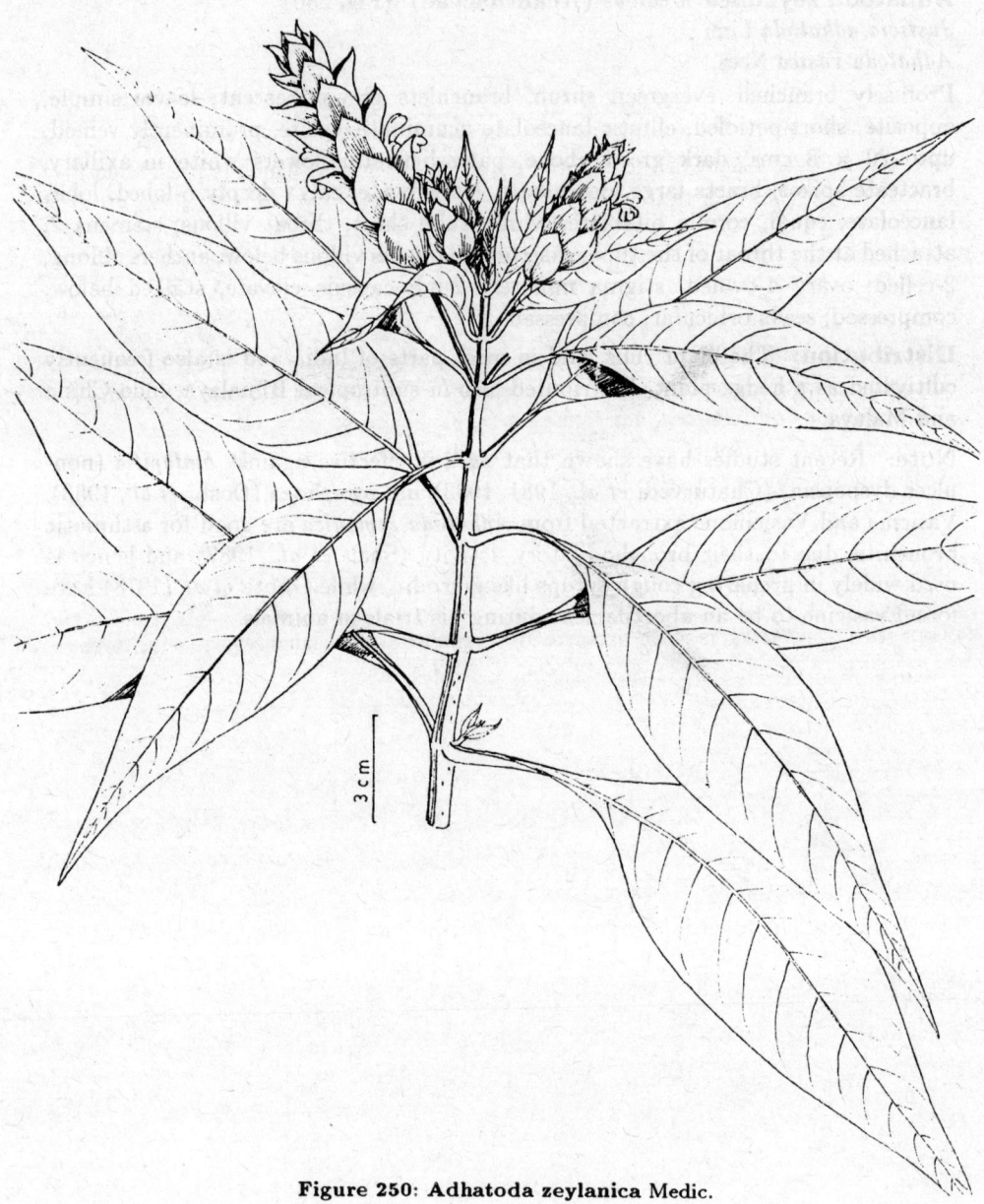

Figure 250: Adhatoda zeylanica Medic.

VIBHĪTAKĪ (Mal. TĀNNI)

Vibhītaki is a constituent of the group *triphala* (three fruits) which is prescribed in a variety of diseases like that which affect the eyes, anaemia, cough, fever, etc. It is bitter, acrid, astringent, laxative, germicidal and antipyretic. It helps abundant growth of hair, cures cough, leprosy, tuberculosis, diseases of the eyes, nose and throat, cleans voice and impurity of blood. The drug is also useful in diarrhoea, dysentery, inflammatory affections of small intestine, dyspepsia and biliousness (Aiyer & Kolammal, 1963. 7: 110; Kurup *et al.*, 1979: 40). Rind of the fruit, which is the officinal part, goes into the composition of *Triphalādi cūrṇaṃ, Triphalādi oil, Daśamūlāriṣṭaṃ, Pārantyādi tailaṃ* and *Triphalādi ghṛtaṃ*, etc.

Terminalia bellirica (Combretaceae), locally called *tānni* is the source of the drug throughout India (see also Rheede, Hort. Malab. 4: 23–24. t. 10. 1683). Ancient texts describe it as the abode of evil spirits or *bhūtās* (*bhūtavṛkṣa*) which bestows our desires (*kalpavṛkṣa*) (cf. Aiyer & Kolammal, 1963. 7: 110). It is believed that going round the tree will cure allergic afflictions from *bhallātaka* (Vern. *cēru*) i.e. *Semicarpus anacardium* and *Holigarna arnottiana* of Anacardiaceae. A paste of the bark or fruit of *vibhītaki* is often prescribed as an antidote for such allergic eruptions.

Terminalia bellirica (*Gaertn.*) *Roxb.* **(Combretaceae)** (Fig. 251)
Myrobalanus bellirica Gaertn.

Deciduous tree; leaves clustered at the ends of branchlets, broadly elliptic to obovate, 10–24 × 5–8 cms, coriaceous, glabrous, entire, apex subacute, or shortly acuminate; flowers small, sessile, yellowish green in axillary spikes; calyx tube constricted above the ovary, pubescent outside; stamens 10; ovary 1-celled; drupe subglobose, 2.5 × 2 cm, softly tomentose, obscurely 5-ridged.

Distribution: The plant is common throughout India in the plains and lower hills chiefly in the deciduous forests upto 900 metres elevation. It is also distributed in Sri Lanka, Nepal, Burma, Thailand, Indochina and Malesia.

Note: The drug has been found to have bronchodilatory, antispasmodic and anti-asthmatic properties (Trivedi, *et al.*, 1982) and to be effective in the treatment of asthma, cough and tropical pulmonary eosinophilia (Sharma, *et al.*, 1987b).

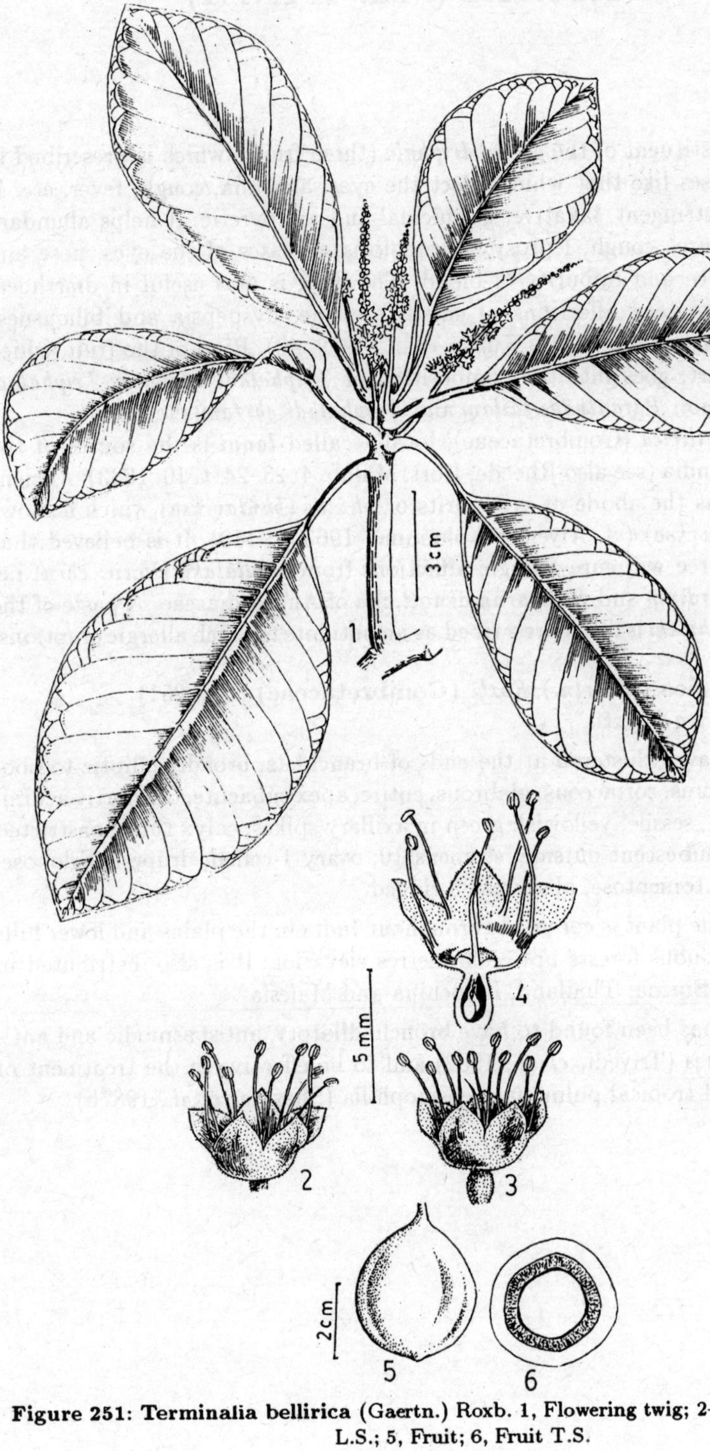

Figure 251: Terminalia bellirica (Gaertn.) Roxb. **1, Flowering twig; 2–3, Flowers; 4, Flower L.S.; 5, Fruit; 6, Fruit T.S.**

VIḌAṄGAḤ (Mal. VIḶĀL)

As the synonyms *viḍaṅga, vēllaṃ* and *kṛmighna* indicate, the drug is highly esteemed as a powerful anthelmintic and is an important ingredient of a number of formulations. In recent times, *viḍaṅga* gained particular importance in view of the wide experimental and clinical trials on its contraceptive potentiality.

Dried berries, which form the officinal part, are light, acrid, astringent, alterative, carminative and nervine tonic and are used for constipation, colic, dyspepsia, flatulence and piles. The drug overcomes diseases due to the morbidity of *kapha* and *vāta* and cures leprosy and other skin diseases. A paste of the seeds is applied locally against ringworm and other cutaneous affections. The seed powder is used as an errhine in cold and headache. Root improves digestion and cures flatulence and colic. Powder made from dried bark of the root is a reputed remedy for tooth ache. (Nadkarni, 1954: 480; Sharma, 1983: 505; Nesamony, 1985: 458). The drug enters into the composition of formulations like *Viḷālvērādi kaṣāyaṃ, Aṇutailaṃ, Abhayāriṣṭaṃ, Gulgulutiktakaṃ kaṣāyaṃ,* etc.

That the drug is the dried berries of fruits of *Embelia ribes* Burm. f. (Myrsinaceae) is widely accepted. (Kirtikar & Basu, 1918: 724; Nadkarni, 1954: 478; Chopra *et al.*, 1956: 106; Kurup *et al.*, 1979: 229; Kapoor & Mitra 1979: 76; Dey, 1980: 160; Chunekar, 1982: 52; Sharma, 1983: 503). This is a forest species and the procurement of the drug is difficult. So, the dried berries of *E. acutipetalum*, (*E. tsjeriam-cottam*), closely allied to the former, and a common shrub in the plains is often found marketted as *viḍaṅga*. This is reported to have properties more or less similar to that of *E. ribes* (Chunekar, 1972: 369; Sharma, 1983: 504). Detailed pharmacognosy and pharmacology of both the plants have been carried out and discussed (Anonymous, 1982: 1046–1057). Rheede has illustrated both under the names *Poovalli* (Hort. Malab. 7: 79. t. 42. 1688 and *Tsjeriam-cottam* (Hort. Malab. 5: 21–22. t. 11. 1685) respectively. The two plants can be identified as follows.

Embelia ribes *Burm. f.* **(Myrsinaceae)** (Fig. 252)
E. glandulifera Wight.

Climbing shrubs; leaves simple, alternate, bifarious, narrowly elliptic to lanceolate, obtusely acute, 4.5–9 × 2–3 cm, chartaceous with scattered, minute, sunken glands; flowers small, white or greenish white in terminal or axillary panicled spikes; calyx 5-lobed; corolla puberulous; stamens 5, exserted; fruits globose, 4 mm across.

Distribution: The plant is found in N. Circars, hills of Vizagapatam, W. Ghats, in all districts, in evergreen forests at elevations upto about 4,000 ft. Distributed also in Sri Lanka, Malaya and S. China

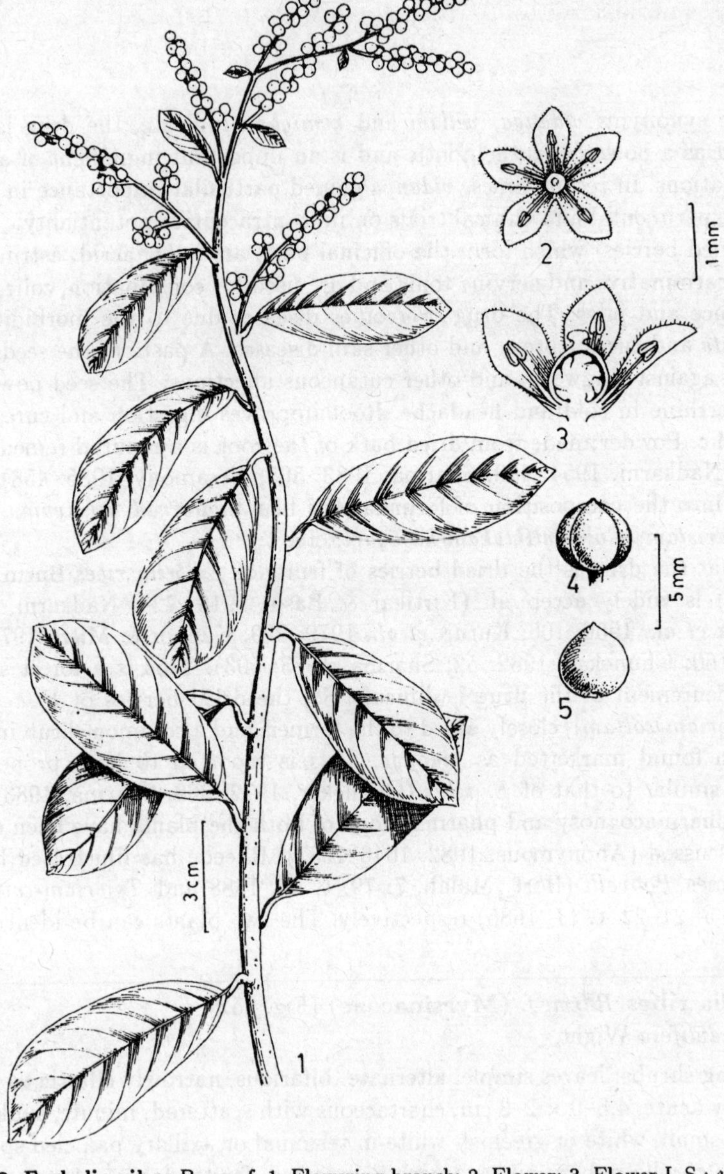

Figure 252: Embelia ribes Burm. f. 1, Flowering branch; 2, Flower; 3, Flower L.S.; 4, Fruit; 5, Seed.

Embelia acutipetalum *(Lam. ex Hassk.) S.M. & M.R. Almeida* **(Myrsinaceae)**

E. tsjeriam-cottam A.DC. (Fig. 253)

E. robusta Roxb.

E. basaal (Roem. & Schult.) A.DC.

Erect, shrub; leaves simple, alternate, broadly elliptic to obovate, cuneate, abruptly acuminate, dentate, upto 14 × 6.5 cms, green above, pale and reticulate beneath; flowers greenish white in axillary simple racemes; petals papillose within; stamens exserted, orbicular, mucronate, glandular on the back; fruits red.

Distribution: The plant grows in most deciduous forest and in plains in the districts in the circars and Deccan; along W. Ghats upto about 3,000 ft.

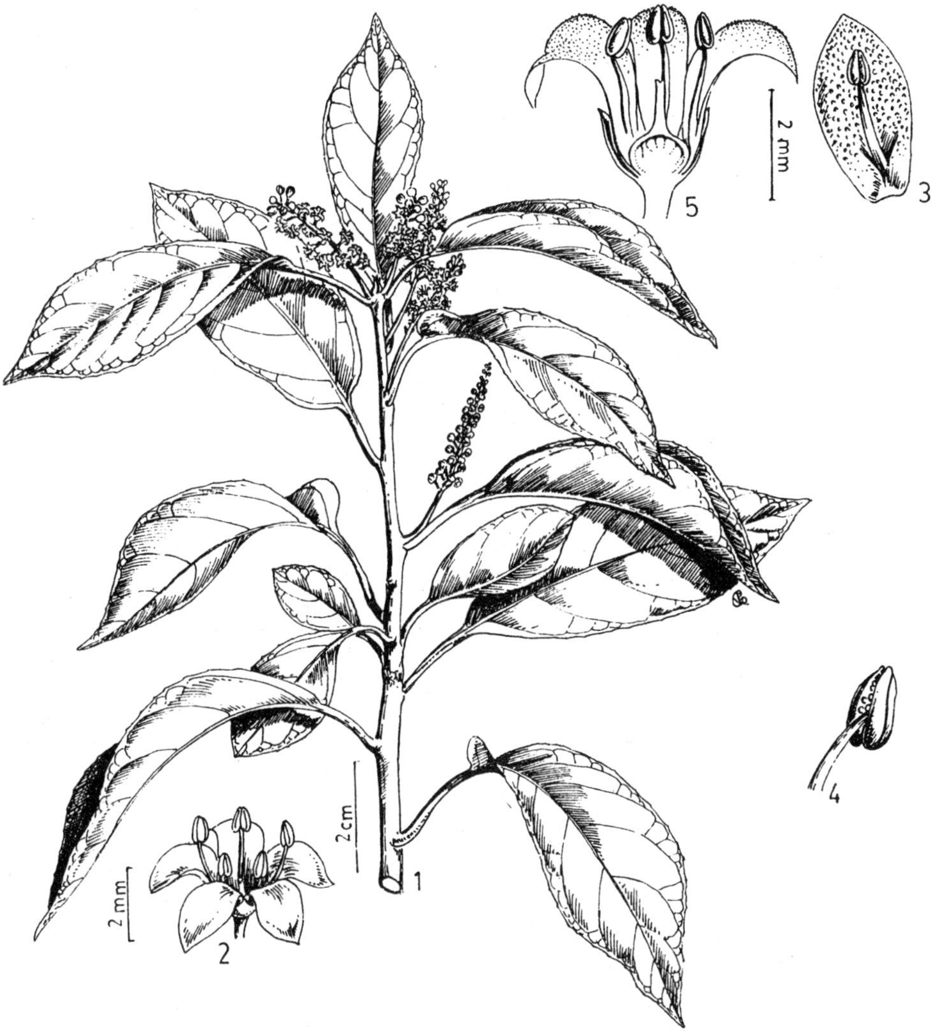

Figure 253: **Embelia acutipetalum** (Hassk.) S.M. & M.R. Almeida. 1, Twig; 2, Flower; 3, A stamen and a petal; 4, A single stamen; 5, Flower L.S.

Note: Fruits of *Embelia ribes* were found to have anthelmintic property (Paul and Vatsa, 1980). The antifertility effect of Embelin isolated from *Embelia ribes* berries had been clinically proved by Seth *et al.* (1982), Bhargava and Dixit (1985a); Kokate *et al.* (1985) etc. who found it to exhibit antispermatogenic and antiimplantation activity.

VIDĀRĪ (Mal. PĀLMUTUKKU)

Vidāri is an important constituent of many Āyurvēdic formulations and according to the texts, the drug source is the subterranean tubers (*vārāhīkanda, vidārikanda*) of a woody climber (*vṛkṣavalli*) which have the shape of the tusk of a boar (*vārāhī, gṛṣṭi*) or conical and curved like a pitcher (*caṛmakārālukō*) with abundant milky juice (*kṣīravalli, kṣīrakanda, payasvini*). The drug is sweet (*svādukanda*), cooling in action, restorative, aphrodisiac, galactagogue, tonic, diuretic and demulcent. It promotes strength and complexion, improves voice, promotes breast milk and semen, overcomes vitiated *pitta* and *vāta* and cures burning sensation. The drug is recommended in all cases of general debility and rheumatism (Aiyer & Kolammal, 1962. 5: 34–35). The important preparations using the drug are *Vidāryādi ghṛtaṃ, Daśamūlariṣṭaṃ, Cyavanapṛāśaṃ*, etc.

Āyurvēdic texts mention two varieties of this drug and attribute different synonyms and virtues to them. They are (1) *vidāri* (also called *svādukanda, kṛōṣṭṛī, sṛgālika*, etc.) and *kṣīravidāri* (also called *kṣīravalli, payasvini, ikṣugandhā*, etc.). Kerala physicians also recognise these two varieties under the vernacular names *mutukku* or *karimutukku* and *pālmutukku* respectively. They differ by the copious milky sap in the tubers of the latter, which is preferred in medicine.

The botanical identity of these drugs has been a matter of debate. Most authors have equated *vidāri* with *Pueraria tuberosa* (Papilionaceae) and *kṣīravidari* with *Ipomoea* (Convolvulaceae) (Anonymous, 1978a: 256; 246; Chunekar, 1982: 388; Sharma, 1983: 738–739).

Kerala physicians also accept *Ipomoea mauritiana*, locally called *pālmutukku* as the plant source of *kṣīravidāri*. Studies on the market samples in Kerala reveal that in addition to *Ipomoea mauritiana*, the large spherical tubers of *Adenia hondaḷa* (Passifloraceae) which is known as *mutukku* or *karimutukku* in vernacular are also sold in the market under the name *vidāri*. That this has been in practice, at least since the seventeenth century, is obvious from Rheede's account of these drugs (Hort. Malab. 8: 39–40. t. 20. 1688 *"Modecca"* & 11: 101–102. t. 49. 1692. *"Palmodecca"*). The tubers of *Adenia hondala* are reported to be poisonous and it may be an adulterant or an unauthorised substitute.

More interestingly, a market survey made by Chaudhuri *et al.* (1981) and Nair *et al.* (1983) in Gujarat, Karnataka and Tamil Nadu revealed that the decorticated stem of *Cycas circinalis*, a gymnosperm, is being marketted there as *vidāri*.

The three most widely used plants as source of this drug can be identified as follows.

Ipomoea mauritiana *Jacq.* **(Convolvulaceae)** (Fig. 254)
Convolvulus paniculatus Linn.
Ipomoea paniculata (Linn.) *R. Br.*
Ipomoea digitata auct. non Linn.

Large, glabrous twining shrub with large tuberous roots; leaves simple, alternate,

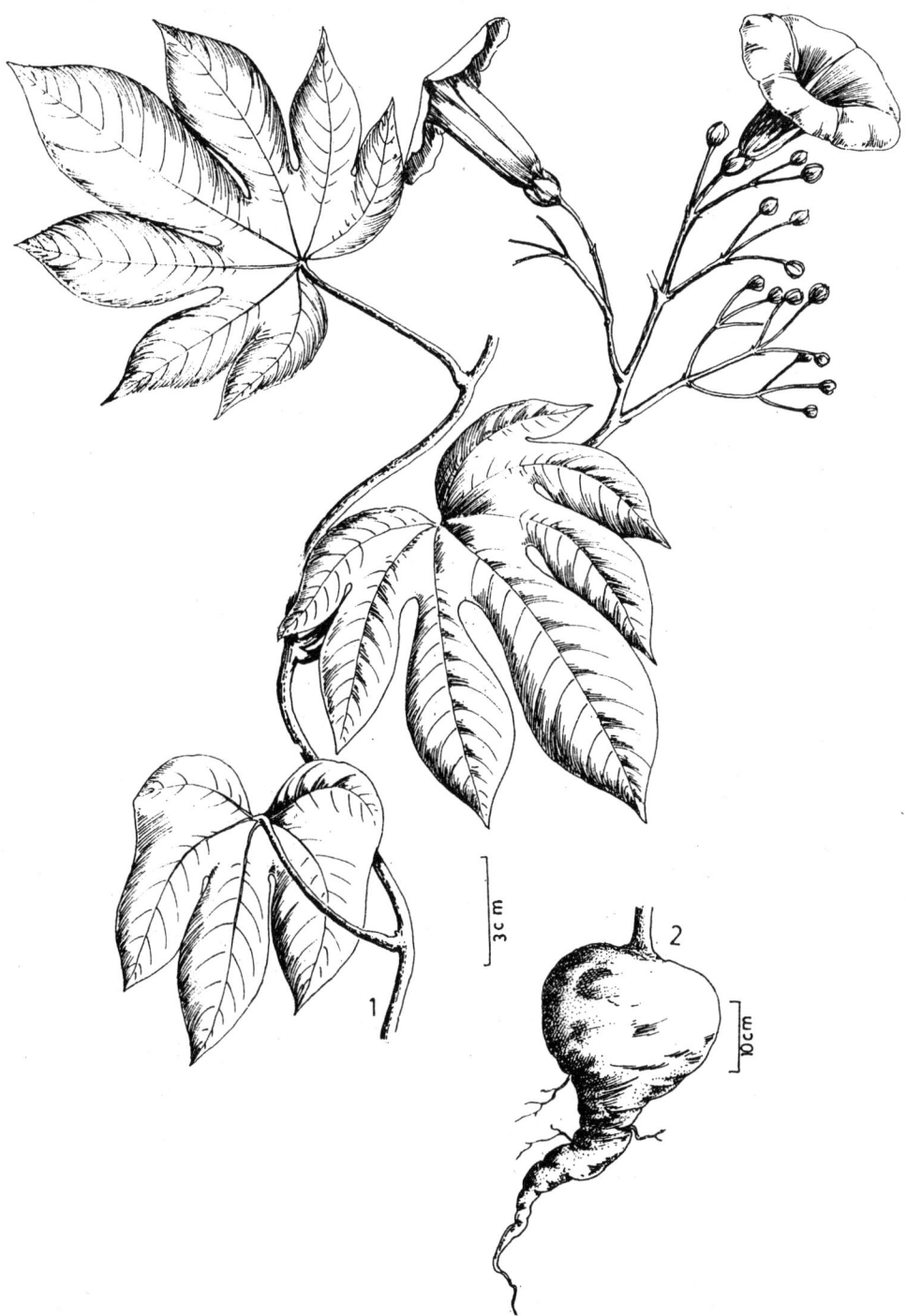

Figure 254: Ipomoea mauritiana Jacq. 1, Habit; 2, Root tuber.

long-petioled, palmately 5–7 lobed, 12–15 cm across; flowers bisexual, large, rose-purple in long pedunculate, axillary cymes; sepals 5, free, nearly equal, slightly enlarging in fruit; corolla funnel-shaped, pink to purple; stamens 5, included, epipetalous; ovary 4-celled with one ovule in each, style simple with a capitate or 2-lobed stigma; capsule ovoid, 4-celled, 4-seeded; seeds woolly.

Distribution: The plant is distributed throughout India. It is common from Bengal to Assam, Deccan, W. Coast, from South Canara to Travancore, climbing over hedges, thickets and small trees.

Adenia hondala (*Gaertn.*) *de Wilde* **(Passifloraceae)** (Fig. 255)
Granadilla hondala Gaertn.
Adenia palmata Engl.
Modecca palmata Poir.

Tendril climber with large tuberous roots; stem thickened at nodes; leaves simple, alternate, palmately 3–5 lobed, 14 × 10 cms, glabrous with two discoid glands at the base of the lamina and one on each sinus between the lobes; stipules hard and horn-like; flowers creamy yellow, unisexual, in axillary monoecious cymes; calyx tube campanulate, lobes 4–5; petals 4–5 attached to the base of the calyx tube. Male flowers: stamens 4–5, filaments united into a cup below, anthers long, ovary rudimentary; Female flowers: staminodes 4–5, ovary subsessile, ovules numerous attached to parietal placenta; fruit a 3-valued capsule, 5 cms long.

Distribution: The plant is found in the hills of Carnatic, Western Ghats and W. Coast.

Pueraria tuberosa (*Willd.*) *DC.* **(Papilionaceae)** (Fig. 256)
Hedysarum tuberosum Roxb. ex. Willd.

Lianae with large, tuberous roots; leaves pinnately 3-foliolate, leaflets broadly ovate, inequilateral, to 8 × 5 cm; flowers pale violet in axillary panicles, usually appear when the plant is leafless; calyx tube campanulate, lobes ovate tomentose; corolla papilionaceous, exserted, petals clawed; stamens diadelphous, filaments incurved; ovary subsessile, oblong, angular, ovules many, style incurred, stigma capitate; pods upto 8 cm long, covered with bristly hairs.

Distribution: The plant grows in the hill forests of N. Circars, Deccan and W. Ghats upto about 3,000 ft down to Travancore.

Note: Pattanshetty *et al.* (1983) have made comparative pharmacognostic studies of *Pueraria tuberosa, Cycas circinalis* and *Ipomoea mauritiana* equated with this drug by various practitioners.

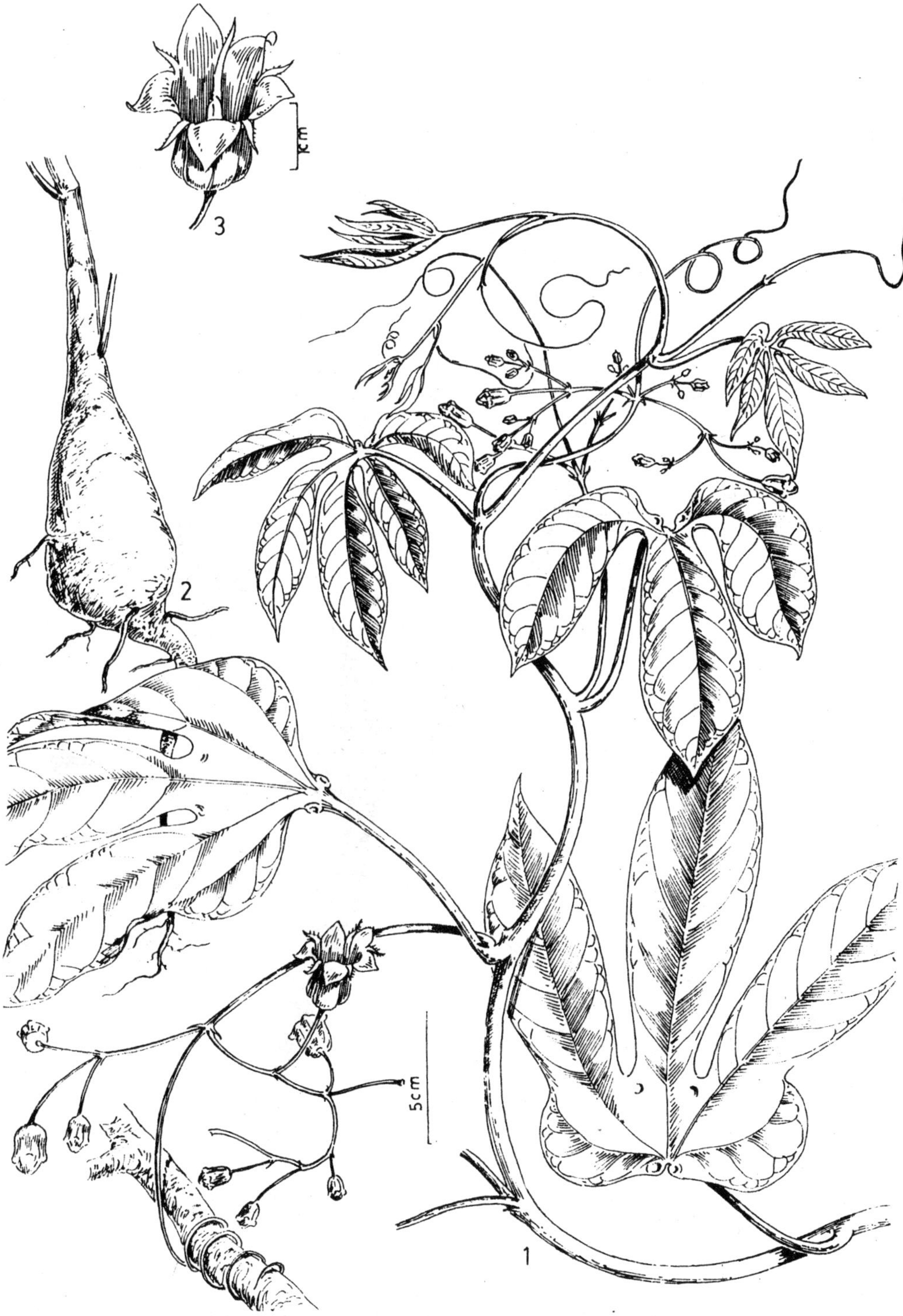

Figure 255: Adenia hondala (Gaertn.) de Wilde. 1, Habit; 2, Root tuber; 3, Flower.

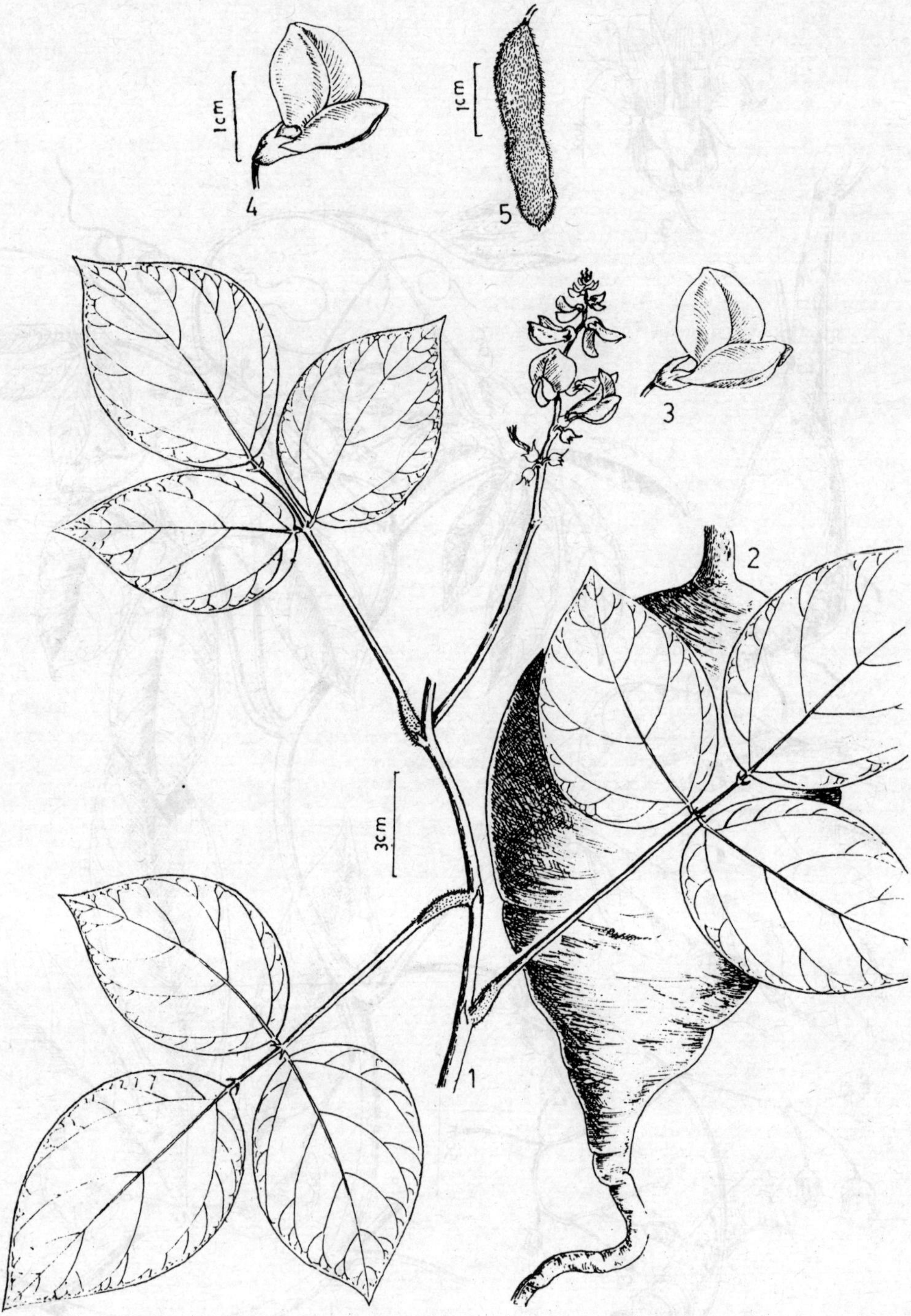

Figure 256: **Pueraria tuberosa** (Willd.) DC. 1, Flowering twig; 2, Root tuber; 3–4, Flowers; 5, Pod.

VILVAḤ (Mal. KŪVAḶAM)

Vilva is considered as an auspicious (*maṅgalya, atimaṅgalya*) tree by the Hindus. All parts of the plant like root, bark, leaves and fruits are highly medicinal. The root is one of the ingredients of the group *daśamūla*, the ten roots, used in Āyurvēda. *Vilva* is astringent, cooling, carminative, laxative, restorative, febrifuge and stomachic and is used in colitis, dysentery, diarrhoea, flatulence, difficult micturition, fever, vomiting and colic. The tender fruit is bitter, astringent, antilaxative, digestive and promotes digestion and strength, overcomes *vāta*, colics and diarrhoea (Kolammal, 1978. 2: 61, Kurup *et al.*, 1979: 42) *Daśamūla-kaṭutrayādi kaṣāyaṃ*, *Vilvādi lēhaṃ*, *Asanavilvādi tailaṃ*, *Amṛtāriṣṭaṃ* etc. are some of the preparations using the drug.

Except for the trifoliate nature of the leaves (*triśikha*), the synonyms are not indicative of the identity of the plant. But there is no confusion with regard to the plant source. *Aegle marmelos* (Linn.) Corr. of Rutaceae, known as *kūvaḷaṃ* in vernacular is the accepted source of the drug throughout India. (See also Rheede, Hort. Malab. 3: 37–38, t. 37. 1682.)

Aegle marmelos (*Linn.*) *Corr.* **(Rutaceae)** (Fig. 257)

Armed tree, spines axillary, straight, single or paired; leaves alternate, 3-foliolate, leaflets elliptic, lanceolate or oblong-obovate obtuse, terminal one 4.5 × 2.5 cm, lateral ones smaller, glabrous, margin subcrenulate; flowers white, sweet-scented in axillary panicles; calyx tube cupular, lobes 4 or 5; petals 5, white, oblong, thick, gland-dotted, spreading; stamens many, inserted around the disc; ovary ovoid, 10-celled with many ovules; berry ovoid, 8 × 6 cm, woody; seeds many.

Distribution: The plant is found throughout India. Also reported from Burma, Indochina, Baluchistan.

Note: The pharmacognosy of the root bark and stem bark of *Aegle marmelos* had been studied in detail by Prakash and Prasad (1969). The hypoglycaemic activity of the root bark of *Aegle marmelos* has been clinically proved by Vyas *et al.* (1979) and Karunanayake *et al.* (1984).

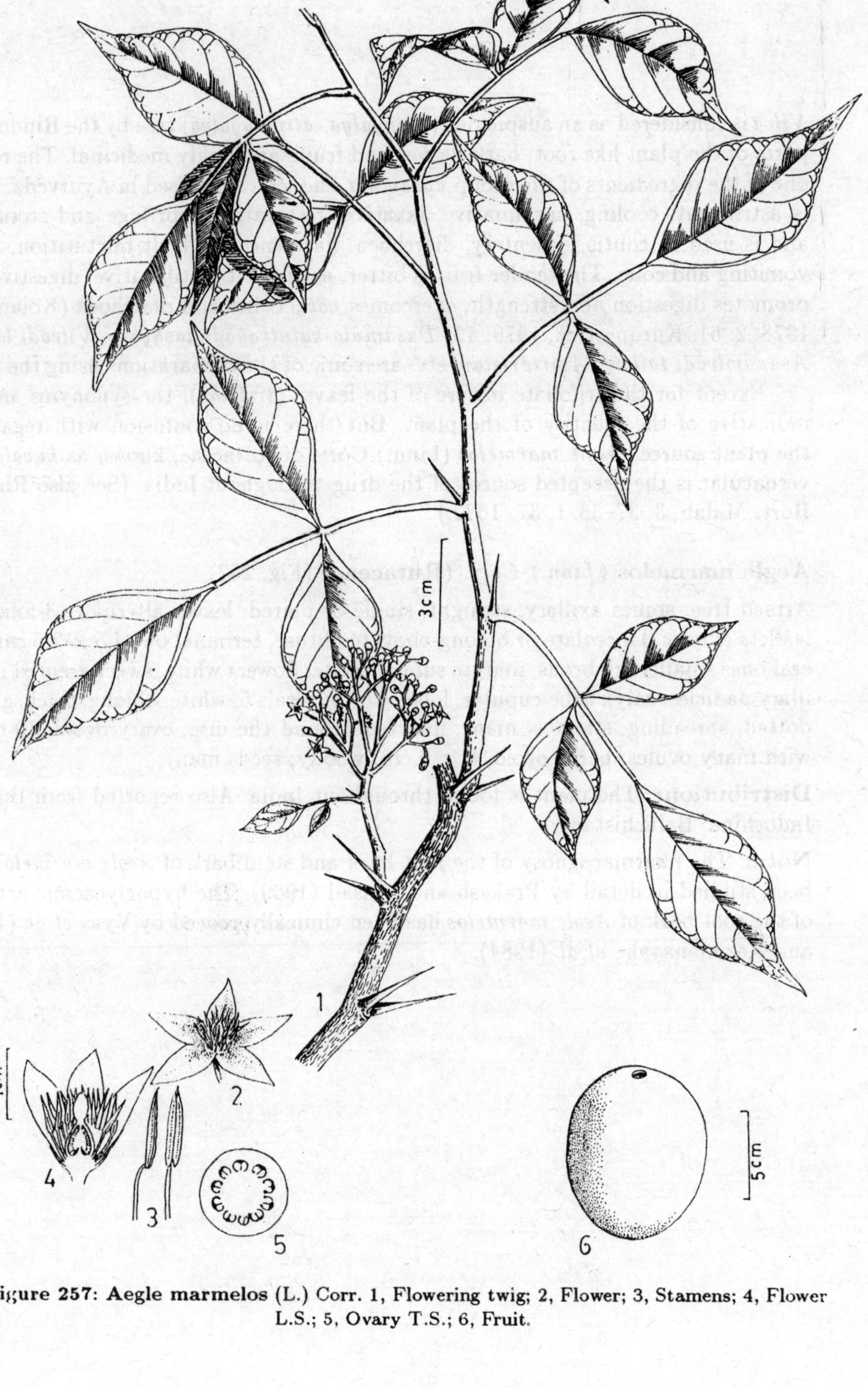

Figure 257: Aegle marmelos (L.) Corr. 1, Flowering twig; 2, Flower; 3, Stamens; 4, Flower L.S.; 5, Ovary T.S.; 6, Fruit.

VIṢĀṆIKĀ (Mal. ĀṬṬUKOṬṬAPPĀLA)

The drug is reported to cure cough, dyspnoea, ulcers, *pitta, kapha* and pain in the eyes. The fruits are bitter, carminative and used in leprosy, diabetes, bronchitis, worms, ulcers and poisons (Chunekar, 1982: 443). Suśruta describes the drug as a destroyer of *madhumēha* (glycosuria) and other urinary disorders. Root has long been reputed as a remedy for snake-bite. Leaves triturated and mixed with castor oil are applied to swollen glands and to enlargement of internal viscera as the liver and spleen (Nadkarni, 1954: 598–599). According to Sharma (1983: 105) the drug is used to strengthen the function of heart, cure jaundice, piles, urinary calculi, difficult micturition and intermittent fevers. The drug enters into the composition of preparations like *Ayaskṛti, Varuṇādi kaṣāyaṃ, Varuṇādi ghṛtaṃ, Mahākalyāṇaka ghṛtaṃ*, etc.

The synonyms do not indicate any morphological feature of the plant except that the fruits resemble the horns of sheep, (*mēṣaśṛṅgi*).

Mēṣaśṛṅgī is equated with *Gymnema sylvestre* R. Br. (Asclepiadaceae) by most of the authors on Indian materia medica (Kirtikar & Basu, 1918: 823, Vaidya K.M., 1936: 10, Nadkarni, 1954: 596; Chopra *et al.*, 1956: 129; Chunekar, 1982: 443; Sharma, 1983: 103). However, this plant is locally called *cakkarakkolli* or *madhunāśini* because of the property of its leaves to neutralise the taste of sugar. Kerala physicians do not use this plant as the source of the drug *mēṣaśṛṅgī*.

The term *mēṣaśṛṅga* is included in the *Sālasāradi gaṇa* of Suśruta (S.S.Su. 38. 12). All the plants given in this group of drugs or *gaṇa* are big trees and so some people consider *mēṣaśṛṅga* also as a tree different from *mēṣaśṛṅgī*. *Mēṣaśṛṅga* has been identified as a tree very much like *putrañjīva* (cf. Vaidya Bapalal, 1982: 50). The repeated reference to the use of its bark and flowers also supports the fact that it should be a tree species contrary to the general belief that it is a climber (Singh & Chunekar, 1972: 321). The drug *mēṣaśṛṅgi* has been included in *Varuṇādi gaṇa* by Suśruta, which includes trees, shrubs, herbs and climbers. Based on these reasons, people consider *mēṣaśṛṅga* and *mēṣaśṛṅgi* as two different drugs, the former equated with *Dolichandrone falcata* (Bignoniaceae), the pods of which are like the horns of sheep as the name implies and the latter with *Gymnema sylvestre* belonging to Asclepiadaceae (Vaidya Bapalal, 1982: 51, 52). Moreover, this tree is known as *mēḍhāśṛṅgi* in Maratti and Gujarati, meaning the horn of a sheep.

Suśruta mentions *mēṣaśṛṅgī* and *ajaśṛṅgī* separately in his *Varuṇādi gaṇa* and so they cannot be considered as synonyms but as two different drugs having similar medicinal properties. The inclusion of *ajaśṛṅgi* in the *Vallīpañcamūla* group (S.S.Su 38. 72) indicates that it is a twiner-climber and not a tree species like *mēṣaśṛṅga* (Singh & Chunekar, 1972: 322) Vāgbhaṭa has replaced both of these by the term *viṣāṇika* in his *Varuṇādi gaṇa*.

According to *Pāṭhya* commentator (Vol. 1: 82) and Parameśwara (Vol. II: 72) both *mēṣaśṛṅgi* and *viṣāṇika* are *āṭṭukoṭṭappāla*. *Bhiṣagārya* describes two varieties of *mēṣaśṛṅgi (Abhidhānamañjari*, p. 71. Nos. 221 & 222) calling them as *āṭṭukoṭṭappāla*, the smaller variety and *valiya āṭṭukoṭṭappāla*, the larger variety respectively (cf. Mooss, 1980: 53). This distinction is, however, not in vogue in Kerala, nor do the Kerala physicians make a distinction between *mēṣaśṛṅga* and *mēṣaśṛṅgī*.

In practice, in Kerala, different plants are used as the source of the drug, but *Dolichandrone falcata* is seldom found used. Instead, *Vallaris solanacea* (Apocynaceae), *Cryptolepis buchanani* (Periplocaceae), *Aristolochia bracteolata* (*Aristolochiaceae*) are all used in different places as the source of *āṭṭukoṭṭappāla*.

The various plant sources of the drug can be identified as follows.

Vallaris solanacea (*Roth*) *Kuntze* **(Apocynaceae)** (Fig. 258)

Large twining shrub; leaves simple, opposite, elliptic-oblong or lanceolate, acuminate, 8.5 × 2.5 cm, glabrous; flowers creamy white in axillary cymes; calyx cupular; corolla rotate, tube very short; stamens 5, attached at the throat of the tube, anthers connate by their connectives around the stigma; follicles linear, 12 cm long; seeds oblong, beaked at one end with a tuft of silky white coma.

Distribution: South and South East Asia. In India the plant is common in southern part in dry forests. It is also frequently cultivated in hedges and in gardens along the Malabar coast.

Cryptolepis buchanani *Roem. & Schult.* **(Asclepiadaceae)** (Fig. 217)

Glabrous twining shrub; leaves elliptic-oblong, shortly acuminate, 18 × 6.5 cms, lateral veins close and parallel, green above, glaucous beneath; calyx lobes 5, lanceolate; corona scales 5, clavate; pollen masses in pairs, granular; follicles 2, narrowed to the tip, divaricate.

Distribution: India, Sri Lanka, Burma and China. In India, it is distributed throughout the peninsular part. Rheede (Hort. Malab. 9: 17–18 t. 11. 1689) has described this plant under the vernacular name, *Katupal-valli*.

Aristolochia bracteolata *Ham.* **(Aristolochiaceae)** (Fig. 259)

A. bracteata Retz.

Prostrate or diffuse perennial herb; leaves simple, alternate, broadly ovate-obtuse or reniform, cordate at base with a wide sinus, 4.5 × 4.5 cm, 5 nerved from base, glaucous on either side; flowers solitary, axillary; perianth greenish, inflated below, then contracted in a cylindrical tube, expanding terminally in a dilated oblique purple limb; stamens 6, included in the dilated part of the perianth tube; ovary inferior, style columnar, thick, 6-lobed; fruit capsular, 12-ribbed, oblong-ellipsoid; seeds flat, covered with round glands on one side.

Distribution: India, Sri Lanka, Arabia and tropical Africa. In India the plant grows in N. Circars, Deccan and Carnatic; on dry, especially black cotton soil.

Dolichandrone falcata (*DC.*) *Seemann* **(Bignoniaceae)** (Fig. 260)

Spathodea falcata Wallich ex DC.

Small, deciduous tree; leaves opposite, pinnate, leaflets usually 7, orbicular-obovate or obcordate, 2–3 × 2–3.25 cm, charataceous, glabrescent to thinly pubescent on either side, base rounded to acute, apex truncate, shortly acute; flowers white in terminal panicles; calyx spathaceous; stamens 4; capsule compressed, falcate, 20–30 × 1.5 cm.

Distribution: Peninsular India.

Note: Pharmacognostical studies on *Vallaris solanacea* had been carried out by Wahi *et al.* (1980). Dhawan and Patnaik (1985) have found that the plant contains several new cardiovascular glycosides including O-acetyl solanoside.

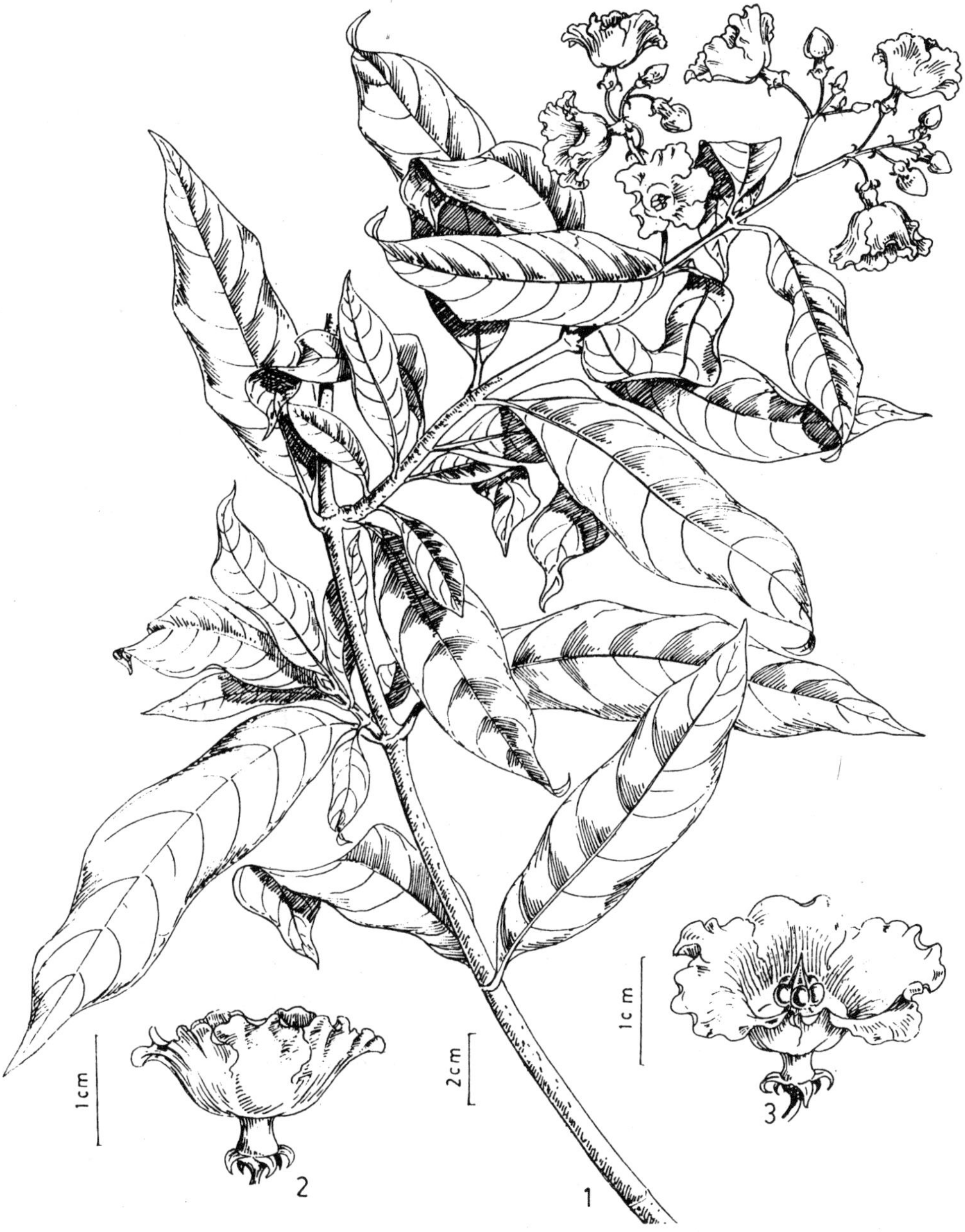

Figure 258: **Vallaris solanacea** (Roth) Kuntze. 1, Flowering twig; 2–3, Flowers.

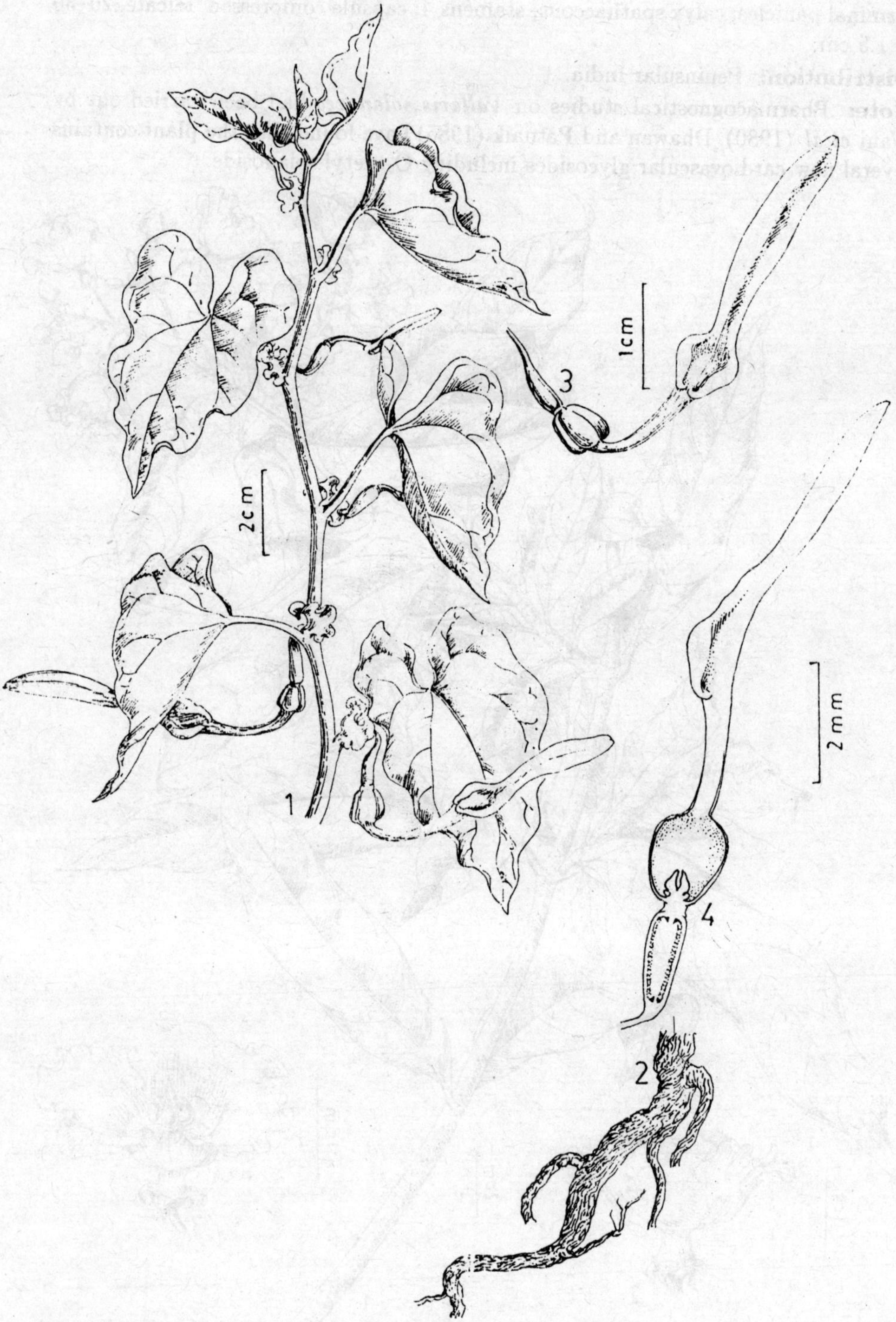

Figure 259: Aristolochia bracteolata Ham. 1, Habit; 2, Roots; 3, Flower; 4, Flower L.S.

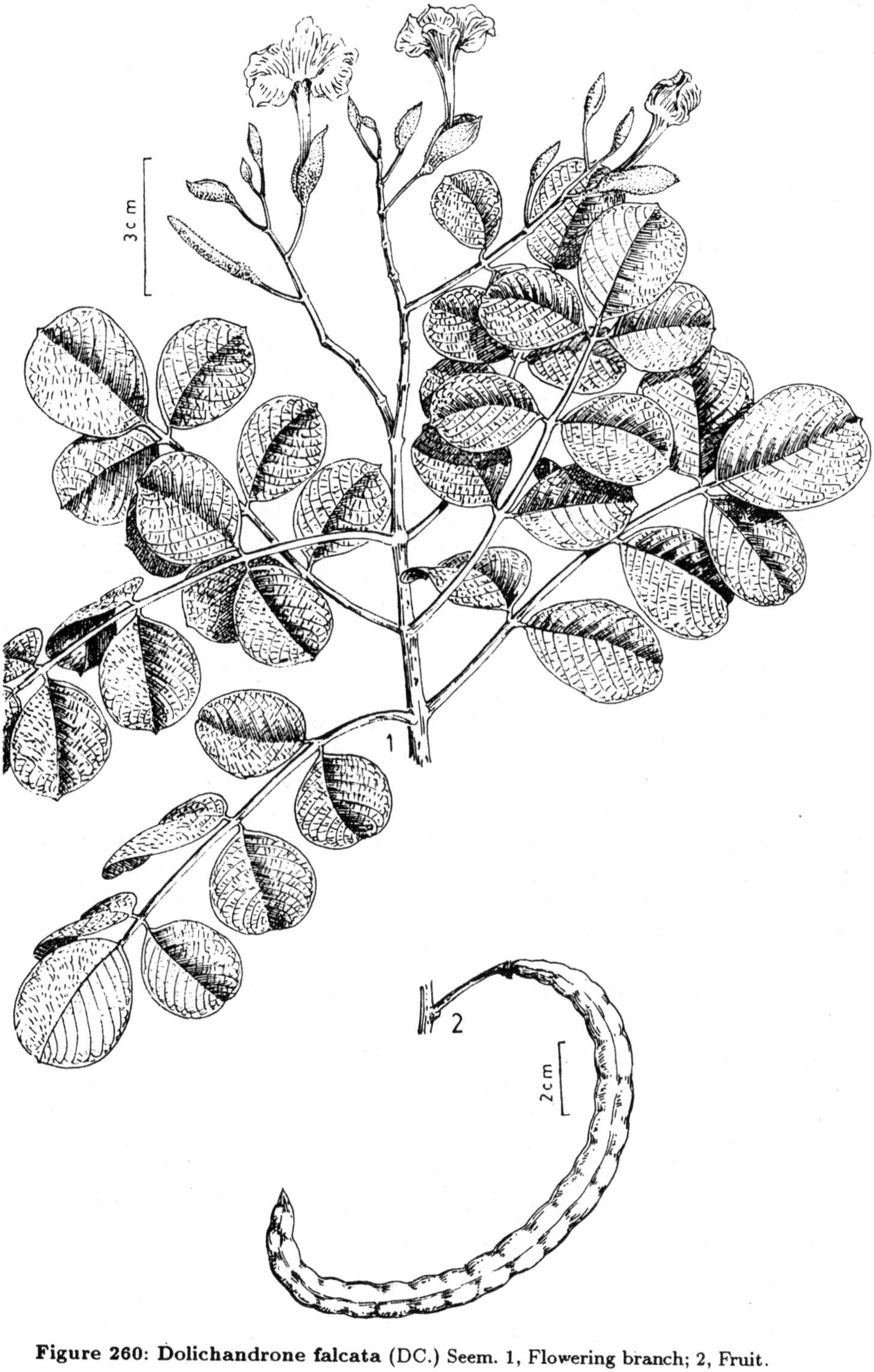

Figure 260: **Dolichandrone falcata** (DC.) Seem. 1, Flowering branch; 2, Fruit.

VIṢṆUKṚĀNTĀ (Mal. VIṢṆUKṚĀNTI)

The drug is considered a specific for all kinds of fevers. The entire plant is used in medicine. It is acrid and bitter in taste. It alleviates diseases due to the derangement of *vāta* and ***kapha*** and is considered a powerful brain stimulant toning up the intellectual prowess, and an aphrodisiac. The drug is also useful in nervous debility and dysentery. It's flowers are reported to be good for uterine bleeding and roots, for gastric and dueodinal ulcers (Aiyer & Kolammal, 1963. 6: 1; Mooss, 1978: 95). The important preparations are *Mṛtasañjīvani, Āraṇyatulasīmūlādi kaṣāyaṃ*, etc.

According to the texts, the plant blossoms all round the year (*āsphotā*) and has leaves which resemble the young ones of a rat (*girikarṇī*). The plant is believed to have great potency to cure ailments, bestowed by *Viṣṇu* (*viṣṇukrāntā*) (Aiyer & Kolammal, 1963. 6: 1).

There is some confusion, regarding the identity of the drug. *Bhāvaprakāśa Nighaṇṭu* treats *viṣṇukrāntā* as the same as *aparājitā* which is later equated with *Clitoria ternatea* L. of Papilionaceae (Chunekar, 1982: 342), the *śaṅkhapuṣpī* of Kerala physicians. *Dhanvantarinighaṇṭu* identifies *viṣṇukrāntā* as the white-flowered variety of *śaṅkhapuṣpī* whereas *Rājanighaṇṭu* considers it as the blue-flowered variety. Vaidya (1936: 543) is also of opinion that of the three varieties of *śaṅkhapuṣpī* viz. white-flowered, red-flowered and blue-flowered, the blue-flowered is called *viṣṇukrāntā* (Mooss, 1978: 73).

In Kerala, however, *viṣṇukrāntā* and *śaṅkhapuṣpī* are treated as separate drugs, the former being equated with *Evolvulus alsinoides* L. (Convolvulaceae) and the latter with *Clitoria ternatea* L. of Papilionaceae (see also notes under *śaṅkhapuṣpī*).

Two varieties i.e. the blue-flowered and the white-flowered, having similar properties, are mentioned in the texts. In Kerala, the blue-flowered *Evolvulus alsinoides* alone is used as *viṣṇukrānti*. That has been the accepted practice in Kerala is evident from the fact that Rheede describes and portrays this under the name *Vistnu-clandi* (Hort. Malab. 11.131—132, t. 64. 1692).

Evolvulus alsinoides (*Linn.*) *Linn.* **(Convolvulaceae)** (Fig. 261)
Convolvulus alsinoides Linn.

Diffuse, densely hispid, perennial herb with a woody root-stock and many spreading branches; leaves alternate, broadly ovate or elliptic-acute to 2 × 1 cms, hairy on both sides; flowers blue, solitary on axillary filiform peduncles; calyx of 5 subequal lanceolate, densely hairy sepals; corolla rotate, limb plicate and subentire; stamens 5, epipetalous, filaments filiform, anthers oblong; ovary superior, 2-celled, 4-ovuled, styles 2, each cleft into two linear branches ending in simple stigmas; fruit a globose 4-valved capsule.

Distribution: A pantropical species, this plant is found wild in most parts of India in the plains. It grows on open ground, by roadsides, grassy lands and other waste places.

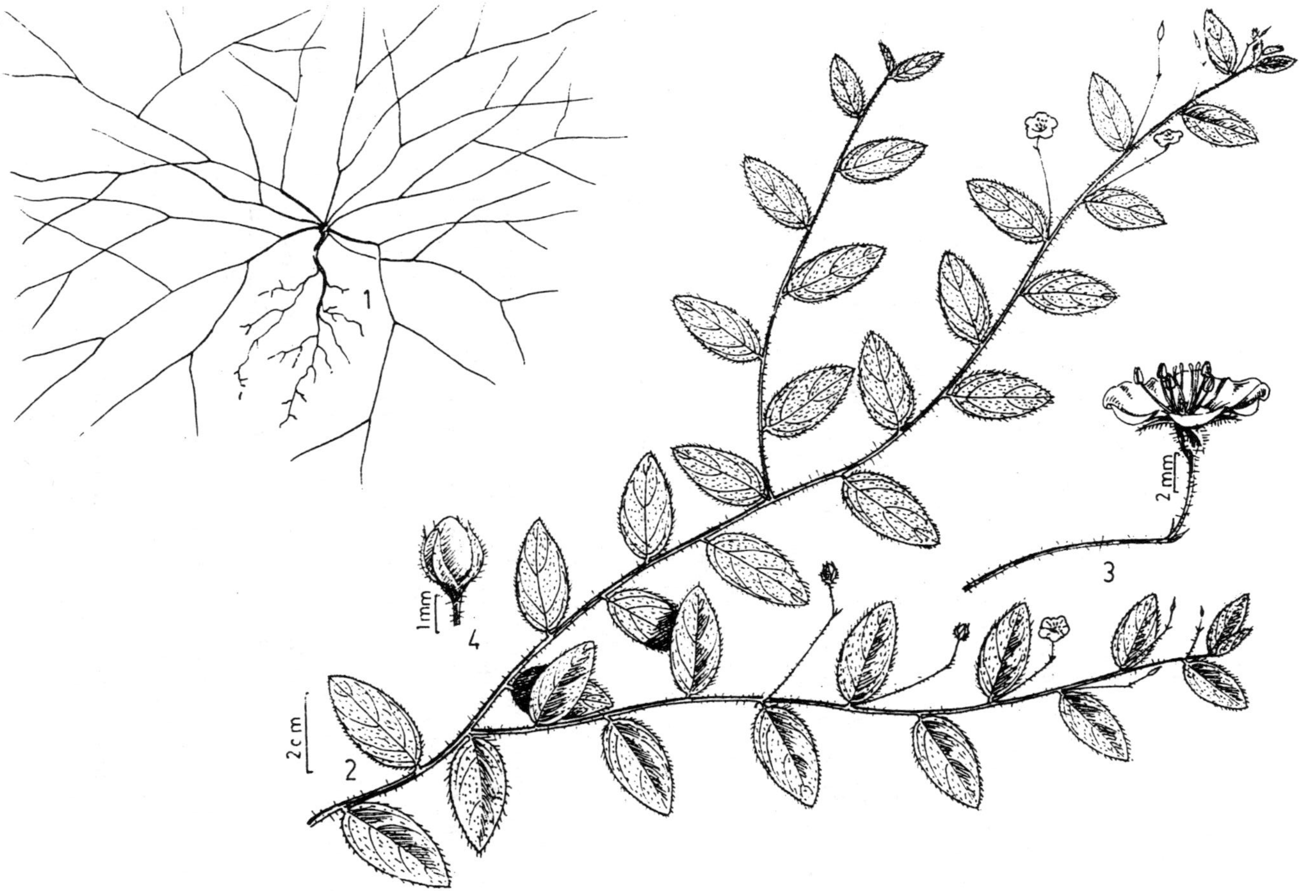

Figure 261: **Evolvulus alsinoides** (L.) L. 1, Habit (diagrammatic); 2, Flowering branch; 3, Flower; 4, Fruit.

VṚŚCIKĀḶĪ (Mal. TĒḶKKAṬA)

The drug is known by the local name *tēḷkkaṭa* which is the literal translation of the Sanskrit word *vṛścikāḷi* which means the tail of the scorpion. It is a constituent of the *Vidāryādi gaṇa* and *Aṛkādi gaṇa* of Vāgbhaṭa. The drug is reported to be bitter and that it pacifies all the three morbidities, cleanses wounds and is useful in worms, skin diseases, poisoning, asthma, cough, anaemia, insanity and epilepsy (Singh & Chunekar, 1972: 377). The roots which are errhine, enter into the composition of preparations like *Vidāryāsavaṃ, Vidāryādi ghṛtaṃ, Vidāryādilēhaṃ*, etc.

Commentaries on Āyurvēdic materia medica have identified the plant source of this drug differently. *Ḍalhaṇa,* the commentator on Suśrutha Samhita (S.S.Su. 38.4) has described it as a climber with leaves resembling those of *pāṭha*, spinous fruits looking like the horns of sheep (*mēṣaśṛṅga*) and bunches of white flowers. Singh & Chunekar (1972: 377) and Vaidya Bapalal (1982: 287) have opined that this description is most appropriate for *Pergularia extensa* (Jacq.) N.E. Brown (Now *P. daemia* (Forsk.) Choiv.) of Asclepiadaceae. However, in Kerala, this plant, commonly known as *vēlipparutti*, is used as a different drug *kurūṭaka* and is described elsewhere.

This has also been equated with *durālabha (Tragia involucrata* L., Euphorbiaceae) by many others, despite the fact that the name *vṛścikāḷi* does not figure anywhere in the verses pertaining to *durālabha* (see Kirtikar & Basu, 1918: 1173; Vaidya, K.M. 1936: 532; Nadkarni, 1954: 1226; Chopra *et al.*, 1956: 246). This is the view held in the Ayurvedic Formulary of India also (see Anonymous, 1978a: 256). Kerala physicians, however, consider *durālabha* (described elsewhere) and *vṛścikāḷi* to be different drugs.

Pāṭhya commentator and Parameśwara equate *vṛścikāḷi* with *tēḷkkaṭa* or *tēkkaṭa* of Kerala physicians (both meaning the same thing). This has been identified as *Heliotropium indicum* L. of Boraginaceae (Mooss, 1980: 31). The inflorescence of this plant, a scorpioid cyme, very closely resembles the tail of the scorpion. Rheede (Hort. Malab. 10: 95–96. t. 48. 1690) has described it under the name *Bena-patsja*, meaning a summer herb.

Our field studies have revealed that in Kerala, another species of the same genus namely *Heliotropium keralens* Siv. & Mani. often grows intermixed with *Heliotropium indicum* and it is also used as the source of the drug. The two can be distinguished by flower colour, the former having white flowers while the latter has pink flowers (see also Sivarajan & Indu, 1985).

The important characters of the two species are described below.

Heliotropium indicum *Linn.* **(Boraginaceae)** (Fig. 262)

Branched herb, stem and branches hirsute; leaves simple, long-petioled, ovate, acute or obtuse, to 14.5 × 6.8 cms base narrowed into the petiole, margin undulate, sparsely strigose along nerves on either side; flowers small, pink in long terminal spikate, scorpioid cymes; calyx lobes 5, linear-lanceolate, sparsely scabrous with-

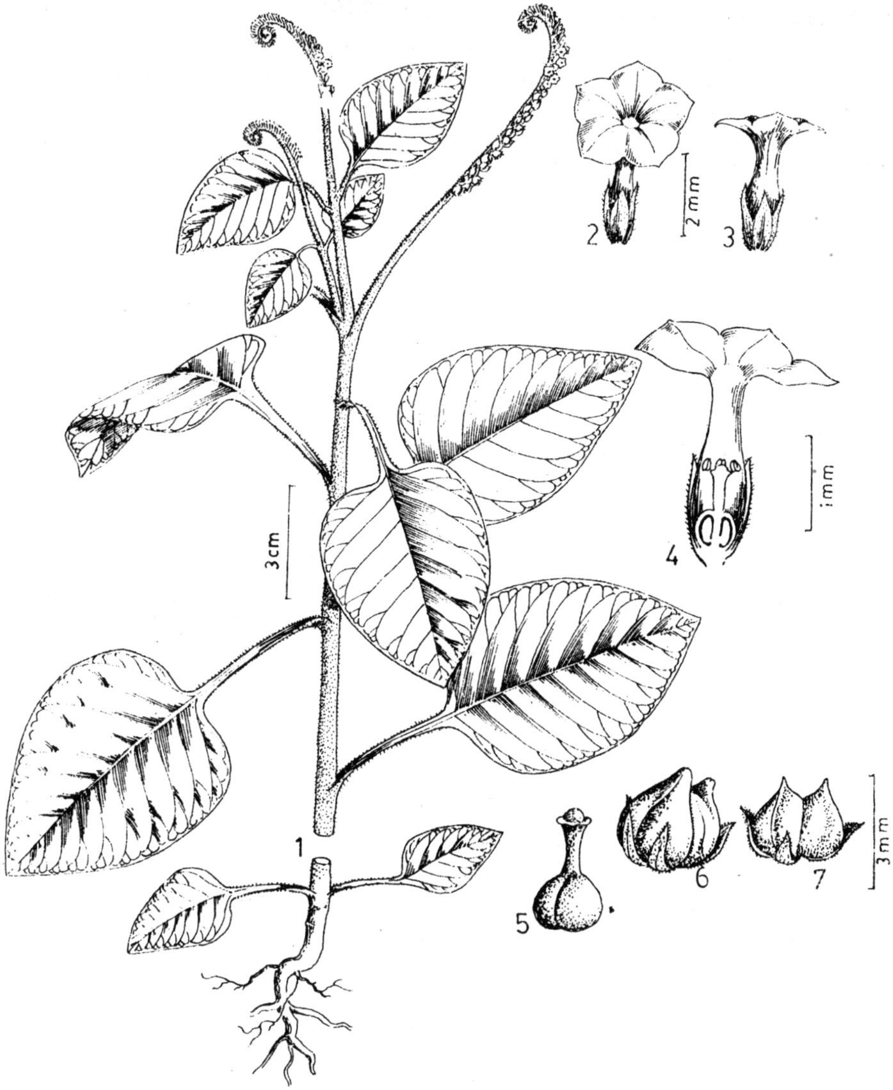

Figure 262: Heliotropium indicum L. 1, Habit; 2–3, Flowers; 4, Flower L.S.; 5, Pistil; 6–7, Fruits.

out; corolla salver-shaped, tube much exceeding the calyx, minutely hairy, lobes 5, broadly ovate, obtuse; stamens 5, anthers lanceolate; ovary globose, style 0.7 mm, disciform above, stigma obtuse; nutlets combined in pairs, ribbed prominently.

Distribution: A common weed in sandy fields and waste places in all plains districts in India. It is also reported from Africa, tropical Himalaya, India, Burma, east to W & S. China, Malesia and America.

Heliotropium keralens *Siv. & Mani.* **(Boraginaceae)**

Erect herb; leaves ovate, obtuse or acute; flowers white in terminal, spicate, scorpioid cymes; corolla tube as long as or slightly longer than the calyx, with long, setose, bulbous-based hairs outside; fruit ribbed, 2-partite at the tip.

Distribution: A very common weed in the paddy fields and sandy low lands in Kerala, often found growing intermixed with *H. indicum*.

REFERENCES

Adwankar, M.K. and Chitnis, M.P. 1982. *In vivo* anticancer activity of RC-18, a plant isolate from *Rubia cordifolia* against a spectrum of experimental tumour models. *Chemotherapy* 28(4): 291–293.

Adwankar, M.K., Chitnis, M.P., Khandalekar, D.D. and Bhadsavale, C.G. 1979. Anticancer activity of the extracts of *Rubia cordifolia* L. *Ind. Jour. Exp. Biol.* 18(1): 102.

Afaq, S.H., Khan, M.M.A., Sumiullah and Alfridi, M.M.R.K. 1985. Predicting solasodine content in fruits of Mako (*Solanum nigrum*) by leaf nitrogen estimation. *Jour. Res. Ind. Med.* (Jan–June): 13–15.

Agrawal, S.S. 1981. Some CNS effects of *Hydrocotyle asiatica* L. *Jour. Res. Ayur. Siddha* 11(2): 144–149.

Aguye, A., Sannusi, A., Tayo, R.A.A. and Dhusnurmath, S.R. 1985. Acute toxicity studies with *Jatropha curcas* L. *Human Toxicol.* 5(4): 269–274.

Ahmad, J. and Siddique, T.O. 1987. Pharmacognostical and elementological studies on *Curcuma longa. Hamdard Med.* 30(1–2): 113–130.

Aiyer, K.N. and Kolammal, M. 1960–1966. *Pharmacognosy of Ayurvedic drugs*, Trivandrum, Nos. 4–9.

Aiyer, M.N., Namboodiri, A.N. and Kolammal, M. 1957. *Pharmacognosy* of *Ayurvedic drugs*, Trivandrum, No. 3.

Akerole, O., Heywood, V.H. and Synge, H. (Eds.) 1991. *Conservation of Medicinal Plants*, Cambridge.

Akhtar, M.S., Athar, M.A. and Yaqub, M. 1981. Effect of *Momordica charantia* on blood glucose level of normal and alloxan diabetic rabbits. *Planta Med.* 42(3): 205–212.

Alam, K., Susan, T. and Purushothaman, K.K. 1986. Antipyretic activity of *dhatakipushpa* in albino rats. *Arogya Journ. Health Sci.* 12(2): 131–133.

Amalraj, V.A., Velayudhan, K.C. and Abraham, Z. 1991. Threatened Medicinal Plants of Western Ghats. In: *Proc. Symp. on Rare, Endangered and Endemic Plants of Western Ghats* (30–31, Aug. 1991), Thiruvananthapuram.

Anand, K.K., Sharma, M.L., Singh, B. and Ray Ghatak, B.J. 1978. Anti-inflammatory, antipyretic and analgesic properties of bavachinin, a flavone isolated from seeds of *Psoralea corylifolia* L. *Ind. Jour. Exp. Biol.* 16(11): 1216–1217.

Anandakumar, A., Rajendran, V., Balasubramaniam, M. and Muralidharan, R. 1984. *Kutajabija*—its pharmacognosy. *Anc. Sci. Life* 3(4): 203–206.

Anonymous. 1948–1976. *The Wealth of India*, New Delhi.

Anonymous. 1951, 1978. *Pharmacognosy of Ayurvedic drugs.* Trivandrum, Nos. 1 and 2.

Anonymous. 1978 a. *The Ayurvedic Formulary of India*, Delhi.

Anonymous. 1978 b. Management of intestinal amoebiasis by an indigenous drug *kantakikaranja* (*Caesalpinia crista* L.). *Jour. Res. Ind. Med. Yoga & Homeop.* 13(1): 140–142.

Anonymous. 1978 c. Hypocholesterolemic effect of bark of *Pterocarpus marsupium* Roxb. (*Bijaka*): an experimental study. *Jour. Res. Ind. Med. Yoga & Homeop.* 13(1): 137–139.

Anonymous. 1987. *Clinical and experimental studies on the efficacy of 777 oil—Siddha preparation in the treatment of Kalanjagapadai (Psoriasis)*, Madras.

Ansari, M.A. and Prasad, S. 1970. Pharmacognostical studies on roots of *Tribulus terrestris* L. *Jour. Res. Ind. Med.* 4(2): 193–200.

Ansari, M.S., Gupta, R.C. and Prasad, S. 1971. Pharmacognostical studies on *Solanum surattense* Burm. (*Kantakari*) *J. Res. Indian Med.* 6(2) 143–158.

Anshuman, P.S., Singh, K.P. and Aasra, K.G. 1984. Effect of *vardhaman pippali (Piper longum)* on patients with respiratory disorders. *Sachitra Ayurved* 37(1): 47–49.

Antarkar, D.S., Chinwalla, T., Bhat, N. and Vadhya, A.B. 1983. Anti-inflammatory activity of *Rubia cordifolia* L. in rats. *Ind. Jour. Pharmacol.* 15(3): 185–188.

Arora, R.B., Kesar, D.K., Saigal, S.K., Ahmed, J., Roy, S., Ali, T. and Qadri, I.Z. 1987. Development of a drug, *ajmaloon*, from *Rauwolfia serpentina* for hypertension. *Hamdard Med.* 30(1–2): 185–208.

Arora, R.C., Agarwal, N., Arora, S. and Garg, R. 1986. *Acorus calamus*—a lipid lowering agent. *Jour. Res. Edn. Ind. Med.* 5(2): 33–55.

Atal, C.K. and Sethi, P.D. 1962. *Wrightia tinctoria* bark, an adulterant of *kurchi*. *Jour. Pharm. Pharmacol.* 14: 41–45.

Atal, C.K., Bhatia, A.K. and Singh, R.P. 1982. Role of *Woodfordia fruticosa* Kurz. in the preparation of *asavas* and *arishtas*. *Jour. Res. Ayur. Siddha* 3(3 & 4): 193–199.

Atiane, A., Iqbal, M. and Ghouse, A.K.M. 1985. Folk medicinal uses of *Ficus benghalensis* L. and *Punica granatum* L. in northern Uttar Pradesh. *Bull. Med. Ethnobot. Res.* 6(1): 42–46.

Austin, D.A. 1986. Nomenclature of the *Ipomoea nil* complex (Convolvulaceae). *Taxon* 35: 355–358.

Bagi, M.K., Kalyani, G.A., Dennis, T.J., Kumar, A.K. and Kakrani, H.K. 1984. A preliminary pharmacological screening of *Abutilon indicum*: Analgesic property. *Indian Drugs* 22(2): 69–72.

Bambhole, V.D. and Jiddewar, G.G. 1984. Evaluation of *Cyperus rotundus* in the management of obesity and high blood pressure of human subjects. *Nagarjun* 27(5): 110–113.

Bambhole, V.D. and Jiddewar, G.G. 1985. Anti-obesity effect of *Iris versicolor* and *Holoptelia integrifolia*. *Sachitra Ayurved* 37(9): 557–561.

Banu, N., Patel, V., Chansouria, J.P.N., Malhotra, O.P. and Udupa, K.N. 1982. Role of *amalaki (Emblica officinalis) rasayana* in experimental peptic ulcer. *Jour. Res. Edn. Ind. Med.* 1(1): 29–34.

Bhalla, T.N., Gupta, M.B. and Bhargava, K.P. 1971. Anti-inflammatory and biochemical study of *Boerhaavia diffusa*. *Jour. Res. Ind. Med.* 6(1): 11–15.

Bharadwaja, T.N. 1980. Recent advances in our knowledge of the water-fern *Marsilea*. *Aspect. Pl. Sci.* 3: 39–62.

Bhargava, S.K. 1986. Anti-fertility effects of the flavanoids of *Vitex negundo* L. seeds in dogs. *Planta Med. Phytother.* 20(2): 188–198.

Bhargava, S.K., Dixit, V.P. and Khanna, P. 1984. Anti-fertility effect of embelin in female rats. *Fitoterapia* 55(5): 302–304.

Bhargava, S.K. and Dixit, V.P. 1985a. Anti-fertility effects of embelin in female rats. *Planta. Med. Phytother.* 19(1): 29–34.

Bhargava, S.K. and Dixit, V.P. 1985b. Anti-fertility effects of plumbagin in female rats. *Planta Med. Phytother.* 19(1): 29–34.

Bhatnagar, S.K. and Verma, S.K. 1986. Effects of 50% ethanol extract of *Calotropis procera* Ait. f. on ulcers caused by assorted types of carcinoma. *Jour. Econ. Tax. Bot.* 8(2): 489–490.

Bhattacharya, C. 1981. Clinical experiences with *nirgundi (Vitex negundo). Rheumatism* 16(3): 111–117.

Bhattacharya, S.B., Parikh, A.K., Debnath, P.K., Pandey, V.B. and Neogy, N.C. 1973. Pharmacological studies with the alkaloids of *Costus speciosus (kemuka). Jour. Res. Ind. Med.* 8(1): 10–19.

Bisset, N.G. 1972. The Asian species of *Strychnos.* Part I. *Strychnos* as a source of the drug *Lignum colubrinum. Lloydia* 35: 95–116.

Boyuan, Hu Ji Yaoyuan. 1986. A research on anti-carcinogenic activation of *Acorus calamus* of alpha asarone on human carcinoma cells. *Chin. Jour. Integ. Trad. West. Med.* 6(8): 480–483.

Brenan, J.P.M. 1958. New and noteworthy Cassias from tropical Africa. *Kew Bull.* 13: 231–252.

Brinda, P., Rukmani, B. and Purushothaman, K.K. 1981. Pharmacognostic studies on *Anisomeles malabarica* R. Br. *Bull. Med. Ethnobiol. Res.* 2(4): 74–84.

Brinda, P., B. Sasikala, Bhima Rao R. and Purushothaman, K.K. 1982. Pharmacognostic studies in *Solanum nigrum* L. an Ayurvedic drug. *J. Econ. Tax. Bot.* 3(2): 125–128.

Chakravarthy, B.K., Gupta, S., Gambhir, S.S. and Gode, K.D. 1981. Epicatechin—a novel anti-diabetic drug. *Indian Drugs* 18(5): 184–185.

Chandra, T., Sidique, J. and Somasundaran, S. 1987. Effect of *Eclipta alba* on inflammation and liver injury. *Fitoterapia* 58(1): 23–32.

Chao, K.H., Chung, T.J., Kim, S.J., Lee, T.H. and Yoon, C.M. 1981. Clinical experience of Madecassol (*Centella asiatica*) in the treatment of peptic ulcer. *Korean Jour. Gastroenterol.* 13(1): 49–56.

Chaturvedi, G.N., Krishna Mohan and Ariyawansaldas. 1981. Clinical correlation of *amlapitta* and its treatment with indigenous drug *vasa* (*Adhatoda vasica* Nees). *Nagarjun* 24(8): 170–174.

Chaturvedi, G.N., Rai, N.P., Dhani, R. and Tiwari, S.K. 1983. Clinical trial of *Adhatoda vasica* syrup (*vasa*) in the patients of non-ulcer dyspepsia (*amlapitta*). *Anc. Sci. Life* 3(1): 19–23.

Chaturvedi, G.N., Thomas, G.S., Tiwari, S.K. and Singh, K.P. 1983. Clinical studies on *kalmegh* (*Andrographis paniculata* Nees) in infective hepatitis. *Anc. Sci. Life* 2(4): 208–215.

Chaudhuri, B.G., Mehta, H.G., Vachharajani, Y.R. and Baxi, A.J. 1981. Botanical identity and pharmacognostical studies of commercial *vidari* of Gujarat. *Bull. Med. Ethnobot. Res.* 2(4): 47–61.

Chawla, Y.K., Dubey, P., Singh, R., Nundy, S. and Tandon, B.N. 1987. Treatment of dyspepsia with *amalaki* (*Emblica officinalis* Linn.), an Ayurvedic drug. *Vagbhata* 5(3): 24–26.

Chopra, R.N., Nayar, S.L. and Chopra I.C. 1956. *Glossary of Indian Medicinal Plants*, New Delhi.

Chowdhury, R.R. and Mishra, M. 1987. *Coccinia indica* in type II diabetes mellitus. *Indian Med. Jour.* 81(2): 31–32.

Chunekar, K.C. 1982. *Bhavaprakasanighantu of Sri Bhavamisra. Commentary*, Varanasi (In Hindi).

Croom, E.M. Jr. 1983. Documenting and evaluating herbal medicines. *Economic Botany* 37: 13–27.

Dehanukar, S.A., Karandikar, S.M. and Desai, M. 1984. Efficacy of *Piper longum* in childhood asthma. *Indian Drugs* 21(9): 384–388.

Das, P.K., Rathor, R.S., Lal, R., Tripathi, R.M., Ram, A.K. and Biswas, M. 1974. Anti-inflammatory and anti-arthritis activity of *Crataeva nurvala* Buch.-Ham. *Jour. Res. Ind. Med.* 9(3): 9–16.

Das, S.K., Chandra, A., Agarwal, S.S. and Singh, N. 1983. *Ocimum sanctum* (*tulsi*) in the treatment of viral encephalitis. *Antiseptic* 80(7): 323–327.

Dasgupta, S. 1922. *A History of Indian Philosophy*, Delhi.

Dassanayake, M.D. and Fosberg, F.R. (Eds.). 1980–1987. *A Revised Handbook of Flora of Ceylon*, Vols. I–VI, New Delhi.

Datta, S.K. and Datta, P.C. 1983. Pharmacognostic study of *Jatropha* stem bark. *Bull. Med. Ethnobot.* 2(3): 336–345.

Datta, P.C. and Sen, A. 1969. Pharmacognosy of *Oldenlandia corymbosa Linn. Quart. J. Crude Drug. Res.* 9: 1365.

Deb, D.B. 1989. *Solanum melongena, S. incanum* versus *S. insanum* (Solanaccae). *Taxon* 38: 138–139.

Deodhar, S.D., Sethi, R. and Srimal, R.C. 1980. Preliminary study on anti-rheumatic activity of curcumin. *Indian Jour. Med. Res.* 71 (April): 632–634.

Deshpande, P.J., Sahu, M. and Kumar, P. 1982. *Crataeva nurvala* Hook. and Forst. (*varuna*)—the Ayurvedic drug of choice in urinary disorders. *Indian Jour. Med. Res.* 76 (Dec., suppl.): 46–53.

Deshpande, V.Y., Mendulkar, K.N. and Sadre, N.L. 1980. Male anti-fertility activity of *Azadirachta indica* in mice. A preliminary report. *Jour. Post-grad. Med.* (Bombay) 26(3): 167–170.

Dev, V. and Wasir, H.S. 1985. Digitalis poisoning by an indigenous plant cardiac glycoside (*Thevetia neriifolia—pilakaner*). *Ind. Heart Jour.* 37(5): 321–322.

De Wilde, W.J.J.O. 1967. A new combination and a new species in *Saraca* L. *Blumea* 15: 393–395.

Dey, A.C. 1980. *Indian Medicinal Plants*, Dehra Dun.

Dey, D. and Das, M.N. 1980. Pharmacognostic studies of *Acorus calamus. Proc. 67th Session, Indian Sci. Congress*, Calcutta.

Dey, D. and Das, M.N. 1985. Drug characterisation of *Vernonia cinerea* Less, by pharmacognostic analysis. *Jour. Res. Edn. Ind. Med.* 4(3–4): 33–34.

Dhawan, B.N. and Patnaik, G.K. 1985. Investigation in some new cardio-active glycosides from *Vallaris solanacea. Indian Drugs* 22(6): 288–290.

Dhir, G.G., Mohan, G., Verma, R.B. and Mishra, S.S. 1982. Studies on the antifungal activity of *Pterocarpus marsupium*. A clinical evaluation. *Ind. Jour. Dermatol. Venerol. Leprol* 48(3): 154–156.

Dixit, S.P. and Achar, M.P. 1979. *Bhringaraja* in the treatment of infective hepatitis. *Curr. Med. Pract.* 23(6): 237–242.

Dixit, S.P. and Achar, M.P. 1983. *Bhumyamalaki* (*Phyllanthus niruri* L.) and jaundice in children. *Jour. Natl. Integ. Med. Assoc.* 25(8): 269–272.

Dixit, P. and Jain, H.C. 1985. Anti-atherosclerotic factor of *Aloe barbadense* ethanolic extract in dogs. *Adv. Biosci.* 4(1): 95–99.

Dixit, V.P., Joshi, S. and Kumar, A. 1983. Possible anti-spermatogenic activity of *Gloriosa superba* (E to H extract) in male gerbil (*Mriones hurrianae* Jerdon). A preliminary study. *Comp. Physiol. Ecol.* 8(i): 117–122.

Doshi, J.J., Patel, V.K. and Bhatt, V.H. 1983. Effect of *Adhatoda uasica* massage in pyorrhoea. *Int. Jour. Crude Drug Res.* 21(4): 173–176.

Dube, C.B., Kumar, D. and Srivastav, P.S. 1982. A trial of *bhringaraja ghanasatwavati* on the patients of hepatocellular jaundice. *Jour. Natl. Integ. Med. Assoc.* 24(9): 265–269.

Dubey, S.D., Singh, R.S., Sen, S.P. and Kumar, N. 1982. Study on indigenous drug *sitivara* (*Celosia argentea* L.). *Med. Surg.* 22 (10–11): 9–12.

Dutta, A. and Sukul, N.C. 1982. Filaricidal properties of a wild herb *Andrographis paniculata*. *Jour. Helminthol.* 56(2): 81–84.

Dwivedi, R.N., Pandey S.P. and Tripathi, V.J. 1977. Role of *japapushpa* (*Hibiscus rosa-sinensis*) in the treatment of arterial hypertension. A trial study. *Jour. Res. Ind. Med. Yoga & Homeop.* 12(4): 31–36.

Farnsworth, N.R. 1979. The present and future of pharmacognosy. *Amer. Jour. Pharmaceut. Edn.* 43: 239–243.

Farnsworth, N.R. 1984a. How can the well be dry when it is filled with water. *Economic Botany* 38: 4–13.

Farnsworth, N.R. 1984b. The role of medicinal plants in drug development. In Alfred Benson Symposium 20. *Natural Products and Drug Development.* Copenhagen, pp. 17–30.

Farnsworth, N.R. and Bingel, A.S. 1977. Problems and prospects of discovering new drugs from higher plants by pharmacological screening. In: (eds. H. Wagner & P. Wolff), *New Natural Products and Plant Drugs with pharmacological, biological or therapeutic activity*, New York, pp. 1–22.

Farnsworth, N.R. and Morris, R.W. 1976. Higher plants—the sleeping giant of drug development. *Amer. Jour. Pharm.* 147: 46–52.

Farnsworth, N.R. and Soejarto, D.D. 1985. Potential consequences of plant extinction in the United States on the current and future availability of prescription drugs. *Economic Botany* 39: 231–240.

Gaitonde, B.B., Joglekar, S.N., Kulkarni, H.J. and Naber, S.D. 1977. Anti-inflammatory, analgesic and anti-pyretic activity of an indigenous medicinal plant, *Oxalis corniculata* L. *Jour. Res. Ind. Med. Yoga & Homeop.* 12(2): 12–17.

Gamble, J.S. 1915–1936. *Flora of the Presidency of Madras*, London.

Gardner, E.G. 1960. *History of Biology*. Minneapolis.

Ghosh, D., Thejmoorth, P. and Veluchamy, G. 1985. Anti-inflammatory, analgesic and antipyretic activities of 777 oil—a Siddha medicine. *Bul. Med. Ethnobot. Res.* 6(2–4): 141–154.

Girij, J., Sakthi Devi, T.K. and Meerarani, S. 1984. Effect of ginger on serum cholesterol levels. *Ind. Jour. Nutr. Diet.* 21(2): 433–436.

Gopakumar, K. 1986. Studies on South Indian market samples of Ayurvedic drugs—V. *Anc. Sci. Life* 6(1): 30–34.

Gowri, N., Srinivasan, K. and Venkataraghavan, S. 1982. Clinical study of AC-4, an Ayurvedic compound preparation as an oral contraceptive. *Anc. Sci. Life* 2(2): 79–83.

Gulati, O.D. and Pandey, D.C. 1982. Anti-inflammatory activity of *Tinospora cordifolia. Rheumatism* 17(2): 76–83.

Gupta, O.P., Ghatak, H.J.R. and Atal, C.K. 1978. Vasicine alkaloid of *Adhatoda vasica*, a promising uterotonic abortifacient. *Indian Jour. Exp. Boil.* 16(10): 1075–1077.

Gupta, R.C. 1985. Pharmacognostic studies on *dravanti*. Part I—*Jatropha curcas*, L. *Proc. Indian Acad. Sci.* (Pl.Sci.) 94(1): 65–82.

Gupta, R.C. 1988. Pharmacobotanical studies on *'shvetsharpunkha'*—A comparative diagnostic account of *Tephroria villosa* Pers. and *T. purpurea* (linn.) Pers. form *albiflora* S.R. Paul et R.C. Gupta *Anc. Sci. Life.* 7(3&4): 207–218.

Gupta, R.C., Singh, P.M., Prasad, G.C. and Udupa, K.N. 1981. Probable mode of action of *sankhapuspi* in the management of thyrotoxicosis. *Anc. Sci. Life* 1(1): 46–54.

Gupta, R.S., Sharma, Nuthan and Dixit, V.P. 1990. Calotropin—a novel compound for fertility control. *Anc. Sci. Life* 9(4): 224–230.

Gupta, S.C., Bajaj, U.K. and Sharma, V.N. 1976. Cardiovascular effects of *Eclipta alba* Hassk (*Bhringaraja*). *Jour. Res. Ind. Med. Yoga & Homeop.* 11(3): 91–93.

Henry, A.N., Vivekanandan, K. and Nair, N.C. 1978. Rare and threatened flowering plants of South India. *J. Bombay nat. Hist. Soc.* 75: 684–697.

Hooker, J.D. 1872–1897. *The Flora of British India.* London.

Indap, M.A., Ambaye, R.Y. and Gokhale, S.V. 1983. Anti-tumour and pharmacological effects of the oil from *Semecarpus anacardium* L. *Ind. Jour. Physiol. Pharmacol.* 27(2): 83–91.

Itokawa, H., Morita, H., Sumitomo, T., Totsuka, N. and Takeya, K. 1987. Antitumour principles from *Alpinia galanga. Planta Med.* 53 (1): 32–33.

Jain, J.P. 1980. A clinical trial of *kantakari* (*Solanum xanthocarpum*) in cases of *tamakswasa* (some respiratory diseases). *Jour. Res. Ayur. Siddha* 1(3): 447–460.

Jain, J.P., Bhatnagar, L.C. and Parsai, M.R. 1979. Clinical trials of *haridra* (*Curcuma longa*) in cases of *tamakswasa* and *kasa*. *Jour. Res. Ind. Med. Yoga & Homeop.* 14(2): 110–120.

Jain, J.P. and Naqvi, S.M.A. 1986. A clinical trial of *palash* (*Butea monosperma* (Lam.) Kuntze (syn. *B. frondosa* Koen. ex. Roxb.) in worm infestations (*krimi roga*). *Jour. Res. Ayur. Siddha* 7(1–2): 13–22.

Jain, P.K., Verma, R., Kumar, N. and Kumar, A. 1985. Clinical trial of *arka-mulatwak*—bark of *Calotripis procera*—a preliminary study. *Jour. Res. Ayur. Siddha* 6(1, 3 & 4): 88–91.

Jeffrey, C. 1980. Further notes on Cucurbitaceae V. The Cucurbitaceae of the Indian sub-continent. *Kew Bull.* 34: 789–809.

Joubert, P.H., Brown, J.M.M., Hay, I.T. and Sebata, P.D.B. 1984. Acute poisoning with *Jatropha curcas* in children. *S. Afr. Med. Jour.* 65(18): 729–730.

Kalyanagurunathan, P., Sulochana, N. and Murugesh, N. 1985. *In vitro* haemolytic effect of the flowers of *Sesbania grandiflora*. *Fitoterapia* 56(3): 188–189.

Kannabiran, B. and Krishnamurthy, K.H. 1972. Pharmacognostic study of *Anisomeles malabarica* L. *(Bhutankusha)*. *Jour. Res. Ind. Med.* 7(4): 43–49.

Kannappareddy, M., Viswanathan, S., Thirugnana Sambantham, P., Santha Ramachandran and Kameswaran, L. 1986. Effect of *Leucas aspera* on experimental inflammation and mast cell degranulation. *Anc. Sci. Life* 5(3): 168–171.

Kapoor, S.L. and Mitra, R. 1979. *Herbal drugs in Indian Pharmaceutical industry*, Lucknow.

Karnick, C.R. 1983. Effect of mantras on human beings and plants. *Anc. Sci. Life* 2(3): 141–147.

Karnick, C.R. and Joshi, S.N. 1986. Studies on standardisation of Ayurvedic crude drugs. Series 1-*Asparagus racemosus* Willd. (*Satavari*). *Nagarjun* 30(1): 21–22.

Karnick, C.R. and Pathak, N.N. 1983. Clinical trials of crude drug *Tephrosia purpurea* L. on adenoids and acute tonsillitis. *Jour. Natl. Integ. Med. Assoc.* 25(10): 333–334.

Karunanayake, E.H., Welihinda, J., Sirimanne, S.R. and Sinna Dorai, G. 1984. Oral hypoglycaemic activity of some medicinal plants of Sri Lanka. *J. Ethnopharmacol.* 11(2): 223–231.

Khan Azad, A.K., Akhtar, S. and Mahtab, H. 1980. Treatment of diabetes mellitus with *Coccinia indica*. *Brit. Med. Jour.* 280(6220): 1044.

Khan, S.S. and Chaghtai, S.A. 1982. Ethnobotanical study of some plants used for curing skin affections. *Anc. Sci. Life* 1(14): 236–238.

Khanna, A. 1987. Theoretical foundations to ancient Indian Medicine. Part I. *Anc. Sci. Life* 7(2): 69–75.

Khanna, S., Gupta, S.R. and Grover, J.K. 1986. Effect of long-term feeding of *tulsi* (*Ocimum sanctum*) on reproductive performance of adult albino rats. *Ind. Jour. Exp. Biol.* 24(5): 302–304.

Khare, A.K., Srivastava, M.C., Sharma, M.K. and Tewari, J.P. 1984. Anti-fertility activity of Neem oil in rabbits and rats. *Probe* 23(2): 90–94.

Khare, A.K., Srivastava, M.A., Tewari, J.P., Puri, J.N., Singh, S. and Ansari, N.A. 1982. A preliminary study of anti-inflammatory activity of *Ipomoea turpethum (Nishoth)*. *Indian Drugs* 19(6): 224–228.

Khoshoo, T.N. 1986. *Environmental priorities in India and sustainable development*, New Delhi.

Khosla, R.L. and Prasad, S. 1971. Pharmacognostical studies on *guduchi (Tinospora cordifolia* Miers). *Jour. Res. Ind. Med.* 6(3): 261–269.

Kirtikar, K.R. and Basu, B.D. 1918. *Indian Medicinal Plants*, Allahabad.

Kishore, P., Pandey, P.N., Pandey, S.N. and Dash, S. 1980. Treatment of duodinal ulcer with *Asparagus racemosus* L. *Jour. Res. Ayur. Siddha* 1(3): 409–416.

Kiso, Y., Suzuki, Y., Watanabe, N., Oshima, Y. and Hikino, H. 1983. Anti-hepatotoxic principles of *Curcuma longa* rhizomes. *Planta Med.* 49(3): 185–187.

Kokate, C.K., Ashok Kumar, R., Rao, P.D., Rambhan, D. and Rao, M.Y. 1985. Studies on *Embelia ribes.* Anti-fertility activity of embelin and its derivatives. *Jour. Res. Edn. Ind. Med.* 4(3–4): 5–7.

Kolammal, M. 1979. *Pharmacognosy of Ayurvedic drugs.* Trivandrum, No. 10.

Koushik, A.K. and Singh, R.H. 1982. Clinical evaluation of *medhya rasayana* compound in cases of non-depressive anxiety neurosis. *Anc. Sci. Life* 2(1): 11–16.

Krishnamurthy, J.R., Kalaimani, S. and Veluchamy, G. 1981. Clinical study of *vetpalai* (*Wrightia tinctoria* L.) oil in the treatment of *Kalanjagapadai* (Psoriasis) *Journ. Res. Ayur. Siddha* 2(1): 58–66.

Krishnan Vaidyar, K.V. and Gopala Pillai, S. 1974. *Sahasrayogam-Sujanapriya commentary*, Alleppey. (in Malayalam)

Kumar, P., Singh, L.M. and Deshpande, P.J. 1982. Clinical study with *Crataeva nurvala* in urinary tract infection. *Jour. Sci. Res. Plant. Med.* 3(2 & 3): 75–79.

Kuppurajan, K., Seshadri, C., Revathy, R. and Venkataraghavan, S. 1986. Hypoglycemic effect of *Coccinia indica* in diabetes mellitus. *Nagarjun* 29(5): 1–4.

Kurup, P.N.V., Ramdas, V.N.K. and Joshi, P. 1979. *Handbook of Medicinal Plants*, New Delhi.

Kuttan, R., Sudheeran, P.C. and Joseph, C.D. 1987. Turmeric and curcumin as topical agents in cancer therapy. *Tumori* 73(1): 29–31.

Lahon, L.C., Lhanikor, H.N. and Ahmed, N. 1979. Preliminary study of local anaesthetic activity of *Euphorbia neriifolia* L. *Ind. Jour. Pharmacol.* 11(3): 239–249.

Laping, J. 1984. Pluralism in the Ayurvedic system of medicine. *Anc. Sci. Life* 4(2): 83–87.

Lee, E.B., Shin, K.H. and Woo, W.S. 1984. Pharmacological study on piperine. *Arch. Pharm. Res.* 7(2): 127–132.

Madan, C.L. and Nayar, S.L. 1959. Pharmacognostic study of the leaf and root of *Vitex negundo* L. *Jour. Sci. Indust. Res.* 18 C(1): 10–14.

Mahadihassan, S. 1980. A comparative study of the early system of Indian cosmology and the Tridosha humoral doctrine. *Ind. Jour. Hist. Sci.* 15: 223–229.

Mahadihassan, S. 1986. A scientific interpretation of the Tridosha doctrine of Humorology. *Anc. Sci. Life* 6(1): 42–46.

Mahadihassan, S. 1989. The Tridosha doctrine traced to breath as soul. *Anc. Sci. Life* 9(1): 25–25.

Majumdar, A. Kaviraj. 1989. Ayurveda and modern medicine. *Anc. Sci. Life.* 8(3&4): 117–190.

Matthew, K.M. 1981–84. *The Flora of Tamilnadu Carnatic*, Thiruchirappalli.

Mehra, P.N., Jolly, S.S. and Puri, H.S. 1968. Pharmacognosy of *Fumaria indica* (Hassk.) Pugsley and its adulterants. *Indian J. Pharm.* 30(12): 284. (Abstr.)

Mehrotra, P.K. and Kamboj, V.P. 1978. Hormonal profile of coronardine hydrochloride—an antifertility agent of plant origin. *Planta Med.* 33(4): 345–349.

Mehta, B.K., Dubey, A., Bokadias, M.M. and Mehta, S.C. 1983. Antifertility activity of *Butea monosperma*. *Acta Cienc. Indica* 19C(4): 218–220.

Meir, P. and Yaniz, Z. 1985. An *in vitro* study on the effect of *Momordica charantia* on glucone uptake and glucose metabolism in rats. *Planta Med.* 1: 12–16.

Menon, V.M.K. 1976. *Ashtangahrudayam: Suthrasthanam.* Commentary, Kottayam (In Malayalam).

Mhaiskar, V.B., Pandya, D.C. and Karmarkar, K.B. 1980. Clinical evaluation of *Tinospora cordifolia* in *amavata* and *sandhigata vata*. *Rheumatism* 16(1): 35–39.

Moosa, J.S. 1985. A study on the crude anti-diabetic drugs used in Arabian folk-medicine. *Int. Jour. Crude Drug. Res.* 23(3): 137–145.

Moosad, T.C.P. 1983. *Amarakosam—Commentary.* Kottayam (In Malayalam)

Mooss, N.S. (Ed.) 1950. *Ashtangahridayasamhita with the Vakya-pradeepika commentary of Parameswara*, Kottayam.

Mooss, N.S. 1952. Studies on Medicinal plants—Some reference to Gojihva - *Jour. Ayur.* 1952: 1–6.

Mooss, N.S. 1976. *Single Drug Remedies*, Kottayam.

Mooss, N.S. 1978. *Ayurvedic Flora Medica*, Kottayam.

Mooss, N.S. 1980. *Ganas of Vahata*, Kottayam.

Mooss, N.S. 1984a. Identification of *canda*. *Anc. Sci. Life* 4(1): 56–57.

Mooss, N.S. 1984b. Identification of *kebuka*. *Anc. Sci. Life* 4(2): 100–102.

Mooss, P.T.N. 1981. Scarcity of the raw drugs (in Malayalam). *Proceedings of the Seminar on Medicinal Plants*, Peechi. pp: 44–45.

Mukhopadhyay, A., Basu, N., Ghatak, N. and Gujral, P.K. 1982. Anti-inflammatory and irritant activities of curcumin analogues in rats. *Agents Actions* 12(4): 508–515.

Murthy, K.S., Rao, D.N., Rao, D.K. and Murthy, L.B.G. 1978. Preliminary study on hypoglycaemic and anti-hyperglycaemic effects of *Azadirachta indica*. *Ind. Jour. Pharmacol.* 10(3): 247–250.

Nadkarni, A.K. 1954. *Indian Materia Medica*, Bombay.

Nair, B.K.H., Nair, C.P.R., Ramiah, N., Kurup, P.B., Chandramouli, G., Chandralekha, Pillai, K.G.B. and Pai, K.N. 1977. *Cassia fistula* in pyoderma—a clinical trial. *Jour. Res. Ind. Med. Yoga & Homeop.* 12(4): 16–21.

Nair, C.P.R. 1984. Single drugs in the treatment of skin diseases. *Vagbhata* 2(3): 21–30.

Nair, K. Vasudevan, Indira Balachandran, S.N. Yoganarasimhan and K. Gopakumar. 1986. Studies on some South Indian market samples of Ayurvedic drugs—V. *Anc. Sci. Life* 6(1) 30–34.

Nair, K.V., Yoganarasimhan, S.N., Kesavamurthy, K.R. and Mary, Z. 1982. Studies on some South Indian market samples of Ayurvedic drugs—I. *Anc. Sci. Life* 2(3): 71–78.

Nair, K.V., Yoganarasimhan, S.N., Kesavamurthy, K.R. and Santha, T.R. 1983. Studies on some South Indian market samples of Ayurvedic drugs II. *Anc. Sci. Life* 3(2): 60–66.

Nair, N.C. 1967. On the identity of *Boerhaavia punarnava* Saha *et* Krishnamurthy. *Bull. Bot. Surv. India* 9: 283.

Nair, R.B., Ravi Sankar, B., Vijayan, N.P., Saraswathy, V.N. and Sasikala, C.K. 1985. Anti-inflammatory effect of *Strobilanthes heyneanus (sahachara)*—biochemical study. *Bull. Med. Ethnobot. Res.* 6(2–4): 196–206.

Nair, R.B. and Santhakumari, G. 1986. Anti-diabetic activity of the seed kernal of *Syzygium cumini* Linn. *Anc. Sci. Life* 6(2): 80–84.

Nambiar, V.P.K., Sasidharan, N., Renuka, C. and Balagopalan, M. 1986. *Studies on the medicinal plants of Kerala forests*, Peechi.

Namboodiri, P.K.N., Menon, T.V., Vijayan, N.P. and Vijayakumar, D. 1985. The role of *snehapana* in *pakshavadha* (Hemiplegia)—a study. *Jour. Res. Ayur. Siddha* 6(1, 3 & 4): 44–58.

Nanda, G.C., Tewari, N.S. and Kishore, P. 1985. Clinical studies on the role of *sunthi* in the treatment of *grahaniroga J. Res. Ayur. Siddha* 6(1, 3 & 4): 78–87.

Narayana Swamy, V. 1981. Origin and development of Ayurveda. *Anc. Sci. Life* 1(1): 1–7.

Nayar, R.C. 1979. A review of the Ayurvedic drug, *sariba. J. Res. Ind. Med. Yoga & Homeop.* 14(2): 69–79.

Nayar, R.C., Pattanshetty, J.K., Mary, Z. and Yoganarasimhan, S.N. 1978. Pharmacognostical studies on the root of *Decalepis hamiltonii* Wt. & Arn. and comparison with *Hemidesmus indicus* (L.) R.Br. *Proc. Ind. Acad. Sci.* 87B (2): 37–48.

Nesamony, S. 1985. *Oushadhasasyangal.* Trivandrum (In Malayalam).

Nicolson, Dan. H., Suresh, C.R. and Manilal, K.S. 1988. *An interpretation of Van Rheede's Hortus Malabaricus*, Konigstein.

Ojewole Jao and Adesina, S.K. 1985. Isolation, identification and some cardiovascular actions of a purine nucleoside from the roots of *Boerhaavia diffusa. Fitoterapia* 56(1): 31–36.

Ojha, J.K., Bajpai, H.S. and Sharma, P.V. 1978. Hypoglycaemic effect of *Pterocarpus marsupium* Roxb. *Jour. Res. Ind. Med. Yoga & Homeop.* 13(4): 12–16.

Pakrashi, A. and Shaha, C. 1978. Effect of methyl ester of aristolic acid from *Aristolochia indica* L. on fertility of female mice. *Experimentia* 34(9): 1192–1193.

Pal, Madhabendra Nath, 1989, 1990. Ayurveda: An international perspective I–III. *Anc. Sci. Life* 8: 235–240; 9:1–6 & 9: 140–146.

Pandya, N.B. 1983. Fundamental principles of Ayurveda. *Anc. Sci. Life* 2(4): 176–180.

Panicker, C.K.B. 1989. Basic principles and practices of Ayurveda. *Presented at the I Int. Conf. on Holistic Health and Medicine* (Nov. 8–12), Bangalore.

Parikh, M.D., Mistry, P.R. and Bhatt, N.S. 1984. Need for an integrated system of medicine—A proposal for its attainment. *Anc. Sci. Life* 4(2): 79–82.

Patel, S.M. and Vasavada, S.A. 1985. Studies on *Ficus racemosa* Linn. Part I Antiulcer activity. *Bull. Med. Ethnobot. Res.* 6(1): 17–26.

Pattanshetty, J.K., Raj, P.V., Abraham, K. and Holla, B.V. 1983. Comparative fluorescence and chromatographic studies of the plants used as *vidari. Anc. Sci. Life* 2(4): 190–193.

Patwardhan, B., Saraf, M.N. and David, S.B. 1988. Toxicity of *Semecarpus anacardium* extract. *Anc. Sci. Life* 8(2): 106–109.

Paul, R. and Vatsa, S.R. 1980. Clinical trial of an Ayurvedic herb in worm infestation. *Nagarjun* 23 (11): 234–235.

Phadke, U.R., Ghooi, R.B. and Bhide, M.B. 1983. Studies on Anaphylaxis. V. *Butea monosperma (palas)* as a potential antiasthmatic agent. *Bull. Hoffk. Inst.* 10(3): 67–76.

Pillai, N.G.K., Menon, T.V., Pillai, G.B., Rajasekharan, S. and Nair, C.R.R. 1981. Effects of plumbagin in *charmakeela* (common warts): A case report. *Jour. Res. Ayur. Siddha* 2(2): 122–126.

Pillai, N.G.K., Pillai, K.G.B., Kurup, P.B. and Nair, C.P.R. 1983. *Ropana guna* of *nimbatikta* in *dushta vrana*—A case report. *Vagbhata* 1(6): 37–38.

Pillai, N.R., Ghosh, D., Uma, R. and Anandakumar, A. 1980. Hypoglycaemic activity of *Coccinia indica* W. & A. *Bull. Med. Ethnobot. Res.* 1(2): 234–242.

Pillai, N.R., Alam, M. and Purushothaman, K.K. 1981. Sterility studies with gangetin in albino rats. *Jour. Res. Ayur. Siddha* 2(4): 349–356.

Pillai, N.R. and Santhakumar, G. 1984. Effects of nimbidin on acute and chronic gastroduodenal ulcer models in experimental animals. *Planta Med.* 50(2): 143–146.

Pillai, N.R., Sugathan, D. and Santhakumari, G. 1980. Analgesic and antipyretic actions of nimbidin. *Bull. Med. Ethnobot. Res.* 1(3): 393–400.

Pillai, N.R., Moorthy, T., Alam, M. and Dasan, K.K.S. 1980. Comparative antipyretic studies on *Amritarishtam* and *Tinospora cordifolia* in albino rats. *Nagarjun* 23 (12): 262–263.

Pillai, N.R. and Vijayamma, N. 1985. Some pharmacological studies on *Cardiospermum halicacabum* L. *Anc. Sci. Life* 5(1): 32–36.

Pradeep, A.K. and Sivarajan, V.V. 1991. *Hibiscus hispidissimus*, the correct name for *H. furcatus* DC. non Willd. and *H. aculeatus* Roxb. non Walter (Malvaceae). *Taxon* 40: 634–637.

Prakash, A. and Prasad, S. 1969a. Pharmacognostical studies on the bark of *Aegle marmelos* Correa. *Jour. Res. Ind. Med.* 4(1): 97.

Prakash, A. and Prasad, S. 1969b. Pharmacognostical studies on the bark of *Oroxylum indicum* Vent. (*Shyonaka*). *Jour. Res. Ind. Med.* 4(1): 73–81.

Prakash, A., Prasad, S., Wahi, S.P. and Wahi, A.K. 1978. Pharmacognostical study of *Bauhinia variegata* L. *Jour. Res. Ind. Med. Yoga & Homoeop.* 13(1): 84–89.

Prakash, C. 1981. A note on preliminary study on *Acorus calamus* L. in the treatment of bronchial asthma. *J. Res. Ayur. Siddha* 1(2): 329–330.

Prakash, D. and Prasad, S. 1971. Pharmacognostical studies on *Cassia tora* L. *Jour. Res. Ind. Med.* 6(3): 270–280.

Prasad, G. 1985. Action of *Calotropis procera* on migraine *J. Natl. Integ. Med. Assoc.* 27(6): 7–10.

Prasad, G.C., Gupta, R.C., Srivastava, D.N., Tandon, A.D., Wahi, R. and Udupa, K.N. 1974. Effect of *sankhapushpi* on experimental stress. *Jour. Res. Ind. Med.* 9(2): 19–27.

Prasad, K.V.S.R.G., Sankarasubramanian, S. and Guruswamy, M.N. 1986. Pharmacological studies on the roots of *Aerva lanata*. *Arogya Jour. Health Sci.* 12: 6–13.

Prasad, S., Khosa, R.L., Wahi, A.K. and Bhardwaj, R.C. 1967. Pharmacognostic studies on *bharngi* root (Part I): Roots of *Clerodendrum serratum* and *C. indicum* Kuntze. *Jour. Res. Ind. Med.* 1(2): 223–229.

Rahman, H., Tyeb, K.M. and Saleemuddin, M. 1985. Hypoglycaemic activity of *Tephrosia purpurea* seeds. *Ind. Jour. Med. Res.* 81: 418–421.

Raghunathan, K. and Sharma, P.V. 1969. Effect of *Tinospora cordifolia* Miers (*guduchi*) on alloxan induced hyperglycaemia. *Jour. Res. Ind. Med.* 3(2): 203–209.

Raghunathan, S. and Mitra, R. (Eds.) 1982. *Pharmacognosy of indigenous drugs.* New Delhi, Vols. 1 and 2.

Rajasekharan, S., Kalavathi, N., Sivanandan, G., Thyagarajan, R., Sundaram, M. and Veluchamy, G. 1984. Clinical evaluation of Siddha drugs in the treatment of *manjal kamalai* (infective hapatitis) Part I. *Kovai* (*Coccinia grandis* W. & A.). *Jour. Res. Ayur. Siddha* 5(1–4): 18–24.

Rajasekharan, S., Pillai, N.G.K.P., Kurup, P.B., Pillai, K.G.B. and Nair, C.P.R. 1980. Effect of nimbidin in Psoriasis—A case report. *Jour. Res. Ayur. Siddha* 1(1): 52–58.

Ramabhimaiah, S., Stalin, D. and Kalaskar, N.J. 1984. Pharmacological investigations on the water soluble fraction of methanol extract of *Boerhaavia diffusa* root. *Indian Drugs* 21(8): 343–344.

Ramaswamy, A.S., Periasamy, S.M. and Basu, N. 1970. Pharmacological studies on *Centella asiatica* L. (*Brahmamanduki*) *Jour. Res. Ind. Med.* 4(2): 160–173.

Rao, A., Srinivasan, K. and Rao, K.T. 1973. The effect of *mandukaparni* (*Centella asiatica*) on the general mental ability (*medhya*) of mentally retarded children. *Jour. Res. Ind. Med.* 8(4): 9–15.

Rao. G.P. and Singri, B.P. 1979. A rare alkaloid from *Tabernaemontana heyneana* Wall. *Ind. Jour. Chem.* 17 B(4): 414–415.

Rao, N.H. 1981. *Bhallatakavati* in *amavata* conditions. *Rheumatism* 16(1) 24–29.

Rao, P.P. 1984. Certain autonomic effects of *Tephrosia purpurea. Nagarjun* 27(7): 179–181.

Ravindran, P.A. 1986. Integrated medicine—a need or a must? *New Wave of Trad. Lines* 3(3): 10–13.

Ravisankar, B., Nair, B.R. and Sasikala, C.K. 1985. Pharmacological evaluation of *Vitex negundo* (*nirgundi*) leaves. *Bull. Med. Ethnobot. Res.* 6(1): 72–92.

Ray, N. and Datta, P.C. 1981. Pharmacognostic study of the bark of *Saraca indica. Quart. Jour. Crude Drug Res.* 19(2–3): 97–102.

Reddy, K., Viswanathan, S., Sanbantham, T.P., Santha, R. and Kameswaran, L. 1986. Effect of *Leucas aspera* on experimental inflammation and mast cell degranulation. *Anc. Sci. Life* 5(3): 168–171.

Rheede, H.A. Van 1678–1703. *Hortus Indicus Malabaricus*, Amsterdam, Vols I–XII.

Saha, J.C. and Krishnamurthy, K.H. 1961. Identity of *swetapunarnava*—*Boerhaavia punarnava* Sp. Nov. of Ayurveda. *J. Sci. Industr. Res.* 21 C: 249–255.

Santha, T.R. and Gopakumar, K. 1988. Macro and microscopical studies on the root and leaf of *Glycosmis arborea* (Roxb.) DC. *Aryavaidyan* 2(1): 35–40.

Santha, T.R., Pattan Shetty, J.K., Gopakumar, K. and Vijayalakshmi, B. 1988. Pharmacognostical studies on the leaves of *sahachara—Nilgirianthus heyneanus* (Nees) Bremek. *Indian Drugs* 25(9): 366–371.

Santha, T.R., Shetty, J.K.P. and Gopakumar, K. 1988. Pharmacognostical studies on the root of *sahachara Nilgirianthus heyneanus* (Nees) Bremek. (Acanthaceae). *Anc. Sci. Life* 7(3 & 4): 139–144.

Santhakumari, G., Pillai, N.R. and Nair, R.B. 1981. Diuretic activity of *Cardiospermum halicacabum* L. in rats. *Jour. Sci. Res. Plant. Med.* 2(1 & 2): 32–34.

Santhakumari, G., Pillai, N.R., Pillai, R.G. and Nair, R.B. 1985. Hypoglycaemic potential of *Murraya koenigii* Spreng. *Bull. Med. Ethnobot. Res.* 6(2–4): 189–195.

Sanyal, M., Roy, S.K. and Dutta, P.C. 1984. Pharmacognostic evaluation of *Embelia ribes* fruit drug. *J. Econ. Tax. Bot.* 5(5): 1235–1239.

Satyavati, G.V., Prasad, D.N., Sen, S.P. and Das, P.K. 1969. Investigations into the uterine activity of *Saraca indica* L. (*Ashoka*). *Jour. Res. Ind. Med.* 4(1): 37–45.

Satyavati, G.V., Raina, M.K. and Sharma, M. (Eds.) 1976, 1987. *Medicinal Plants of India*, New Delhi, Vols. 1 and 2.

Saxena, R.C. 1980. *Cyperus rotundus* in conjunctivities. *J. Res. Ayur. Siddha* 1(1): 115–120.

Seth, S.D., Johri, N. and Sundaram, K.R. 1982. Anti-spermatogenic effect of embelin from *Embelia ribes*. *Ind. Jour. Pharmacol.* 14(2): 207–211.

Sethi, N., Nath, D. and Singh, R.K. 1986. Teratological study of an indigenous anti-fertility medicine, *Hibiscus rosa-sinensis* in rats. *Arogya Jour. Health Sci.* 12: 86–88.

Sethi, N., Nath, D., Shukla, S.C. and Dayal, R. 1988. Abortifacient activity of a medicinal plant, *Moringa oleifera* in rats. *Anc. Sci. Life* 7(3 & 4): 172–174.

Shah, A.C., Pajankar, S.D., Nabar, S.T., Trivedi, A.M. and Deshmukh, S.N. 1987. A double blind study of "Wintry"—a new bronchodilator in asthmatic bronchitis. *Indian Pract.* 40(4): 263–268.

Shah, C.S. and Shah, N.S. 1967. Pharmacognosy of *Trichosanthes cucumerina* L. *Jour. Res. Ind. Med.* 1(2): 230–235.

Sharma, A., Jaiswal, A.N., Kumar, S., Chaturvedi, S. and Tewari, P.V. 1985. Role of *brahmi* (*Centella asiatica*) in educable mentally retarded children. *Jour. Res. Edn. Ind. Med.* 4(1–2) 55–57.

Sharma, G. 1983. Anti-asthmatic efficacy of *Ocimum sanctum*. *Sachitra Ayurved.* 35(10): 665–668.

Sharma, G.D., Upadhyay, B.N. and Tripathi, S.N. 1982. A clinical trial of *Euphorbia prostrata* W. Ait. and *E. thymifolia* L. in the treatment of bronchial asthma (*tamakaswasa*). *Jour. Res. Ayur. Siddha* 3(3 & 4): 109–118.

Sharma, G.P. and Sharma, P.V. 1971. Effect of *dugdhika* on *shwasa roga* (bronchial asthma)—A clinical study. *Jour. Res. Ind. Med.* 6(2): 118–124.

Sharma, G.P. and Sharma, P.V. 1972. Experimental studies on anti-spasmodic and bronchodilator actions of *dugdhika* (*Euphorbia thymifolia* L. and *E. prostrata* W. Ait). *Jour. Res. Ind. Med.* 7(4): 24–28.

Sharma, J.D., Jha, R.K., Gupta, I.R.A., Jain, P. and Dixit, V.P. 1987. Anti-androgenic properties of neem-seed oil (*Azadirachta indica*) in male rat and rabbit. *Anc. Sci. Life* 7(1): 30–38.

Sharma, K., Puri, S. Ajit and Sannd, B.N. 1971. Role of *kantakari* (*Solanum xanthocarpum*) in *shwas* and *kas*—Bronchial asthma and non-specific cough. *Jour. Res. Ind. Med.* 6(2): 200–201.

Sharma, M.K., Khare, A.K. and Feroz, H. 1983. Effect of neem oil on blood sugar levels of normal, hyperglycaemic and diabetic animals. *Nagarjun* 26(10): 247–250.

Sharma, P.C. and Kapoor, L.D. 1970. Pharmacognostic study of *Nerium indicum* Mill. *Jour. Res. Ind. Med.* 5(1): 39–47.

Sharma, P.V. 1983. *Dravyaguna vijnana*, Varanasi (in Hindi)

Sharma, R., Chaturvedi, C. and Tewari, P.V. 1987a. Efficacy of *Bacopa monnieri* in revitalising intellectual functions in children. *Jour. Res. Edn. Ind. Med.* 6(1–2): 1–10.

Sharma, R., Chaturvedi, C. and Tewari, P.V. 1987b. Management of tropical pulmonary eosinophilia in children with Ayurvedic drugs. *Jour. Res. Edn. Ind. Med.* 6(1–2): 11–17.

Sharma, S.D., Upadhyay, B.N. and Tripathi, S.N. 1986. A new Ayurvedic compound for the management of Ischaemic Heart disease (*hrydroga*). *Anc. Sci. Life* 5(3): 161–167.

Sharma, V.N., Singh, V. and Prabhu, S. 1969. Anti-inflammatory activity of *Ricinus communis* L. (*eranda*). *Jour. Res. Ind. Med.* 4(1): 47–52.

Shastri, M.S. 1981. Effects of *eranda* in *amavata*. *Rheumatism* 16(4): 149–152.

Shaw, B.P. and Jana, P. 1982. Clinical assessment of *sigru* (*Moringa oleifera* Lam.) on *mutrakrichra* (lower urinary tract infection). *Nagarjun* 25(10): 231–235.

Shaw, B.P. and Tripathi, A.K. 1982. Clinical assessment of *palasha beej* (seeds of *Butea monosperma*) on *Ascaris lumbricoides*. *Nagarjun* 26(3): 53–56.

Sheehan, E.W., Zemaitis, M.A., Slatkin, D.J. and Schiff Jr. 1983. A constituent of *Pterocarpus marsupium*—epicatechin, as a potential anti-diabetic agent. *Jour. Nat. Prod.* 46(2): 232–234.

Shoj, N., Umeyama, A., Saito, N., Takemoto, T. and Kajiwara, O. 1986. Dehydropiperonaline, an amide-possessing coronary vascodilating activity isolated from *Piper longum* L. *Jour. Pharm. Sci.* 75(12): 1188–1189.

Sijoria, K.K. and Prasad, G.C. 1979. Effect of *Bauhinia purpurea* in *galgand* (thyroid). *J. Res. Ind. Med. Yoga & Homeop.* 14(3-4): 67–73.

Singh, B.N. and Sharma, P.V. 1971. Effect of *amalaki* on *amlapitta*. *Jour. Res. Ind. Med.* 5(2): 223–230.

Singh, G.A., Narayanan, S. and Mahadevan, G. 1988. Phytochemistry and pharmacognosy of *shankhapushpi*—Four varieties. *Anc. Sci. Life* 7(3 & 4): 149–156.

Singh, K.P. 1986. Clinical studies on Amoebiasis and Giardiasis: Evaluating the efficacy of *kutaja* (*Holarrhena antidysenterica*) in *Entamoeba histolytica* cyst passers. *Anc. Sci. Life* 5(4): 228–231.

Singh, K.P. and Singh, R.H. 1986. Clinical trial on *satavari* (*Asparagus racemosus* Willd.) in duodinal ulcer disease. *Jour. Res. Ayur. Siddha* 7(3–4): 91–100.

Singh, M.P., Singh, R.H. and Udupa, K.N. 1982. Antifertility activity of a benzene extract of *Hibiscus rosa-sinensis* flowers on female albino rats. *Planta Med.* 44(3): 171–174.

Singh, N., Kulshrestha, V.K. and Kohli, R.P. 1970. Cardiovascular pharmacology of *Nerium indicum*. *Jour. Res. Ind. Med.* 5(1): 32–37.

Singh, N., Misra, N., Singh, S.P. and Kohli, R.P. 1979. *Melia azadirachta* in some common skin disorders. *Antiseptic* 76 (11): 677–680.

Singh, N., Nath, R., Singh, S.P. and Kohli, R.P. 1980. Clinical evaluation of anthelmintic activity of *Melia azadirachta*. *Antiseptic* 77(5): 274–276.

Singh, N., Singh, S.P., Nath, R., Singh, D.R., Gupta, M.L., Kohli, R.P. and Bhargava, K.P. 1986. Prevention of Urethane-induced lung adenomas by *Withania somnifera* (L.) Dunal, in albino mice. *Int. Jour. Crude Drug Res.* 24(2): 90–100.

Singh, P. and Srivastava, G.N. 1980. Pharmacognostic study of leaf and stem of *Costus speciosus* (Koen.) Sm. *Bull. Med. Ethnobot. Res.* 1(2): 203–212.

Singh, R.H. and Singh, K.P. 1990. Perspectives in plant drug research. *Anc. Sci. Life* 9(3): 154–158.

Singh, R.H. and Malaviya, P.C. 1978. Studies of the psychotropic effect of an indigenous rasayana drug *aswagandha* (*Withania somnifera* Dunal) Part I. *Jour. Res. Ind. Med. Yoga & Homoeop.* 13(1): 15–24.

Singh, R.H. and Mehta, A.K. 1977. Studies on Psychotropic effect of the *medhya rasayana* drug *shankhupushpi* (*Convolvulus pluricaulis* Chois) Part I (Clinical studies). *Jour. Res. Ind. Med. Yoga & Homeop.* 12(3): 18–25.

Singh, R.H., Singh, L. and Sen, P.O. 1979. Studies on the anti-anxiety effect of the *medhya rasayana* drug *brahmi* (*Bacopa monniera* L.) Part II. Experimental studies. *Jour. Res. Ind. Med. Yoga & Homeop.* 14(3–4): 1–6.

Singh, R.H., Shukla, S.P and Mishra, B.K. 1981. The psychotropic effect of *medhya rasayana* drug *mandukaparni* (*Hydrocotyle asiatica*) an experimental study—Part II. *Jour. Res. Ayur. Siddha* 2(1): 1–10.

Singh, R.H. and Tripathy, R.K. 1982. A conceptual and clinical study on the scope of *medhya-rasāyana* and *vājīkarana* therapy in *mānasaroga* with special reference to the anti-anxiety and anti-depressant activity of certain drugs. *Jour. Res. Edn. Ind. Med.* 1(1): 23–28.

Singh, S.P. 1985. Regulation of fertility in male through an indigenous plant *Semecarpus anacardium*. *Jour. Res. Edn. Ind. Med.* 4(3–4): 9–20.

Singh, T.B. and Chunekar, K.C. 1972. *Glossary of vegetable drugs in Brhttrayı*. Varanasi.

Singhal, P.C. and Joshi, L.D. 1983. Glycemic and cholesterolemic role of ginger and til. *J. Sci. Res. Plant. Med.* 4(3): 32–34.

Sinha, A.K. 1984. Philosophical presuppositions of Ayurveda and Modern Medicine. *Anc. Sci. Life* 3(3): 123–128.

Sinha, K.C. and Riar, S.S. 1985. Neem oil—an ideal contraceptive. *Biol. Mem.* 10(1 & 2): 107–114.

Sinha, K.C., Riar, S.S., Bardhan, J., Thomas, P., Kain, A.K. and Jain, R.D. 1984. Anti-implantation effect of neem oil. *Ind. Jour. Med. Res.* 80: 708–710.

Sinha, K.C., Riar, S.S., Tiwari, R.S., Dhawan, A.K., Bardhan, J., Thomas, P., Kain, A.K. and Jain, R.K. 1984. Neem oil as a vaginal contraceptive. *Ind. Jour. Med. Res.* 79: 131–136.

Sinha, P., Wahi, S.P. and Prasad, R.R. 1984. Pharmacognostical studies in *Euphorbia thymifolia* L. *Bull. Med. Ethnobot. Res.* 5(3–4): 159–170.

Sinha, P., Gupta, I., Tank, R. and Dixit, V.P. 1986. Anti-fertility plant agents: *Syzygium cumini* seed extract as a potential source for male contraception. *Adv. Biosci.* 5(1): 69–73.

Sivarajan, V.V. 1985. The integration quagmire. *New Wave of Trad. Lines* 2(4): 9–12

Sivarajan, V.V. 1988. Indian Medicine and Medicinal Plants: a taxonomic dilemma. *Symb. Bot Ups.* 18: 197–206.

Sivarajan, V.V. 1991. Causes and consequences of forest destruction: The Indian Scenario. *Aryavaidyan* 4(3): 159–167.

Sivarajan, V.V. and Balachandran, I. 1983a. Plant resources for Ayurveda: An outlook for the future. *Anc. Sci. Life* 3(1): 45–47.

Sivarajan, V.V. and Balachandran, I. 1983b. Botanical notes on the identity of certain herbs used in Ayurvedic medicine in Kerala I. *Thamalaki Anc. Sci. Life* 1(2): 103–105.

Sivarajan, V.V. and Balachandran, I. 1985. Botanical notes on the identity of certain herbs used in Ayurvedic medicines in Kerala II. *Anc. Sci. Life* 4(4): 217–219.

Sivarajan, V.V and Balachandran, I. 1986a. Botanical notes on the identity of certain herbs used in Ayurvedic medicines in Kerala III. *Hribera* and *Amragandha. Anc. Sci. Life* 5(4): 250–254.

Sivarajan, V.V and Balachandran, I. 1986b. Needs and priorities in Ayurvedic research—A botanical approach. *Jour. Res. Edn. Ind. Med.* 4(1): 33–38.

Sivarajan, V.V. and Balachandran, I. 1987a. In pursuit of new herbal sources for Indian medicine. *Anc. Sci. Life* 7(1): 39–44.

Sivarajan, V.V. and Balachandran, I. 1987b. Botanical notes on the identity of certain herbs used in Ayurvedic Medicine in Kerala IV. *Sooranam. Anc. Sci. Life* 6(3): 155–158.

Sivarajan, V.V. and S.D. Biju 1990. Taxonomic and nomenclatural notes on the *Hedyotis corymboaa-diffusa* complex. *Taxon.* 39: 665–674.

Spjut, R.W. 1985. Limitations of a random screen: Search for new anticancer drugs in Higher plants. *Economic Botany* 39: 266–288.

Spjut, R.W. and Perdue, Jr. R.E. 1976. Plant folklore: A tool for predicting sources of anti-tumour activity? *Cancer Treatment Reports* 60: 979–985.

Srinivas, C. and Prabhakaran, K.V.S. 1987. Clinical bacteriological study of *Curcuma longa* on conjuctivitis. *Antiseptic* 84(3): 166–168.

Srivastava, M.A., Singh, S.W., Tewari, J.P. and Kant, V. 1967. Anthelmintic activity of *Psoralea corylifolia* seeds. *Jour. Res. Ind. Med.* 2(1): 11–15.

Srivastava, Y., Bhatt, H.V., Gupta, O.P. and Gupta, P.S. 1983. Hypoglycemia induced by *Syzygium cumini* L. seeds in diabetes mellitus. *Asian Med. Jour.* 26(7): 489–491.

Sudhir, S., Budhiraja, R.D., Miglani, G.P., Arora, B., Gupta, L.C. and Garg, K.N. 1986. Pharmacological studies of leaves of *Withania somnifera*. *Planta Med.* 1: 61–63.

Suresh, A., Anandan, T., Sivanandan, G. and Veluchamy, G. 1985. A pilot study of *Naayuruvikuzhithailam* in *Eraippunoi* (bronchial asthama). *J. Res. Ayur. Siddha* 6(2) 171–176.

Symon, D.E. 1981. A revision of the genus *Solanum* in Australia. *Jour. Adelaide Bot. Gard.* 4: 1–367.

Tajuddin, S.A. and Tariq, M. 1983. Anti-inflammatory activity of *Andrographis paniculata* Nees (*Chirayata*). *Nagarjun* 27(1): 13–14.

Takahashi, M., Konno, C. and Hikino, H. 1985. Isolation and hypoglycemic activity of saccharans, A.B.C.D.E. and F. glycans of *Saccharum officinarum* stalks. *Planta Med.* 3: 258–260.

Tewari, K.M., Prasad, D.N., Chaturvedi, C. and Das, P.K. 1967. Preliminary studies on uterine activity of *Gloriosa superba* L. and its adulterant *Costus speciosus* Sm. *Jour. Res. Ind. Med.* 1(2): 196–202.

Tewari, P.V., Chaturvedi, C. and Dixit, S.N. 1970. Antifertility effect of betel leaf stalk—A preliminary experimental study. *Jour. Res. Ind. Med.* 4(2): 143–151.

Thakur, C.P. and Mandal, K. 1984. Effect of *Emblica officinalis* in cholesterol-induced atherosclerosis in rabbits. *Ind. J. Med. Res.* 79: 142–146.

Thakur, D.K., Misri, S.K. and Choudhuri, P.C. 1982. Antifungal activity of *Leucas aspera* Spr. against experimental dermatomycosis in mice. *J. Res. Punjab. Agric. Univ.* 19(3): 265–266.

Togunashi, V.S., Venkataram, B.S. and Yoganarasimhan, S.N. 1976. Discussion and identification of *amlavetasa*. *Nagarjun* 20(3): 15–17.

Togunashi, V.S., Yoganarasimhan, S.N. and Venkataraman, B.S. 1978. New source for *sariba* and identification of *swetasariba*. *J. Res. Ind. Med. Yoga & Homeop.* 13(4): 75–80.

Tripathi, S.N., Tiwari, C.M., Jaiswal, L.C., Upadhyaya, B.N. and Pandey, P. 1979. Role of *Semicarpus anacardium* (*bhallataka*) in the management of rheumatoid arthritis. *Jour. Res. Ind. Med. Yoga & Homoeop.* 14(2): 33–43.

Tripathi, V.N., Tewari, S.K., Gupta, J.P. and Chaturvedi, G.N. 1983. Clinical trial of *haritaki* (*Terminalia chebula*) in treatment of simple constipation. *Sachitra Ayurved* 35(11): 733–740.

Trivedi, V.P., Nesamony, S. and Sharma, V.K. 1978. A clinical study of the effect of tincture *raktakarveer patra* (*Nerium indicum* L.) on the respiratory tract involvement in the case of conjestive heart failure. *Jour. Net. Integ. Med. Assoc.* 20(6): 161–168.

Trivedi, V.P., Nesamony, S. and Sharma, V.K. 1982. A clinical study of the antitussive and antiasthmatic effects of *vibhitakyadi churna* in the cases of *kasa-swasa*. *Jour. Res. Ayur. Siddha* 3(1 & 2): 1–8.

Tyler, V.E. 1986. Plant drugs in twenty-first century. *Economic Botany* 40: 279–288.

Udupa, K.N. 1983. Ayurveda for the service of common man. *Anc. Sci. Life* 2(3): 117–121.

Upadhyay, B.N., Singh, T.N., Tewari, C.M., Jaiswal, L.C. and Tripathi, S.N 1986. Experimental and clinical evaluation of *Semecarpus anacardium* nut (*bhallataka*) in the treatment of *amavata* (Rheumatoid arthritis). *Rheumatism* 21(3): 70–87.

Upadhyaya, G.L. and Pant, M.C. 1986. Effects of water and ether extracts of bitter-gourd powder on blood sugar and serum cholesterol level in albino rabbits. *Jour. Diabet. Assoc. India* 26(1): 17–19.

Usman Ali, S., Pillai, G.S., Nair, V.K. and Chelladurai, V. 1981. Contribution to the exact botanical identity of *brahmi* and *mandookaparni*. *Bull. Med. Ethnobot. Res.* 2(1): 23–36.

Vaidya, K.M. 1936. *The Ashtangahridayakosha with the Hridayaprakasha Commentary*, Trichur (in Sanskrit).

Vaidya, Baplal. 1982. *Some controversial drugs in Indian Medicine*, Varanasi.

Vimaladevi, M., Satyanarayana, S. and Rao, S.A. 1986. Effect of *Phyllanthus niruri* on the diuretic activity of *punarnava* tablets. *Jour. Res. Edn. Ind. Med.* 5(1): 11–13.

Vohra, S.B., Shah, S.A., Naqvi, S.A.H., Ahmad, S. and Khan, M.S.Y. 1983. Studies on *Trianthema portulacastrum*. *Planta Med.* 47(2) 106–108.

Vyas, D.S., Sharma, V.N., Sharma, H.K. and Khanna, N.K. 1979. Preliminary study on antidiabetic properties of *Aegle marmelos* and *Enicostemma littorale*. *Jour. Res. Ind. Red. Yoga & Homoeop.* 14: 3.

Wadhwa, V., Singh, M.M., Gupta, D.N., Singh, C. and Kamboj, V.P. 1986. Contraceptive and hormonal properties of *Achyranthes aspera* in rats and hamsters. *Planta Med.* 3: 231–233.

Wahi, A.K., Khosa, R.L. and Mukherjee, A.K. 1979. Diagnostic characters of *sariba*. *J. Res. Indian. Med. Yoga & Homeop.* 14(2): 166–169.

Wahi, S.P., Wahi, A.K. and Jaiswal, D.K. 1974. Pharmacognostical studies on *Hibiscus rosa-sinensis* L. *Jour. Res. Ind. Med.* 9(4): 84–95: 1974.

Wahi, A.K., Khosa, R.L. and Mukherjee, A.K. 1980. Pharmacognostical studies on *Vallaris solanacea* O. Ktze. *Bull. Med. Ethonobot. Res.* 1(4): 506–524.

Weiss, M.G. 1987. Karma and Ayurveda. *Anc. Sci. Life* 6(3): 129–134.

Yang, L.L., Yen, K.Y., Konno, C., Oshima, Y., Kiso, Y. and Hikino, H. 1986. Anti-hepatotoxic principles of *Wedelia chinensis* herbs. *Planta Med.* 6: 499–500.

Zhou, L.F. and Lei, H.P. 1984. The effects of gossypol acetic acid on the uterus and ovary. *Acta Pharm. Sin.* 19(3) 220–223.

Zia-Ul-Haque, A., Qasi, M.H. and Hamdard, M.E. 1983. Studies on the anti-fertility properties of active components isolated from the seeds of *Abrus precatorius* L. *Pak. Jour. Zool.* 15(2): 129–139.

Index to Latin Binomials

(Species described in the text are given in bold, and those that are not are in normal letters. Synonyms are given in italics)

Index to Sanskrit Names

(The names under which the drugs are described, are given in bold)

Index to Malayaḻam Names

(The names under which the drugs are described, are given in bold)

Index to Illustrations